Platelet Glycoprotein IIb/IIIa Inhibitors in Cardiovascular Disease

CONTEMPORARY CARDIOLOGY

CHRISTOPHER P. CANNON, MD
SERIES EDITOR

Platelet Glycoprotein IIb/IIIa Inhibitors in Cardiovascular Disease, Second Edition, edited by *A. Michael Lincoff, MD, 2003*

Nuclear Cardiology Basics: How to Set Up and Maintain a Laboratory, edited by *Frans J. Th. Wackers, MD, Wendy Bruni, CNMT, and Barry L. Zaret, MD, 2003*

Minimally Invasive Cardiac Surgery, Second Edition, edited by *Mehmet C. Oz, MD, and Daniel J. Goldstein, MD, 2003*

Cardiovascular Health Care Economics, edited by *William S. Weintraub, MD, 2003*

Heart Failure: A Clinician's Guide to Ambulatory Diagnosis and Treatment, edited by *Mariell L. Jessup, MD, FACC, FAHA, and Evan Loh, MD, FACC, FAHA, 2003*

Cardiac Repolarization: Basic and Clinical Research, edited by *Ihor Gussak, MD, PhD, Charles Antzelevitch, PhD, co-edited by Stephen C. Hammill, MD, Win-Kuang Shen, MD, and Preben Bjerregaard, MD, DMSc, 2003*

Management of Acute Coronary Syndromes, Second Edition, edited by *Christopher P. Cannon, MD 2003*

Aging, Heart Disease, and Its Management: Facts and Controversies, edited by *Niloo M. Edwards, MD, Mathew S. Maurer, MD, and Rachel B. Wellner, MPH, 2003*

Peripheral Arterial Disease: Diagnosis and Treatment, edited by *Jay D. Coffman, MD and Robert T. Eberhardt, MD, 2003*

Essentials of Bedside Cardiology: With A Complete Course in Heart Sounds and Murmurs on CD, Second Edition, by *Jules Constant, MD, FACC, 2003*

Primary Angioplasty in Acute Myocardial Infarction, edited by *James E. Tcheng, MD, 2002*

Cardiogenic Shock: Diagnosis and Treatment, edited by *David Hasdai, MD, Peter B. Berger, MD, Alexander Battler, MD, and David R. Holmes, Jr., MD, 2002*

Management of Cardiac Arrhythmias, edited by *Leonard I. Ganz, MD, 2002*

Diabetes and Cardiovascular Disease, edited by *Michael T. Johnstone, MD and Aristidis Veves, MD, DSC, 2001*

Blood Pressure Monitoring in Cardiovascular Medicine and Therapeutics, edited by *William B. White, MD, 2001*

Vascular Disease and Injury: Preclinical Research, edited by *Daniel I. Simon, MD, and Campbell Rogers, MD 2001*

Preventive Cardiology: Strategies for the Prevention and Treatment of Coronary Artery Disease, edited by *JoAnne Micale Foody, MD, 2001*

Nitric Oxide and the Cardiovascular System, edited by *Joseph Loscalzo, MD, PhD and Joseph A. Vita, MD, 2000*

Annotated Atlas of Electrocardiography: A Guide to Confident Interpretation, by *Thomas M. Blake, MD, 1999*

PLATELET GLYCOPROTEIN IIB/IIIA INHIBITORS IN CARDIOVASCULAR DISEASE

Second Edition

Edited by

A. MICHAEL LINCOFF, MD

Department of Cardiovascular Medicine,
The Cleveland Clinic Foundation,
Cleveland, OH

 HUMANA PRESS
TOTOWA, NEW JERSEY

© 2003 Humana Press Inc.
999 Riverview Drive, Suite 208
Totowa, New Jersey 07512

www.humanapress.com

Production Editor: Jessica Jannicelli.
Cover design by Patricia F. Cleary.
Cover Illustration by Marion Tomasko.

For additional copies, pricing for bulk purchases, and/or information about other Humana titles, contact Humana at the above address or at any of the following numbers: Tel.: 973-256-1699; Fax: 973-256-8341, E-mail: humana@humanapr.com; or visit our Website: www.humanapress.com

This publication is printed on acid-free paper. ∞
ANSI Z39.48-1984 (American National Standards Institute) Permanence of Paper for Printed Library Materials.

Printed in the United States of America. 10 9 8 7 6 5 4 3 2 1

Library of Congress Cataloging-in-Publication Data

Platelet glycoprotein IIb/IIIa inhibitors in cardiovascular disease / edited by A. Michael Lincoff.-- 2nd ed.
    p. ; cm. -- (Contemporary cardiology)
  Includes bibliographical references and index.
  ISBN 1-58829-185-5 (alk. paper) eISBN 1-59259-376-3.
    1. Coronary heart disease--Chemotherapy. 2. Coronary heart disease--Pathophysiology.
  3. Platelet glycoprotein GPIIb-IIIa complex--Inhibitors--Therapeutic use--Testing. I.
Lincoff, A. Michael. II. Contemporary cardiology (Totowa, N.J. : unnumbered)
  [DNLM: 1. Cardiovascular Diseases--drug therapy. 2. Platelet Glycoprotein GPIIb-IIIa
Complex--antagonists & inhibitors. WG 166 P716 2003]
  RC685.C6P585 2003
  616.1'061--dc21
                                                                            2002191923

Preface

One of the most important developments in the field of cardiovascular medicine over the last two decades has been recognition of the key role played by arterial thrombosis in the pathogenesis of acute coronary syndromes, ischemic complications of percutaneous coronary revascularization, and coronary and peripheral atherosclerosis. The pharmacologic armamentarium directed against vascular thrombosis has thus expanded substantially during that time, with development of new fibrinolytic agents, low-molecular-weight heparins, direct thrombin inhibitors, antagonists to platelet activation, and the platelet glycoprotein IIb/IIIa inhibitors. Though clinical investigations of these compounds have been marked by failures as well as successes, there is little doubt that enhanced antithrombotic therapies have markedly improved the outcome of patients undergoing coronary revascularization or with acute coronary syndromes.

Glycoprotein IIb/IIIa receptor antagonists were introduced into clinical practice to overcome the limitations of approaches that inhibit only individual pathways of platelet activation. Multiple mechanisms of platelet activation in response to different agonists converge on the platelet membrane glycoprotein IIb/IIIa complex, the "final common pathway" of platelet aggregation. The clinical hemorrhagic syndrome caused by a rare inherited defect in this receptor (Glanzmann's thrombasthenia), characterized by mucocutaneous and postsurgical bleeding, but infrequent spontaneous organ (particularly central nervous system) bleeding, suggested that therapeutic inhibition of this receptor might be a potent, yet well-tolerated means of treating thrombotic disorders. The first agent directed against the receptor, a monoclonal antibody fragment developed by Coller that blocks the interaction of glycoprotein IIb/IIIa with adhesion molecules, received marketing approval in 1995. On the basis of unequivocal efficacy demonstrated during extensive systematic controlled clinical trial evaluations, three parenteral glycoprotein IIb/IIIa inhibitors are presently available for the management of patients undergoing percutaneous coronary revascularization or with unstable ischemic syndromes.

In 1999, we published the first edition of this text, a comprehensive, definitive, and detailed overview of the preclinical and clinical development of the class of glycoprotein IIb/IIIa receptor antagonists. Since that time, new trials have evaluated the relative efficacy of different agents, expanded our understanding of the roles of these drugs in the management of acute coronary syndromes, critically assessed the efficacy of oral agents, and explored the interaction between glycoprotein IIb/IIIa antagonists and other antithrombotic and mechanical interventional therapies. The goals of this second edition, as with the first, are to elucidate the theoretical basis for inhibition of platelet aggregation in the treatment of coronary syndromes, to synthesize the evidence demonstrating the efficacy of glycoprotein IIb/IIIa blockade in inhibiting ischemic complications of coronary intervention and the acute coronary syndromes, and to provide guidelines for the use of this class of agents in the clinical management of cardiovascular disease. In every case, chapters have been contributed by acknowledged experts in the field, including the pioneers in the discovery and characterization of cell surface adhesion molecules and the glycoprotein IIb/IIIa receptor, as well as the principal investigators of the major clinical trials. The most current data are included, with the intent to provide a comprehensive body of knowledge of the contemporary "state of the art" in this field.

The first section of *Platelet Glycoprotein IIb/IIIa Inhibitors in Cardiovascular Disease, Second Edition* outlines the basic pathophysiology underlying the theoretical usefulness and development of this class of agents. In Chapter 1, the role of thrombosis and platelet activity in the pathophysiology of acute ischemic syndromes or complications of coronary intervention are reviewed, providing the underpinnings for antithrombotic therapy in cardiovascular disease. Platelet adhesion, the essential reaction for the hemostatic function of platelets, is discussed in Chapter 2, followed by a detailed description of the structure and functions of the glycoprotein IIb/IIIa receptor in Chapter 3. The "bench to bedside" development of the first agent directed against this receptor is recounted in Chapter 4, along with a summary of the pharmacologic properties of the other parenteral compounds of this class.

The second section concentrates on the adjunctive use of glycoprotein IIb/IIIa blockade during percutaneous coronary revascularization. The three agents that have been evaluated for this indication (abciximab, eptifibatide, and tirofiban) are discussed in Chapters 5–7, focusing on data derived from the pivotal Phase III and IV studies. A summary overview then follows, integrating the results of the major trials in this setting, comparing the different agents, and providing practical guidelines for clinical use.

The third section focuses on glycoprotein IIb/IIIa blockade in the management of the acute coronary ischemic syndromes. Chapters 9–11 detail the roles of these agents as adjuncts to medical and revascularization therapies for unstable angina. Chapters 12 and 13 discuss the use of glycoprotein IIb/IIIa antagonists with mechanical or pharmacologic (fibrinolytic) reperfusion therapies for ST-segment-elevation myocardial infarction.

The fourth section explores practical issues with the use of these agents and provides a view into future applications in the treatment of vascular disease. Medico-economic aspects are analyzed in Chapter 14. Chapters 15 and 16 describe techniques for monitoring the efficacy of platelet inhibition and provide preliminary data regarding the interaction of glycoprotein IIb/IIIa antagonists with other inhibitors of platelet function or the coagulation cascade. The unexpected failure of chronic oral glycoprotein IIb/IIIa therapy in a series of large-scale trials is discussed in Chapter 17. Chapter 18 speculates on the possibility that clinical benefit may be derived from these agents through mechanisms other than platelet inhibition, such as antiinflammatory effects. The potential efficacy and established risks of glycoprotein IIb/IIIa blockade in relation to cerebrovascular disease are explored in Chapters 19 and 20. Finally, advances made in the management of vascular thrombosis and new directions for progress in this field are summarized in Chapter 21.

I am most appreciative of the superb contributions by the chapter authors of this book, who drew on their considerable expertise, first-hand experience, and perspectives to produce a truly comprehensive discussion of this field. Additionally, the publisher and production staff at Humana Press made exceptional efforts for the timely completion of this project. Marion Tomasko and Robin Moss deserve recognition for their imaginative book cover artwork.

I would also like to recognize the continued support, tolerance, and understanding of my wife Debra and our children, Gabrielle, Aaron, and Jacob.

A. Michael Lincoff, MD

CONTENTS

Preface v

Contributors ix

PART I BASIC PRINCIPLES

1 Thrombosis in Acute Coronary Syndromes and Coronary
  Interventions 3
  Thaddeus R. Tolleson and Robert A. Harrington

2 Platelet Adhesion 23
  Edward F. Plow

3 Glycoprotein IIb/IIIa in Platelet Aggregation and Acute
  Arterial Thrombosis 39
  Patrick Andre and David R. Phillips

4 Glycoprotein IIb/IIIa Antagonists: *Development of Abciximab
  and Pharmacology of Abciximab, Tirofiban,
  and Eptifibatide* 73
  Barry S. Coller

PART II GLYCOPROTEIN IIB/IIIA BLOCKADE DURING CORONARY
  INTERVENTION

5 Abciximab During Percutaneous Coronary Intervention:
  EPIC, EPILOG, and EPISTENT Trials 105
  A. Michael Lincoff

6 Eptifibatide in Coronary Intervention: *The IMPACT
  and ESPRIT Trials* 125
  Jean-Pierre Dery, J. Conor O'Shea, and James E. Tcheng

7 Tirofiban in Interventional Cardiology: *The RESTORE
  and TARGET Trials* 147
  Nicholas Valettas and Howard C. Herrmann

8 Overview of the Glycoprotein IIb/IIIa Interventional Trials 167
  A. Michael Lincoff and Eric J. Topol

PART III GLYCOPROTEIN IIB/IIIA BLOCKADE FOR ACUTE
  ISCHEMIC SYNDROMES

9 The Use of Abciximab in Therapy-Resistant Unstable Angina:
  *Clinical and Angiographic Results of the CAPTURE Pilot
  Trial and the CAPTURE Study* 203
  Marcel J. B. M. van den Brand and Maarten L. Simoons

10 Unstable Angina Trials: *PARAGON, PURSUIT, PRISM,
  PRISM-PLUS, and GUSTO-IV* 233
  David J. Moliterno

11 Platelet Glycoprotein IIb/IIIa Inhibitors and an Invasive
Strategy 263
Christopher P. Cannon

12 Glycoprotein IIb/IIIa Receptor Blockade in Myocardial
Infarction: *Adjunctive Therapy to Percutaneous
Coronary Interventions* 275
Franz-Josef Neumann

13 Glycoprotein IIb/IIIa Receptor Blockade in Acute Myocardial
Infarction: *Adjunctive Therapy to Fibrinolysis* 289
Sorin J. Brener

PART IV PRACTICAL ISSUES AND FUTURE APPLICATIONS

14 Economics of Glycoprotein IIb/IIIa Inhibition 305
Daniel B. Mark

15 Platelet Monitoring and Interaction of Glycoprotein IIb/IIIa
Antagonists with Other Antiplatelet Agents 321
Steven R. Steinhubl

16 Platelet Glycoprotein IIb/IIIa Antagonists: *Their Interaction
with Low-Molecular-Weight Heparins and Direct
Thrombin Inhibitors* 341
Amol S. Bapat, Naji Yazbek, and Neal S. Kleiman

17 Oral Agents 365
L. Kristin Newby

18 Platelet Glycoprotein IIb/IIIa Inhibitors: *Effects Beyond
the Platelet* 383
Dean J. Kereiakes and Pascal J. Goldschmidt-Clermont

19 Cerebrovascular Interventions 397
Leslie Cho and Jay S. Yadav

20 Cerebrovascular Aspects of Glycoprotein IIb/IIIa Receptor
Inhibitors 409
Cathy A. Sila

21 Evolution of Drug Development in Evidence-Based Medicine:
Summary and the Future 425
David E. Kandzari, David F. Kong, and Robert M. Califf

Index 459

CONTRIBUTORS

PATRICK ANDRE, PhD • *Millennium Pharmaceuticals Inc., South San Francisco, CA*

AMOL S. BAPAT, MD • *The Methodist DeBakey Heart Center, Baylor College of Medicine, Houston, TX*

SORIN J. BRENER, MD • *Department of Cardiovascular Medicine, The Cleveland Clinic Foundation, Cleveland, OH*

ROBERT M. CALIFF, MD • *Duke Clinical Research Institute, Duke University Medical Center, Durham, NC*

CHRISTOPHER P. CANNON, MD • *Cardiovascular Division, Department of Medicine, Brigham and Women's Hospital and Harvard Medical School, Boston, MA*

LESLIE CHO, MD • *Department of Cardiovascular Medicine, The Loyola University Medical Center, Chicago, IL*

BARRY S. COLLER, MD • *Laboratory of Blood and Vascular Biology, Rockefeller University, New York, NY*

JEAN-PIERRE DERY, MD • *Duke Clinical Research Institute, Duke University Medical Center, Durham, NC*

PASCAL J. GOLDSCHMIDT-CLERMONT, MD • *Division of Cardiology, Duke University Medical Center, Durham, NC*

ROBERT A. HARRINGTON, MD • *Division of Cardiology, Duke Clinical Research Institute, Duke University Medical Center, Durham, NC*

HOWARD C. HERRMANN, MD • *Cardiovascular Division, Hospital of the University of Pennsylvania, University of Pennsylvania Health System, Philadelphia, PA*

DAVID E. KANDZARI, MD • *Duke Clinical Research Institute, Duke University Medical Center, Durham, NC*

DEAN J. KEREIAKES, MD • *The Lindner Center for Research and Education, Ohio Heart Health Center, Ohio State University, Cincinnati, OH*

NEAL S. KLEIMAN, MD • *The Methodist DeBakey Heart Center, Baylor College of Medicine, Houston, TX*

DAVID F. KONG, MD • *Duke Clinical Research Institute, Duke University Medical Center, Durham, NC*

A. MICHAEL LINCOFF, MD • *Department of Cardiovascular Medicine, The Cleveland Clinic Foundation, Cleveland, OH*

DANIEL B. MARK, MD, MPH • *Duke Clinical Research Institute, Duke University Medical Center, Durham, NC*

DAVID J. MOLITERNO, MD • *Department of Cardiovascular Medicine, The Cleveland Clinic Foundation, Cleveland, OH*

FRANZ-JOSEF NEUMANN, MD • *Heart Center, Bad Krozingen, Germany*

L. KRISTIN NEWBY, MD • *Duke Clinical Research Institute, Duke University Medical Center, Durham, NC*

J. CONOR O'SHEA, MD • *Duke Clinical Research Institute, Duke University Medical Center, Durham, NC*

DAVID R. PHILLIPS, PhD • *Millennium Pharmaceuticals Inc., South San Francisco, CA*

EDWARD F. PLOW, PhD • *Joseph J. Jacobs Center for Thrombosis and Vascular Biology, Department of Molecular Cardiology, The Cleveland Clinic Foundation, Cleveland, OH*

CATHY A. SILA, MD • *Section of Stroke and Neurologic Intensive Care, Department of Neurology, The Cleveland Clinic Foundation, Cleveland, OH*

MAARTEN L. SIMOONS, MD • *University Hospital Rotterdam, Rotterdam, The Netherlands*

STEVEN R. STEINHUBL, MD • *Division of Cardiology, University of North Carolina, Chapel Hill, NC*

JAMES E. TCHENG, MD • *Duke Clinical Research Institute, Duke University Medical Center, Durham, NC*

THADDEUS R. TOLLESON, MD • *Division of Cardiology, Duke Clinical Research Institute, Duke University Medical Center, Durham, NC*

ERIC J. TOPOL, MD • *The Cleveland Clinic Foundation, Cleveland, OH*

NICHOLAS VALETTAS, MASc, MD • *Cardiovascular Division, Hospital of the University of Pennsylvania, University of Pennsylvania Health System, Philadelphia, PA*

MARCEL J. B. M. VAN DEN BRAND, MD • *University Hospital Rotterdam, Rotterdam, The Netherlands*

JAY S. YADAV, MD • *Department of Cardiovascular Medicine, The Cleveland Clinic Foundation, Cleveland, OH*

NAJI YAZBEK, MD • *The Methodist DeBakey Heart Center, Baylor College of Medicine, Houston, TX*

I BASIC PRINCIPLES

1

Thrombosis in Acute Coronary Syndromes and Coronary Interventions

Thaddeus R. Tolleson, MD
and Robert A. Harrington, MD

CONTENTS

INTRODUCTION
HISTORY
COMPONENTS OF THE THROMBOTIC PROCESS
THE PROCESS OF THROMBUS FORMATION
REFERENCES

INTRODUCTION

Acute coronary syndromes (ACS), including unstable angina, non-ST elevation myocardial infarction, and ST-elevation myocardial infarction, are the most commonly encountered clinical scenarios faced by clinical cardiologists today, accounting for over 650,000 hospitalizations annually *(1)*. The pathophysiology of ACS is now well described, beginning with disruption of an atheromatous plaque, with subsequent platelet aggregation and thrombus formation. The resulting clinical syndromes vary and depend on multiple related factors.

The treatment of ischemic coronary disease, including ACS, by percutaneous interventions has dramatically increased over the past decade. The number of coronary artery lesions treated by percutaneous coronary interventions now exceeds well over one million annually. Although the success rate is now greater than 90%, acute periprocedural occlusion continues to complicate approx 6% of all procedures *(1)*. The vast majority of acute occlusions are a result of, at least in part, intracoronary thrombosis.

Although the inciting event leading to plaque rupture is different in ACS and percutaneous interventions (spontaneous vs iatrogenic rupture), the resulting arterial pathophysiology is similar for both events. The complex interaction of the exposed endothelium, atherosclerotic plaque, inflammatory factors, platelets, and coagulation cascade results

From: *Contemporary Cardiology: Platelet Glycoprotein IIb/IIIa
Inhibitors in Cardiovascular Disease, 2nd Edition*
Edited by: A. M. Lincoff © Humana Press Inc., Totowa, NJ

in thrombosis with compromise of vessel patency in a percentage of patients. Thus, in both ACS and percutaneous interventions, therapies targeting thrombosis have proved efficacious, even as new therapies are developed and undergoing clinical trials. This chapter discusses the pathophysiologic mechanisms responsible for these interactions.

HISTORY

In 1912, Herrick, an American physician, concluded from his clinical experience and research that the common feature in acute myocardial infarction was sudden occlusion of a coronary artery (2). Although not readily accepted at first, Herrick's observations slowly gained acceptance over the next 50 yr. The clinical syndromes of acute myocardial infarction were described and linked to coronary thrombosis by Levine and Brown in Boston (3), as well as Parkinson and Bedford in Europe (4). Not long after, two groups of researchers in the United States described the clinical syndrome now known as unstable angina and again linked its pathophysiology to coronary thrombus (5,6). Heparin was used in some form as early as the 1920s (7), and by the late 1930s, was being used to treat venous thrombosis (8). Irving Wright (9) is generally credited with being the first American physician to treat a patient with heparin and was probably the first to use dicoumarol therapeutically as well (10). He subsequently headed up the American Heart Association Trial of anticoagulation in acute myocardial infarction in 1948, which showed a significant mortality benefit in the treated group (11).

Clinical experience with acetylsalicylic acid (ASA) for treatment of acute myocardial infarctions actually began in the 1940s. Craven, an otorhinolaryngologist in private practice in California, noted that his tonsillectomy patients who chewed excessive amounts of Aspergum for pain relief had excessive bleeding (9). He then began to treat all his older male patients with ASA to prevent myocardial infarction. He subsequently published two papers, reporting on over 8400 treated patients in whom he found no myocardial infarction (12,13). However, his work appears to have been largely ignored at the time.

Although thrombolytic therapy is often viewed as a relatively recent advance in the treatment of ACS, reports of the proteolytic activity of urine (later known as urokinase) were first described as early as 1861 (14). The first report of myocardial infarction being treated with a thrombolytic agent, streptokinase, was in 1958 by Sherry and Fletcher (15).

At the end of the 1950s, with these important clinical findings known, the medical community appeared poised to make significant advances in the treatment of ACS. Instead, in a remarkable turnaround in conceptual understanding and therapeutic approach, physicians began to use less anticoagulation in treating the acute ischemic syndromes over the next two decades. Several key factors probably contributed to this, including misinterpretation of autopsies and the conclusion that coronary thrombus follows, rather than precedes, myocardial infarction; inadequate clinical trials employing nonrandomized designs with insufficient sample sizes; and increasing focus on approaches to limiting infarct size by reducing oxygen demand.

In 1969, Gifford and Feinstein (16) reviewed the trials of anticoagulation in acute myocardial infarction, noting the numerous design deficiencies and the paucity of randomized data. Although numerous trials of thrombolytic therapy were conducted between 1960 and 1980, none demonstrated a definitive benefit of therapy. Thus, by the early 1980s, the role of thrombosis in acute coronary syndromes, and hence, the value of anticoagulation and thrombolytic therapy remained controversial.

In a landmark paper, DeWood *(17)* showed that total coronary occlusion was present in 87% of patients in the early hours of transmural myocardial infarction. His group believed that patients in the early hours of infarction were best treated by emergency bypass surgery; hence, these patients all had coronary arteriography in the acute phase of their infarction. Subsequent autopsy studies further elucidated the now reemerging concept of thrombosis as the predominant cause of ACS *(18,19)*. Ambrose et al. *(20)* then correlated the progression from stable angina to unstable coronary syndromes with angiographic evidence of intraluminal thrombus. Falk *(21)* showed through pathologic studies that patients experiencing sudden death, preceded by episodes of unstable symptoms, often had occlusive thrombus composed of layers of platelet thrombi in various stages of organization.

As the pathophysiologic mechanism of ACS became better understood, treatment strategies to alter the natural course of this event soon followed. Thus, the understanding of thrombosis as the underlying mechanism in unstable coronary syndromes, as well as in acute occlusion following percutaneous coronary interventions, led to new therapeutic developments aimed at preventing or inhibiting this phenomenon. Once these therapies reached the clinical phase, randomized controlled clinical trials formed the basis of evaluating their efficacy.

COMPONENTS OF THE THROMBOTIC PROCESS

Fissuring or rupture of an atherosclerotic plaque, with subsequent thrombus formation reducing or obliterating coronary blood flow, is accepted as the primary mechanism responsible for the development of unstable angina and myocardial infarction. The pathologic response that follows rupture of an atherosclerotic plaque is similar to the physiologic response to any vascular injury. Whether in acute coronary syndromes or coronary interventions, the process that ultimately results in arterial thrombosis involves the complex interactions of five components of the thrombotic process: (1) the endothelium, (2) the atherosclerotic plaque, (3) inflammatory factors, (4) platelets, and (5) the coagulation cascade.

The Endothelium

The vascular endothelium controls normal vessel responsiveness and thromboresistance (Fig. 1). It is a multifunctional organ system composed of metabolically active and physiologically responsive component cells that meticulously regulate blood flow. The endothelium forms an obligate monolayer that lines the entire arterial tree, representing the principal barrier between the blood and the arterial wall. As an active site of protein synthesis, endothelial cells synthesize, secrete, modify, and regulate connective tissue components, vasodilators, vasoconstrictors, anticoagulants, procoagulants, fibrinolytics, proteins, and prostanoids.

The most important function of the vascular endothelium is to prevent the initiation and development of nonphysiologic thrombi. The endothelium normally provides a nonthrombogenic surface because of its surface coat of heparin sulfate and its capacity to form prostaglandin derivatives, particularly prostacyclin (PGI_2), a potent vasodilator and effective inhibitor of platelet aggregation *(22)*. Endothelial cells also produce the most potent natural vasodilator known, endothelium-derived relaxing factor, a thiolated form of nitric oxide *(23)*. EDRF formation by the endothelium is critical in maintaining a balance between

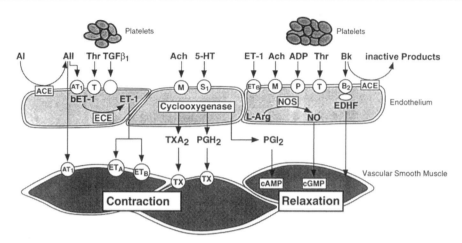

Fig. 1. Endothelium-derived vasoactive substances. The endotheliurn is a source of relaxing (right part) and contracting factors (left part). AI/AH = angiotensin I/II; Ach = acetylcholine; ADP = adenosine diphosphate; Bk = bradykinin; cAMP/cGMP = cyclic adenosine/guanosinie monophosphate; ECE = endothelin-converting enzyme; EDHF = endothelium-derived hyperpolarizing factor; ET-1 = endothelin-1; bET-1 = big endothelin-1; 5-HT = 5-hydroxy-tryptamine (serotonin); L-Arg = L-arginine; NO = nitric oxide; PGH_2 = prostaglandin H_2; PGI_2 = prostacyclin; $TGF\beta_1$ = transforming growth factor-β_1; Thr = thrombin; TXA_2 = thromboxane A_2. Circles represent receptors: B_2 = bradykinergic receptor; M = muscarinic receptor; P = purinergic receptor; T = thrombin receptor; S = serotonergic receptor. (From ref. *74*.)

vasoconstriction and vasodilation in the process of arterial homeostasis *(24)*. Endothelial cells also secrete a number of vasoactive agents (such as endothelin, angiotensin-converting enzyme, and platelet-derived growth factor) that mediate vasoconstriction *(25)*. In addition, these cells also secrete agents that are effective in lysing fibrin clots, including plasminogen and procoagulant materials, such as von Willebrand factor (Table 1) *(26)*.

In addition to the numerous substances produced and subsequently secreted, endothelial cells also possess receptors for many different molecules on their surface. These include receptors for low-density lipoprotein (LDL) *(27)*, growth factors, and various pharmacologic agents. This receptor-ligand interaction on the surface of the endothelial cell serves as the initial substrate for thrombus formation. In addition, the interaction of endothelial cells with cellular elements of the blood (specifically platelets, macrophages, and thrombin) is critical in pathologic thrombus formation in acute coronary syndromes and coronary interventions.

Atherosclerotic Plaque Formation

Our understanding of the pathophysiology of coronary atherosclerosis has changed dramatically in the last few years. The types of atherosclerotic lesions, the mechanisms of progression of coronary atherosclerosis with plaque instability and rupture, and the subsequent thrombotic phenomenon leading to ACS have now been more clearly elucidated. In 1995, a report from the Committee on Vascular Lesions of the Council on Arteriosclerosis of the American Heart Association *(28)* presented a new classification for atherosclerosis in which lesions are divided into six types (Figs. 2 and 3).

Table 1
The Endothelial Cell and Hemostasis

Product	Properties
Ectonucleotidases	Surface enzymes that regulate breakdown of platelet-active and vasoactive nucleotides
Nitric oxide	Labile-secreted inhibitor of platelet aggregation and adhesion; vasodilator
Plasminogen activator inhibitor	Secreted, circulating and matrix-bound inhibitor of tPA
Platelet-activating factor	Secreted and cell surface-associated platelet and leukocyte stimulant
Prostacyclin	Labile-secreted inhibitor of platelet aggregation; vasodilator
Tissue factor (thromboplastin)	Procoagulant only expressed on activated endothelium
Tissue plasminogen activator (tPA)	Stored and secreted regulator of fibrinolysis
Thrombomodulin	Surface-expressed anticoagulant
von Willebrand factor and clotting factor VIII	Stored and secreted cofactor for platelet adhesion

From ref. 77.

Type I lesions consist mainly of adaptive thickening secondary to smooth muscle cell proliferation in lesion-prone locations in coronary arteries. Type II lesions consist of both macrophages and smooth muscle cells with extracellular lipid deposits, and type III lesions consist of smooth muscle cells surrounded by some extracellular fibrils and lipid deposits. This type III lesion, or fatty streak, is the earliest grossly detectable lesion of atherosclerosis (29). By age 25, most individuals in Western society have fatty streaks, which consist of an accumulation of lipid (mainly oxidized LDL) within macrophages or foam cells, mostly in the extracellular space of the intima. Type IV lesions are confluent cellular lesions with a great deal of extracellular lipid, whereas type V lesions consist of an extracellular lipid core covered by a thin fibrous cap. The type VI, or complicated lesion, occurs as a result of rupture or fissure of a nonseverely stenotic type IV or V lesion. Depending on changes in the geometry of the disrupted plaque, particularly on whether the subsequent thrombus completely occludes the artery, the event may be catastrophic, resulting in myocardial infarction and/or death, or clinically silent (30).

In the last few years, a number of studies have demonstrated that arteriographically mild coronary lesions may be associated with significant progression to severe stenosis or total occlusion (31–33). These lesions may account for as many as two-thirds of the patients in whom unstable angina or other acute coronary syndromes develop (Table 2).

The nonlinear and episodic progression seen in coronary artery lesions probably results from disruption of type IV and V lesions, with subsequent thrombus formation leading to either acute coronary syndromes or asymptomatic plaque growth. Following plaque disruption, hemorrhage into the plaque, luminal thrombosis, or vasospasm may cause sudden flow obstruction, giving rise to new or changing symptoms. The magnitude of thrombotic response following plaque rupture may depend on the thrombogenicity of the exposed plaque components, local flow conditions determined by the severity and geometry of the luminal stenosis, and the systemic thrombotic-thrombolytic milieu at the time of plaque rupture (34).

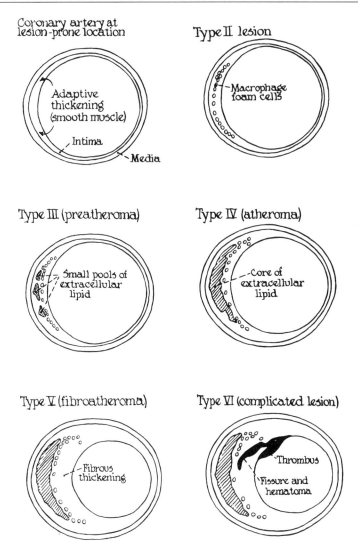

Fig. 2. Cross-sections of identical, most proximal part of six left anterior descending coronary arteries. The morphology of the intima ranges from adaptive intimal thickening always present in this lesion-prone location to a type VI lesion in advanced atherosclerotic disease. Other cross-sections show sequence of atherosclerotic lesion types that may lead to type VI. Identical morphologies may be found in other lesion-prone parts of the coronary and many other arteries. (From ref. *28*.)

What factors predispose a percentage of these plaques to become unstable and rupture? Understanding this requires a closer look at the makeup of these lesions. Plaques are composed of a variable amount of lipid core and a connective tissue matrix cap. The lipid component is derived mainly from plasma LDL, which has been oxidized and subsequently taken up by monocyte-derived macrophages, now known as foam cells. Within the core is a soft, hypocellular, and avascular pool containing cholesterol *(35,36)*. The composition of the cholesterol is critically important, as an atheromatous pool containing cholesterol esters is soft and prone to disruption *(37)*. Once plaque rupture occurs, the

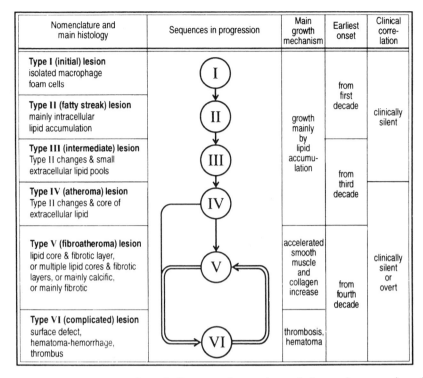

Nomenclature and main histology	Sequences in progression	Main growth mechanism	Earliest onset	Clinical corre-lation
Type I (initial) lesion isolated macrophage foam cells	I	growth mainly by lipid accumu-lation	from first decade	clinically silent
Type II (fatty streak) lesion mainly intracellular lipid accumulation	II			
Type III (intermediate) lesion Type II changes & small extracellular lipid pools	III		from third decade	
Type IV (atheroma) lesion Type II changes & core of extracellular lipid	IV			
Type V (fibroatheroma) lesion lipid core & fibrotic layer, or multiple lipid cores & fibrotic layers, or mainly calcific, or mainly fibrotic	V	accelerated smooth muscle and collagen increase	from fourth decade	clinically silent or overt
Type VI (complicated) lesion surface defect, hematoma-hemorrhage, thrombus	VI	thrombosis, hematoma		

Fig. 3. Flow diagram in center column indicates pathways in evolution and progression of human athero-sclerotic lesions. Roman numerals indicate histologically characteristic types of lesions enumerated in Table 2 and defined at left of the flow diagram. The direction of arrows indicates sequence in which characteristic morphologies may change. From type I to type IV, changes in lesion morphology occur primarily because of increasing accumulation of lipids. The loop between types V and VI illustrates how lesions increase in thickness when thrombotic deposits form on their surfaces. Thrombotic deposits may form repeatedly over varied time spans in the same location and may be the principal mechanism for gradual occlusion of medium-sized arteries. (From ref. *28*.)

thrombogenic components of this pool (tissue factor, collagen, foam cells, and so on) provide a substrate for subsequent thrombus formation.

The process of plaque disruption can best be understood in terms of factors that increase the vulnerability of the plaque to rupture and stresses or strains imposed on the plaque, referred to as triggers. Plaque vulnerability to rupture is dependent on a number of interrelated factors, including the size of the lipid pool, the thickness of the fibrous cap, and the inflammatory state of the plaque and surrounding vascular tree (Fig. 4).

LIPID CONTENT OF THE PLAQUE

The size and consistency of the atheromatous lipid core are important factors for the stability of a plaque. In general, the bigger the lipid core, the more vulnerable (rupture-prone) is the plaque *(38)*. Data from Ambrose et al. *(20)* suggest that in ulcerated, ruptured plaques, the size of the lipid pool exceeds 40% of the total plaque area in >90% of cases. At body temperature, the cholesterol is in liquid or crystaline form *(39)*; the ratio of liquid to crystaline cholesterol has been hypothesized to influence the propensity for plaque disruption *(40)*.

Table 2
Angiographic Severity of Culprit Coronary Artery Stenosis
Before the Development of Acute Coronary Syndromes[a]

		Percentage of patients with diameter stenosis of culprit vessel		
		<50%	50–70%	>70%
Clinical presentation				
Unstable angina				
Ambrose et al. (3)	N = 25	72	16	12
Acute myocardial infarction				
Ambrose et al. (3)	N = 23	48	30	22
Little et al. (82)	N = 41	66	31	3
Giroud et al. (50)	N = 92	78	9	13
Nobuyoshi et al. (94)	N = 39	59	15	26
Average of pooled results		65	20	15

[a]From ref. 34. References in table are found in ref. 34.

THICKNESS OF THE FIBROUS CAP

As this highly thrombogenic lipid core underlies the fibrous cap, the integrity of the fibrous cap determines the stability of an atherosclerotic plaque. Disruption of the fibrous cap usually occurs at the point where the cap is thinnest, most commonly at the border of the plaque with the normal wall or in the center of the cap overlying a lipid pool (41).

A dense, fibrous extracellular matrix is the main component of the fibrous cap of atherosclerotic plaques. The principal constituents of this extracellular matrix are types I and III collagen (a triple helical coil derived from specific procollagen precursors), elastin, and proteoglycans (Fig. 5) (42). Interferon-β (IFN-β) elaborated by activated T-cells reduces collagen synthesis by causing smooth muscle cell apoptosis and by specifically inhibiting collagen synthesis in smooth muscle cells. Additionally, the matrix metalloproteinases, such as collagenase and stromelysin, which facilitate intercellular matrix degradation, are released by lipid-laden macrophages under the influence of cytokines such as IFN-β, macrophage colony-stimulating factor (M-CSF), macrophage chemoattractant protein-1 (MCP-1), and interleukin-1 (IL-1). These metalloproteinases can also be expressed by endothelial and smooth muscle cells in the plaque, after being activated by cytokines (23). Libby (42) has shown that cytokines do not appear to affect the synthesis of tissue inhibitors of matrix metalloproteinases. This lab has also helped to define the role of another important cytokine, IFN-γ. Among the cells found in human atherosclerotic plaques, only activated T-lymphocytes can elaborate IFN-γ. This interferon markedly decreased the ability of human smooth muscle cells to express the interstiial collagen genes when exposed to transforming growth factor-β, the most potent stimulus for interstitial collagen gene expression known for these cells (25).

INFLAMMATORY MARKERS

Inflammatory processes are now known to play an integral role in the formation of atherosclerotic plaques (43,44). Elevated plasma levels of several markers of the inflammatory

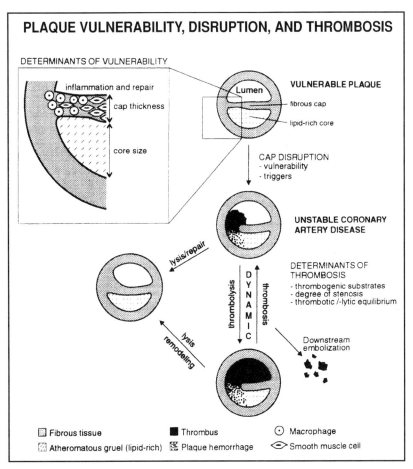

Fig. 4. Schematic illustrating pathophysiologic mechanisms. (Reprinted with permission from ref. *75*.)

cascade have been shown to predict future risk of plaque rupture *(45)*. From the initial phases of leukocyte recruitment to eventual rupture of vulnerable atherosclerotic plaques, inflammatory mediators appear to play a key role in the pathogensis in atherosclerosis.

Endothelial leukocyte adhesion molecules such as intercellular adhesion molecule (ICAM), vascular adhesion molecule (VCAM), and selectin have been shown to play a role in the early stages of atherogenesis *(46,47)*. Both macrophages and endothelial cells produce ICAM in response to inflammatory cytokines such as IL-1, tumor necrosis factor (TNF-α, and IFN-γ, whereas VCAM expression is mainly restricted to endothelial cells. Endothelial cells stimulated by cytokines also produce MCP-1, monocyte CSF, and IL-6, which further amplify the inflammatory cascade *(48)*. VCAM-1 expression has been demonstrated to precede macrophage and T-lymphocyte recruitment to atheromatous plaques *(49)*. C-reactive protein (CRP) is now thought to contribute directly to the pro-inflammatory state, rather than merely being a bystander marker of vascular inflammation. CRP stimulates monocyte release of inflammatory cytokines such as IL-1, IL-6, and TNF-α and also induces expression of ICAM-1 and VCAM-1 by endothelial cells *(50)*. CRP has been localized directly within atheromatous plaque, where it precedes and mediates monocyte recruitment; it is also an activator of complement *(51)*.

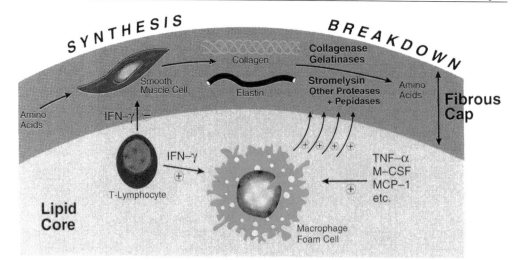

Fig. 5. Black and white diagram showing metabolism of collagen and elastin in the plaque's fibrous cap. The vascular smooth muscle cell synthesizes the extracellular matrix protein, collagen, and elastin from amino acids. In the unstable plaque, interferon-γ (1FN-γ) secreted by activated T-cells may inhibit collagen synthesis, interfering with the maintenance and repair of the collagenous framework of the plaque's fibrous cap. The activated macrophage secretes proteinases that can break down both collagen and elastin to peptides and eventually amino acid. This breakdown of these structural molecules of the extracellular matrix can weaken the fibrous cap, rendering it particularly susceptible to rupture and precipitation of acute coronary syndromes. IFN-γ secreted by the T-lymphocytes can in turn activate the macrophage. Plaques also contain other activators of macrophages, including tumor necrosis factor-α (TNF-α), macrophage colony-stimulating factor (M-CSF), and macrophage chemo-attractant protein-1 (MCP-1), among others. From ref. *42.*

The inflammatory response may be promoted at several different sites. Although many inflammatory markers are derived from the liver, including CRP, fibrinogen, and serum amyloid A, low levels may also be derived from other sources including the endothelium itself. Production of inflammatory markers is stimulated by circulating cytokines such as IL-6 and TNF-α, which in turn may also be generated from a variety of systemic sources, including adipose tissue, which is a potent source of cytokines, and inflammatory cells either in the atherosclerotic lesion in the arterial wall or elsewhere *(52).* The trigger for the inflammatory response remains unclear, however. Numerous studies of infectious etiologies, although intriguing, have thus far failed to prove conclusively a cause-and-effect relationship with the systemic inflammatory response.

TRIGGERS OF PLAQUES RUPTURE

Events triggering plaque rupture have been intensely investigated. Coronary plaques are constantly stressed by a variety of mechanical and hemodynamic forces that may trigger disruption of vulnerable plaques *(53).* These include plasma catecholamine surges and increased sympathetic activity *(54),* blood pressure surges, exercise *(55),* changes in heart rate and contractility affecting the angulation of coronary arteries, coronary vasospasm *(56),* and various hemodynamic forces *(57,58).* Hence, plaque rupture is a function of both internal plaque changes (vulnerability) and external stresses (triggers). Vulnerability is more important than triggers in determining the risk of a future event, because

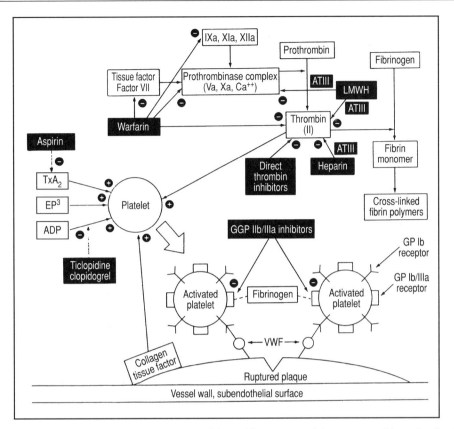

Fig. 6. Interaction between antiplatelet and antithrombin agents and the process of thrombosis. ADP = adenosine diphosphate; ATIII = antithrombin III; Epi = epinephrine; GPIb receptor = glycoprotein Ib receptor; GPIIb/IIIa receptor = glycoprotein IIb/IIIa receptor; GPIIb/IIIa inhibitors = glycoprotein IIb/IIIa inhibitors; LMWH = low-molecular-weight heparin; TxA$_2$ = thromboxane A$_2$; VWF = von Willebrand factor. (Reprinted with permission from ref. *76*.)

if no vulnerable plaques are present in the coronary arteries, there is no rupture-prone substrate for a potential trigger to affect *(59)*.

Platelets

Once plaque rupture occurs, exposing thrombogenic substances to flowing blood, the interaction of platelets and coagulation factors, namely, thrombin, determines the magnitude and extent of thrombosis at the site (Fig. 6). Platelet deposition occurs almost instantaneously after deep arterial injury. Triggered by damage to the vessel wall and local exposure of the subendothelial matrix, platelets adhere to subendothelial collagen. At least two rheologic factors potentiate early platelet binding to the subendothelium. First, platelets are unevenly distributed in flowing arterial blood. Owing to the dynamics of laminar flow and the relative densities of the blood corpuscles, platelets tend to concentrate at the periphery, directly adjacent to the endothelium *(60)*. This enhances maximal platelet-collagen interaction and facilitates binding in areas of endothelial injury. Second, through poorly understood mechanisms, high shear stress is known to increase activation of platelets *(61)*. Platelets traveling through an area rendered acutely stenotic

Table 3
Platelet Granule Content

α- Granules	Dense granules	Lysosomes
Fibrinogen	Serotonin	Glucose-6 phosphatase
Thrombospondin	Calcium	Acid phosphatase
β-thromboglobulin	ATP	Platele factor 3
Platelet factor 4	ADP	B-*N*-acetyl-galactosominidase
Albumin	Pyrophosphate	α-Arabinosidase
Von Willebrand factor		
Fibronectin		
Factor V		
β$_2$-Macroglobulin		
Vitronectin		
α$_1$-Proteinase inhibitor		
Histidine-rich glycoprotein		
Platelet-derived growthfactor		

From ref. *77*.

by plaque rupture are transiently exposed to high shear stress forces and may become activated. Adherence is mediated primarily by the von Willebrand factor (vWF), a multimeric glycosylated protein that is synthesized in endothelial cells and secreted into the subendothelium, where it binds to collagen *(61)*. Coverage of the exposed site by platelets depends on the recognition of adhesive proteins by specific platelet-membrane glycoproteins, many of which are integrins *(62)*.

The glycoprotein (GP)Ib receptor, which exists in a complex with GPIX and GPV on the platelet surface, binds von Willebrand factor and is the principal glycoprotein involved in the initial contact between platelets and the vessel wall *(63)*. Because GPIB is a constitutively expressed integrin, resting platelets can bind vWF and thereby adhere to collagen without first being activated. Platelets then continue accruing at the site of endothelial cell denudation until the entire area of injury is covered by a platelet monolayer, anchored to the subendothelium via the GPIb-vWF bond.

Platelet activation follows adhesion and can be initiated by several mechanical and chemical stimuli. The presence of thrombin and the adhesion of platelets to collagen and other components of the subendothelial matrix are among the strongest stimulators of platelet activation. Although they are capable of little or no protein synthesis, platelets contain, sequestered in their granules, numerous prepacked extraordinarily potent molecules (Table 3) *(64)*. Once bound and subsequently activated, these platelets release the contents of their storage granules, which contain, in addition to potent growth factors (mitogens), various other substances such as serotonin, ADP, thromboxane A$_2$, and epinephrine, which are capable of activating additional nearby platelets. Irrespective of the agonist, the final common pathway leading to the formation of the platelet plug is platelet aggregation. These activated platelets, however, do not bind via the aforementioned GPIb-vWF interaction, as these sites are already occupied by the initial platelet monolayer. Instead, further platelet recruitment depends on the expression of a second platelet receptor, the GPIIb/IIIa receptor complex (Fig. 7).

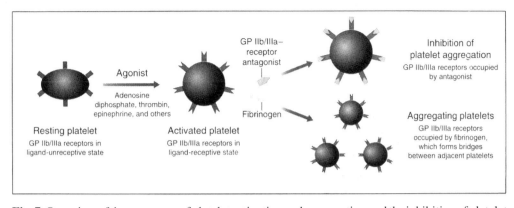

Fig. 7. Overview of the processes of platelet activation and aggregation and the inhibition of platelet aggregation by inhibitors of glycoprotein (GP)IIb/IIIa receptors. Platelet activation causes changes in the shape of platelets and conformational changes in GPIIb/IIIa receptors, transforming the receptors from a ligand-unreceptive to a ligand-receptive state. Ligand-receptive GPIIb/IIIa receptors bind fibrinogen molecules, which form bridges between adjacent platelets and facilitate platelet aggregation. Inhibitors of GPIIb/IIIa receptors also bind to GPIIb/III receptors, blocking the binding of fibrinogen and thus preventing platelet aggregation. From ref. *61.*)

The GPIIb/IIIa receptor belongs to the integrin family of heterodimeric adhesion molecules, which are formed by the noncovalent interaction of a series of α and β-subunits *(65)*. Integrins are found on virtually all cell types and mediate a diversity of physiologic responses. Multiple integrins (Ia/IIa, Ic, IIa, receptor for laminin, and others) are present on the surface of the platelet and play a role in platelet adhesion *(66)*. The GP IIb-IIIa receptor is the most abundant on the platelet surface, with approx 50,000 copies per platelet. Although clearly the most clinically important interaction is with fibrinogen, the receptor has also been shown to bind other adhesive proteins involved in aggregation, such as fibronectin, vitronectin, and vWF *(67,68)*.

The recognition specificity of the GPIIb/IIIa receptor is defined by two peptide sequences. The Arg-Gly-Asp (RGD) sequence was initially identified as the adhesive sequence in fibronectin, but it is also present in fibrinogen, vWF, and vitronectin. All these ligands contain at least one RGD sequence, whereas fibrinogen contains two RGD sequences per half-molecule *(42)*. The second sequence involved is the Lys-Gln-Ala-Gly-Asp-Val sequence, located at the extreme carboxy terminus of the γ-chain of fibrinogen *(69,70)*. Unlike the RGD sequence, this sequence is found only in fibrinogen. Electron microscopic and immunologic studies suggest that this second sequence is the predominant site for fibrinogen/GPIIb/IIIa binding *(71,72)*.

Resting platelets do not express GPIIb/IIIa in a configuration suitable for ligand binding, but upon platelet activation this complex undergoes a conformational change that allows it to bind fibrinogen avidly *(73)*. Once activated, the original platelet monolayer recruits additional platelets, eventually forming a platelet plug via GPIIb/IIIa/fibrinogen/GPIIb/IIIa bridging. This process replicates itself as new platelets enter the injured vascular bed, become activated, expressing GPIIb/IIIa receptors in the appropriate conformation, and become incorporated into the growing plug. The area of previously denuded endothelium is thereby quickly covered by the growing platelet plug. Left unchecked with no compensatory mechanisms, this process would lead to arterial lumen occlusion. This

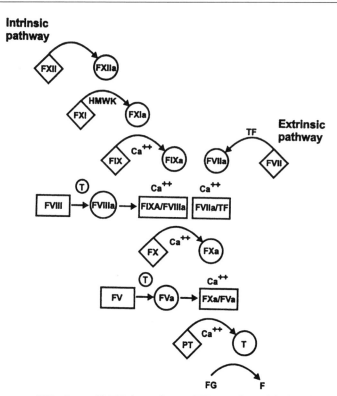

Fig. 8. Platelet structure. FX = factor X; TF tissue factor; PT = prothrombin; T = thrombin; F = fibrin; FG = fibrinogen; HMWK = high-molecular-weight kininogens; Ca^{++} = calcium. (Reprinted with permission from ref. *77*.)

is prevented as neighboring endothelial cells secrete antiaggregatory agents including prostacyclin, endothelium-derived relaxation factor, or nitric oxide, as it is now known, and ADPase *(34)*.

The Coagulation Cascade

The initial flow obstruction after arterial injury is usually caused by platelet aggregation. However, a pure platelet thrombus is highly unstable and may be easily dislodged unless it is subsequently reinforced by fibrin crosslinking. Therefore, both platelets and fibrin play intimate roles in thrombus formation.

Following arterial injury, in vivo coagulation is initiated by the tissue factor (TF)-dependent pathway. This system becomes activated when TF comes in contact with circulating factor VII, a plasma zymogen (Fig. 8). Recall that the coenzyme TF is found on the surface of macrophages, fibroblasts, smooth muscle cells, and activated endothelial cells. The atherosclerotic plaque itself also contains abundant TF, which is synthesized by lipid-laden foamy macrophages and is predominantly localized in the necrotic core of the plaque *(69)*.

The TF/VII complex undergoes limited autoactivation, generating the more potent TF/VIIa complex. This process then replicates, leading to a self-amplification of the TF/VIIa complex *(35)*. After self-amplification, the TF/VIIa complex then forms an additional complex with plasma coagulation factor X on the surface of activated platelets. This is thought to occur on activated platelets because the platelet membranes contain essential phospholipids that are in the correct configuration to support coagulation. Once

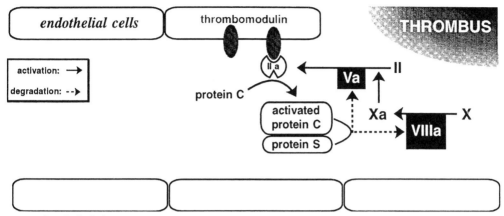

subendothelial matrix

Fig. 9. Feedback mechanism for the inactivation of factors Va and VIIIa. Thrombin (IIa) bound to thrombomodulin specifically activates protein C. Activated protein C, in concert with protein S, efficiently cleaves and thus inactivates the coagulation factors VIIIa and Va required for the assembly of the ternary complexes to accelerate the thrombin generation. This potent feedback mechanism may be essential to confine excessive thrombin generation to severely injured, deendothelialized parts of the blood vessel. (From ref. *54*.)

factor X is converted to Xa by limited proteolysis, it disengages from the complex and then reassembles on the platelet with factor V to form the so-called prothrombinase complex (Xa/V). However, in its inactive form, this complex is inefficient in converting prothrombin to thrombin. The mechanism of thrombin-mediated positive feedback is not fully understood, but moderate levels of thrombin may be capable of activating factor V to a more potent cofactor, factor Va *(70)*. This then assembles with Xa to form the Xa/Va prothrombinase complex, with dramatically more thrombin-generating capability *(72)*. Increased levels of thrombin also enhance the conversion of factor VIII to VIIIa, which then combines with factor IXa on the platelet surface, dramatically increasing the conversion of factor X to Xa, and subsequently generating even more prothrombinase complex.

Each of the reactions following the TF-VII interaction occurs on the surface of activated platelets. Hence, thrombin-mediated platelet activation can be considered another of the positive feedback mechanisms responsible for the dramatic increase in thrombin generation leading to clot formation. More intense platelet recruitment increases the available platelet surface area, thus enhancing thrombin generation. Thrombin presumably plays a key role in additional platelet recruitment, as thrombin itself is the most potent physiologic activator of platelets *(35)*.

Similar to the mechanisms that limit platelet growth to areas of endothelial injury, there are also mechanisms to limit thrombin generation and subsequent fibrin formation *(74)*. The two principal inhibitors are the heparin sulfate-antithrombin III (ATIII) system and the thrombomodulin-protein C-protein S system. ATIII binds circulating thrombin, inactivates it, and eventually clears it through the reticuloendothelial system. Once bound by heparin, ATIII undergoes a conformational change that greatly enhances its affinity for thrombin *(75)*.

In the presence of ongoing thrombin generation, neighboring endothelial cells increase their concentration of a membrane-bound protein receptor, thrombomodulin (Fig. 9).

This protein is capable of modifying the function (specificity) of thrombin. Whereas the preferred substrates for free thrombin are factors V and VIII, fibrinogen, and possibly factor XI, thrombin associated with endothelial cell thrombomodulin alters its affinity so that it binds specifically (and virtually exclusively) to a plasma protein referred to as protein C (35). Limited proteolysis of protein C by thrombomodulin-bound thrombin activates protein C, which then associates with protein S. This complex is then able to inhibit factors Va and VIIIa, abolishing the procoagulant properties of these cofactors.

THE PROCESS OF THROMBUS FORMATION

Although it is conceptually useful to view the components of the thrombotic process individually, it must be understood that these processes occur simultaneously and in concert. As mentioned previously, without the appropriate substrate (a vulnerable plaque), the various triggers known to be associated with unstable coronary syndromes are of no clinical consequence. Once plaque rupture does occur, the response to this perturbation is multifactorial, with the final clinical outcome dependent on the interplay of the components described above, namely, the (dysfunctional) endothelium, the procoagulant constituents of the exposed plaque, activated platelets, inflammatory processes, and TF-dependent coagulation mediated primarily by thrombin *(76)*. It appears as if most ruptured plaques are resealed by a small mural thrombus, and only infrequently does a major luminal thrombus evolve. The factors that seem to determine the thrombotic response include (1) the character and extent of the exposed thrombogenic substrate; (2) local flow disturbances secondary to degree of stenosis and surface irregularities; and (3) thrombotic-thrombolytic equilibrium at the time of rupture *(63)*, incorporating the dynamic interaction between activated platelets and components of the coagulation cascade *(77)*.

Based on these mechanisms of thrombus formation and propagation, treatment strategies utilizing an understanding of the molecular pathophysiology of this process continue to be developed. These then form the underpinnings of randomized controlled trials to evaluate the clinical outcomes of these therapies in populations of patients undergoing percutaneous interventions or with acute coronary syndromes.

REFERENCES

1. Hillis WS. The continuing debate: conservative or interventional therapy for unstable coronary artery disease. Am J Cardiol 1997;80:51E–54E.
2. Herrick JB. Clinical features of sudden obstruction of the coronary arteries. JAMA 1912;59:2015–2020.
3. Levine SA, Brown CL. Coronary thrombosis: its various clinical features. Medicine 1929;8:245–418.
4. Parkinson J, Bedford DE. Cardial infarction and coronary thrombosis. Lancet 1928;14:195–239.
5. Sampson JJ, Eliaser M. The diagnosis of impending acute coronary artery occlusion. Am Heart J 1937; 13:676–686.
6. Feil H. Preliminary pain in coronary thrombosis. Am J Med Sci 1937;193:42–48.
7. Howell WH. Heparin, an anticoagulant. Am J Physiol 1922;63:434–435.
8. Best CH. Heparin and thrombosis. Harvey Lectures 1940;Nov:66–90.
9. Wright IS. Experience with anticoagulants. Circulation 1959;19:110–113.
10. Cairns JA. The acute coronary ischemic syndromes—the central role of thrombosis. Can J Cardiol 1996; 12:901–907.
11. Wright IS, Marple CD, Beck DF. Report of the committee for the evaluation of anticoagulants in the treatment of coronary thrombosis with myocardial infarction. Am Heart J 1948;36:801–815.
12. Craven LL. Acetylsalicylic acid, possible preventive of coronary thrombosis. Ann West Med Surg 1950; 4:95.

13. Craven LL. Experiences with aspirin in the nonspecific prophylaxis of coronary thrombosis. Miss V Med J 1953;75:38–44.
14. Mueller RL, Scheidt S. History of drugs for thrombotic disease. Discovery, development, and directions for the future. Circulation 1994;89:432–449.
15. Sherry S. The origin of thrombolytic therapy. J Am Coll Cardiol 1989;14:1085–2092.
16. Gifford RH, Feinstein AR. A critique of methodology in studies of anticoagulant therapy for acute myocardial infarction. N Engl J Med 1969;280:351–357.
17. DeWood MA. Prevalence of total coronary occlusion during the early hours of transmural myocardial infarction. N Engl J Med 1980;303:897–901.
18. Davies MJ, Thomas A. Thrombosis and acute coronary artery lesions in sudden cardiac ischemic death. N Engl J Med 1984;310:1137–1140.
19. Moise A, Theroux P, Taeymans Y, et al. Unstable angina and progression of coronary atherosclerosis. N Engl J Med 1983;309:685–689.
20. Ambrose JA, Winters SL, Stern A, et al. Angiographic morphology and the pathogenesis of unstable angina pectoris. J Am Coll Cardiol 1985;5:609–616.
21. Falk E. Why do plaques rupture? Circulation 1992;86:111-30–111-42.
22. Moncada S. Differential formation of prostacyclin by layers of the arterial wall: an explanation for the antithrombotic properties of vascular endothelium. Thromb Res 1977;11:323.
23. Braunwald E. Heart Disease, 5th ed. WB Saunders, Philadelphia, 1997, p. 1108.
24. Furchgott RF. Role of endothelium in responsiveness of vascular smooth muscle. Circ Res 1983;53:557.
25. Yanagisawa M. A novel potent vasoconstrictor peptide produced by vascular endothelial cells. Nature 1988;332:411.
26. Jaffe EA, Hoyer LW, Nahcman RL. Synthesis of antihemophilic factor antigen by cultured human endothelial cells. J Clin Invest 1973;52:2757.
27. Steinberg D. Lipoproteins and atherosclerosis: a look back and a look ahead. Arteriosclerosis 1983;3:283.
28. Stary HC, Chandler AB, Dinsmore RE, et al. A definition of advanced types of atherosclerotic lesions and a histopathological classification of atherosclerosis: a report from the Committee on Vascular Lesions of the Council on Arteriosclerosis, American Heart Association. Circulation 1995;92:1355–1374.
29. Fuster V, Badimon JJ, Chesebro JH, Fallon JT. Plaque rupture, thrombosis, and therapeutic implications. Haemostasis 1996;26(Suppl 4):269–284.
30. Fuster V. Mechanisms leading to myocardial infarction: insights from studies of vascular biology. Lewis A. Conner Memorial Lecture. Circulation 1994;90:2126–2146.
31. Ambrose JA, Tannenbaum M, Alexpoulos D, et al. Angiographic progression of coronary artery disease and the development of myocardial infarction. J Am Coll Cardiol 1988;12:56–62.
32. Little WC, Constantinescu M, Applegate RJ, et al. Can coronary angiography predict the site of a subsequent myocardial infarction in patients with mild-to-moderate coronary artery disease. Circulation 1982;78:1157–1166.
33. Falk E, Shah PK, Fuster V. Coronary plaque disruption. Circulation 1995;92:657–671.
34. Shah PK. Pathophysiology of plaque rupture and the concept of plaque stabilization. Cardiol Clin 1996; 14:17–29.
35. Shah PK. New insights into the pathogenesis and prevention of acute coronary syndromes. Am J Cardiol 1997;79:17–23.
36. Lundberg B. Chemical composition and physical state of lipid deposits in atherosclerosis. Atherosclerosis 1985;56:93–110.
37. Falk E, Shah PK, Fuster V. Coronary plaque disruption. Circulation 1996;92:657–671.
38. Davies MJ, Richardson PD, Woolf N, Katz DR, Mann J. Risk of thrombosis in human atherosclerotic plaques: role of extracellular lipid, macrophage, and smooth muscle cell content. Br Heart J 1993;69: 377–381.
39. Loree HM, Tobias BJ, Gibson LJ, Kamm RD, Small DM, Lee RT. Mechanical properties of midel atherosclerotic lesions lipid pools. Arterioscler Thromb 1994;14:230–234.
40. Richardson RD, Davies MJ, Born GVR. Influence of plaque configuration and stress distribution on fissuring of coronary atherosclerotic plaques. Lancet 1989;2:941–944.
41. Crea F, Biasucci LM. Role of inflammation in the pathogenesis of unstable coronary artery disease. Am J Cardiol 1997;80:10E–16E.
42. Libby P. Molecular basis of the acute coronary syndromes. Circulation 1995;91:2844–2850.
43. Ross R. The pathogenesis of atherosclerosis: a perspective for the 1990s. Nature 1993;362:801–808.
44. Ross R. Atherosclerosis—an inflammatory disease. N Engl J Med 1999;340:115–126.

45. Blake GJ, Ridker PM. Novel clinical markers of vascular wall inflammation. Circ Res 2001;89:763–771.
46. Davies MJ, Gordon JL, Gearing AJ, et al. The expression of the adhesion molecules ICAM-1, VCAM-1, PECAM, and E-selectin in human atherosclerosis. J Pathol 1993;171:223–229.
47. Adams DH, Shaw S. Leucocyte-endothelial interactions and regulation of leucocyte migration. Lancet 1994;343:831–836.
48. Bevilacqua MP, Gimbrone MA, Jr. Inducible endothelial functions in inflammation and coagulation. Semin Thromb Hemost 1987;13:425–433.
49. Sakai A, Kume N, Nishi E, Tanoue K, Miyasaka M, Kita T. P-selectin and vascular cell adhesion molecule-1 are focally expressed in aortas of hypercholesterolemic rabbits before intimal accumulation of macrophages and T lymphocytes. Arterioscler Thromb Vasc Biol 1997;17:310–316.
50. Pasceri V, Willerson JT, Yeh ET. Direct proinflammatory effect of C-reactive protein on human endothelial cells. Circulation 2000;102:2165–2168.
51. Torzewski M, Rist C, Mortensen RF, et al. C-reactive protein in the arterial intima: role of C-reactive protein receptor-dependent monocyte recruitment in atherogenesis. Arterioscler Thromb Vasc Biol 2000; 20:2094–2099.
52. Blake GJ, Ridker PM. Novel clinical markers of vascular wall inflammation. Circ Res 2001;89:763–771.
53. Falk E, Fernandez-Ortiz A. Role of thrombosis in atherosclerosis and its complications. Am J Cardiol 1995;75:5B–11B.
54. Fiore LD, Deykin D. Mechanisms of hemostasis and arterial thrombosis. Cardiol Clin 1994;12:399–409.
55. Weiss HJ, Turitto VT, Baumgartner HR. Effect of shear rate on platelet interaction with subendothelium in citrated and native blood. J Lab Clin Med 1978;92:750–756.
56. Weiss HJ, Turitto VT, Baumgartner HR. Effect of shear rate on platelet interaction with subendothelium in citrated and native blood. J Lab Clin Med 1978;92:750–756.
57. Lefkovits J, Plow EF, Topol EJ. Platelet glycoprotein IIb/IIIA receptors in cardiovascular medicine. N Engl J Med 1995;23:1553–1559.
58. Kroll MH, Harris TS, Moake JL, Handin RI, Shafer AI. von Willebrand factor binding to platelet GpIB initiates signals for platelet activation. J Clin Invest 1991;88:1568–1573.
59. Pepper DS. Macromolecules released from platelet storage organelles. Thromb Haemost 1980;42: 1667–1670.
60. Hynes RO, Integrins. A family of cell surface receptors. Cell 1987;48:549–554.
61. Lefkovits J, Plow EF, Topol EJ. Platelet glycoprotein IIB-IIA receptors in cardiovascular medicine. N Engl J Med 1995;332:1553–1559.
62. Ruggeri ZM, De Marco L, Gatti L, Bader R, Montgomery RR. Platelets have more than one binding site for von Willebrand factor. J Clin Invest 1983;72:1–12.
63. Phillips DR, Charo IF, Parise LV, Fitzgerald LA. The platelet membrane glycoprotein IIB-IIIA complex. Blood 1988;71:831–843.
64. Topol EJ. Platelet glycoprotein IIB-IIIA receptor antagonists in coronary artery disease. Eur Heart J 1996; 17:9–18.
65. Klociwiak M, Timmons S, Hawiger J. Recognition site for the platelet receptor is present on the 15-residue carboxy-terminal fragment of the gamma chain of human fibrinogen and is not involved in the fibrin polymerization reaction Thromb Res 1983;29:249–255.
66. Weisel JW, Nagaswami C, Vilair G, Bennett JS. Examination of the platelet membrane glycoprotein IIB-IIIA complex its interaction with fibrinogen and other ligands by electron microscopy. J Biol Chem 1992; 267:16,637–16,643.
67. D'Souza SE, Ginsberg MH, Matsueda GR, Plow EF. A discrete sequence in a platelet integrin is involved in ligand recognition. Nature 1991;350:66–68.
68. Shattil SJ, Hoxie JA, Cunningham M. Changes in the platelet membrane glycoprotein IIB-IIIA complex during platelet activation. J Biol Chem 1985;260:11,107–11,111.
69. Wilcox JN, Smith KM, Schwartz SM, Gordon D. Localization of tissue factor in the normal vessel wall and in the atherosclerotic plaque. Proc Natl Acad Sci USA 1989;86:2839–2843.
70. Ofosu FA, Sie P, Modi GJ, et al. The inhibition of thrombin-dependent positive feedback reactions is critical to the expression of the anticoagulant effect of heparin. Biochem J 1987;243:579.
71. Lindahl AK, Wildgoose P, Lumsden AS, et al. Active site-inhibited factor VIIa blocks tissue factor activity and prevents arterial thrombus formation in baboons (Abstr.) Circulation 1993;88:2240.
72. Pieters J, Lindhout T. The limited importance of factor Xa inhibition of the anticoagulant property of heparin in thromboplastin activated plasma. Blood 1988;72:2048–2054.

73. Rosenberg RD, Damus PS. The purification and mechanism of action of human antithrombin-heparin cofactor. J Biol Chem 1973;248:579–583.
74. Ruschitzka FT, Noll G, Luscher TF. The endothelium in coronary artery disease [Review]. Cardiology 1997;88:3.
75. Kristensen SD, Ravn HB, Flak E. Insights into the pathophysiology of unstable coronary artery disease. Am J Cardiol 1997;80:7E.
76. Alexander JH, Harrington RA. Antiplatelet and antithrombin therapies in the acute coronary syndromes. Curr Opin Cardiol 1997;12:427–434.
77. Rock G, Wells P. New concepts in coagulation. Crit Rev Clin Lab Sci 1997;34:475–481.

2

Platelet Adhesion

Edward F. Plow, PhD

Contents

Introduction
Substrate Proteins for Platelet Adhesion
Platelet Adhesion Receptors
Acknowledgments
References

INTRODUCTION

Platelets are born from megakaryocytes and are bred to adhere. As such, these anuclear particles represent one of the most highly specialized cells within the body. This functional dedication to adhesion is essential in order to prevent excessive bleeding from sites of vascular injury. The rapidity with which platelets seal an injured vessel is a remarkable testament to their adhesive specialization and is essential to the maintenance and/or restoration of vascular integrity. As with many physiologic systems, an overly exuberant cellular response can have major pathophysiologic consequences. In the case of platelet adhesion, the out-of-control response can be devastating, thrombosis, leading to life-threatening or debilitating pathologies.

Platelet attachment and spreading reactions, together referred to as platelet adhesion, are essential for the hemostatic function of platelets. Platelet adhesion depends primarily on the interaction of these cells with components of the subendothelial matrix that become exposed as a consequence of injury to the endothelial cell lining of the vessel wall. Engagement of these substrates is mediated by an array of adhesion receptors that are displayed on the cell surface. Platelet-platelet interaction (platelet aggregation) is essential for formation of a platelet-rich thrombus and thereby regulates the thrombotic properties of platelets. Platelet aggregation depends primarily on the engagement of the plasma proteins, fibrinogen and von Willebrand factor (vWF), by the cell surface glycoprotein GPIIb/IIIa (integrin $\alpha_{IIb}\beta_3$). Hence, at a theoretical level, it appears possible to block the thrombotic function of platelets without severely compromising their hemostatic function by blockade of GPIIb/IIIa. Direct support for this supposition can be derived from the clinical observation that patients with Glanzmann's thrombasthenia, who lack functional GPIIb/IIIa, exhibit only episodic bleeding events. This set of observations provided a rationale and an impetus for the development of GPIIb/IIIa antagonists.

From: *Contemporary Cardiology: Platelet Glycoprotein IIb/IIIa
Inhibitors in Cardiovascular Disease, 2nd Edition*
Edited by: A. M. Lincoff © Humana Press Inc., Totowa, NJ

From one perspective, this volume can be viewed as a testimonial to the principle that the adhesion and aggregation functions of platelets are sufficiently separable that GPIIb/IIIa can be targeted for antithrombotic therapy. This chapter focuses on the mechanisms underlying platelet adhesion. The major receptor systems and their ligands will be discussed briefly. GPIIb/IIIa and its role in platelet aggregation are considered in Chapter 3. Unfortunately, the adhesive and aggregation functions of platelets are not entirely separable, and a bleeding risk appears to be intrinsic to total blockade of GPIIb/IIIa, particularly in the context of an invasive procedure. This overlap between risk and efficacy may reflect the requirement for some platelet aggregation for effective hemostasis, or to the role of GPIIb/IIIa not only in platelet aggregation but also in platelet adhesion. At one level, it has been the severity of the bleeding risk relative to the antithrombotic efficacy that has shaped the development of GPIIb/IIIa antagonism.

SUBSTRATE PROTEINS FOR PLATELET ADHESION

The Subendothelial Matrix

In addition to serving as a physical barrier, endothelial cells synthesize and elaborate components, notably prostaglandin I_2 (PGI$_2$), nitric oxide (NO), and enzyme(s) that degrade ADP *(1,2)*, which prevent platelet activation and adhesion. Also present on endothelial cell surfaces are potent anticoagulant molecules, such as thrombomodulin and the tissue factor pathway inhibitor (TFPI), which influence thrombin specificity or production and hence the availability of this potent platelet agonist *(3)*. Heparin sulfate and other proteoglycans on the endothelial cell surface combine with antithrombin III to neutralize thrombin and other coagulation proteases, which directly or indirectly affect the availability of thrombin. When the endothelium is disrupted, these platelet-suppressive activities are abolished, and components of the subendothelium that support platelet adhesion and activation become exposed. As discussed shortly, a variety of subendothelial cell constituents serve as substrates for platelet attachment and spreading. Furthermore, the matrix is a mutable surface. It can be remodeled as a consequence of its interaction with plasma proteins and/or by proteolysis, and these alterations influence its capacity to support platelet adhesion. Another relevant consideration is that, since the phenotypic properties of endothelial cells from different blood vessels varies, the composition of the matrix they deposit will vary as well. Accordingly, certain proteins may play a dominant role in supporting platelet adhesion in certain blood vessels. Moreover, even at the same anatomic location, the composition of the atherosclerotic plaque and the nature of the fissure or injury to the endothelium will expose different substratum. Thus, certain plaques, even when ruptured may have greater or lesser tendencies to support platelet adhesion and thrombus formation.

Some of major subendothelial matrix proteins that support platelet attachment and/or spreading reactions are listed in Table 1. From the extent of this list, it is clear that platelets can adhere to a variety of substrates once the endothelium has been disrupted. Not all the adhesive proteins listed in Table 1 support the same spectrum of platelet responses. For example, under some conditions, platelets attach to but do not spread on laminin *(4)*, whereas vWF and fibronectin appear to support both cell attachment and spreading *(5–7)*. Certain collagen types not only support the attachment and spreading of platelets but also evoke platelet secretion *(8)*. In turn, the secretory response, which can be induced by a variety of platelet agonists, directly influences the adhesive properties of platelets by altering

Table 1
Major Subendothelial Proteins That Support Platelet Adhesion

Matrix constituent	Comment
Collagens	Large family of proteins that can support platelet adhesion aggregation and secretion
von Willebrand factor	Large multimeric protein critical for the hemostatic function of platelets
Fibronectins	Dimeric or multimeric proteins that support attachment and spreading of platelets
Thrombospondins	Trimeric or higher multimeric proteins exhibiting both adhesive and antiadhesive properties for platelets
Laminins	Proteins supporting platelet adhesion

Table 2
Origins of Platelet Adhesive Proteins

Adhesive protein	Matrix	Plasma	Platelets
von Willebrand factor	+	+	+
Fibronectin	+	+	+
Thrombospondin-1	+	−	+
Vitronectin	*	+	+
Fibrinogen	*	+	+
Laminin	+	−	−
Collagen	+	−	−

*Constituent of provisional matrices.

their surface. Specifically, as a consequence of the secretory response, certain adhesion receptors become expressed (e.g., P-selectin [9]), and the density and/or distribution of others becomes altered (e.g., GPIIb/IIIa [10], GPIb/IX [11]). Of the multiple forms of collagen, types I, III, IV, and VI are regarded as being particularly important in supporting platelet adhesion (12,13).

Although endothelial disruption is the primary stimulus for platelet adhesion, platelets can interact with activated endothelial cells (14) and neutrophils, which in turn can interact with matrix or endothelial adherent platelets (15,16). There is a body of literature suggesting that such cell–cell interactions may play an important role in thrombus formation (15,16). Furthermore, circulating platelet–leukocyte complexes in the blood may be diagnostic of ongoing thrombotic events (17–19). Although not interacting directly with platelets, erythrocytes also exert a marked effect on adhesion of platelet to the vessel wall (20). Thus, the subendothelial matrix, and perhaps even intact endothelium, provide multiple substrates and mechanisms to support platelet adhesion, and other vascular cells can modulate these interactions.

Nonmatrix Sources of Matrix Proteins

In addition to the subendothelial matrix, proteins that support platelet adhesion can be derived from two other biologically relevant sources: blood, which comes in contact with the injured vessel; and platelet α-granules, which secrete their content of adhesive proteins when stimulated by agonists. The sources of key platelet adhesive proteins are listed in Table 2. Some of the platelet adhesive proteins (e.g., vWF and fibronectin) reside in all three locations. Fibrinogen and vitronectin are present in platelets and plasma but are not synthesized by endothelial cells. However, they are components of the provisional matrix formed at sites of vascular injury and are, therefore, particularly relevant substrates for platelet adhesion. It should be noted that the molecular forms of the adhesive proteins derived from these different sources are not identical. For example, the degree of vWF multimerization differs for the plasma and platelet forms (21), and the splicing variants of fibronectin differ depending on their sites of synthesis (22). As still yet another variable, a number of these adhesive proteins interact with one another. For example, vWF, fibronectin, and thrombospondin-1 (TSP-1) all bind to collagen (23–25). These interactions may indirectly bridge platelets to a matrix protein or may modulate the adhesive properties of the matrix. Although TSP-1 can be synthesized by many cell types in vitro, the platelet appears to be its primary source in vivo. Members of the thrombospondin gene family, including TSP-1, have been identified as risk factors for premature atherosclerosis (26).

Shear and Platelet Adhesion

Shear rate developed by flowing blood varies with vessel caliber. Local turbulence may develop as blood flows across the irregularities of an atherosclerotic plaque or a developing thrombus (27). Variations in the fluid dynamics of blood greatly influence platelet adhesion (28–30). Over the past two decades, more and more studies of platelet adhesion have been conducted under flow conditions to help ensure the biologic relevance of the analyses. Shear is particularly important in defining the contribution of vWF to platelet adhesion. In in vitro experiments, a role of vWF in platelet adhesion is readily demonstrable at high but not at low shear or under static conditions (6,31). By contrast, a role for fibronectin in supporting platelet adhesion can be demonstrated both high and low shear (32). Nevertheless, patients with von Willebrand disease have a major bleeding syndrome, which indicates the importance of vWF and shear in supporting platelet function. The development of vWF-deficient mice has attested to the importance of vWF in supporting platelet adhesion and thrombus formation (33), although evidence for still other mechanisms of platelet thrombus formation exists in mice that lack not only vWF but also fibrinogen (34). Shear may exert its influence on platelet/vWF adhesion by affecting the conformation of the adhesive protein or its platelet receptor, GPIb, or both (30,35,36). Also coming into play in the complex interrelationship between shear and vWF is the multimeric structure of vWF; the higher multimers of vWF are hemostatically more active (37).

PLATELET ADHESION RECEPTORS

The individual adhesive proteins discussed above interact with platelets by serving as ligands for specific cell-surface receptors. The major platelet adhesion receptors are listed in Table 3. Several nomenclature systems have been used to identify the same membrane proteins of the platelet. The original nomenclature was based on electrophoretic mobility, giving rise to GPI, -II, -III, and so on, with GPI having the highest molecular weight. As gel separation and protein detection systems became more sophisticated, several proteins were discerned with similar electrophoretic mobilities (e.g., GPI became GPIa, GPIb, and GPIc). Several of the membrane proteins exist on the platelet surface as noncovalent complexes; thus, GPIb/IX, GPIc/IIa, and GPIIb/IIIa should be viewed as single-membrane proteins with multiple subunits. Despite these ambiguities, the nomenclature

Table 3
Major Platelet Adhesion Receptors

Receptor	Common alternative designations	Major adhesive ligands
GPIa/IIa	$\alpha_2\beta_1$, VLA-2	Collagen
GPIb/IX/V		vWF
GPIc/IIa	$\alpha_5\beta_1$, VLA-5, fibronectin receptor	Fibronectin
GPIIb/IIIa	$\alpha_{IIb}\beta_3$	Fibrinogen, vWF, fibronectin, vitronectin, thrombospondin
GPIV	GPIIIb, CD36	Collagen, thrombospondin
GPVI		Collagen
$\alpha_6\beta_1$		Laminin
$\alpha_V\beta_3$	Vitronectin receptor	Vitronectin, fibrinogen, fibronectin, vWf thrombospondin, osteopontin

Abbreviations: GP, glycoprotein; vWF, von Willebrand factor; VLA, very late antigen.

based on electrophoretic properties remains the most widely used. Other nomenclature systems have arisen from the fact that several platelet membrane proteins are present and have been assigned different names on other cell types. This is the basis for the very late antigen (VLA), which is now rarely used, and leukocyte differentiation (CD) designations, which receive sporadic usage in the platelet literature. Some receptors are also identified on the basis of their function (e.g., the vitronectin and the fibronectin receptors). Such functional designations have major limitations since multiple membrane proteins can function as receptors for the same ligand (e.g., vitronectin [$\alpha_{IIb}\beta_3$ and $\alpha_V\beta_3$], fibronectin [$\alpha_{IIb}\beta_3$ and $\alpha_5\beta_1$], and several platelet membrane proteins can function as collagen receptors [*see* the Platelet Collagen Receptors section]). Beyond creating a nomenclature complexity (nightmare), the functional redundancy of the platelet receptors enables the cell to establish multiple contacts with a single matrix constituent. In turn, a single ligand may initiate several distinct functional responses by engaging multiple receptors.

Platelet Integrins

Many of the adhesive protein receptors on platelets, including GPIIb/IIIa, are integrins. The integrins are a broadly distributed family of heterodimeric cell surface molecules that share certain structural, immunochemical, and functional properties *(38–44)*. A prototypic integrin structure is illustrated in Fig. 1A. The β-subunits, of which eight are known currently, are highly homologous to one another, exhibiting extensive (35–45%) identity at the primary amino acid sequence level. The α-subunits, of which 15 are presently known, are also similar to one another but exhibit less extensive sequence identity. The α-subunits are synthesized as single-chain polypeptides, but some, such as GPIIb (α_{IIb}), are proteolytically processed to a two-chain, disulfide-linked form *(45–48)*. Each α-subunit has a short cytoplasmic tail, a single transmembrane segment, and a large extracellular portion, which contains several cation binding sites. Each β-subunit is the product of a separate gene and combines in a noncovalent complex with an α-subunit to form an adhesive protein receptor. Each β-subunit also spans the membrane once and typically has a short cytoplasmic tail.

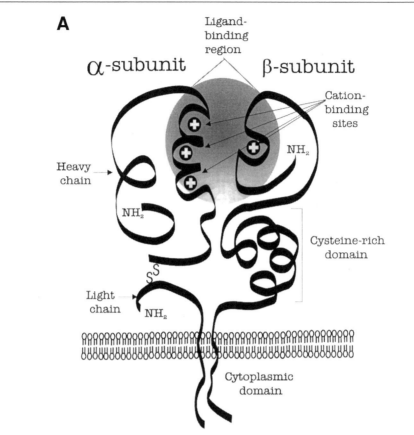

A

α-subunit

Ligand-
binding
region

β-subunit

Cation-
binding
sites

Heavy
chain

NH₂

NH₂

Cysteine-rich
domain

Light
chain   NH₂

Cytoplasmic
domain

Fig. 1. (A) Schematic depiction of the structure of a prototypic integrin adhesion receptor.

The extracellular domain is formed as a complex between the α- and β-subunits, and high-affinity binding of adhesive proteins depends on contributions from both subunits. The crystal structure of the extracellular domain of integrin $\alpha_V\beta_3$ has recently been reported *(49)*. Each subunit is composed of a series of structural motifs, which are strung together into stalks that can extend at some distance from the cell membrane. A single β-subunit can combine with several α-subunits, with each complex having distinct functional properties. The cytoplasmic tails of the subunits also appear to interact with each other *(50,51)* and link to the cytoskeleton and to signaling pathways. These intracellular interactions determine the roles of integrins in cell adhesion, cell spreading, and signal transduction. Key to the regulation of the ligand binding function of many integrins is their activation state. Stimulation of cells by a variety of agonists can generate intracellular signals that are transmitted from within the cell to the extracellular domain of integrins, enhancing their affinity for ligands (inside-out signaling). Similarly, occupancy of integrins can generate signals that are transmitted across the membrane and initiate intracellular responses (outside-in signaling). Such bidirectional signaling, as it relates to GPIIb/IIIa function, is discussed separately in Chapter 3 and reviewed elsewhere *(43,52)*. Other integrins that are present on platelets can undergo activation on other cell types and on platelets *(53–56)*, but the importance of such activation to the hemostatic function of platelets is uncertain.

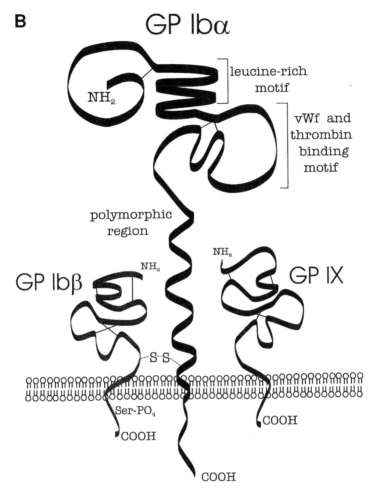

B

GP Ibα

NH$_2$

leucine-rich
motif

vWf and
thrombin
binding
motif

polymorphic
region

NH$_2$

NH$_2$

GP Ibβ

GP IX

S–S

Ser-PO$_4$

COOH

COOH

COOH

Fig. 1. (B) Schematic depiction of the GPIb/IX complex on the platelet surface. (Adapted from ref. *30*)

Table 4
Platelet Integrins

Integrin	Ligands
$\alpha_2\beta_1$	Collagen
$\alpha_5\beta_1$	Fibronectin
$\alpha_{IIb}\beta_3$	Fibrinogen, fibronectin, vitronectin, von Willebrand factor, thrombospondin, factor XIII, prothrombin
$\alpha_V\beta_3$	Vitronectin, fibrinogen, von Willebrand factor, thrombospondin, fibronectin, prothrombin, osteopontin
$\alpha_6\beta_1$	Laminin

Platelets express two major β-subunits, β_1 and β_3 (β_2 has been reported to be present at low levels) and five α-subunits (Table 4). Of the integrins expressed on blood cells, GPIIb/IIIa ($\alpha_{IIb}\beta_3$) is the most narrowly distributed and is restricted predominantly to platelets/megakaryocytes. GPIIb/IIIa may contribute to the association of platelets with tumor cells *(57–59)*, an interaction important to the metastatic dissemination of neoplastic cells *(60,61)*; and certain tumors have been reported to express GPIIb/IIIa *(59)*. Particularly relevant to the consideration of GPIIb/IIIa blockade is its sister receptor, $\alpha_V\beta_3$, which shares the same β_3 subunit *(62–64)*. The ligand repertoires of $\alpha_{IIb}\beta_3$ and $\alpha_V\beta_3$ are overlapping but not identical, and monoclonal antibodies and low-molecular-weight antagonists (e.g., tirofiban and eptifibatide) have been developed, which are selective for each of the β_3 integrins *(65,66)* [although there are data that suggest crossreactivity even of these drugs *(67)*]. In contrast, abciximab reacts equally with $\alpha_V\beta_3$ and GPIIb/IIIa *(68)*. $\alpha_V\beta_3$ is expressed at low levels on platelets (50–500 copies) *(69,70)*, in contrast to GPIIb/IIIa (40,000–80,000 copies) *(71)*. However, in vitro studies have ascribed a functional role of $\alpha_V\beta_3$ in platelet adhesion *(53,72)*. Furthermore, $\alpha_V\beta_3$ is broadly distributed and is present at high copy numbers on many vascular cells including endothelial cells, smooth muscle cells, and certain leukocytes *(64,73)*. Its role in the biology of these cells includes contributions to angiogenesis, chemotaxis, cell adhesion and migration *(64,74,75)*. Thus, crossreactivity of GPIIb/IIIa antagonists with $\alpha_V\beta_3$ is an important consideration, although the consequences of such crossreactivity (beneficial or deleterious) are uncertain.

Role of GPIb/IX in Platelet Adhesion

GPIb/IX is critical to the hemostatic function of platelets. Patients with Bernard-Soulier syndrome lack GPIb/IX and have a marked bleeding diathesis *(76,77)*. The major role of GPIb/IX in hemostasis can be traced to its function as a receptor for vWF *(28,30, 78–81)*. vWF is composed of multiple functional domains, including domains involved in binding to GPIb *(82,83)* and to matrix collagen *(84)*. Thus, vWF in the matrix may directly mediate platelet adhesion, and the plasma and/or platelet forms of the molecule may bridge the cells to other matrix components. In vitro, vWF does not interact directly with GPIb on platelets. An interaction can be measured in the presence of ristocetin *(85)*, an antibiotic, or botrocetin *(86)*, a snake venom peptide. High shear serves as the physiologic counterpart of these agonists *(31)*. High shear alters the conformation of vWF and/or GPIb/IX, permitting their productive interaction *(35,87–89)*. Such high shear stress can be attained in the microcirculation or in stenotic arteries.

GPIb/IX is multifunctional, as it can also serve as a binding site for thrombin *(90–92)*. It is also a target for certain of the drug-induced platelet antibodies and bears several allo-antigens *(30)*. The full primary structures of both GPIb and GPIX were determined from cDNA cloning approaches *(93,94)*. GPIb is composed of a heavy chain (α) and a light chain (β), and both span the platelet membrane once (Fig. 1B). GPIbα associates with actin binding protein *(95)*, thereby establishing a linkage with the cytoskeleton of the platelet *(96)*. The extracellular portion of the α-chain is highly susceptible to proteolysis, and a large proteolytic fragment, glycocalicin, can be detected in the plasma of some patients with thrombocytopenic disorders *(97)*. GPIX is a small, single-chain polypeptide with a molecular weight of 20,000. All three subunits of the GPIb/IX complex are structurally related and contain leucine-rich structural motifs *(36)*. GPV is also deficient in Bernard-Soulier platelets and forms a loose association with GPIb/IX *(98)*, but its role in the function of GPIb/IX is uncertain. A potential regulatory role of GPV in controlling platelet responses to thrombin has been suggested from data in GPV-deficient mice *(99)*.

An important consequence of occupancy of GPIb/IX by vWF is the induction of intracellular signaling events, which ultimately lead to activation of GPIIb/IIIa and then platelet aggregation *(100)*. GPIb/IX has been shown to associate with 14.3.3 *(101)*, a protein that has been implicated in signaling pathways in many cells. Also, the cytoplasmic tails of the GPIb/IX complex are subject to phosphorylation of specific serine residues *(102)*, modifications that may control its interactions with actin binding protein *(95)* and, consequently, with the cytoskeleton and signaling pathways. Recent data indicate that vWF/ GPIb/IX may play a significant role not only in platelet adhesion and activation of GPIIb/ IIIa but also in mediating direct platelet-platelet interactions *(103)*. Thus, vWF may engage GPIb/IX activating GPIIb/IIIa, which may then engage the RGD sequence in the vWF that is already platelet-bound. The occupancy of GPIIb/IIIa may induce further platelet activation, leading to occupancy by fibrinogen and thrombus growth.

Platelet Collagen Receptors

If functional redundancy is an indication of importance, then collagen must be a particularly important substrate for platelet adhesion [reviewed in refs. *12* and *13*]. In addition to the bridging of collagen to platelets via vWF *(see* previous section) and fibronectin, no fewer than three other distinct collagen receptors, GPIa/IIa (integrin $\alpha_2\beta_1$) *(104)* GPIV *(105,106)*, and GPVI *(107)*, exist on platelets. Natural deficiencies of all three of these receptors have been reported to reduce platelet adhesion to collagen *(108–110)*, and the deficiencies of GPIa/IIa and GPVI lead to bleeding phenotypes. Cooperativity between these receptors, rather than overlap in function, may explain their role in platelet adhesion to collagen *(111)*. GPIa/IIa and GPIV *(105)* are involved in the initial adhesion of platelets to collagen (although the relative contribution of these receptors is controversial *[109, 112]*), and GPVI is primarily involved in platelet activation and aggregation induced by collagen. GPVI forms a complex with the Fc receptor γ-chain, and this interaction is necessary for cell surface expression of GPVI *(113,114)*. Collagen structure also plays a significant role in influencing platelet reactivity *(115,116)*. The triple helical structure of collagen *(117)* is important in triggering platelet adhesion and secretory responses, as is the degree of multimerization (monomeric vs fibrillar collagen). Superimposed on these variables are differential effects of shear rates on platelet adhesion to collagens *(118)*. These variables are considered in detail in several articles and reviews *(12,13,111)*.

GPIIb/IIIa as an Adhesion Receptor

In addition to its role in platelet aggregation, GPIIb/IIIa is a platelet adhesion receptor. This adhesive function reflects the capacity of GPIIb/IIIa to recognize multiple ligands, which are present in matrices. These ligands include fibronectin *(119)*, thrombospondin *(120)*, and vWF *(121)*. Fibrin(ogen) *(122)* and vitronectin *(123)*, which deposit at sites of vascular injury, also support platelet adhesion via GPIIb/IIIa. Without exception, all these ligands have alternative and/or cooperative platelet adhesion receptors. As an illustrative example, TSP-1 is recognized by GPIIb/IIIa *(120)* and $\alpha_V\beta_3$ *(72)*, with both integrins probably recognizing an RGD sequence within the ligand. GPIV recognizes a distinct site within thrombospondin *(124–126)*, and the integrin-associated protein cooperates with GPIIb/ IIIa to develop a tight interaction of thrombospondin with the platelet surface *(127,128)*. Also, without exception, recognition of these adhesive ligands by GPIIb/IIIa is blocked by the same set of monoclonal antibodies *(129)* to the receptor and by the RGD and fibrinogen γ-chain ligand peptides *(130–133)*. Accordingly, although the subject has not been explored systematically in the literature, it is a reasonable prediction that the GPIIb/IIIa antagonists will block recognition of these adhesive substrates and also block the binding of soluble ligands to the receptor. With the availability of other platelet receptors to recognize these ligands, such blockade may not compromise hemostasis; however, numerous in vitro studies [e.g., *(134–136)*] conducted under both static and flow conditions have demonstrated a role of GPIIb/IIIa in platelet adhesion to various substrates. Thus, some of the limitations of GPIIb/IIIa blockade may arise from the effects of the antagonists on platelet adhesion. Such effects would enhance bleeding and thereby limit the dose of GPIIb/IIIa antagonists that could be administered.

ACKNOWLEDGMENTS

The author wishes to thank Dr. Tatiana V. Byzova for preparation of the figures and Ms. Jane Rein for preparation of the manuscript.

REFERENCES

1. Marcus AJ, Safier LB, Broekman MJ, et al. Thrombosis and inflammation as multicellular processes. Significance of cell-cell interactions. Thromb Haemost 1995;74:213–217.
2. Marcus AJ, Broekman MJ, Drosopoulos JHF, et al. The endothelial cell ecto-ADPase responsible for inhibition of platelet function is CD39. J Clin Invest 1997;99:1351–1360.
3. Bombeli T, Mueller M, Haeberli A. Anticoagulant properties of the vascular endothelium. Thromb Haemost 1997;77:408–423.
4. Ill CR, Engvall E, Ruoslahti E. Adhesion of platelets to laminin in the absence of activation. J Cell Biol 1985;99:2140–2145.
5. Grinnell F, Hays DG. Cell adhesion and spreading factor. Similarity to cold insoluble globulin in human serum. Exp Cell Res 1978;115:221–229.
6. Sakariassen KS, Bolhuis PA, Sixma JJ. Human blood platelet adhesion to artery subendothelium is mediated by factor VIII-von Willebrand factor bound to the subendothelium. Nature 1979;279:636–638.
7. Leytin VL, Gorbunova NA, Misselwitz F, Novikov ID, Podrez EA, Plyusch OP. Step-by-step analysis of adhesion of human platelets to a collagen-coated surface. Defect in initial attachment and spreading of platelets in von Willebrand's disease. Thromb Res 1984;34:51–63.
8. Brass LF, Bensusan HB. The role of collagen quaternary structure in the platelet: collagen interaction. J Clin Invest 1974;54:1480–1487.
9. Stenberg PE, McEver R-P, Shuman MA, Jacques YV, Bainton DF. A platelet alpha-granule membrane protein (GMP-140) is expressed on the plasma membrane after activation. J Cell Biol 1985;101:880–886.
10. Niija K, Hodson E, Bader R, et al. Increased surface expression of the membrane glycoprotein IIb/IIIa complex induced by platelet activation. Relationship to the binding of fibrinogen and platelet aggregation. Blood 1987;70:475–482.
11. Michelson AD, Adelman B, Barnard MR, Carroll E, Handin RI. Platelet storage results in a redistribution of glycoprotein Ib molecules. Evidence for a large intraplatelet pool of glycoprotein Ib. J Clin Invest 1988;81:1734–1740.
12. Kehrel B. Platelet receptors for collagens. Platelets 1995;6:11–16.
13. Sixma JJ, van Zanten GH, Saelman EUM, et al. Platelet adhesion to collagen. Thromb Haemost 1995;74:454–459.
14. Bombeli T, Schwartz BR, Harlan JM. Adhesion of activated platelets to endothelial cells: evidence for a GPIIbIIIa-dependent bridging mechanism and novel roles for endothelial intercellular adhesion molecule 1 (ICAM-1), $\alpha_V\beta_3$ integrin, and GPIba. J Exp Med 1998;187:329–339.
15. Diacovo TG, Roth SJ, Buccola JM, Bainton DF, Springer TA. Neutrophil rolling, arrest, and transmigration across activated, surface-adherent platelets via sequential action of P-selectin and the β_2 integrin CD11b/CD18. Blood 1996;88:146–157.
16. Weber C, Springer TA. Neutrophil accumulation on activated, surface-adherent platelets in flow is mediated by interaction of Mac-1 with fibrinogen bound to $\alpha_{IIb}\beta_3$ and stimulated by platelet-activating factor. J Clin Invest 1997;100:2085–2093.

17. Neri Serneri GG, Prisco D, Martini F, et al. Acute T-cell activation is detectable in unstable angina. Circulation 1997;95:1806–1812.

18. Kirchhofer D, Riederer MA, Baumgartner HR. Specific accumulation of circulating monocytes and polymorphonuclear leukocytes on platelet thrombi in a vascular injury model. Blood 1997;89: 1270–1278.

19. Ott J, Neumann FJ, Gawaz M, Schmitt M, Schomig A. Increased neutrophil-platelet adhesion in patients with unstable angina. Circulation 1996;94:1239–1246.

20. Sixma JJ, de Groot PG. Platelet adhesion. Br J Haematol 1990;75:308–312.

21. Lopez-Fernandez M, Ginsberg MH, Ruggeri ZM, Batlle FJ, Zimmerman TS. Multimeric structure of platelet factor VIII/von Willebrand factor: the presence of larger multimers and their reassociation with thrombin-stimulated platelets. Blood 1982;60:1132–1138.

22. Paul JI, Schwarzbauer JE, Tamkun JW, Hynes RO. Cell-type-specific fibronectin subunits generated by alternative splicing. J Biol Chem 1986;261:12,258–12,265.

23. Santoro SA, Cowan JF. Adsorption of von Willebrand factor by fibrillar collagen. Implications concerning the adhesion of platelets to collagen. Coll Relat Res 1982;2:31–43.

24. Engvall E, Ruoslahti E, Miller EJ. Affinity of fibronectin to collagens of different genetic types and to fibrinogen. J Exp Med 1978;147:1584–1595.

25. Mumby SM, Raugi GJ, Bornstein P. Interactions of thrombospondin with extracellular matrix proteins: selective binding to type V collagen. J Cell Biol 1984;98:646–652.

26. Topol EJ, McCarthy J, Gabriel S, et al. Single nucleotide polymorphisms in multiple novel thrombospondin genes may be associated with familial premature myocardial infarction. Circulation 2001; 104:2641–2644.

27. Strony J, Beaudoin A, Brands D, Adelman B. Analysis of shear stress and hemodynamic factors in a model of coronary artery stenosis and thrombosis. Am J Physiol 1993;265:H1787–H1796.

28. Girma J-P, Meyer D, Verweij CL, Pannekoek H, Sixma JJ. Structure-function relationship of human von Willebrand factor. Blood 1987;70:605–611.

29. Kroll MH, Hellums JD, McIntire LV, Schafer AI, Moake JL. Platelets and shear stress. Blood 1996; 88:1525–1541.

30. Lopez JA. The platelet glycoprotein Ib-IX complex. Blood Coagul Fibrinolysis 1994;5:97–119.

31. Weiss HJ, Turitto VT, Baumgartner HR. Effect of shear rate on platelet interaction with subendothelium in citrated and native blood. I. Shear rate-dependent decrease of adhesion in von Willebrand's disease and the Bernard-Soulier syndrome. J Lab Clin Med 1978;92:750–764.

32. Houdijk PM, Sixma JJ. Fibronectin in artery subendothelium is important for platelet adhesion. Blood 1985;65:698–604.

33. Denis C, Methia N, Frenette PS, et al. A mouse model of severe von Willebrand disease: defects in hemostasis and thrombosis. Proc Natl Acad Sci USA 1998;95:9524–9529.

34. Ni H, Denis CV, Subbarao S, et al. Persistence of platelet thrombus formation in arterioles of mice lacking both von Willebrand factor and fibrinogen. J Clin Invest 2000;106:385–392.

35. Peterson DM, Stathopoulos NA, Giorgio TD, Hellums JD, Moake JL. Shear-induced platelet aggregation requires von Willebrand factor and platelet membrane glycoproteins Ib and IIb-IIIa. Blood 1987; 69:625–628.

36. Roth GJ. Developing relationships: arterial platelet adhesion, glycoprotein Ib, and leucine-rich glycoproteins. Blood 1991;77:5–19.

37. Ruggeri ZM. Structure and function of von Willebrand factor: relationship to von Willebrand's disease. Mayo Clin Proc 1991;66:847–861.

38. Hynes RO. Integrins: a family of cell surface receptors. Cell 1987;48:549–550.

39. Parise LV. The structure and function of platelet integrins. Curr Opin Cell Biol 1989;1:947–952.

40. Ruoslahti E. Integrins. J Clin Invest 1991;87:1–5.

41. Hynes RO. Integrins: versatility, modulation, and signaling in cell adhesion. Cell 1992;69:11–25.

42. Ginsberg MH, Du X, O'Toole TE, Loftus JC, Plow EF. Platelet integrins. Thromb Haemost 1993;70: 87–93.

43. Shattil SJ, Ginsberg MH. Perspective series: cell adhesion in vascular biology. Integrin signaling in vascular biology. J Clin Invest 1997;100:S91–S95.

44. Plow EF, Haas TA, Zhang L, Loftus J, Smith JW. Ligand binding to integrins. J Biol Chem 2000;275: 21,785–21,788.

45. Bray PF, Rosa J-P, Lingappa VR, Kan YW, McEver R-P, Shuman MA. Biogenesis of the platelet receptor for fibrinogen: evidence for separate precursors for glycoproteins IIb and IIIa. Proc Natl Acad Sci USA 1986;83:1480–1484.

46. Poncz M, Eisman R, Heidenreich R, et al. Structure of the platelet membrane glycoprotein IIb. Homology to the alpha subunits of the vitronectin and fibronectin membrane receptors. J Biol Chem 1987; 262:8476–8482.

47. Loftus JC, Plow EF, Frelinger AL, III, et al. Molecular cloning and chemical synthesis of a region of platelet glycoprotein IIb involved in adhesive function. Proc Natl Acad Sci USA 1987;84:7114–7118.

48. Loftus JC, Plow EF, Jennings LK, Ginsberg MH. Alternative proteolytic processing of platelet membrane GPIIb. J Biol Chem 1988;263:11,025–11,028.

49. Xiong JP, Stehle T, Diefenbach B, et al. Crystal structure of the extracellular segment of integrin alphaV beta3. Science 2001;294:339–345.

50. Haas TA, Plow EF. The cytoplasmic domain of $\alpha_{IIb}\beta_3$: a ternary complex of the integrin α and β subunits and a divalent cation. J Biol Chem 1996;271:6017–6026.

51. Hughes PE, Diaz-Gonzalez F, Leong L, et al. Breaking the integrin hinge. A defined structural constraint regulates integrin signaling. J Biol Chem 1996;271:6571–6574.

52. Shattil SJ, Ginsberg MH, Brugge JS. Adhesive signaling in platelets. Curr Opin Cell Biol 1994;6: 695–704.

53. Bennett JS, Chan C, Vilaire G, Mousa SA, DeGrado WF. Agonist-activated $\alpha_V\beta_3$ on platelets and lymphocytes binds to the matrix protein osteopontin. J Biol Chem 1997;272:8137–8140.

54. Byzova TV, Plow EF. Activation of $\alpha_V\beta_3$ on vascular cells controls recognition of prothrombin. J Cell Biol 1998;143:2081–2092.

55. Hughes PE, Pfaff M. Integrin affinity modulation. Trends Cell Biol 1998;8:359–364.

56. Hogg N, Leitinger B. Shape and shift changes related to the function of leukocyte integrins LFA-1 and Mac-1. J Leukoc Biol 2001;69:893–898.

57. Grossi IM, Hatfield JS, Fitzgerald LA, Newcombe M, Taylor JD, Honn KV. Role of tumor cell glycoproteins immunologically related to glycoproteins Ib and IIb/IIIa in tumor cell-platelet and tumor cell-matrix interactions. FASEB J 1988;2:2385–2395.

58. Boukerche H, Berthier-Vergnes O, Tabone E, Dore J-F, Leung LLK, McGregor JL. Platelet-melanoma cell interaction is mediated by the glycoprotein IIb-IIIa complex. Blood 1989;74:658–663.

59. Honn KV, Chen YQ, Timar J, Onoda JM, et al. $\alpha_{IIb}\beta_3$ integrin expression and function in subpopulations of murine tumors. Exp Cell Res 1992;201:23–32.

60. Gasic GJ, Gasic TB, Stewart CC. Antimetastatic effects associated with platelet reduction. Proc Natl Acad Sci USA 1968;61:46–52.

61. Karpatkin S, Pearlstein E, Ambrogio C, Coller BS. Role of adhesive proteins in platelet tumor interaction in vitro and metastasis formation in vivo. J Clin Invest 1988;81:1012–1019.

62. Plow EF, Loftus JC, Levin EG, Fair DS, Dixon D, Forsyth J, Ginsberg MH. Immunologic relationship between platelet membrane glycoprotein relationship between platelet membrane glycoprotein GPIIb/IIIa and cell surface molecules expressed by a variety of cells. Proc Natl Acad Sci USA 1986;83: 6002–6006.

63. Fitzgerald LA, Steiner B, Rall SC Jr, Lo SS, Phillips DR. Protein sequence of endothelial glycoprotein IIIa derived from a cDNA clone. J Biol Chem 1987;262:3936–3939.

64. Byzova TV, Rabbani R, D'Souza S, Plow EF. Role of integrin $\alpha_V\beta_3$ in vascular biology. Thromb Haemost 1998;80:726–734.

65. Phillips DR, Scarborough RM. Clinical pharmacology of eptifibatide. Am J Cardiol 1997;80:11B–20B.

66. Barrett JS, Murphy G, Peerlinck K, et al. Pharmacokinetics and pharmacodynamics of MK-383, a selective non-peptide platelet glycoprotein-IIb/IIIa receptor antagonist, in healthy men. Clin Pharmacol Ther 1994;56:377–388.

67. Lele M, Sajid M, Wajih N, Stouffer GA. Eptifibatide and 7E3, but not tirofiban, inhibit alpha(v)beta(3) integrin-mediated binding of smooth muscle cells to thrombospondin and prothrombin. Circulation 2001;104:582–587.

68. Tam SH, Sassoli PM, Jordan RE, Nakada MT. Abciximab (ReoPro, chimeric 7E3 Fab) demonstrates equivalent affinity and functional blockade of glycoprotein IIb/IIIa and $\alpha_V\beta_3$ integrins. Circulation 1998; 98:1085–1091.

69. Lam SC, Plow EF, D'Souza SE, Cheresh DA, Frelinger AL III, Ginsberg MH. Isolation and characterization of a platelet membrane protein related to the vitronectin receptor. J Biol Chem 1989;264:3742–3749.

70. Coller BS, Cheresh DA, Asch E, Seligsohn U. Platelet vitronectin receptor expression differentiates Iraqi-Jewish from Arab patients with Glanzmann thrombasthenia in Israel. Blood 1991;77:75–83.

71. Wagner CL, Mascelli MA, Neblock DS, Weisman HF, Coller BS, Jordan RE. Analysis of GPIIb/IIIa receptor number by quantification of 7E3 binding to human platelets. Blood 1996;88:907–914.

72. Lawler J, Hynes RO. An integrin receptor on normal and thrombasthenic platelets that bind thrombo-spondin. Blood 1989;74:2022–2027.
73. Smyth SS, Joneckis CC, Parise LV. Regulation of vascular integrins. Blood 1993;81:2827–2843.
74. Brooks PC, Clark RA, Cheresh DA. Requirement of vascular integrin $\alpha_v\beta_3$ for angiogenesis. Science 1994;264:569–571.
75. Liaw L, Skinner MP, Raines EW, et al. The adhesive and migratory effects of osteopontin are mediated via distinct cell surface integrins: role of $\alpha_v\beta_3$ in smooth muscle cell migration to osteopontin *in vitro*. J Clin Invest 1995;95:713–724.
76. Nurden AT, Didry D, Rosa JP. Molecular defects of platelets in Bernard-Soulier syndrome. Blood Cells 1983;9:333–258.
77. George JN, Nurden AT, Phillips DR. Molecular defects in interactions of platelets within the vessel wall. N Engl J Med 1984;311:1084–1088.
78. Ruggeri ZM, Zimmerman TS. von Willebrand factor and von Willebrand disease. Blood 1987;70:895–904.
79. Kroll MH, Harris TS, Moake JL, Handin RI, Schafer AI. von Willebrand factor binding to platelet GpIb initiates signals for platelet activation. J Clin Invest 1991;88:1568–1573.
80. Yuan Y, Dopheide SM, Ivanidis C, Salem HH, Jackson SP. Calpain regulation of cytoskeletal signaling complexes in von Willebrand factor-stimulated platelets. Distinct roles for glycoprotein Ib-V-IX and glycoprotein IIb-IIIa (integrin $\alpha_{IIb}\beta_3$) in von Willebrand factor-induced signal transduction. J Biol Chem 1997;272:21,847–21,854.
81. Savage B, Cattaneo M, Ruggeri ZM. Mechanisms of platelet aggregation. Curr Opin Hematol 2001;8:270–276.
82. Miyata S, Goto S, Federici AB, Ware J, Ruggeri ZM. Conformational changes in the A1 domain of von Willebrand factor modulating the interaction with platelet glycoprotein Ibα. J Biol Chem 1996;271:9046–9053.
83. Cruz MA, Handin RI, Wise RJ. The interaction of the von Willebrand factor-A1 domain with platelet glycoprotein Ib/IX. J Biol Chem 1993;268:21,238–21,245.
84. Roth GJ, Titani K, Hoyer LW, Hickey MJ. Localization of binding sites within human von Willebrand factor for monomeric type III collagen. Biochemistry 1986;25:8357–8361.
85. Howard MA, Firkin BG. Ristocetin—a new tool in the investigation of platelet aggregation. Thromb Haemost 1971;26:362–369.
86. Read MS, Smith SV, Lamb MA, Brinkhous KM. Role of botrocetin in platelet agglutination: formation of an activated complex of botrocetin and von Willebrand factor. Blood 1989;74:1031–1035.
87. Roth GJ. Platelets and blood vessels: the adhesion event. Immunol Today 1992;13:100–105.
88. Denis C, Williams JA, Lu X, Meyer D, Baruch D. Solid-phase von Willebrand factor contains a conformationally active RGD motif that mediates endothelial cell adhesion through the $\alpha_v\beta_3$ receptor. Blood 1993;82:3622–3630.
89. Kroll MH, Hellums JD, Guo Z, et al. Protein kinase C is activated in platelets subjected to pathological shear stress. J Biol Chem 1993;268:3520–3524.
90. Okumura T, Jamieson GA. Platelet glycocalicin: a single receptor for platelet aggregation induced by thrombin or ristocetin. Thromb Res 1976;8:701–706.
91. Moroi M, Goetze A, Dubay E, Wu C, Hasitz M, Jamieson GA. Isolation of platelet glycocalicin by affinity chromatography on thrombin-sepharose. Thromb Res 1982;28:103–114.
92. Andrews RK, Shen Y, Gardiner EE, Dong JF, Lopez JA, Berndt MC. The glycoprotein Ib-IX-V complex in platelet adhesion and signaling. Thromb Haemost 1999;82:357–364.
93. Lopez JA, Chung DW, Fujikawa K, Hagen FS, Davie EW, Roth GJ. The alpha and beta chains of human platelet glycoprotein Ib are both transmembrane proteins containing a leucine-rich amino acid sequence. Proc Natl Acad Sci USA 1988;85:2135–2139.
94. Hickey MJ, Williams SA, Roth GJ. Human platelet glycoprotein IX: an adhesive prototype of leucine-rich glycoproteins with flank-center-flank structures. Proc Natl Acad Sci USA 1989;86:6773–6777.
95. Andrews RK, Fox JEB. Interaction of purified actin-binding protein with the platelet membrane glycoprotein Ib-IX complex. J Biol Chem 1991;266:7144–7147.
96. Cunningham JG, Meyer SC, Fox JEB. The cytoplasmic domain of the α-subunit of glycoprotein (GP) Ib mediates attachment of the entire GP Ib-IX complex to the cytoskeleton and regulates von Willebrand factor-induced changes in cell morphology. J Biol Chem 1996;271:11,581–11,587.
97. Steinberg MH, Kelton JG, Coller BS. Plasma glycocalicin: an aid in the classification of thrombocytopenic disorders. N Engl J Med 1987;317:1037–1042.

98. Modderman PW, Admiraal LG, Sonnenberg A, von Dem Borne AE. Glycoproteins V and Ib-IX form a noncovalent complex in the platelet membrane. J Biol Chem 1992;267:364–369.

99. Ni H, Ramakrishnan V, Ruggeri ZM, Papalia JM, Phillips DR, Wagner DD. Increased thrombogenesis and embolus formation in mice lacking glycoprotein V. Blood 7-15-2001;98:368–373.

100. DeMarco L, Girolami A, Russell S, Ruggeri ZM. Interaction of asialo von Willebrand factor with glycoprotein Ib induces fibrinogen binding to the glycoprotein IIb/IIIa complex and mediates platelet aggregation. J Clin Invest 1985;75:1198–1203.

101. Du X, Fox JE, Pei S. Identification of a binding sequence for the 14-3-3 protein within the cytoplasmic domain of the adhesion receptor, platelet glycoprotein Ibα. J Biol Chem 1996;271:7362–7367.

102. Wardell MR, Reynolds CC, Berndt MC, Wallace RW, Fox JEB. Platelet glycoprotein Ib is phosphorylated on serine-166 by cyclic AMP-dependent protein kinase. J Biol Chem 1989;264:15,656–15,661.

103. Goto S, Ikeda Y, Saldivar E, Ruggeri ZM. Distinct mechanisms of platelet aggregation as a consequence of different shearing flow conditions. J Clin Invest 1998;101:479–486.

104. Santoro SA. Identification of a 160,000 dalton platelet membrane protein that mediates the initial divalent cation-dependent adhesion of platelets to collagen. Cell 1986;46:913–920.

105. Tandon NN, Kralisz U, Jamieson GA. Identification of GPIV (CD36) as a primary receptor for platelet-collagen adhesion. J Biol Chem 1989;264:7576–7583.

106. Nakamura T, Jamieson GA, Okuma M, Kambayashi J, Tandon NN. Platelet adhesion to native type I collagen fibrils. Role of GPVI in divalent cation-dependent and -independent adhesion and thromboxane A2 generation. J Biol Chem 1998;273:4338–4344.

107. Moroi M, Jung SM, Shinmyozu K, Tomiyama Y, Ordinas A, Diaz-Ricart M. Analysis of platelet adhesion to a collagen-coated surface under flow conditions: the involvement of glycoprotein VI in the platelet adhesion. Blood 1996;88:2081–2092.

108. Nieuwenhuis HK, Akkerman JWN, Houdijk WPM, Sixma JJ. Human blood platelets showing no response to collagen fail to express surface glycoprotein Ia. Nature 1985;318:470–472.

109. Diaz-Ricart M, Tandon NN, Carretero M, Ordinas A, Bastida E, Jamieson GA. Platelets lacking functional CD36 (glycoprotein IV) show reduced adhesion to collagen in flowing whole blood. Blood 1993;82:491–496.

110. Moroi M, Jung SM, Okuma M, Shinmyozu K. A patient with platelets deficient in glycoprotein VI that lack both collagen-induced aggregation and adhesion. J Clin Invest 1989;84:1440–1445.

111. Verkleij MW, Morton LF, Knight CG, de Groot P, Barnes MJ, Sixma JJ. Simple collagen-like peptides support platelet adhesion under static but not under flow conditions: interaction via α2β1 and von Willebrand factor with specific sequences in native collagen is a requirement to resist shear forces. Blood 1998;91:3308–3816.

112. Saelman EUM, Kehrel B, Hese KM, de Groot PG, Sixma JJ, Nieuwenhuis HK. Platelet adhesion to collagen and endothelial cell matrix under flow conditions is not dependent on platelet glycoprotein IV. Blood 1994;83:3240–3244.

113. Watson SP. Collagen receptor signaling in platelets and megakaryocytes. Thromb Haemost 1999;82: 365–376.

114. Clemetson KJ, Clemetson JM. Platelet collagen receptors. Thromb Haemost 2001;86:189–197.

115. Morton LF, Fitzsimmons CM, Rauterberg J, Barnes MJ. Platelet-reactive sites in collagen. Collagens I and III possess different aggregatory sites. Biochem J 1987;248:483–487.

116. Santoro SA, Walsh JJ, Staatz WD, Baranski KJ. Distinct determinants on collagen support α2β1 integrin-mediated platelet adhesion and platelet activation. Cell Regul 1991;2:905–913.

117. Morton LF, Hargreaves PG, Farndale RW, Young RD, Barnes MJ. Integrin α2β1-independent activation of platelets by simple collagen-like peptides: collagen tertiary (triple-helical) and quaternary (polymeric) structures are sufficient alone for α2β1-independent platelet reactivity. Biochem J 1995;306: 337–344.

118. Saelman EUM, Nieuwenhuis HK, Hese KM, et al. Platelet adhesion to collagen types I through VIII under conditions of stasis and flow is mediated by GPIa/IIa (α2β1-integrin). Blood 1994;83: 1244–1250.

119. Ginsberg MH, Forsyth J, Lightsey A, Chediak J, Plow EF. Reduced surface expression and binding of fibronectin by thrombin-stimulated thrombasthenic platelets. J Clin Invest 1983;71:619–624.

120. Karczewski J, Knudsen KA, Smith L, Murphy A, Rothman VL, Tuszynski GP. The interaction of thrombospondin with platelet glycoprotein GPIIb-IIIa. J Biol Chem 1989;264:21,322–21,326.

121. Ruggeri ZM, Bader R, DeMarco L. Glanzmann thrombasthenia. Deficient binding of von Willebrand factor to thrombin-stimulated platelets. Proc Natl Acad Sci USA 1982;79:6038–6041.

122. Hantgan RR. Fibrin protofibril and fibrinogen binding to ADP-stimulated platelets: evidence for a common mechanism. Biochim Biophys Acta 1988;968:24–35.

123. Thiagarajan P, Kelley KL. Exposure of binding sites for vitronectin on platelets following stimulation. J Biol Chem 1988;263:3035–3038.

124. Asch AS, Barnwell J, Silverstein RL, Nachman RL. Isolation of the thrombospondin membrane receptor. J Clin Invest 1987;79:1054–1061.

125. Asch AS, Silbiger S, Heimer E, Nachman RL. Thrombospondin sequence motif (CSVTCG) is responsible for CD36 binding. Biochem Biophys Res Commun 1992;182:1208–1217.

126. Catimel B, Leung L, El Ghissasi H, Mercier N, McGregor J. Human platelet glycoprotein IIIb binds to thrombospondin fragments bearing the *C*-terminal region, and/or the type I repeats (CSVTCG motif), but not to the *N*-terminal heparin-binding region. Biochem J 1992;284:231–236.

127. Gao AG, Lindberg FP, Dimitry JM, Brown EJ, Frazier WA. Thrombospondin modulates $\alpha_v\beta_3$ function through integrin-associated protein. J Cell Biol 1996;135:533–544.

128. Chung J, Gao AG, Frazier WA. Thrombospondin acts via integrin-associated protein to activate the platelet integrin $\alpha_{IIb}\beta_3$. J Biol Chem 1997;272:14,740–14,746.

129. Plow EF, McEver R-P, Coller BS, Woods VL, Marguerie GA, Ginsberg MH. Related binding mechanisms for fibrinogen, fibronectin, von Willebrand factor and thrombospondin on thrombin-stimulated human platelets. Blood 1985;66:724–727.

130. Plow EF, Srouji AH, Meyer D, Marguerie G, Ginsberg MH. Evidence that three adhesive proteins interact with common recognition site on activated platelets. J Biol Chem 1984;259:5388–5391.

131. Plow EF, Pierschbacher MD, Ruoslahti E, Marguerie GA, Ginsberg MH. The effect of Arg-Gly-Asp-containing peptides on fibrinogen and von Willebrand factor binding to platelets. Proc Natl Acad Sci USA 1985;82:8057–8061.

132. Hantgan RR, Endenburg SC, Cavero I, et al. Inhibition of platelet adhesion to fibrin(ogen) in flowing whole blood by arg-gly-asp and fibrinogen gamma-chain carboxy terminal peptides. Thromb Haemost 1992;68:694–700.

133. Cherny RC, Honan MA, Thiagarajan P. Site-directed mutagenesis of the arginine-glycine-aspartic acid in vitronectin abolishes cell adhesion. J Biol Chem 1993;268:9725–9729.

134. Weiss HJ, Hawiger J, Ruggeri ZM, Turitto VT, Thiagarajan P, Hoffmann T. Fibrinogen-independent platelet adhesion and thrombus formation of subendothelium mediated by glycoprotein IIb-IIIa complex at high shear rate. J Clin Invest 1989;83:288–297.

135. Hantgan RR, Hindriks G, Taylor RG, Sixma JJ, de Groot PG. Glycoprotein Ib, von Willebrand factor, and glycoprotein IIb:IIIa are all involved in platelet adhesion to fibrin in flowing whole blood. Blood 1990;76:345–353.

136. Agbanyo FR, Sixma JJ, de Groot PG, Languino LR, Plow EF. Thrombospondin-platelet interactions. Role of divalent cations, wall shear rate, and platelet membrane glycoproteins. J Clin Invest 1993;92:288–296.

3

Glycoprotein IIb/IIIa in Platelet Aggregation and Acute Arterial Thrombosis

Patrick Andre, PhD and David R. Phillips, PhD

CONTENTS

INTRODUCTION
GPIIb/IIIa IN THROMBOGENESIS
GPIIb/IIIa STRUCTURE
LIGAND BINDING PROPERTIES OF GPIIb/IIIa
STIMULUS-INDUCED GPIIb/IIIa ACTIVATION
OUTSIDE-IN GPIIb/IIIa SIGNAL TRANSDUCTION
GPIIb/IIIa POLYMORPHISMS AS A CARDIOVASCULAR RISK FACTOR
GPIIb/IIIa IN INFLAMMATION
ADDITIONAL FUNCTIONS FOR GPIIb/IIIa
NEW PERSPECTIVES FOR GPIIb/IIIa IN ANTITHROMBOTIC THERAPIES
GLOSSARY
REFERENCES

INTRODUCTION

Glycoprotein (GP) IIb/IIIa antagonists have been shown to therapeutically regulate platelet function to prevent, for example, the thrombotic complications associated with coronary artery disease *(1)*. Moreover, it is now suggested that the modulation of GPIIb/IIIa affects not only platelet aggregation and thrombosis, but also inflammation, which might ultimately result in a reduction of recurrent thrombotic events. Three main reasons explain why GPIIb/IIIa ($\alpha_{IIb}\beta_3$ integrin) *(2)* is an ideal platelet target for the treatment of acute arterial thrombosis and why the development of GPIIb/IIIa antagonists has been successful. First, GPIIb/IIIa is on the "final common pathway" *(3)* mediating platelet aggregation, a process central to acute arterial thrombosis, irrespective of the agonist used to induce platelet activation. Second, GPIIb/IIIa is a platelet-specific glycoprotein, the most abundant protein on the platelet surface. Third, the dynamic nature of GPIIb/IIIa allows it to affect a variety of platelet responses, therefore allowing GPIIb/IIIa antagonists to modulate

From: *Contemporary Cardiology: Platelet Glycoprotein IIb/IIIa*
Inhibitors in Cardiovascular Disease, 2nd Edition
Edited by: A. M. Lincoff © Humana Press Inc., Totowa, NJ

a variety of platelet functions including those involved in coagulation, inflammation, fibrinolysis, and vascular cell proliferation.

The function of GPIIb/IIIa in platelet aggregation is often initiated by inside-out signaling events, which cause expression of the receptor function of GPIIb/IIIa for soluble fibrinogen. On unstimulated platelets, GPIIb/IIIa has low affinity for soluble fibrinogen, i.e., it is in an "inactive" conformation. However, after stimulation of platelets by a variety of agonists, agonists generated at sites of vascular injury such as occurs during percutaneous interventions or upon rupture of an atherosclerotic plaque (i.e., thrombin, ADP, fibrillar collagens), GPIIb/IIIa undergoes a rapid conformational change such that it can now bind soluble fibrinogen. Upon binding to GPIIb/IIIa, the bivalent fibrinogen as well as other adhesive proteins including fibronectin, vitronectin, and von Willebrand factor (vWf) can further mediate platelet aggregation by crosslinking the surfaces of activated platelets via GPIIb/IIIa. The binding of vWf may have a unique role in mediating aggregation since it is considered to be the key ligand mediating platelet aggregation under conditions of high shear such as would occur in coronary arteries.

A second signaling reaction of GPIIb/IIIa is also involved in platelet aggregation. When fibrinogen interacts with GPIIb/IIIa on the platelet surface, or otherwise becomes immobilized on artificial surfaces, it undergoes a conformational change that allows it to bind to "inactive" GPIIb/IIIa on unstimulated platelets. This binding results in "outside-in" signals being transduced via GPIIb/IIIa, which, in turn, can lead to further platelet activation including the activation of other GPIIb/IIIa molecules on the platelet surface, the induction of platelet secretion, and the consolidation and stabilization of platelet aggregates. These events also occur when fibrinogen is immobilized on the vessel wall. The signaling pathway initiated by ligand binding to GPIIb/IIIa appears to involve the phosphorylation of two tyrosines on the cytoplasmic domain of GPIIIa *(4,5)*. Proteins have been identified that bind to tyrosine-phosphorylated GPIIIa and are currently being evaluated for their potential roles in GPIIb/IIIa signal transduction. These outside-in signaling events including GPIIIa tyrosine phosphorylation are also involved in processes such as clot retraction, in which GPIIb/IIIa serves as the transmembrane link between extracellular fibrin and intracellular cytoskeletal proteins.

Recent studies have shown that GPIIb/IIIa, in addition to its role in platelet aggregation and thrombosis, also interacts with CD40L, thereby having a role in inflammation *(6)*. CD40L is an inflammatory mediator that has recently been identified on platelets. This protein is shed during platelet stimulation, generating a soluble cleavage product termed sCD40L. GPIIb/IIIa is involved in this process in two ways. First, cleavage can be blocked by GPIIb/IIIa antagonists, indicating a role for GPIIb/IIIa in CD40L shedding and in the generation of this proinflammatory product. Second, sCD40L also binds directly to GPIIb/IIIa, promoting platelet thrombosis.

This chapter summarizes recent studies pertaining to the structure and function of GPIIb/IIIa. The themes to be developed are twofold. First, GPIIb/IIIa is not a static receptor, but one whose adhesive functions respond to, and initiate signal transduction processes within the platelet and whose distribution changes during platelet stimulation. Second, whereas the central role of GPIIb/IIIa in aggregation indicates that it is an attractive target for effective therapeutic regulation of platelet aggregation and thrombosis, the role of GPIIb/IIIa in the generation of inflammatory mediators suggests that GPIIb/IIIa antagonists may also function in the inhibition of inflammation.

GPIIb/IIIa IN THROMBOGENESIS

Perhaps the most well-studied function of GPIIb/IIIa is that of platelet aggregation. These studies have resulted in the development of the central tenant of platelet biology: platelet stimulation induces the activation of the receptor function of GPIIb/IIIa for fibrinogen and vWF, the binding of which mediates platelet aggregation. However, recent data now show that through secondary activities, GPIIb/IIIa is also required to stabilize platelet aggregates and arterial thrombi. Without these secondary events involving both direct and indirect roles of GPIIb/IIIa, stable thrombosis does not occur. These observations highlight new functions for GPIIb/IIIa in platelet biology and new considerations in the use of GPIIb/IIIa antagonists for the treatment of acute coronary thrombosis.

GPIIb/IIIa in Platelet Aggregation

On unstimulated discoid platelets such as those that normally exist in the circulation, GPIIb/IIIa is distributed among the plasma membrane (approx 80,000 copies per platelet), the α-granule membrane (approx 40,000 copies per platelet), and the dense body membrane (trace amounts) *(7,8)*. Only limited receptor functions have been attributed to GPIIb/IIIa on the surface of unstimulated platelets. The primary one is to bind immobilized fibrinogen—a reaction that may assist in the recruitment of platelets to damaged vessel walls or to platelet aggregates *(9)*. However, following platelet stimulation, which also may involve α-granule secretion, there is an up to 50% increase in the GPIIb/IIIa expressed on the surface membranes of platelets. The amount of GPIIb/IIIa recruited to the platelet surface during platelet stimulation is a function of the strength of the platelet agonist. Potent agonists like thrombin cause most of the α-granule GPIIb/IIIa to be recruited with prebound fibrinogen to the platelet surface, whereas weak agonists like ADP only marginally increase the platelet surface GPIIb/IIIa *(10,11)*. The GPIIb/IIIa on the surface of activated platelets becomes a receptor for the soluble forms of several adhesive proteins, most prominantly fibrinogen and vWf. The affinity of fibrinogen for GPIIb/IIIa on stimulated platelets (K_d approx 500 nmol/L) and the high concentration of fibrinogen in plasma (approx 11 µmol/L) predicts that GPIIb/IIIa will rapidly become saturated with fibrinogen upon platelet stimulation. The binding of fibrinogen (a bivalent ligand) and vWf (a polyvalent ligand) to the GPIIb/IIIa on stimulated platelets is responsible for the initial platelet aggregation.

GPIIb/IIIa also shuttles between the plasma membrane and the α-granule membrane, which is independent of platelet stimulation *(12)*. This shuttling allows for the packaging of fibrinogen in α-granules during megakaryocytopoiesis *(13)* and for the uptake of GPIIb/IIIa ligands in mature platelets *(14)*. The function of GPIIb/IIIa shuttling in circulating platelets could potentially allow for the uptake of GPIIb/IIIa antagonists during antithrombotic therapy *(15)*. Indeed, it has been demonstrated that abciximab accumulates in α-granules within 3 h following the initiation of therapy, and as fast as 5 min in vitro, suggesting a possible mechanism for localization of this antagonist during thrombosis *(16)*. It is not yet known whether eptifibatide or aggrastat also accumulate in α-granules. The α-granule pool of GPIIb/IIIa is functionally important to platelet aggregation. Indeed, thrombin stimulation of platelets in which the plasma membrane GPIIb/IIIa molecules have been rendered inactive can still induce sufficient functional GPIIb/IIIa to the platelet surface to support platelet aggregation *(17)*.

Clinical studies have shown that thrombin-induced, but not ADP-induced, platelet aggregation is rapidly restored following discontinuation of infusion of high-affinity GPIIb/IIIa antagonists like the Fab fragment, abciximab, or L-738,167, a synthetic GPIIb/IIIa antagonist *(18,19)*. In these trials, the unbound pool of these antagonists, but not the platelet-bound pool, is rapidly cleared. Since thrombin, but not ADP, induces maximal surface expression of the α-granule pool of GPIIb/IIIa, thrombin-induced aggregation is more rapidly restored. P-selectin is another α-granule protein that becomes expressed on the surface of activated platelets *(20)*. FACS analysis has shown that thrombosis associated with percutaneous intervention or unstable angina increases the amount of platelet-associated P-selectin, implying that these indications increase the amount of activated platelets within the circulation, and also providing an assay to measure such platelets *(21)*.

GPIIb/IIIa in Thrombus Stability

In a simple aggregation reaction, such as that occurring with a stirred suspension of platelets activated by agonists like as collagen, ADP, or thrombin in a cuvette during laboratory analysis, it is likely that fibrinogen, which is bivalent, bridges the surfaces of activated platelets and is sufficient to stabilize platelet-platelet contacts (Fig. 1). Aggregation reactions under flow such as that occurring during thrombosis and hemostasis within the vasculature are much more complicated, primarily because the effects of shear require the involvement of additional factors both to induce thrombus growth and to stabilize platelet-platelet interactions. There are multiple pathways in which GPIIb/IIIa is involved in thrombus stability, only four of which will be described.

First, the initial reversible binding of fibrinogen to GPIIb/IIIa becomes irreversible *(22)*. Although the mechanism of converting a reversible fibrinogen interaction to one that is irreversible is not known, the lack of this conversion might explain the destabilization of the arterial thrombi observed in the fibrinogen-deficient mice *(23)*.

Second, GPIIb/IIIa outside-in signaling is partly induced by the tyrosine phosphorylation of the cytoplasmic domain of GP IIIa (*see* below). One consequence of outside-in signaling during platelet aggregation is the release of autocrine factors from platelet storage organelles, which are required to induce further platelet activation to stabilize aggregates. Such factors include ADP and serotonin, two dense body constituents, and Gas6, a protein released from α-granules. Although the roles of ADP and serotonin in aggregate stability are well known, the function of Gas6 is new and was discovered by observations showing that Gas6-deficient mice produce only loosely packed thrombi *(24)*. It is also of interest that the long form of the leptin receptor has been detected in platelets, and high concentrations of leptin have been noted to potentiate platelet aggregation *(25,26)*. Moreover, it has been proposed that the conversion from the reversible to the irreversible binding of fibrinogen to GPIIb/IIIa is facilitated by the factor XIIIa-catalyzed coupling of secreted serotonin to fibrinogen on the platelet surface, thus permitting the high-affinity binding of derivatized protein to serotonin receptors *(27)*.

Third, sCD40L generated from stimulated platelets plays a cofactor role in the production of stable arterial thrombi. GPIIb/IIIa is not only involved in the processing of CD40L to sCD40L, it also serves as the sCD40L receptor (*see* below).

Fourth, the generation of thrombin on the surface of platelet aggregates not only provides an additional platelet stimulus, but also catalyzes the formation of fibrin, both of which cause increased aggregate stability. The generation of the procoagulant surface is another consequence of outside-in GPIIb/IIIa signaling.

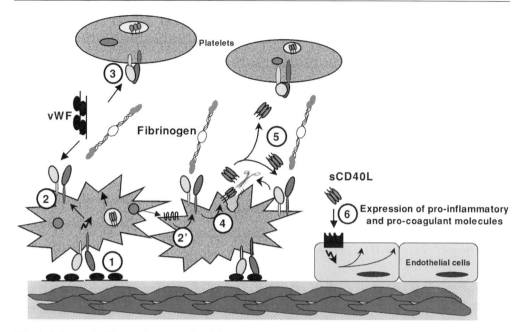

Fig. 1. Schematic illustrating the role of GPIIb/IIIa in the multiple steps leading to thrombus formation under high shear rate. On resting discoid platelets, the GPIIb/IIIa is present in an "inactive" conformation and is unable to bind soluble fibrinogen. **1,** Upon vessel wall injury, von Willebrand factor (vWF) binds to the exposed collagen and undergoes a conformational change that allows the platelet to adhere via an interaction with the GPIbα. Other receptors such as $\alpha_2\beta_1$ and GPVI participate in platelet adhesion. GPIIb/IIIa becomes activated and mediates final spreading onto the thrombogenic surface. **2,** The platelet undergoes a shape change, and the GPIIb/IIIa expressed on the luminal side is activated such that it can now bind its soluble ligands, fibrinogen and vWf. **3,** Those ligands will now be able to sustain the recruitment of unactivated platelets (platelet aggregation) via GPIbα and GPIIb/IIIa. 2', Activated platelets also release their granules contents and are procoagulant. Released ADP and newly synthesized thrombin will be able to accentuate platelet recruitment further by activating other GPIIb/IIIa. **4,** α-Granules containing intracellular GPIIb/IIIa are present in both resting and stimulated platelets. The contents of the α-granules are released as a consequence of outside-in signaling, resulting in the secretion of factors involved in inflammation, vascular remodeling, platelet recruitment, and coagulation. CD40L is expressed during this process. **5,** The surface-expressed CD40L is rapidly cleaved, and the soluble form of CD40L (sCD40L) further enhances thrombosis via its binding to GPIIb/IIIa and also activates endothelium, inducing the expression of proinflammatory and procoagulant proteins. The cleavage mechanism of CD40L is GPIIb/IIIa-dependent and can be blocked by GPIIb/IIIa antagonists.

More generally, aggregation and stabilization cofactors released from activated/aggregated platelets will undoubtefully become a major center of scientific interest, as both CD40L- and Gas6-deficient mice exhibit a normal bleeding time, even though they have abnormal thrombosis. In addition, since serotonin is now believed to enhance the binding of prothrombotic ligands on activated platelets *(27)*, it is highly likely that other molecules will emerge as key players of the aggregation and stability processes.

GPIIb/IIIa STRUCTURE

GPIIb/IIIa is a member of the integrin family of adhesion receptors. All integrins consist of two subunits, termed α and β (Fig. 2). In mammals, the integrin family is quite large,

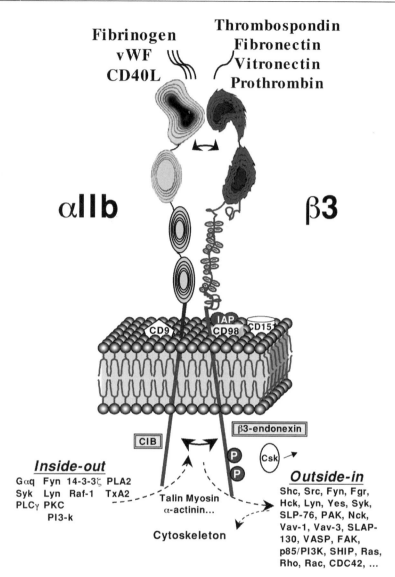

Fig. 2. Schematic diagram of GPIIb/IIIa and its interacting proteins. **GPIIb/IIIa structure:** The schematic for the extracellular domain is adapted from the crystal structure of $\alpha_v\beta_3$ *(65)*, which is anticipated to be similar to that of GPIIb/IIIa *(30)*. The ligand binding domain of the complex exists at the contact between the distal, amino terminal domains of each subunit at the top of the figure. Each subunit has a single transmembrane domain with short cytoplasmic tails. *GPIIb/IIIa ligands:* The known physiologic ligands of GPIIb/IIIa (i.e., fibrinogen, vWf, and CD40L) are indicated. GPIIb/IIIa antagonists function by competing for the binding of these proteins. *Intramembraneous GPIIb/IIIa binding proteins:* Four transmembrane proteins have been shown to form intramembraneous complexes with GPIIb/IIIa: CD9, CD151, CD98, and integrin-associated protein (IAP). *Cytoplasmic GPIIb/IIIa binding proteins:* Proteins known to bind to the cytoplasmic domains of GPIIb/IIIa include CIB (to GPIIb), β3-endonexin (to GPIIIa), and several cytoskeletal proteins (i.e., talin, myosin, α-actinin). *Proteins involved in GPIIb/IIIa signaling:* Signaling proteins involved in the activation of the receptor function of GPIIb/IIIa (Inside-out) and in mediating platelet activation in response to GPIIb/IIIa ligands (Outside-in) are indicated. *GPIIIa phosphorylation sites:* The two cytoplasmic tyrosines phosphorylated during outside-in GPIIb/IIIa signaling are indicated.

consisting of at least 16 α subunits (one of which is GPIIb, or αIIb in the integrin nomenclature) and 8 β-subunits (e.g., GPIIIa, also termed β3). Although the tissue distribution of GPIIb/IIIa is quite limited, being restricted to platelets and other cells of the megakaryocytic lineage, the β subunit of this integrin, i.e., β3, is widely distributed and complexed with an α-subunit, αv, generating the $\alpha_v\beta_3$ integrin. The limited tissue distribution of GPIIb/IIIa permits specific targeting of platelets by GPIIb/IIIa antagonists.

The GPIIb subunit of GPIIb/IIIa consists of two disulfide-linked subunits, GPIIbα (M_r = 125 kDa) and GPIIbβ (M_r = 22 kDa), which are formed when the precursor GPIIb polypeptide undergoes cleavage into a heavy and light chain. In contrast, GPIIIa (M_r = 105 kDa) is a single polypeptide that contains intrachain disulfide linkages. In both cases the proteins have large extracellular domains, single transmembrane domains, and relatively short cytoplasmic domains (47 amino acids for GPIIIa and 20 for GPIIb). The extracellular structure of GPIIb/IIIa can be inferred from the crystal structure of $\alpha_v\beta_3$, the integrin predicted to have the highest similarity to GPIIb/IIIa (identical β-subunits, highly homologous α-subunits). This structure consists of 12 domains assembled into an ovoid head, which contains the binding site for fibrinogen *(28)*, and two legs, which anchor the integrin to the membrane. X-ray crystallography has shown that the binding pocket for the RGD (arginine-glycine-aspartic acid) peptide sequence, used by many of the adhesive proteins that bind GPIIb/IIIa, and mimicked by many GPIIb/IIIa antagonists, appears to reside in the head at the juncture of the MIDAS domain of GPIIIa and the β-propeller domain of GPIIb. Although the direct identification of the RGD binding site on GPIIb/IIIa predicts where fibrinogen, vWF, CD40L, and other proteins bind GPIIb/IIIa, it is recognized that the binding of such ligands will be more complex and possibly involve additional domains within the head of GPIIb/IIIa. Nuclear magnetic resonance (NMR) analysis of GPIIb/IIIa cytoplasmic tails has also been performed and reveals that they are both relatively flexible *(29)*.

LIGAND BINDING PROPERTIES OF GPIIb/IIIa

Although fibrinogen, vWf, and sCD40L are ligands for GPIIb/IIIa, these molecules utilize different sequences to bind to the GPIIb/IIIa, and their binding is regulated differently. Fibrinogen consists of six polypeptide chains, two α, two β, and two γ, arranged in a symmetric, bivalent orientation. Because peptides containing the Arg-Gly-Asp (RGD) sequence were the first identified antagonists of fibrinogen binding and because the fibrinogen α-chain has two RGD sequences, it was initially assumed that one or both of

---

Fig. 2. (*Continued*) **GPIIb/IIIa signaling:** *Inside-out signaling:* Signaling events originating from different agents such as collagen, thrombin, ADP, or vWF bound to collagen and transmitted by the indicated "Inside-out" signaling proteins lead to the activation of the receptor function of GPIIb/IIIa for soluble ligands (i.e., fibrinogen, vWf, CD40L). Although the mechanism for GPIIb/IIIa activation is not known, possible candidate GPIIb/IIIa binding proteins for this function include CIB, β_3-endonexin, and talin. *Outside-in signaling:* Upon platelet aggregation, a process mediated by the binding of fibrinogen, vWf, and CD40L to GPIIb/IIIa, the cytoplasmic domain of GPIIIa becomes tyrosine phosphorylated on residues 747 and 759, allowing the association of GPIIb/IIIa with the cytoskeletal protein myosin. Aggregation also initiates signaling events transmitted by the indicated outside-in signaling proteins, which serve to induce platelet secretion reactions, further GPIIb/IIIa activation to produce stable aggregates, and clot retraction. Outside-in signaling is mediated, in part, by the tyrosine phosphorylation of GPIIIa. For abbreviations, *see* Glossary.

these sequences were used to bind GPIIb/IIIa (reviewed in ref. *30*). Surprisingly, however, mutations of either RGD sequence in recombinant fibrinogen has no effect on fibrin-
ogen-GPIIb/IIIa interactions as measured either by platelet aggregation *(31)* or platelet
adhesion to immobilized fibrinogen *(32)*. An additional sequence in fibrinogen that binds
GPIIb/IIIa is the carboxy-terminal hexapeptide on the γ- chain, Lys-Gln-Ala-Gly-Asp-
Val (KQAGDV), an activity first identified by Hawiger and coworkers *(33)*.

This sequence is contained within both outer nodules of fibrinogen, the structural
entity of fibrinogen that binds GPIIb/IIIa *(28)*. Several lines of evidence indicate that this
is the GPIIIb/IIIa binding domain of fibrinogen: antibodies to this sequence block fibrinogen binding *(34)*; fibrinogen lacking this sequence does not support platelet aggregation; and a bleeding diathesis is induced when mouse fibrinogen is mutated so that it
lacks this sequence *(35)*. Novel technologies such as Laser Tweezers have now revealed
the interaction strength between fibrinogen and its receptor GPIIb/IIIa *(36)*. Fibrin also binds
to GPIIb/IIIa but appears to utilize a different sequence than fibrinogen in that fibrin harboring a deletion truncation of the γ-chain QAGDV sequence is still capable of supporting clot retraction *(37)*. Since clot retraction depends on the fibrin adhesive property of
GPIIb/IIIa, this finding suggests that conversion of fibrinogen to fibrin exposes a different GPIIb/IIIa binding site.

Although the binding of soluble fibrinogen to GPIIb/IIIa requires prior activation of
the integrin, fibrinogen immobilized on surfaces or bound to the GPIIb/IIIa on the surface
of aggregated platelets is fully capable of binding to GPIIb/IIIa on unstimulated platelets.
It thus appears that fibrinogen bound to the GPIIb/IIIa on the surface of an aggregated
platelet undergoes a conformational change into an "activated" form that is capable of
mediating further cellular interactions. One is to bind the GPIIb/IIIa on unstimulated
platelets *(38)*, which, through a process known as "outside-in" signaling, induces platelet
binding and subsequent stimulation. Another is to bind Mac-1 on neutrophils to initiate
the adhesion of these cells *(39)*. Thus these activities of bound fibrinogen are important
as they allow for the recruitment of unstimulated platelets and neutrophils, respectively,
into a growing thrombus. Both reactions, the interaction of bound fibrinogen with the GPIIb/
IIIa on unstimulated platelets and the activation of GPIIb/IIIa by vWf, serve to promote
thrombus growth by mechanisms mediated primarily through the binding of adhesive proteins to GPIIb/IIIa.

Adhesive proteins other than fibrinogen that bind to GPIIb/IIIa, e.g. vWf, fibronectin,
and vitronectin, most likely do so by the RGD sequences contained within their primary
amino acid structures. Of these proteins, the binding of vWf is unique and has features
that make it ideally suited to mediate platelet adhesion and aggregation under conditions
of high shear, as can be found in stenosed coronary arteries. vWf is a large, disulfide-linked
multimer of approx 220 kDa subunits that has two motifs that bind to receptors on platelets; in addition to the RGD (residues 1744–1746), which binds to GPIIb/IIIa , it also has
an A1 domain, a disulfide-linked loop (residues 449–728) that binds the GPIb/IX/V complex *(40)*. Both motifs in soluble vWf are refractory to unstimulated platelets; however,
the conformational change vWf undergoes when it is immobilized on subendothelial
structures, is exposed to conditions of high shear, or even when exposed to the antibiotic
ristocetin or the snake venom protein botrocetin activates it to bind to the GPIb/IX/V complex on the platelet surface, an interaction mediated by the A1 domain. GPIb/IX/V is a
signaling receptor, and vWf binding induces platelet activation including the activation

of the receptor function of GPIIb/IIIa, which allows it to bind the RGD sequence on vWf and also to bind fibrinogen *(41,42)*. The ability of vWf to support platelet aggregation under conditions of high shear *(43)* may be related to these dual-binding motifs, repeated on each subunit of vWf, which together would be expected to bind with much higher affinity than either would singly and are thus more capable of binding platelets under conditions of high shear than is fibrinogen. The finding that aggregation initiated by platelet adhesion to vWf is GPIIb/IIIa-dependent and is more important at high shear *(44)* suggests that agonist-induced aggregation (e.g., thrombin- or ADP-induced) may be more important at low shear. This may, in part, explain why GPIIb/IIIa antagonists are more effective at preventing arterial thrombosis than are agonist inhibitors like ticlopidine and clopidogrel *(45)*, since high shear conditions such as occurs in coronary arteries would increase the importance of GPIIb/IIIa binding to vWf with subsequent GPIIb/IIIa activation—an interaction blocked by GPIIb/IIIa antagonists but not by the inhibitors that affect ADP-induced platelet stimulation. It may also explain why direct thrombin inhibitors caused bleeding as detected by cerebral hemorrage at doses required to inhibit arterial thrombosis, whereas GPIIb/IIIa antagonists apparently do not *(46)*.

The sequence used by sCD40L to bind to GPIIb/IIIa is Lys-Gly-Asp (KGD). KGD is a known GPIIb/IIIa recognition motif that was discovered by the specific binding of barbourin, a snake venom disintegrin, to GPIIb/IIIa *(47)*. The disintegrins are a family of proteins found in snake venoms and other hemataophagous organisms that normally express the RGD motif, which causes them to be potent antagonists of the adhesive protein binding activity of GPIIb/IIIa and other integrins (e.g., $\alpha_v\beta_3, \alpha_5\beta_1$) *(48,49)*. Barbourin is a unique disintegrin, as it expresses a Lys-Gly-Asp (KGD) sequence that causes this disintegrin to bind specifically to GPIIb/IIIa and inhibits its ligand binding activity *(47)*. Conservative mutations of this sequence, for example, aspartic acid to glutamic acid (converting the KGD to KGE), cause a loss of binding. This finding was utilized in the synthesis of the cyclic heptapeptide eptifibatide *(50,51)*. The role of the KGD sequence in sCD40L binding to GPIIb/IIIa was established by observations showing that mutation of the KGD in sCD40L to KGE caused a loss of GPIIb/IIIa binding, and a loss of the platelet effects of this protein *(6)*. sCD40L is the first of the many endogenous GPIIb/IIIa ligands that is known to use the KGD sequence for integrin recognition.

The synthetic GPIIb/IIIa antagonists constitute a wide variety of structures but as a class do have a common structural feature, a positive and negative charge separated by a distance of 10–20 Å *(52)*, a distance similar to that between the positive charge of arginine and the negative charge of aspartic acid on RGD *(53)*, to the positive and negative charge on KGD, and possibly even to that of the positive charge on lysine and the negative charge of aspartic acid on the KQAGDV sequence as it exists in a helical conformation *(54)*. Although it is tempting to speculate that these similarities indicate that synthetic GPIIb/IIIa antagonists bind to the RGD or KQAGDV binding site(s) and are classical competitive inhibitors of fibrinogen binding, data are not yet available to support this competitive mode of inhibition.

Ca²⁺ in GPIIb/IIIa Function

The primary amino acid sequence of GPIIb/IIIa predicts five divalent cation binding sites on the GPIIb/IIIa complex: the four EF hands on GP IIb and the one MIDAS domain on GPIIIa. Five divalent cations binding to GPIIb/IIIa have indeed been observed, and the affinities of these sites for Ca^{2+} predict that all are occupied by this divalent cation when platelets are suspended in plasma *(55,56)*. Divalent cation binding is reversible, and reductions in the amount of extracellular cations remove Ca^{2+} from GPIIb/IIIa, dramatically affecting its structure, its binding of adhesive proteins, and its binding of antagonists. For exam-ple, suspension of platelets in solutions containing ionized calcium concentrations of 40–50 µmol/L, such as those achieved in citrate-anticoagulated blood, causes partial removal of Ca^{2+} from GPIIb/IIIa, inducing a loss of fibrinogen binding activity *(57)*. At <1 µmol/L Ca^{2+}, as would occur for example in an EDTA-containing buffer, and at 37°C (but to a lesser extent at 25°C), GPIIb dissociates from GPIIIa within the plane of the plasma membrane *(58)*. Dissociated subunits irreversibly lose their structure and their ability to bind fibrinogen and accordingly can no longer mediate platelet aggregation *(59)*. The close proximity of the second EF hand of GPIIb and the MIDAS domain of GPIIIa to the site responsible for binding RGD ligands may account for observations suggesting that binding of Ca^{2+}, RGD ligands, and some GPIIb/IIIa antagonists (e.g., eptifibatide) are mutually competitive *(60)*. Thus, platelet assays relying on GPIIb/IIIa function may not be valid when performed in buffers containing less than the 1.1 mmol/L Ca^{2+} normally found in plasma.

One illustration of this effect was seen in the pharmacodynamic analysis of eptifibatide. The reduced Ca^{2+} caused by citrate anticoagulation actually increased the binding of eptifibatide but decreased the binding of fibrinogen. The combined result of these two effects is that the apparent inhibitory activity of eptifibatide is markedly overestimated in this condition, an event that led to a dose giving 40–50% inhibition of platelet aggregation at steady state, versus the 80% inhibition that had been targetted in the IMPACT II trial *(61)*. The same effect of citrate has been reported for abciximab and tirofiban *(62)* and may also have contributed to the suboptimal doses of these drugs achieved in clinical development.

Crystallographic analysis has shown that an additional binding site for divalent cations is induced upon binding of RGD-containing peptides to $\alpha_v\beta_3$. The function of this additional cation binding is not known, nor is it known whether this also occurs in GPIIb/IIIa.

GPIIb/IIIa LIBS Epitope Expression

Ligand binding to GPIIb/IIIa (e.g., adhesive proteins, GPIIb/IIIa antagonists, antibodies) induces a conformational change in the receptor, resulting in the formation of neoepitopes, collectively termed ligand-induced binding sites (LIBS) epitopes *(63,64)*. The change in integrin structure upon ligand binding has been directly observed in $\alpha_v\beta_3$ by crystallographic analysis, which showed that the formation of RGD-integrin complexes induces a profound change in the structure of the integrin *(65)*. The change in structure undoubtedly accounts for the neoepitopes generated when fibrinogen or GPIIb/IIIa antagonists bind GPIIb/IIIa. The response of GPIIb/IIIa to ligands has proved variable in that although all ligands and antibodies induce LIBS expression *(66)*, the LIBS epitopes expressed are different. For example, whereas tirofiban, eptifibatide, and abciximab all induce the binding of the LIBS antibody termed LIBS-1 *(67)*, abciximab fails to induce expression of the epitope for D-3, although the large size of abciximab may have sterically hindered D-3 access *(68)*. LIBS epitope expression is now recognized as a possible cause of thrombocytopenia following exposure to GPIIb/IIIa antagonists *(69–71)*. The incidence of thrombocytopenia is low (from 0.1 to 2% or more depending on the GPIIb/IIIa antagonists used) and varies between the different GPIIb/IIIa antagonists *(72)*. Antibodies directed against

LIBS epitopes (revealed by the drug-dependent binding to GPIIb/IIIa), which secondarily cause platelet clearance by an immune mechanism, have been observed, for example, in chimpanzee and Rhesus monkeys in response to both L-738, 167, and L-739,758 *(73)* in clinical trials in roxifiban *(74)* and in other studies in response to abciximab *(75,76)*.

STIMULUS-INDUCED GPIIb/IIIa ACTIVATION

The activation of the receptor function of GPIIb/IIIa (i.e., inside-out GPIIb/IIIa signaling) is known to occur in response to a wide spectrum of physiologic and pathophysiologic conditions (e.g., vascular trauma to initiate normal hemostasis; atherosclerotic plaque rupture or percutaneous intervention to initiate thrombosis). It is not surprising, therefore, that the stimulus pathways resulting in GPIIb/IIIa activation are redundant. Redundancy is found on at least two levels. First, GPIIb/IIIa activation occurs in response to multiple agonists. A host of soluble agonists, including thrombin and ADP, several adhesive proteins in the extracellular matrix including collagen, vWf, and fibrinogen, and even high shear act on distinct receptors and are each capable of initiating signal transduction pathways to induce activation of the receptor function of GPIIb/IIIa for soluble adhesive proteins (reviewed in refs. *77* and *78*). This multiplicity of agonists broadens the physiologic conditions capable of initiating platelet aggregation, which causes thrombosis and hemostasis.

Second, it is now appreciated that many of the primary agonists, e.g., thrombin, collagen, and ADP, act on multiple receptors (Table 1). Indeed, it appears that there may be a synergy between the different receptors with more than one receptor needing to be activated by a particular agonist for successful platelet activation to occur. In one example, ADP activates at least three receptors on platelets: the recently cloned *P2Y12* (P2Y$_{ADP}$ or P2T$_{AC}$), which inhibits adenylylcyclase and induces platelet aggregation *(79)*; P2Y1 (P2Y$_{ADP}$ or P2T$_{PLC}$), which is coupled to phospholipase C and mediates mobilization of Ca^{2+} from intracellular stores and platelet shape change; and a ligand-gated ion channel similar to P2X1 that allows for rapid Ca^{2+} influx. The indirectly acting thienopyridine-based platelet inhibitors clopidogrel and ticlopidine and the directly acting ATP-based antagonist ARL 66096 all target P2Y12 and inhibit ADP-induced GPIIb/IIIa activation *(79–81)*. In another example, collagen is now known to bind to at least two receptors, the integrin $\alpha_2\beta_1$ and a membrane glycoprotein termed GPVI *(82–84)*. The two receptors are interdependent, as antibodies against either receptor will block collagen-induced platelet activation *(85,86)*, and individuals lacking either receptor are defective in collagen-induced GPIIb/IIIa activation and have a bleeding diathesis *(87–89)*. $\alpha_2\beta_1$ appears to be the high-affinity receptor, which tethers collagen so that it can bind GPVI to initiate a signal transduction reaction culminating in GPIIb/IIIa activation.

A third example is thrombin. It is uniformly recognized that proteolysis of PAR1 by thrombin initiates signal transduction reactions within platelets and GPIIb/IIIa activation *(90)*. However, the inability of PAR1 antagonists to block thrombin-induced human platelet stimulation completely *(91)* and the differences between thrombin-induced responses compared with those induced by TRAP, peptide agonists of PAR1 *(92)*, suggest that the thrombin responsiveness of platelets may be partly mediated by a receptor in addition to PAR1. Possible candidates for a second thrombin receptor include PAR4 and the GPIb/IX/V complex, which contains a thrombin cleavage site (in GPV) and a high-affinity thrombin binding site (in GPIbα) and is known to have thrombin signaling capabilities *(93–97)*.

Table 1

Agonist	Receptor	Platelet signaling
Adenosine	$P2Y_1$ ($P2T_{PLC}$)	Gq-coupled, activation of PLC_β
diphosphate (ADP)	$P2Y_{12}$ ($P2T_{AC}$)	Gi-coupled, inhibition of adenylate cyclase
	P2X1	Ligand-gated ion channel, increase in intracellular Ca^{2+} levels
Thrombin	PAR 1	Gi-coupled, inhibition of adenylate cyclase, activation of non-receptor tyrosine kinases, G protein
	PAR 4	Coupled receptor kinases, PLC_β, PI3K, K^+ channel
		Gq, activation of PLC_β
		$G_{12/13}$-coupled, activation of Rho proteins
Collagen	$\alpha_2\beta_1$	Tyrosine phosphorylation and activation of Syk, phosphorylation of $PLC_{\gamma2}$
PLC	GP VI	Associated with Fcγ, activation linked to Syk
Epinephrine	α_2	Gz-coupled, inhibition of adenylate cyclase, activation of PLC
Serotonin	5-HT receptor	Gq-coupled
Thromboxane (TXA_2)	TPα	Gq and $G_{12/13}$-coupled, activation of PLCβ
vWF	GPIb/IX/V	Association with 14-3-3 εf, calmodulin
	complex	Coupled with Fc receptor γ-chain, association with tyrosine kinases (Fyn, Lyn), activation of Syk, PI3K
Immobilized fibrinogen	GPIIb/IIIa	Activation of tyrosine kinases (e.g., Src, and Syk, activation of PLC, PI3K, SHIP
sCD40L	GPIIb/IIIa	Required for aggregate stability
Leptin	Leptin receptor	Aggregate stability cofactor
Gas6	Axl, Sky	Aggregate stability cofactor
Eph kinase/ephrin	Ephrin/Eph kinase	Aggregate stability cofactors

The second level of redundancy is the signal transduction pathways from agonist receptor stimulation through GPIIb/IIIa activation, as different receptors use overlapping signal transduction pathways. For example, many of the agonist receptors on platelets are heptahelical receptors (e.g., PAR1, thromboxane receptor, ADP receptor), which as a class are known to be coupled to G proteins, a heterotrimeric family of signaling molecules consisting of α-, β-, and γ-subunits that signal by dissociating into Gα (a GTPase) and β-γ-dimers, both of which can propagate signals (98). Support for the direct involvement of Gαq in GPIIb/IIIa inside-out signaling is provided by observations showing that platelets from mice made deficient in this α-subunit have defective platelet aggregation in response to ADP and thrombin (99). Gαq-deficient mice also have defective thrombosis in response to collagen and have prolonged bleeding times. Interestingly, Gabbeta et al. (100) found that the platelets from a patient with defective GPIIb/IIIa activation in response to thrombin or ADP were partially deficient in Gαq. Recently, platelets from G$\alpha2^{-/-}$ mice have also been found to be defective for ADP-dependent inhibition of adenylyl cyclase, integrin activation, and aggregation (101).

Receptors for collagen or for vWf activate different intracellular signaling pathways that ultimately result in GPIIb/IIIa activation. GPVI is normally bound to another membrane protein termed Fcγ *(102)*. Binding of collagen to GPVI causes phosphorylation of the two tyrosine residues in the ITAM domain on the cytoplasmic face of Fcγ. Phosphorylated Fcγ then recruits Syk to the membrane so that it can be phosphorylated, activating its tyrosine kinase so that it, in turn, can phosphorylate downstream effectors (e.g., phospholipase Cγ) to propagate the signal through to GPIIb/IIIa activation. Platelets from mice in which either the Syk or the Fcγ genes are disrupted are now known to have defective collagen-induced signaling *(103)*. More recently, a direct association of Fyn and Lyn with the proline-rich domain of GPVI via their SH3 domain has been shown to regulate intracellular signaling *(104)*. GPIbα, the receptor for activated vWf, is also coupled to the Fc receptor γ-chain, Fyn and Lyn *(105)*.

The cytoplasmic domains of GPIbα and GPV in the GPIb/IX/V complex also bind protein 14-3-3ζ *(94,106,107)*, an adapter protein that binds Raf-1 and PKC, both serine/threonine kinases known to couple receptors to signaling pathways, and to phosphatidyl inositol 3-kinase *(108)*. Shear conditions in which the thrombotic process happens also directly influenced signaling events leading to GPIIb/IIIa activation. If, under static conditions, binding of GPIbα to immobilized vWF induced a PI 3-kinase-independent intracellular calcium release *(109)*, under conditions of high shear rates, the same kinase is indispensable for the calcium release and promotion of platelet adhesion to immobilized vWF *(95)*. Interestingly, GPIbα also seems to be able to mediate two different types of signaling pathways leading to GPIIb/IIIa activation, whether thrombin or vWF is the agonist *(110)*. These examples indicate that the intracellular signaling pathways within platelets for GPIIb/IIIa activation can have diverse origins.

As of this writing it is unknown how signal transduction pathways initiated by the various agonist receptors are coupled to GPIIb/IIIa activation. However, key players between agonist receptors and GPIIb/IIIa have been identified. Two are phospholipase C (PLC) and protein kinase C (PKC). PLC exists in several isoforms and functions to catalyze the hydrolysis of phosphatidylinositol phosphates to produce inositol phosphate (IP_3), which induces the release of Ca^{2+} from intracellular stores, and diacylglycerol, which markedly enhances the catalytic activity of PKC *(111)*. Phosphatidyl inositol phosphate hydrolysis can be mediated by PLCβ, which is activated by Gαq, or by PLCγ, which can be activated by kinases such as Syk. Support for the role of IP3, Ca^{2+}, and diacylglycerol is derived from studies showing that elevation of the cytoplasmic Ca^{2+} concentration with the calcium ionophore A23187 also induces GPIIb/IIIa activation *(112)* and that the GPIIb/IIIa activation induced by certain platelet agonists can be diminished by PKC inhibitors *(113)*.

Another key player between agonist receptors and GPIIb/IIIa activation is phospholipase A_2 (PLA_2), which catalyzes the release of arachidonic acid from the 2-position of phospholipids. Arachidonate is metabolized to thromboxane A_2 (TXA_2), the final reaction being catalyzed by cyclooxygenase. TXA_2 acts on the TXA_2 receptor, a heptahelical receptor, to propagate the signaling response. The effectiveness of aspirin, a cyclooxygenase inhibitor, in blocking GPIIb/IIIa activation, particularly at low agonist concentrations, demonstrates the importance of this pathway to GPIIb/IIIa signaling *(114)*. However, the ability of high agonist concentrations to overcome the effects of aspirin inhibition, even when cyclooxygenase is completely inhibited, indicates the redundancy of the signal transduction mechanisms for GPIIb/IIIa activation. Less well understood are the proximal events at GPIIb/IIIa that result in its activation. Because chemical modifications of GPIIb/IIIa have not been observed during inside-out GPIIb/IIIa signaling, it has been assumed that signaling induces either the association or dissociation of a regulatory protein(s) to the short cytoplasmic domains of GPIIb/IIIa. Several intracellular proteins have been identified that bind to peptides corresponding to the cytoplamic domains of GPIIb/IIIa including β3-endonexin (to GPIIIa) *(115)*, CIB (to GPIIb *(116,117)*, and several cytoskeletal proteins *(see* below). Of these proteins, the binding of CIB seems most relevant as this protein has been shown to activate GPIIb/IIIa directly via an interaction with the cytoplasmic domain of αIIb *(118)*. This conclusion, however, remains controversial *(119)* and requires further investigation. Three transmembrane proteins have also been shown to bind GPIIb/IIIa, CD9, a member of the tetraspanin class of proteins *(120,121)*, CD47, integrin-associated protein, which may assist in thrombospondin-induced GPIIb/IIIa activation *(122)*, CD98, a potential GPIIb/IIIa modulator *(123)*, and CD151 *(124)*.

Fibrinogen Binding on Unstimulated Platelets

Although GPIIb/IIIa must become activated to bind soluble fibrinogen, this is not the case for fibrinogen immobilized on surfaces (e.g., vessel walls or plastic) or for fibrinogen bound to GPIIb/IIIa. In both instances, binding apparently alters the conformation of fibrinogen so that the γ-chain sequence becomes capable of binding GPIIb/IIIa on unstimulated platelets *(9,38,125,126)*. Importantly, fibrinogen in this instance becomes a platelet agonist, as binding of GPIIb/IIIa by this mechanism initiates an outside-in signal transduction reaction through GPIIb/IIIa, resulting in platelet stimulation (see below for discussion of mechanism).

There are potentially three important physiologic consequences of this reaction. First, it provides a mechanism for platelet aggregation whereby fibrinogen is the primary agonist and the bound fibrinogen is responsible for recruiting and activating platelets by outside-in GPIIb/IIIa signaling. Second, fibrinogen bound to GPIIb/IIIa on surfaces is also capable of binding Mac-1 to mediate the arrest and adhesion of neutrophils *(39)*. Third, fibrinogen is one of the proteins bound to artificial surfaces, including extracorporeal devices such as in-dwelling catheters. The immobilization of fibrinogen on these surfaces, leading to the generation of an active conformation of fibrinogen capable of activating GPIIb/IIIa, may also account for the thrombotic potential of artificial surfaces when exposed to plasma proteins *(9)*, and may explain the thrombocytopenia associated with bypass surgery. This idea is supported by observations showing that GPIIb/IIIa antagonists reduce platelet loss in animal models of cardiopulmonary bypass *(127)*.

OUTSIDE-IN GPIIb/IIIa SIGNAL TRANSDUCTION

The binding of adhesive ligands (e.g., fibrinogen, vWF) to GPIIb/IIIa, together with the resultant clustering of the integrin following adhesion or aggregation, initiates outside-in signaling events leading to further platelet activation. These activation events are required for maximal platelet responses when platelets are activated with ADP or suboptimal amounts of other platelet agonists. Such responses include secretion of the contents of α-granules and dense bodies when platelets are activated with ADP or suboptimal amounts of other agonists as well as activation of the remaining GPIIb/IIIa molecules.

Although outside-in signals are required for maximal platelet aggregation, adhesion, clot retraction, and secretion, in and of themselves they are insufficient to induce these responses: low concentrations of other agonists (e.g., ADP) are required as costimuli. However, since low concentrations of other platelet agonists are normally present at sites of vascular injury such as would occur with plaque rupture or following percutaneous intervention, it can be anticipated that platelet activation via outside-in GPIIb/IIIa signaling occurs in these settings and that GPIIb/IIIa antagonists will have effects on platelet functions like secretion, GPIIb/IIIa activation, and enhancement of coagulation that are normally attributed to the classical platelet agonists such as ADP, thrombin, and collagen. In support of this conclusion, Carroll et al. *(128)* showed that the GPIIb/IIIa antagonist Ro 44-9883 inhibited α-granule secretion when platelet aggregation was induced by ADP or low doses of TRAP or collagen. Studies claiming that GPIIb/IIIa antagonists do not affect these reactions *(129)* were apparently performed under conditions in which aggregation and outside-in GPIIb/IIIa signaling were not involved. The requirement for low levels of other agonists may also allow for a further level of regulation of platelet aggregation by confluent endothelium, which expresses CD39, an ecto-ADPase that acts by metabolizing the ADP released by platelets *(130)*, and thrombomodulin *(131)*, which neutralizes thrombin. A lack of these two activities at sites of disrupted endothelium may facilitate platelet activation through outside-in GPIIb/IIIa signaling. However, the antithrombotic phenotype displayed by the CD39-deficient mice demonstrates the complexity of pro- and antithrombotic activities present at sites of vascular injury *(132)*.

The mechanism by which GPIIb/IIIa propagates outside-in signaling is of extreme importance in understanding GPIIb/IIIa function. Analysis of mutations of GPIIb/IIIa revealed that the extracellular adhesive protein binding pocket and the cytoplasmic domains were crucial for outside-in signaling events. Previous work in our laboratory has identified a postaggregation phosphorylation of the cytoplasmic domain of GPIIIa that appears to act as scaffolds for the recruitment of signaling proteins and propagation of the outside-in signal, and as anchor sites for the cytoskeletal proteins myosin *(133–136)*.

The clear demonstration of a physiologic role for the GPIIIa tyrosine phosphorylation signaling pathway following engagement of GPIIb/IIIa came from the generation of transgenic mice (diYF) in which both tyrosines in the cytoplasmic domain of GPIIIa were replaced by phenylalanines. Inside-out signaling is not affected in diYF mice, as demonstrated by the normal binding of FITC-fibrinogen upon platelet activation, whereas outside-in signaling is impaired, which in turn affects both thrombosis and hemostasis. Indeed, whereas the velocity of platelet aggregation induced by weak agonists is normal in diYF mice, the platelet aggregates spontaneously disaggregate. This defect in aggregation causes the diYF mice to generate unstable hemostatic plugs and to retract clots poorly *(5,134,135)*.

The downstream signaling events induced by outside-in GPIIb/IIIa signaling include protein tyrosine phosphorylation of numerous cytoplasmic proteins, as well as reorganization of the cytoskeletal/contractile apparatus within the platelet. Several of the proteins phosphorylated are tyrosine kinases, including multiple Src family members (e.g., Src, Lyn, Fyn), Syk, and FAK *(137,138)*. The effects of tyrosine kinase inhibitors have highlighted the importance of tyrosine phosphorylation in platelet signaling, as a wide range of tyrosine kinase inhibitors including genistein, erbstatin, the tyrphostins B42 and B46, and piceatannol have been found to inhibit platelet aggregation and secretion *(83,139–141)*. Both Syk and Src become phosphorylated and activated within seconds of fibrinogen binding to GPIIb/IIIa and translocate to the cytoskeleton upon aggregation. Upon fibrinogen binding, Csk, which is a negative regulator of Src under nonstimulated conditions, dissociates from GPIIb-IIIa, which allows the Src activation loop to be phosphorylated *(142)*.

Chemical crosslinking studies have demonstrated that Src is physically associated with GPIIb/IIIa within platelets as is another Src family member, Lyn *(143)*. The lack of any defect in platelet function in platelets from mice in which the gene for Src has been disrupted is probably owing to the redundancy between members of the Src family of tyrosine kinases *(144)*. Indeed, normal aggregation in response to γ-thrombin was observed with Src- and Fyn-deficient platelets, whereas Lyn deficiency reduced the aggregation response *(145)*. In contrast to the phosphorylation of Syk and Src, the FAK tyrosine kinase only becomes phosphorylated and activated upon full spreading or aggregation of platelets and requires agonist costimulation in addition to integrin ligation *(146)*. FAK autophosphorylation at tyrosine 397 leads to its association with Src, which can phosphorylate other tyrosine residues within the protein to provide docking sites for other phosphotyrosine binding proteins including GRB2 *(147)*. Thus, the common theme emerging from the study of outside-in GPIIb/IIIa signaling involves the tyrosine phosphorylation of a series of proteins, including the phosphorylation and activation of tyrosine kinases, followed by the assembly of signaling complexes.

Other second messenger pathways have also been implicated in outside-in GPIIb/IIIa signal transduction events, one of which is the hydrolysis of phosphoinositides. As described earlier, platelet activation leads to activation of phospholipases, leading to the production of inositol 1,4,5-trisphosphate. This polyphosphoinositide can be phosphorylated on the D3 position, subsequent to platelet activation, by at least two types of phosphoinositide 3-kinases (p85/PI3K and PI3Kγ) *(148)*. D3 phosphoinositides have been implicated in actin assembly and filopodial extension in the platelet *(149)*. The activation of p85/PI3K and its translocation to the cytoskeleton are dependent on GPIIb/IIIa outside-in signaling and platelet aggregation *(150)*. Treatment of platelets with the PI3K inhibitor wortmannin results in the reversal of TRAP-induced platelet aggregation and affects aggregation induced by the LIBS6 antibody, although platelet secretion remains unaffected. That wortmannin also inhibited the maintenance of GPIIb/IIIa in its high-affinity conformation suggested that PI3K may be involved in the formation of stable platelet aggregates, possibly by sustaining GPIIb/IIIa in an active state *(151)*. This hypothesis was confirmed by the defect in thrombus formation observed in the PI 3-kinase-deficient mice *(152)*. Another protein involved in this signaling pathway that is also phosphorylated and induced to translocate to the cytoskeleton upon GPIIb/IIIa-mediated platelet aggregation is the inositol 5-phosphatase, SHIP. This 145-kDa protein can dephosphorylate inositol 1,3,4,5-tetra-kisphosphate and phosphatidyl inositol 3,4,5-trisphosphate, leading to the further production of D3 phosphoinositides *(153)*.

The calcium-activated protease calpain also becomes activated during platelet aggregation, possibly indicating that this protein is another second messenger in GPIIb/IIIa signaling *(154–156)*. Indeed, recent studies in the calpain knockout mouse showed that calpain deficiency causes the same aggregation and clot retraction defect as occurred in the diYF mouse *(157)*. A direct link between GPIIb/IIIa and calpain was established by observations showing that calpain-deficient platelets fail to tyrosine phosphorylate the cytoplasmic domain of GPIIIa *(157)* and by observations showing that the cytoplasmic domain of GPIIIa is a calpain substrate and that calpain-mediated hydrolysis of GPIIIa during platelet aggregation leads to inhibition of fibrin clot retraction *(156)*. However, since calpain cleaves several proteins in addition to GPIIIa, it is not clear which hydrolytic event is responsible for this effect *(158)*. The small GTPases including Ras, Rho, Rac, and CDC42 constitute a further class of second messengers that appear to be involved in

GPIIb/IIIa-mediated signaling downstream of calpain. The Rho family (Rho, Rac, CDC42) are important in GPIIb/IIIa-mediated actin assembly *(159,160)*. The role that Ras plays in platelet integrin signaling remains to be established. Although in many cell types Ras is involved in activation of the MAP kinase cascade, it is not clear that this is its role in platelet biology. Indeed, Ras may even act to regulate Rho negatively, since the Ras-associated protein GAP can associate with p190 Rho-GAP, leading to the inactivation of Rho *(161)*.

GPIIb/IIIa Cytoskeletal Interactions

Many of the signaling events described above involve the translocation of proteins to the cytoskeleton, leading to reorganization of the cytoskeleton/contractile apparatus so that it can consolidate a platelet aggregate and retract a clot, processes important to thrombus stability. The binding of fibrinogen and subsequent platelet aggregation result in an increased association of GPIIb/IIIa with cytoplasmic actin filaments and the formation of focal contact-like structures *(162,163)*. Important issues concern (1) how outside-in signaling induces GPIIb/IIIa association with the cytoskeleton and (2) the identity of the cytoskeletal protein used for integrin attachment. It is estimated that approx 30% of GPIIb/IIIa becomes associated with the cytoskeleton following platelet aggregation. GPIIIa tyrosine phosphorylation is involved in this interaction, since tyrosine-phosphorylated GPIIIa is retained preferentially with the cytoskeletal fraction from aggregated platelets *(164)*. Phosphorylated GPIIIa appears to bind to platelet myosin, as phosphorylated GPIIIa cytoplasmic domain peptides but not unphosphorylated peptides have been found to interact selectively with the heavy chain of platelet myosin *(165)*. This suggests a mechanism for regulation of the interaction of GPIIb/IIIa with the platelet cytoskeleton: the cytoplasmic domain of GPIIIa becomes tyrosine phosphorylated upon integrin ligation and platelet aggregation. In addition to the phospho-GPIIIa interacting with signaling proteins (described previously), it also translocates to the cytoskeleton, where the phosphotyrosine residues may direct binding to the contractile protein myosin. GPIIb/IIIa on adherent platelets aligns with cytoplasmic actin filaments *(166)* and, with time, redistributes to the abluminal surface, causing the platelet to become refractory for the recruitment of additional platelets *(167)*. The resultant loss, on the luminal surface, of accessible, activated GPIIb/IIIa may serve to limit the recruitment of platelets to a growing thrombus *(167)*.

Clot retraction is GPIIb/IIIa-dependent: the integrin serves as the transmembrane bridge between extracellular fibrin and the cytoplasmic contractile machinery. The direct binding of GPIIb/IIIa with several purified cytoskeletal proteins in addition to myosin has been demonstrated, e.g., the binding of purified GPIIb and GPIIIa to talin *(168)*, the binding of GPIIb/IIIa incorporated into phospholipid vesicles with α-actinin *(169)*, and the binding of the GPIIIa cytoplasmic domain, in a yeast two-hybrid screen, to skelemin *(170)*. An unsolved problem is the identification of the cytoskeletal interactions that are responsible for the clot retraction process. In this regard, it is of interest that mutations in the cytoplasmic domains of GPIIb/IIIa that affect integrin signaling can also inhibit clot retraction *(171)*, including those mutations involving GPIIIa tyrosine residues (as described previously) *(164,172)*. Since tyrosine mutations would prevent GPIIIa phosphorylation, it is possible that one way such mutations can exert their effect on clot retraction is by preventing the association of phosphotyrosine-GPIIIa with myosin. In support of this idea, tyrosine kinase inhibitors can regulate the cytoskeletal attatchment of GPIIb/IIIa and can inhibit the clot retraction process *(173)*. Furthermore, diYF-deficient mice also presented a defect in fibrin clot retraction *(134)*.

GPIIb/IIIa POLYMORPHISMS
AS A CARDIOVASCULAR RISK FACTOR

Our initial understanding of GPIIb/IIIa structure-function relationships came from the study of patients with Glanzmann's thrombasthenia. This hereditary disease, which results in a life-long bleeding diathesis, is caused by a lack of GPIIb/IIIa function. More than 38 mutations in GPIIb and 27 in GPIIIa have been characterized at the genetic level *(174)*. The identified mutations cause either (1) defective biosynthesis or (2) normal or nearly normal expression of a defective protein owing to a loss of function mutation. Mutations that lead to defective expression of GPIIb/IIIa include those that produce defective proteins caused by early terminations, deletions, or frameshifts, those that generate a GPIIb/IIIa complex that is sensitive to dissociation [e.g., an Arg214Trp point mutation in GP IIIa *(175)*], and those affecting mRNA stability [e.g., Arg53Stop in GPIIb *(176)*] or RNA processing [e.g., an extensive 3-kb insertion in GPIIIa *(177)*]. Loss of function mutations include those that affect the ligand binding and Ca^{2+} binding sites in GPIIb/IIIa and also those that affect GPIIb/IIIa signaling. Some of these latter mutations highlight the importance of the cytoplasmic domains in GPIIb/IIIa function. For example, a patient with a single point mutation in the cytoplasmic domain of GPIIIa where serine 752 is replaced by a proline (S752P) had platelets that expressed nearly normal amounts of GPIIb/IIIa but that failed to aggregate, to spread, or to undergo FAK phosphorylation in response to fibrinogen binding *(178)*. This mutation helped validate the CHO cell expression system as a model for studying GPIIb/IIIa. When transfected into CHO cells with GPIIb, GPIIIa protein bearing S752P also showed a loss of GPIIb/IIIa function with impaired integrin signaling *(171)*.

In addition to the mutations arising in GPIIb/IIIa that lead to Glanzmann's thrombasthenia, there are a number of naturally occuring allotypic variants of GPIIb/IIIa. One of these is the Pl[A] alloantigen system, which has frequently been implicated in syndromes of immune-mediated platelet destruction. The Pl[A1] and Pl[A2] isoforms arise through a Leu33Pro amino acid polymorphism in GPIIIa *(179)*, a polymorphism that has generated considerable interest since it has been postulated that the Pl[A2/2] genotype is a possible risk factor for coronary thrombosis. A correlation between the Pl[A2/2] genotype (found in approx 2% of the Caucasian population) and acute coronary thrombosis was observed in one study (71 patients, 68 controls) *(180)*. This correlation was strongest in patients who had had coronary events at a relatively young age (<60 yr). However, although a number of studies support this putative association between the Pl[A2/2] genotype and an increased chance of coronary disease *(181,182)*, it remains controversial since other investigators have failed to observe such an association *(183–185)*. Although it remains to be established whether the Pl[A2/2] polymorphism is indeed a risk factor indicator for coronary disease, recent studies do suggest that platelet glycoprotein polymorphisms may provide a whole new array of thrombotic risk factors *(186)*. Indeed, it is of particular interest that Greenland Inuits, a population with a low incidence of thrombotic disease, have a lower frequency of the Pl[A2] allele than does the general Caucasian population *(187)*. An increased aggregability in response to ADP and epinephrine stimulation might be associated with Pl[A2]-bearing platelets *(188)*. One study noted that the Pl[A2] polymorphism of β3 enhances outside-in signaling *(189)*; even more interestingly, two recent studies highlight decreased levels of inhibition achieved by abxicimab in platelets with the Pl[A2] polymorphism and enhanced thrombin generation associated with the Pl[A2] polymorphism *(190,191)*. A higher risk of a primary event and

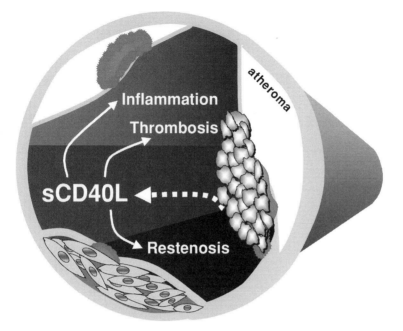

Fig. 3. Model showing the interelations existing among GPIIb/IIIa, thrombosis, inflammation, coagulation, and restenosis. Soluble CD40L (sCD40L) is released from platelet-rich thrombi and contributes to various steps in atherosclerotic lesion progression: (1) inflammation—sCD40L induces the production and release of proinflammatory cytokines from vascular cells and matrix metalloproteinases from resident cells in the atheroma; (2) thrombosis—sCD40L stabilizes platelet-rich thrombi; and (3) restenosis—sCD40L inhibits the reendothelialization of the injured vessel, potentially leading to the activation and proliferation of smooth muscle cells.

myocardial infarction in Pl$^{(A2)}$ carriers compared with noncarriers was observed in patients receiving orbofiban, suggesting that an analysis of the polymorphism might be required upon the use of oral GPIIb/IIIa antagonists *(192)*.

GPIIb/IIIa IN INFLAMMATION

Although the role of GPIIb/IIIa in platelet aggregation is well established, recent findings suggest that GPIIb/IIIa is also involved in vascular inflammation via its interaction with CD40 ligand (CD40L, CD154, gp39), a transmembrane protein in platelets (Fig. 3). CD40L is a member of the TNF-α family of proteins, which was originally identified in T-lymphocytes *(193)*, where it functions in the immune response by binding to its receptor on B-cells, CD40, to mediate a variety of responses including antibody class switching *(194)*. CD40L and its receptor, CD40, have in addition been identified on cells within the vasculature including endothelial cells, smooth muscle cells, monocytes, and macrophages where it has been implicated in various inflammatory responses *(194)*, including expression of inflammatory adhesion receptors [e.g., E-selectin, VCAM-1, and ICAM-1 *(195)*], expression of tissue factor *(196)*, and the release of chemokines (e.g., MCP-1, IL-6, and IL-8]. Studies utilizing blocking monoclonal antibodies and gene targeting have now determined that the CD40L/CD40 system has roles in atherosclerotic lesion progression *(197)*, establishing CD40L as a major mediator of vascular inflammation.

The pioneering studies of Henn and associates have shown not only that CD40L also exists in platelets but that platelets contain most of the circulating protein *(198–200)*. CD40L is cryptic in unstimulated platelets, but platelet agonists cause this protein to become rapidly exposed on the platelet surface, where it is subsequently cleaved, generating a soluble hydrolytic fragment termed sCD40L. Essentially all the sCD40L generated during the clotting of whole blood is derived from platelets *(198,200)*. Although the CD40L expressed on activated platelets is proinflammatory, sCD40L appears to be involved in both thrombosis and inflammation. The prothrombotic activity of sCD40L was demonstrated in mice harboring a CD40L gene deletion. These mice have a thrombosis defect, but infusion of recombinant sCD40L normalizes this deficiency *(6)*, demonstrating the prothrombotic activity of this protein. Other studies have shown that sCD40L is also proinflammatory, capable of inducing chemokine production in peripheral blood mononuclear cells *(201,202)*, PGE_2 production in lung fibroblasts *(203)*, adhesive protein expression in endothelial cells *(195)*, and proliferation of B-lymphocytes *(204)*; yet other studies have failed to observe these activities *(200)*. Thus, sCD40L has the potential of mediating several events within the vasculature. Indeed, elevated levels of sCD40L have been documented in several thrombotic and inflammatory conditions including acute coronary syndromes *(205)*, peripheral arterial occlusive disease *(206)*, and systemic lupus erythematosus *(207)*. Furthermore, elevated levels of sCD40L are associated with an increased cardiovascular risk in women *(208)*.

GPIIb/IIIa is linked to CD40L function in two ways. A primary role for GPIIb/IIIa in CD40L function is demonstrated by observations showing that GPIIb/IIIa antagonists inhibit the release of sCD40L from the surface of activated platelets *(209)*. Thus, the ligand binding activity of GPIIb/IIIa is involved in the release of this proinflammatory protein. An additional role for GPIIb/IIIa is to serve as a receptor for the released sCD40L. Direct binding measurements have shown that sCD40L binds to purified GPIIb/IIIa and to activated platelets in a GPIIb/IIIa-dependent manner. sCD40L is involved in platelet function, as it can serve as a substrate allowing for platelet spreading, it is also required for platelet aggregation under conditions of high shear.

In addition to the linkage of GPIIb/IIIa to CD40L, there are additional ways that GPIIb/IIIa can be linked to vascular inflammation. One example is by modulating the level of several soluble inflammatory markers released from activated platelets. Platelet α-granules contain several proinflammatory proteins in addition to CD40L, e.g., TGF-β, PF4, RANTES, and P-selectin. GPIIb/IIIa is indirectly involved in the activities of each of these proteins, as their release following activation of platelets by weak agonists such as ADP is promoted by the outside-in signaling through GPIIb/IIIa induced by platelet aggregation. In another example, fibrinogen bound to GPIIb/IIIa on the surface of activated platelets is capable of also binding to the β2-integrin Mac-1 and recruiting neutrophils into a growing thrombus *(39)*. In yet another example, the coagulation factors generated by GPIIb/IIIa signaling, including factor Xa and thrombin, are also proinflammatory *(210)*.

One study has tested the hypothesis that GPIIb/IIIa antagonists are antiinflammatory. Increased levels of inflammatory markers including C-reactive protein, IL-6, and TNF-α normally accompany percutaneous coronary revascularization *(211)*: elevations of these markers were found to be prevented by performing the procedure in the presence of abciximab *(212)*. Although the authors of this manuscript suggested that the crossreactivity of abciximab with $\alpha_M\beta_2$ might explain the antiinflammatory effects of this drug, two considerations argue against this conclusion. First, abciximab has low affinity for $\alpha_M\beta_2$ and would have very low receptor occupancy (<5%) on this integrin during the clinical administration of abciximab. Second, a recent study has shown that Integrilin, which does not crossreact with $\alpha_M\beta_2$, also significantly reduced C-reactive protein concentration after angioplasty *(213)*. Third, as outlined above, there are several mechanisms by which GPIIb/IIIa antagonism can be antiinflammatory. Thus, GPIIb/IIIa antagonists can be antiinflammatory by a GPIIb/IIIa mechanism. Additional studies are required to determine whether the clinical benefits of GPIIb/IIIa antagonists are derived not only from their direct inhibition of platelet aggregation, but also from their inhibition of inflammation by their blockade of the release of CD40L and other inflammatory mediators from platelets.

ADDITIONAL FUNCTIONS FOR GPIIb/IIIa

It is well known that the presence of platelets in blood shortens the time required for clot formation. Several studies *(214–216)* have shown that GPIIb/IIIa antagonists reduced tissue factor-induced thrombin formation, indicating that clot formation and GPIIb/IIIa may be linked. This finding raises the interesting possibility that GPIIb/IIIa antagonists may decrease thrombin formation at sites of vascular injury. In support of this suggestion, ex vivo samples have prolonged clot formation time when they were obtained from patients receiving GPIIb/IIIa antagonists *(217)*. Although unstimulated platelets have poor clot-promoting activity, activated, adherent platelets assemble prothrombinase and factor Xase on their surface to greatly enhance the rate of thrombin generation *(218)*. Since aggregation induces platelet activation through outside-in GPIIb/IIIa signaling, one possibility is that GPIIb/IIIa antagonists reduce thrombin formation by their ability to reduce aggregation-induced platelet stimulation. An alternative hypothesis is that prothrombin binding to GPIIb/IIIa on unstimulated platelets may enhance the rate of prothrombin activation *(219, 220)*. On the other hand, it is also likely that GPIIb/IIIa antagonists prolong blood clotting by inhibiting outside-in signaling through GPIIb/IIIa. Either explanation could account for the long clotting times in the platelet-rich plasma from patients with Glanzmann's thrombasthenia *(221)*.

An additional way that GPIIb/IIIa may affect coagulation is by prevention of α-granule secretion. α-Granules contain several proteins involved in blood coagulation including CD40L P-selectin, and factor V. CD40L and P-selectin are both expressed on the surface of activated platelets and subsequently cleaved *(199)*. CD40 ligand has been shown to upregulate the expression of tissue factor in macrophages *(222)*, and soluble P-selectin has been shown to be procoagulant *(223)*. These data suggest a third mechanism by which GPIIb/IIIa antagonists will reduce the ability of ruptured lesions to synthesize thrombin, i.e., by prevention of outside-in signaling through GPIIb/IIIa and the subsequent α-granule secretion.

Platelets provide perhaps the most abundant source of platelet-derived growth factor (PDGF), a growth factor implicated in atherosclerosis and restenosis *(224)*. PDGF is released with other α-granule proteins during platelet stimulation, and it has been speculated that sufficient PDGF is released during thrombosis to affect the vessel wall *(225)*. Tests of this idea using GPIIb/IIIa antagonists in the setting of angioplasty have proved negative in that the large, randomized clinical trials have not shown that the use of these drugs prevents the need for revascularization *(226–228)*. The exception was the EPIC trial using abciximab, which did show a decreased need for revascularization, a result attributed to the $\alpha_v\beta_3$ crossreactivity of abciximab *(229)*. However, since subsequent trials using this drug for the same indication did not reproduce this effect *(226)*, it is now believed that the use of abciximab does not affect this clinical outcome *(46)*. Nonetheless, it remains to be determined whether other aspects of the mitogenic activity of PDGF such as matrix and metalloprotease production *(230,231)* are affected by the use of GPIIb/IIIa antagonists for other clinical indications and whether the need for revascularization is a true indication of a smooth muscle cell proliferative response.

NEW PERSPECTIVES
FOR GPIIb/IIIa IN ANTITHROMBOTIC THERAPIES

Future directions in GPIIb/IIIa research can be expected to continue to focus on extracellular and intracellular domains, providing new insights into the molecular description of how GPIIb/IIIa interacts with its ligands, how GPIIb/IIIa is involved in the various signal transduction pathways, and the therapeutic strategies for the regulation of GPIIb/IIIa function. One can anticipate that the molecular crystal structure of GPIIb/IIIa will follow closely on the recent achievement of the structure of $\alpha_V\beta_3$, thus providing a contour map of the GPIIb/IIIa surface and a precise description of the binding sites of this receptor. Such information will undoubtedly yield new information on the way GPIIb/IIIa interacts with adhesive proteins and may also provide new insights into how therapeutic antagonists block the adhesive protein binding fuction of the integrin. It is now established that physical aggregation is only part of GPIIb/IIIa function and that signaling in platelets facilitates a wide range of reactions such as platelet shape change, consolidation of aggregates, clot retraction, and, perhaps most importantly, the release or expression of vasoactive factors.

These functions of GPIIb/IIIa indicate that it is not only involved in thrombosis and hemostasis but also links platelets and platelet aggregates to coagulation, inflammation, thrombolysis, atherosclerosis, and the proliferation of cells in the vessel wall in a dynamic way, more than would result from simple vessel occlusion. Evidence from both naturally occurring and experimentally induced mutations of GPIIb/IIIa clearly indicates a role for the cytoplasmic domains of GPIIb and GPIIIa in the function of GPIIb/IIIa, both in linking the integrin to the platelet cytoskeleton and in associations with signaling proteins. Post-aggregation tyrosine phosphorylation of the cytoplasmic domain of GPIIIa is the most proximal signaling event in these cascades, and it is reasonable to speculate that targeting this event may offer a new strategy for the pharmacologic intervention of GPIIb/IIIa.

Given that GPIIb/IIIa is not only involved in platelet aggregation, but also has signaling functions that allow it to be vasoactive, it is reasonable to ask whether the clinical benefits of GPIIb/IIIa antagonists achieved in the settings of percutaneous coronary interventions and unstable angina were achieved solely because of the simple inhibition of occlusive thrombi and whether additional therapeutic indications can be treated by GPIIb/IIIa antagonism. Is this the mechanism by which the short-term inhibition of thrombosis with GPIIb/IIIa antagonists (e.g., <20 h) in the setting of percutaneous coronary intervention translated into a prolonged inhibition of the accrual of events (e.g., up to a year or longer), as was observed in EPIC and ESPRIT studies *(232)*? Was this owing to the prevention of release of inflammatory mediators that normally occurred by procedure-induced thrombosis? Another example is the use of GPIIb/IIIa antagonists in the setting of acute myocardial infarction. If GPIIb/IIIa antagonists prove to be effective in this setting of acute myocardial infarction, are they beneficial not only because of the inhibition of thrombo-sis, but also because they prevent the release of vasoactive proteins and proinflammatory mediators? Will more aggressive use of GPIIb/IIIa antagonists in unstable angina more efficiently block the release of inflammatory and other vasoactive mediators and improve the therapeutic benefit by such mechanisms? Might therapeutic indications dependent on vascular inflammatory mediators released from platelets such as sickle cell disease, which is accompanied by elevated sCD40L *(233)*, also be treated with GPIIb/IIIa antagonists? Answers to these questions might affect the future use of GPIIb/IIIa antagonists in a variety of clinical settings.

GLOSSARY

ADP	adenosine diphosphate, a platelet agonist
CD40L	a membrane protein that is a ligand for CD40 and a member of the nerve growth factor superfamily; expressed on activated platelets; CD40L binding to CD40 results in intracellular signaling being initiated
CHO cells	Chinese hamster ovary cells
CIB	calcium and integrin binding protein, a protein that was identified as associating with the cytoplasmic domain of GPIIb using a yeast two-hybrid screen
EF hand	structural motif forming a calcium binding site typified by helices E and F of parvalbumin
FACS	fluorescence-activated cell sorting
FAK	focal adhesion kinase, a cytoplasmic tyrosine kinase
Fcγ	a protein associated with the Fc receptor complexes FcγRIII and FcεRI, which contains an ITAM (*see* below)
GP	glycoprotein
IP_3	inositol triphosphate
ITAM	immune receptor tyrosine activation motif, a consensus motif containing two tyrosine residues that, when phosphorylated, are important in initiating signals through a number of cell surface receptors present on cells of the immune system
K_d	equilibrium dissociation constant
KQAGDV	peptide sequence consisting of the amino acids lysine, glutamine, arginine, glycine, aspartic acid, and valine
LIBS	ligand-induced binding sites, neoepitopes expressed on GPIIb/IIIa following the binding of ligands like fibrinogen and GPIIb/IIIa antagonists and recognized by LIBS antibodies
Mac-1	the leukocyte integrin CD11b/CD18
MIDAS domain	metal ion-dependent adhesion site, a structural motif identified first in integrin α-subunits
M_r	apparent molecular weight of a protein determined by electrophoresis on a reduced SDS-polyacrylamide gel
P2X1	ADP-activated ligand-gated ion channel that directly increases intracellular calcium levels
P2Y1	ADP-activated, Gq-coupled seven-spanning transmembrane recept

PAR1, PAR3	Members of the protease-activated receptor family that function as thrombin receptors in platelets; activated by cleavage of their amino termini, leading to the exposure of a new amino acid sequence that acts as a "tethered ligand" to activate the receptors
PDGF	platelet-derived growth factor
PKC	protein kinase C
Pl^{A2}	a GPIIb/IIIa isotype
PLA_2	phospholipase A_2
PLC	phospholipase C, a phospholipase isoform that when activated can lead to phosphoinositide hydrolysis, diacylglycerol production, and increases in intracellular calcium levels
Raf-1	a serine/threonine kinase
RGD	peptide sequence consisting of the amino acids arginine, glycine, and aspartic acid
SHC/GRB2	two adaptor proteins capable of binding to phosphotyrosine residues of signaling proteins; SHC can associate with GRB2, which can then associate with SOS (*see* below), linking cell surface receptors to the Ras signaling pathway
SOS	son of sevenless, a guanine nucleotide exchange factor that activates Ras
Src-family	a family of at least 11 cytoplasmic tyrosine kinases whose prototypic member is Src
Syk	spleen tyrosine kinase, also known as p72, a tyrosine kinase found in hematopoietic cells; known to bind to phosphorylated tyroinse residues in ITAM motifs via its two SH2 regions
TGF-β	transforming growth factor-β
TRAP	thrombin receptor activation peptide, a peptide corresponding to the amino acid sequence of the "tethered ligand" of the PAR1 thrombin receptor; this peptide can activate PAR1 in the absence of thrombin cleavage
TXA_2	thromboxane A_2
VWF	von Willebrand factor

REFERENCES

1. Lincoff AM, Califf RM, Topol EJ. Platelet glycoprotein IIb/IIIa receptor blockade in coronary artery disease. J Am Coll Cardiol 2000;35:1103–1115.

   Hynes RO. Integrins: versatility, modulation, and signaling in cell adhesion. Cell 1992;69:11–25.

   ᵗᵉʳ BS. Blockade of platelet GPIIb/IIIa receptors as an antithrombotic strategy. Circulation 1995;92: ⁻ʔ80.

   ᵗ. Genetic and pharmacological analyses of Syk function in alphaIIbbeta3 signaling in plate- ⁻·93:2645–2652.

   ⁻ᵉrin tyrosine phosphorylation in platelet signaling. Curr Opin Cell Biol 2001;13:

   ᵉs arterial thrombi by a beta3 integrin-dependent mechanism. Nat Med

   of GPIIb/IIIa receptor number by quantification of 7E3 binding to human .907–914.

   .elet and megakaryocyte dense granules contain glycoproteins Ib and IIb-IIIa. -4057.

9. Shiba E, et al. Antibody-detectable changes in fibrinogen adsorption affecting platelet activation on polymer surfaces. Am J Physiol 1991;260:C965–C974.

10. Gralnick HR, et al. Endogenous platelet fibrinogen surface expression on activated platelets. J Lab Clin Med 1991;118:604–613.

11. Legrand C, Dubernard V, Nurden AT. Studies on the mechanism of expression of secreted fibrinogen on the surface of activated human platelets. Blood 1989;73:1226–1234.

12. Wencel-Drake JD, et al. Localization of internal pools of membrane glycoproteins involved in platelet adhesive responses. Am J Pathol 1986;124:324–334.

13. Handagama P, et al. Endocytosis of fibrinogen into megakaryocyte and platelet alpha-granules is mediated by alpha IIb beta 3 (glycoprotein IIb-IIIa). Blood 1993;82:135–138.

14. Wencel-Drake JD, et al. Arg-Gly-Asp-dependent occupancy of GPIIb/IIIa by applaggin: evidence for internalization and cycling of a platelet integrin. Blood 1993;81:62–69.

15. Pike NB, Lumley P. Uptake of a fibrinogen receptor antagonist by human platelets appears dependent upon GPIIb/IIIa. Thromb Haemost 1995;73:1195.

16. Nurden P, et al. Labeling of the internal pool of GP IIb-IIIa in platelets by c7E3 Fab fragments (abciximab): flow and endocytic mechanisms contribute to the transport. Blood 1999;93:1622–1633.

17. Woods VL Jr, Wolff LE, Keller DM. Resting platelets contain a substantial centrally located pool of glycoprotein IIb-IIIa complex which may be accessible to some but not other extracellular proteins. J Biol Chem 1986;61:15,242–15,251.

18. Kleiman NS, et al. Differential inhibition of platelet aggregation induced by adenosine diphosphate or a thrombin receptor-activating peptide in patients treated with bolus chimeric 7E3 Fab: implications for inhibition of the internal pool of GPIIb/IIIa receptors. J Am Coll Cardiol 1995;26:1665–1671.

19. Cook JJ, et al. Nonpeptide glycoprotein IIb/IIIa inhibitors. 15. Antithrombotic efficacy of L-738,167, a long-acting GPIIb/IIIa antagonist, correlates with inhibition of adenosine diphosphate-induced platelet aggregation but not with bleeding time prolongation. J Pharmacol Exp Ther 1997;281:677–689.

20. Stenberg PE, et al. A platelet alpha-granule membrane protein (GMP-140) is expressed on the plasma membrane after activation. J Cell Biol 1985;101:880–886.

21. Nurden AT, et al. Markers of platelet activation in coronary heart disease patients. Eur J Clin Invest 1994;24(Suppl 1):42–45.

22. Parise LV, et al. Evidence for novel binding sites on the platelet glycoprotein IIb and IIIa subunits and immobilized fibrinogen. Biochem J 1993;289:445–451.

23. Ni H, et al. Persistence of platelet thrombus formation in arterioles of mice lacking both von Willebrand factor and fibrinogen. J Clin Invest 2000;106:385–392.

24. Angelillo-Scherrer A, et al. Deficiency or inhibition of Gas6 causes platelet dysfunction and protects mice against thrombosis. Nat Med 2001;7:215–221.

25. Konstantinides S, et al. Leptin-dependent platelet aggregation and arterial thrombosis suggests a mechanism for atherothrombotic disease in obesity. J Clin Invest 2001;108:1533–1540.

26. Nakata M, et al. Leptin promotes aggregation of human platelets via the long form of its receptor. Diabetes 1999;48:426–429.

27. Dale GL, et al. Stimulated platelets use serotonin to enhance their retention of procoagulant proteins on the cell surface. Nature 2002;415:175–179.

28. Weisel JW, et al. Examination of the platelet membrane glycoprotein IIb-IIIa complex and its interaction with fibrinogen and other ligands by electron microscopy. J Biol Chem 1992;267:16,637–16,643.

29. Ulmer TS, et al. NMR analysis of structure and dynamics of the cytosolic tails of integrin alpha IIb beta 3 in aqueous solution. Biochemistry 2001;40:7498–7508.

30. Phillips DR, et al. The platelet membrane glycoprotein IIb-IIIa complex. Blood 1988;71:831–843.

31. Farrell DH, et al. Role of fibrinogen alpha and gamma chain sites in platelet aggregation. Proc Natl Acad Sci USA 1992;89:10,729–10,732.

32. Farrell DH, Thiagarajan, P. Binding of recombinant fibrinogen mutants to platelets. J Biol Chem 1994; 269:226–231.

33. Kloczewiak M, et al. Platelet receptor recognition site on human fibrinogen. Synthesis and structure-function relationship of peptides corresponding to the carboxy-terminal segment of the gamma chain. Biochemistry 1984;23:1767–1774.

34. Abrams CS, et al. Anti-idiotypic antibodies against an antibody to the platelet glycoprotein (GP) IIb-IIIa complex mimic GP IIb-IIIa by recognizing fibrinogen. J Biol Chem 1992;267:2775–2785.

35. Holmback K, et al. Impaired platelet aggregation and sustained bleeding in mice lacking the fibrinogen motif bound by integrin alpha IIb beta 3. EMBO J 1996;15:5760–5771.

36. Litvinov RI, et al. Binding strength and activation state of single fibrinogen-integrin pairs on living cells. Proc Natl Acad Sci USA 2002;99:7426–7431.

37. Rooney MM, Parise LV, Lord ST. Dissecting clot retraction and platelet aggregation. Clot retraction does not require an intact fibrinogen gamma chain C terminus. J Biol Chem 1996;271:8553–8555.

38. Gawaz MP, et al. Ligand bridging mediates integrin alpha IIb beta 3 (platelet GPIIB- IIIA) dependent homotypic and heterotypic cell-cell interactions. J Clin Invest 1991;88:1128–1134.

39. Weber C, Springer T. Neutrophil accumulation on activated, surface-adherent platelets in flow is mediated by interaction of Mac-1 with fibrinogen bound to aIIbb3 and stimulated by platelet-activating factor. J Clin Invest 1997;100:2085–2093.

40. Montgomery R, Coller B von Willebrand disease. In: Colman R, et al., eds. Hemostasis and Thrombosis: Basic Principles and Clinical Practice. JB Lippincott, Philadelphia, 1994, pp. 134–168.

41. Yuan Y, et al. Calpain regulation of cytoskeletal signaling complexes in von Willebrand factor-stimulated platelets. Distinct roles for glycoprotein Ib-V-Ix and glycoprotein IIb-IIIa (integrin alphaIIb beta3) in von Willebrand factor-induced signal transduction [In Process Citation]. J Biol Chem 1997;272: 21,847–21,854.

42. Savage B, Saldivar E, Ruggeri Z. Initiation of platelet adhesion by arrest onto fibrinogen or translocation on von Willebrand factor. Cell 1996;84:289–297.

43. Chow TW, et al. Shear stress-induced von Willebrand factor binding to platelet glycoprotein Ib initiates calcium influx associated with aggregation. Blood 1992;80:113–120.

44. Goto S, et al. Distinct mechanisms of platelet aggregation as a consequence of different shearing flow conditions. J Clin Invest 1998;101:479–486.

45. Lefkovits J, Topol EJ. The clinical role of platelet glycoprotein IIb/IIIa receptor inhibitors in ischemic heart disease. Cleve Clin J Med 1996;63:181–189.

46. Coller BS. Platelet GPIIb/IIIa antagonists: the first anti-integrin receptor therapeutics. J Clin Invest 1997; 100(11 Suppl):S57–S60.

47. Scarborough RM, et al. Barbourin. A GPIIb-IIIa-specific integrin antagonist from the venom of *Sistrurus m. barbouri*. J Biol Chem 1991;266:9359–9362.

48. Niewiarowski S, et al. Disintegrins and other naturally occurring antagonists of platelet fibrinogen receptors. Semin Hematol 1994;31:289–300.

49. Scarborough RM, et al. Characterization of the integrin specificities of disintegrins isolated from American pit viper venoms. J Biol Chem 1993;268:1058–1065.

50. Scarborough RM, et al. Design of potent and specific integrin antagonists. Peptide antagonists with high specificity for glycoprotein IIb-IIIa. J Biol Chem 1993;268:1066–1073.

51. Phillips DR, Scarborough RM. Clinical pharmacology of eptifibatide. Am J Cardiol 1997;80:11B–20B.

52. Hartman GD, et al. Non-peptide fibrinogen receptor antagonists. 1. Discovery and design of exosite inhibitors. J Med Chem 1992;35:4640–4642.

53. Zablocki JA, et al. Potent inhibitors of platelet aggregation based upon the Arg-Gly-Asp-Phe sequence of fibrinogen. A proposal on the nature of the binding interaction between the Asp-carboxylate of RGDX mimetics and the platelet GP IIb-IIIa receptor. J Med Chem 1992;35:4914–4917.

54. Mayo KH, et al. RGD induces conformational transition in purified platelet integrin GPIIb/IIIa-SDS system yielding multiple binding states for fibrinogen gamma-chain C-terminal peptide. FEBS Lett 1996; 378:79–82.

55. Rivas GA, Gonzalez-Rodriguez J. Calcium binding to human platelet integrin GPIIb/IIIa and to its constituent glycoproteins. Effects of lipids and temperature. Biochem J 1991;276:35–40.

56. Cierniewski CS, et al. Characterization of cation-binding sequences in the platelet integrin GPIIb-IIIa (alpha IIb beta 3) by terbium luminescence. Biochemistry 1994;33:12,238–12,246.

57. Marguerie GA, Edgington TS, Plow EF. Interaction of fibrinogen with its platelet receptor as part of a multistep reaction in ADP-induced platelet aggregation. J Biol Chem 1980;255:154–161.

58. Fitzgerald LA, Phillips DR. Calcium regulation of the platelet membrane glycoprotein IIb-IIIa complex. J Biol Chem 1985;260:11,366–11,374.

59. Fujimura K, Phillips DR. Calcium cation regulation of glycoprotein IIb-IIIa complex formation in platelet plasma membranes. J Biol Chem 1983;258:10,247–10,252.

60. Hu DD, Barbas CF, Smith JW. An allosteric Ca^{2+} binding site on the beta3-integrins that regulates the dissociation rate for RGD ligands. J Biol Chem 1996;271:21,745–21,751.

61. Phillips DR, et al. Effect of Ca^{2+} on GP IIb-IIIa interactions with Integrilin: enhanced GP IIb-IIIa binding and inhibition of platelet aggregation by reductions in the concentration of ionized calcium in plasma anticoagulated with citrate. Circulation 1997;96:1488–1494.

62. Marciniak SJ Jr, Jordan RE, Mascelli MA. Effect of Ca2+ chelation on the platelet inhibitory ability of the GPIIb/IIIa antagonists abciximab, eptifibatide and tirofiban. Thromb Haemost 2001;85:539–543.

63. Kouns WC, et al. A conformation-dependent epitope of human platelet glycoprotein IIIa. J Biol Chem 1990;265:20,594–20,601.

64. Frelinger AL III, et al. Selective inhibition of integrin function by antibodies specific for ligand-occupied receptor conformers. J Biol Chem 1990;265:6346–6352.

65. Xiong JP, et al. Crystal structure of the extracellular segment of integrin alpha Vbeta3. Science 2001; 294:339–345.

66. Abraham DG, et al. Arginine-glycine-aspartic acid mimics can identify a transitional activation state of recombinant alphaIIb beta3 in human embryonic kidney 293 cells. Mol Pharmacol 1997;52:227–236.

67. Dickfeld T, et al. Differential antiplatelet effects of various glycoprotein IIb-IIIa antagonists. Thromb Res 2001;101:53–64.

68. Jennings LK, Haga JH, Slack SM. Differential expression of a ligand induced binding site (LIBS) by GPIIb-IIIa ligand recognition peptides and parenteral antagonists. Thromb Haemost 2000;84: 1095–1102.

69. Ferrari E, et al. Acute profound thrombocytopenia after c7E3 Fab therapy. Circulation 1997;96: 3809–3810.

70. Simpfendorfer C, et al. First chronic platelet glycoprotein IIb/IIIa integrin blockade. A randomized, placebo-controlled pilot study of Xemlifoban in unstable angina with percutaneous coronary interventions. Circulation 1997;96:76–81.

71. Cannon C, et al. Randomized trial of an oral platelet glycoprotein IIb/IIIa antagonist, sibrafiban, in patients after an acute coronary syndrome. Circulation 1998;97:340–349.

72. Vorchheimer DA, Fuster V. Oral platelet glycoprotein IIb/IIIa receptor antagonists: the present challenge is safety. Circulation 1998;97:312–314.

73. Bednar B, et al. Fibrinogen receptor antagonist-induced thrombocytopenia in chimpanzee and rhesus monkey associated with preexisting drug-dependent antibodies to platelet glycoprotein IIb/IIIa. Blood 1999;94:587–599.

74. Billheimer JT, et al. Evidence that thrombocytopenia observed in humans treated with orally bio-available glycoprotein IIb/IIIa antagonists is immune mediated. Blood 2002;99:3540–3546.

75. Berkowitz SD, et al. Acute profound thrombocytopenia after C7E3 Fab (abciximab) therapy. Circulation 1997;95:809–813.

76. Bougie DW, Robbins ED, Aster RH. Antibodies associated with tirofiban-induced thrombocytopenia recognize multiple sites on ligand-occupied GPIIB/IIIA and may be specific for ligand-induced binding sites (LIBS). Blood 2001;98:1861.

77. Shattil S, Kashiwagi H, Pampori N. Integrin signaling: the platelet paradigm. Blood 1998;91:1–14.

78. Shattil SJ, Ginsberg MH, Brugge JS. Adhesive signaling in platelets. Curr Opin Cell Biol 1994;6: 695–704.

79. Hollopeter G, et al. Identification of the platelet ADP receptor targeted by antithrombotic drugs. Nature 2001;409:202–207.

80. Daniel J, et al. Molecular basis for ADP-induced platelet activation. I. Evidence for three distint ADP receptors on human platelets. J Biol Chem 1998;273:2024–2029.

81. Mills DCB. ADP receptors on platelets. Thromb Haemost 1996;76:835–856.

82. Kahmann RD, et al. Platelet function in adolescent idiopathic scoliosis. Spine 1992;17:145–148.

83. Keely PJ, Parise LV. The alpha2beta1 integrin is a necessary co-receptor for collagen-induced activation of Syk and the subsequent phosphorylation of phospholipase Cgamma2 in platelets. J Biol Chem 1996;271:26,668–26,676.

84. Ishibashi T, et al. Functional significance of platelet membrane glycoprotein p62 (GP VI), a putative collagen receptor. Int J Hematol 1995;62:107–111.

85. Sugiyama T, et al. A novel platelet aggregating factor found in a patient with defective collagen-induced platelet aggregation and autoimmune thrombocytopenia. Blood 1987;69:1712–1720.

86. Coller BS, et al. Collagen-platelet interactions: evidence for a direct interaction of collagen with platelet GPIa/IIa and an indirect interaction with platelet GPIIb/IIIa mediated by adhesive proteins. Blood 1989;74:182–192.

87. Handa M, et al. Platelet unresponsiveness to collagen: involvement of glycoprotein Ia-IIa (alpha 2 beta 1 integrin) deficiency associated with a myeloproliferative disorder. Thromb Haemost 1995;73:521–528.

88. Arai M, et al. Platelets with 10% of the normal amount of glycoprotein VI have an impaired response to collagen that results in a mild bleeding tendency. Br J Haematol 1995;89:124–130.

89. Ichinohe T, et al. Collagen-stimulated activation of Syk but not c-Src is severely compromised in human platelets lacking membrane glycoprotein VI. J Biol Chem 1997;272:63–68.

90. Vu TK, et al. Molecular cloning of a functional thrombin receptor reveals a novel proteolytic mechanism of receptor activation. Cell 1991;64:1057–1068.

91. Cook JJ, et al. An antibody against the exosite of the cloned thrombin receptor inhibits experimental arterial thrombosis in the African green monkey. Circulation 1995;91:2961–2971.

92. Henriksen RA, Samokhin, Tracy PB. Thrombin-induced thromboxane synthesis by human platelets. Properties of anion binding exosite I-independent receptor. Arterioscler Thromb Vasc Biol 1997;17: 3519–3526.

93. Clemetson KJ. Platelet activation: signal transduction via membrane receptors. Thromb Haemost 1995; 74:111–116.

94. Andrews R, et al. Binding of the purified 14-3-3z signaling protein to discrete amino acid sequences within the cytoplasmic domian of the platelet membrane glycoprotein Ib-IX-V complex. Biochemistry 1998;37:638–647.

95. Yap CL, et al. Essential role for phosphoinositide 3-kinase in shear-dependent signaling between platelet glycoprotein Ib/V/IX and integrin alpha(IIb)beta(3). Blood 2002;99:151–158.

96. Ramakrishnan V, et al. Increased thrombin responsiveness in platelets from mice lacking glycoprotein V. Proc Natl Acad Sci USA 1999;96:13,336–13,341.

97. Ramakrishnan V, et al. A thrombin receptor function for platelet glycoprotein Ib-IX unmasked by cleavage of glycoprotein V. Proc Natl Acad Sci USA 2001;98:1823–1828.

98. Neer E. Heterotrimeric G proteins: organizers of transmembrane signals. Cell, 1995;80:249–257.

99. Offermanns S, et al. Defective platelet activation in G alpha(q)-deficient mice. Nature 1997;389:183–186.

100. Gabbeta J, et al. Platelet signal transduction defect with Ga subunit dysfunction and diminished Gaq in a patient with abnormal platelet responses. Proc Natl Acad Sci USA 1997;94:8750–8755.

101. Jantzen HM, et al. Impaired activation of murine platelets lacking G alpha(i2). J Clin Invest 2001;108: 477–483.

102. Tsuji M, et al. A novel association of Fc receptor gamma-chain with glycoprotein VI and their co-expression as a collagen receptor in human platelets [In Process Citation]. J Biol Chem, 1997;272: 23,528–23,531.

103. Poole A, et al. The Fc receptor gamma-chain and the tyrosine kinase Syk are essential for activation of mouse platelets by collagen. EMBO J 1997;16:2333–2341.

104. Suzuki-Inoue K, et al. Association of Fyn and Lyn with the proline rich domain of GPVI regulates intracellular signalling. J Biol Chem 2002;277:21,561–21,566.

105. Falati S, Edmead CE, Poole AW. Glycoprotein Ib-V-IX, a receptor for von Willebrand factor, couples physically and functionally to the Fc receptor gamma-chain, Fyn, and Lyn to activate human platelets. Blood 1999;94:1648–1656.

106. Du X, et al. Association of a phospholipase A2 (14-3-3 protein) with the platelet glycoprotein Ib-IX complex. J Biol Chem 1994;269:18,287–18,290.

107. Calverley D, Kavanagh T, Roth G. Human signaling protein 14-3-3z interacts with platelet glycoprotein Ib subunits Iba and Ibb. Blood 1998;91:1295–1303.

108. Dubois T, et al. Structure and sites of phosphorylation of 14-3-3 protein: role in coordinating signal transduction pathways. J Protein Chem 1997;16:513–522.

109. Schoenwaelder SM, et al. RhoA sustains integrin alpha IIbbeta 3 adhesion contacts under high shear. J Biol Chem 2002;277:14,738–14,746.

110. Zaffran Y, et al. Signaling across the platelet adhesion receptor glycoprotein Ib-IX induces alpha IIbbeta 3 activation both in platelets and a transfected Chinese hamster ovary cell system. J Biol Chem 2000; 275:16,779–16,787.

111. Missiaen L, Taylor CW, Berridge MJ. Spontaneous calcium release from inositol trisphosphate-sensitive calcium stores. Nature 1991;352:241–244.

112. Lages B, Weiss H. Evidence for a role of glycoprotein IIb-IIIa, distinct from its ability to support aggregation, in platelet activation by ionophores in the presence of extracellular divalent cations. Blood 1994; 83:2549–2559.

113. Puri R, Colman R. Thrombin- and cathepsin G-induced platelet aggregation: effect of protein kinase C inhibitors. Anal Biochem 1993;210:50–57.

114. Mustard JF, Kinlough-Rathbone RL, Packham MA. Aspirin in the treatment of cardiovascular disease: a review. Am J Med 1983;74:43–49.

115. Shattil SJ, et al. Beta 3-endonexin, a novel polypeptide that interacts specifically with the cytoplasmic tail of the integrin beta 3 subunit. J Cell Biol 1995;131:807–816.

116. Naik UP, Patel PM, Parise LV. Identification of a novel calcium-binding protein that interacts with the integrin alphaIIb cytoplasmic domain. J Biol Chem 1997;272:4651–4654.

117. Barry WT, et al. Molecular basis of CIB binding to the integrin alphaIIb cytoplasmic domain. J Biol Chem 2002;277:28,877–28,883.

118. Tsuboi S. Calcium integrin-binding protein activates platelet integrin alpha IIbbeta 3. J Biol Chem 2002; 277:1919–1923.

119. Vallar L, et al. Divalent cations differentially regulate integrin alphaIIb cytoplasmic tail binding to beta3 and to calcium- and integrin-binding protein. J Biol Chem 1999;274:17,257–17,266.

120. Brisson C, et al. Co-localization of CD9 and GPIIb-IIIa (alpha IIb beta 3 integrin) on activated platelet pseudopods and alpha-granule membranes. Histochem J 1997;29:153–165.

121. Indig FE, Diaz-Gonzalez F, Ginsberg MH. Analysis of the tetraspanin CD9-integrin alphaIIbbeta3 (GPIIb-IIIa) complex in platelet membranes and transfected cells. Biochem J 1997;327:291–298.

122. Chung J, Gao AG, Frazier WA. Thrombspondin acts via integrin-associated protein to activate the platelet integrin alphaIIbbeta3. J Biol Chem 1997;272:14,740–14,746.

123. Fenczik CA, Sethi T, Ramos JW, Hughes PE, Ginsberg MH. Complementation of dominant supression implicates CD98 in integrin activation. Nature 1997;390:81–85.

124. Fitter S, et al. Transmembrane 4 superfamily protein CD151 (PETA-3) associates with beta 1 and alpha IIb beta 3 integrins in haemopoietic cell lines and modulates cell-cell adhesion. Biochem J 1999;338:61–70.

125. Sims PJ, et al. Effect of platelet activation on the conformation of the plasma membrane glycoprotein IIb-IIIa complex. J Biol Chem 1991;266:7345–7352.

126. Kieffer N, et al. Adhesive properties of the beta 3 integrins: comparison of GP IIb-IIIa and the vitronectin receptor individually expressed in human melanoma cells. J Cell Biol 1991;113:451–461.

127. Uthoff K, et al. Inhibition of platelet adhesion during cardiopulmonary bypass reduces postoperative bleeding. Circulation 1994;90:II269–II274.

128. Carroll R, et al. Blocking platelet aggregation inhibits thromboxane A2 formation by low dose agonists but does not inhibit phosphorylation and activation of cytosolic phospholipase A2. Thromb Res 1997; 88:109–125.

129. Tsao P, Forsythe M, Mousa S. Dissociation between the anti-aggregatory and anti-secretory effects of platelet integrin aIIbb3 (GPIIb/IIIa) antagonists, c7E3 and DMP728. Thromb Res 1997;88:137–146.

130. Marcus A, et al. The endothelial cell ecto-ADPase responsible for inhibition of platelet function is CD39. J Clin Invest 1997;99:1351–1360.

131. Esmon N, Carroll R, Esmon C. Thrombomodulin blocks the ability of thrombin to activate platelets. J Biol Chem 1983;258:12,238–12,242.

132. Enjyoji K, et al. Targeted disruption of cd39/ATP diphosphohydrolase results in disordered hemostasis and thromboregulation. Nat Med 1999;5:1010–1017.

133. Law DA, Nannizzi-Alaimo L, Phillips DR. Outside-in integrin signal transduction. Alpha IIb beta 3-(GP IIb IIIa) tyrosine phosphorylation induced by platelet aggregation. J Biol Chem 1996;271: 10,811–10,815.

134. Law DA, et al. Integrin cytoplasmic tyrosine motif is required for outside-in alphaIIbbeta3 signalling and platelet function. Nature 1999;401:808–811.

135. Phillips DR, Nannizzi-Alaimo L, Prasad KS. Beta3 tyrosine phosphorylation in alphaIIbbeta3 (platelet membrane GP IIb-IIIa) outside-in integrin signaling. Thromb Haemost 2001;86:246–258.

136. Cowan KJ, Law DA, Phillips DR. Identification of shc as the primary protein binding to the tyrosine-phosphorylated beta 3 subunit of alpha IIbbeta 3 during outside-in integrin platelet signaling. J Biol Chem 2000;275:36,423–36,429.

137. Shattil SJ, Brugge JS. Protein tyrosine phosphorylation and the adhesive functions of platelets. Curr Opin Cell Biol 1991;3:869–879.

138. Clark EA, Shattil SJ, Brugge JS. Regulation of protein tyrosine kinases in platelets. Trends Biochem Sci 1994;19:464–469.

139. Dillon AMR, Heath MF. The effects of tyrophostins B42 and B46 on equine platelet function and protein tyrosine phosphorylation. Biochem Biophy Res Commun 1995;212:595–601.

140. Salari H, et al. Erbstatin blocks platelet activating factor-induced protein-tyrosine phosphorylation, polyphosphoinositide hydrolysis, protein kinase C activation, serotonin secretion and aggregation of rabbit platelets. FEBS 1990;263:104–108.

141. Hargreaves PG, et al. The tyrosine kinase inhibitors, genistein, and methyl 2,5-dihydroxycinnamate, inhibit the release of (^{3}H)arachidonate from human platelets stimulated by thrombin or collagen. Thromb Haemost 1994;72:634–642.

142. Obergfell A, et al. Coordinate interactions of Csk, Src, and Syk kinases with [alpha] IIb[beta] 3 initiate integrin signaling to the cytoskeleton. J Cell Biol 2002;157:265–275.

143. Dorahy DJ, Berndt MC, Burns GF. Capture by chemical crosslinkers provides evidence that integrin alpha IIb beta 3 forms a complex with protein tyrosine kinases in intact platelets. Biochem J 1995;309: 481–490.

144. Soriano P, et al. Targeted disruption of the c-src proto-oncogene leads to osteopetrosis in mice. Cell 1991;64:693–702.

145. Cho MJ, et al. Role of the Src family kinase Lyn in TxA2 production, adenosine diphosphate secretion, Akt phosphorylation, and irreversible aggregation in platelets stimulated with gamma-thrombin. Blood 2002;99:2442–2447.

146. Shattil SJ, et al. Tyrosine phosphorylation of pp125FAK in platelets requires coordinated signaling through integrin and agonist receptors. J Biol Chem 1994;269:14,738–14,745.

147. Eide BL, Turck CW, Escobedo JA. Identification of Tyr-397 as the primary site of tyrosine phosphorylation and pp60src association in the focal adhesion kinase, pp125FAK. Mol Cell Biol 1995;15: 2819–2827.

148. Zhang J, et al. Phosphoinositide 3-kinase gamma and p85/phosphoinositide 3-kinase in platelets. Relative activation by thrombin receptor or beta-phorbol myristate acetate and roles in promoting the ligand-binding function of alphaIIbbeta3 integrin. J Biol Chem 1996;271:6265–6272.

149. Hartwig JH, et al. D3 phosphoinositides and outside-in integrin signaling by glycoprotein IIb-IIIa mediate platelet actin assembly and filopodial extension induced by phorbol 12-myristate 13-acetate. J Biol Chem 1996;271:32,986–32,993.

150. Guinebault C, et al. Integrin-dependent translocation of phosphoinositide 3-kinase to the cytoskeleton of thrombin-activated platelets involves specific interactions of p85 alpha with actin filaments and focal adhesion kinase. J Cell Biol 1995;129:831–842.

151. Kovacsovics TJ, et al. Phosphoinositide 3-kinase inhibition spares actin assembly in activating platelets but reverses platelet aggregation. J Biol Chem 1995;270:11,358–11,366.

152. Hirsch E, et al. Resistance to thromboembolism in PI3Kgamma-deficient mice. FASEB J 2001;15: 2019–2021.

153. Giuriato S, et al. Tyrosine phosphorylation and relocation of SHIP are integrin-mediated in thrombin-stimulated human blood platelets. J Biol Chem 1997;272:26,857–26,863.

154. Fox JE. On the role of calpain and Rho proteins in regulating integrin-induced signaling. Thromb Haemost 1999;82:385–391.

155. Fox JE. Cytoskeletal proteins and platelet signaling. Thromb Haemost 2001;86:198–213.

156. Du X, et al. Calpain cleavage of the cytoplasmic domain of the integrin beta 3 subunit. J Biol Chem 1995;270:26,146–26,151.

157. Azam M, et al. Disruption of the mouse mu-calpain gene reveals an essential role in platelet function. Mol Cell Biol 2001;21:2213–2220.

158. Schoenwaelder SM, et al. Calpain cleavage of focal adhesion proteins regulates the cytoskeletal attachment of integrin alphaIIbbeta3 (platelet glycoprotein IIb/IIIa) and the cellular retraction of fibrin clots. J Biol Chem 1997;272:1694–1702.

159. Dash D, Aepfelbacher M, Siess W. Integrin alpha IIb beta 3-mediated translocation of CDC42Hs to the cytoskeleton in stimulated human platelets. J Biol Chem 1995;270:17,321–17,326.

160. Tapon N, Hall A. Rho, Rac and Cdc42 GTPases regulate the organization of the actin cytoskeleton. Curr Opin Cell Biol 1997;9:86–92.

161. Dedhar S, Hannigan GE. Integrin cytoplasmic interactions and bidirectional transmembrane signalling. Curr Opin Cell Biol 1996;8:657–669.

162. Phillips DR, Jennings LK, Edwards HH. Identification of membrane proteins mediating the interaction of human platelets. J Cell Biol 1980;86:77–86.

163. Fox JE, et al. On the role of the platelet membrane skeleton in mediating signal transduction. Association of GP IIb-IIIa, pp60c-src, pp62c-yes, and the p21ras GTPase-activating protein with the membrane skeleton. J Biol Chem 1993;268:25,973–25,984.

164. Nannizzi-Alaimo L, Jenkins AL, Law DA, Eigenthaler M, Ginsberg MH, Phillips DR. The tyrosine residues within b3 are phosphorylated only upon platelet aggregation and are required for b3-dependent clot retraction in CHO cells. Blood 1997;90(Suppl):426a (abstract 1892).

165. Jenkins AL, et al. Tyrosine phosphorylation of the beta3 cytoplasmic domain mediates integrin-cyto-skeletal interactions. J Biol Chem 1998;273:13,878–13,885.
166. Simmons SR, Albrecht RM. Self-association of bound fibrinogen on platelet surfaces. J Lab Clin Med 1997;128:39–50.
167. Coller BS, et al. Studies of activated GPIIb/IIIa receptors on the luminal surface of adherent platelets. Paradoxical loss of luminal receptors when platelets adhere to high density fibrinogen. J Clin Invest 1993;92:2796–2806.
168. Knezevic I, Leisner TM, Lam SC. Direct binding of the platelet integrin alphaIIbbeta3 (GPIIb-IIIa) to talin. Evidence that interaction is mediated through the cytoplasmic domains of both alphaIIb and beta3. J Biol Chem 1996;271:16,416–16,421.
169. Otey CA, Pavalko FM, Burridge K. An interaction between alpha-actinin and the beta 1 integrin sub-unit in vitro. J Cell Biol 1990;111:721–729.
170. Reddy KB, et al. Identification and characterization of a specific interaction between skelemin and beta integrin cytoplasmic tails. Circulation Suppl I 1996;94:I–98.
171. Chen YP, et al. A point mutation in the integrin beta 3 cytoplasmic domain (S752→P) impairs bidirec-tional signaling through alpha IIb beta 3 (platelet glycoprotein IIb-IIIa). Blood 1994;84:1857–1865.
172. Blystone SD, et al. Requirement of integrin beta3 tyrosine 747 for beta3 tyrosine phosphorylation and regulation of alphavbeta3 avidity. J Biol Chem 1997;272:28,757–28,761.
173. Schoenwaelder SM, et al. Tyrosine kinases regulate the cytoskeletal attachment of integrin alpha IIb beta 3 (platelet glycoprotein IIb/IIIa) and the cellular retraction of fibrin polymers. J Biol Chem 1994; 269:32,479–32,487.
174. French DL. Glanzmann Thrombasthenia Database. 1999.
175. Djaffar I, Rosa JP. A second case of variant of Glanzmann's thrombasthenia due to substitution of platelet GPIIIa (integrin beta 3) Arg214 by Trp. Hum Mol Genet 1993;2:2179–2180.
176. Kato A, et al. Molecular basis for Glanzmann's thrombasthenia (GT) in a compound heterozygote with glycoprotein IIb gene: a proposal for the classification of GT based on the biosynthetic pathway of glycoprotein IIb-IIIa complex. Blood 1992;79:3212–3218.
177. Djaffar I, Caen JP, Rosa JP. A large alteration in the human platelet glycoprotein IIIa (integrin beta 3) gene associated with Glanzmann's thrombasthenia. Hum Mol Genet 1993;2:2183–2185.
178. Chen YP, et al. Ser-752→Pro mutation in the cytoplasmic domain of integrin beta 3 subunit and defective activation of platelet integrin alpha IIb beta 3 (glycoprotein IIb-IIIa) in a variant of Glanzmann thrombasthenia. Proc Natl Acad Sci USA 1992;89:10,169–10,173.
179. Newman P, Derbes R, Aster R. The human platelet alloantigens, PlA1 and PlA2, are associated with a leucine33/proline33 amino acid polymorphism in membrane glycoprotein IIIa, and are distinguish-able by DNA typing. J Clin Invest 1989;83:1778–1781.
180. Weiss EJ, et al. A polymorphism of a platelet glycoprotein receptor as an inherited risk factor for cor-onary thrombosis. N Engl J Med 1996;334:1090–1094.
181. Walter DH, et al. Platelet glycoprotein IIIa polymorphisms and risk of coronary stent thrombosis. Lancet 1997;350:1217–1219.
182. Carter A, et al. Association of the platelet PlA polymorphism of glycoprotein IIb/IIIa and the fibrino-gen Bb 448 polymorphism with myocardial infarction and extent of coronary disease. Circulation 1997; 96:1424–1431.
183. Herrmann SM, et al. The Leu33/Pro polymorphism (PlA1/PlA2) of the glycoprotein IIIa (GPIIIa) receptor is not related to myocardial infarction in the ECTIM Study. Etude Cas-Témoins de l'Infarctus du Myocarde. Thromb Haemost 1997;77:1179–1181.
184. Samani NJ, Lodwick D. Glycoprotein IIIa polymorphism and risk of myocardial infarction. Cardiovasc Res 1997;33:693–697.
185. Bennett JS, et al. Effect of the Pl(A2) alloantigen on the function of beta(3)-integrins in platelets. Blood 2001;97:3093–3099.
186. Murata M, et al. Coronary artery disease and polymorphisms in a receptor mediating shear stress-depen-dent platelet activation. Circulation 1997;96:3281–3286.
187. de Maat MP, et al. PlA1/A2 polymorphism of platelet glycoprotein IIIa and risk of cardiovascular disease. Lancet 1997;349:1099–1100.
188. Feng D, et al. Increased platelet aggregablilty associated with platelet GPIIIa PLA2 polymorphism. Circulation 1997;96a:I-412 (abstract 2301).
189. Vijayan KV, et al. The Pl(A2) polymorphism of integrin beta(3) enhances outside-in signaling and adhesive functions. J Clin Invest 2000;105:793–802.

190. Wheeler GL, et al. Reduced inhibition by abciximab in platelets with the PlA2 polymorphism. Am Heart J 2002;143:76–82.

191. Undas A, et al. Pl(A2) polymorphism of beta(3) integrins is associated with enhanced thrombin generation and impaired antithrombotic action of aspirin at the site of microvascular injury. Circulation 2001;104:2666–2672.

192. O'Connor FF, et al. Genetic variation in glycoprotein IIb/IIIa (GPIIb/IIIa) as a determinant of the responses to an oral GPIIb/IIIa antagonist in patients with unstable coronary syndromes. Blood 2001; 98:3256–3260.

193. Graf D, et al. Cloning of TRAP, a ligand for CD40 on human T cells. Eur J Immunol 1992;22:3191–3194.

194. Mach F, et al. Functional CD40 ligand is expressed on human vascular endothelial cells, smooth muscle cells, and macrophages: implications for CD40-CD40 ligand signaling in atherosclerosis. Proc Natl Acad Sci USA 1997;94:1931–1936.

195. Hollenbaugh D, et al. Expression of functional CD40 by vascular endothelial cells. J Exp Med 1995; 182:33–40.

196. Slupsky JR, et al. Activated platelets induce tissue factor expression on human umbilical vein endothelial cells by ligation of CD40. Thromb Haemost 1998;80:1008–1014.

197. Mach F, et al. Reduction of atherosclerosis in mice by inhibition of CD40 signalling. Nature 1998;394: 200–203.

198. Viallard JF, et al. Increased soluble and platelet-associated CD40 ligand in essential thrombocythemia and reactive thrombocytosis. Blood 2002;99:2612–2614.

199. Henn V, et al. CD40 ligand on activated platelets triggers an inflammatory reaction of endothelial cells. Nature 1998;391:591–594.

200. Henn V, et al. The inflammatory action of CD40 ligand (CD154) expressed on activated human platelets is temporally limited by coexpressed CD40. Blood 2001;98:1047–1054.

201. Aukrust P, et al. Enhanced levels of soluble and membrane-bound CD40 ligand in patients with unstable angina. Possible reflection of T lymphocyte and platelet involvement in the pathogenesis of acute coronary syndromes. Circulation 1999;100:614–620.

202. Kiener PA, et al. Stimulation of CD40 with purified soluble gp39 induces proinflammatory responses in human monocytes. J Immunol 1995;155:4917–4925.

203. Zhang Y, et al. CD40 engagement up-regulates cyclooxygenase-2 expression and prostaglandin E2 production in human lung fibroblasts. J Immunol 1998;160:1053–1057.

204. Mazzei GJ, et al. Recombinant soluble trimeric CD40 ligand is biologically active. J Biol Chem 1995; 270:7025–7028.

205. Garlichs CD, et al. Patients with acute coronary syndromes express enhanced CD40 ligand/CD154 on platelets. Heart 2001;86:649–655.

206. Tsakiris DA, et al. Platelets and cytokines in concert with endothelial activation in patients with peripheral arterial occlusive disease. Blood Coagul Fibrinolysis 2000;11:165–173.

207. Kato K, et al. The soluble CD40 ligand sCD154 in systemic lupus erythematosus. J Clin Invest 1999; 104:947–955.

208. Schonbeck U, et al. Soluble CD40L and cardiovascular risk in women. Circulation 2001;104:2266–2268.

209. Nannizzi-Alaimo L, et al. Cardiopulmonary bypass induces release of soluble CD40 ligand. Circulation 2002;105:2849–2854.

210. Gillis S, Furie B, Furie B. Interactions of neutrophils and coagulation proteins. Semin Hematol 1997;34: 336–342.

211. Liuzzo G, et al. Enhanced inflammatory response to coronary angioplasty in patients with severe unstable angina. Circulation 1998;98:2370–2376.

212. Lincoff AM, et al. Abciximab suppresses the rise in levels of circulating inflammatory markers after percutaneous coronary revascularization. Circulation 2001;104:163–167.

213. Merino Otermin A, et al. [Eptifibatide blocks the increase in C-reactive protein concentration after coronary angioplasty]. Rev Esp Cardiol 2002;55:186–189.

214. Reverter JC, et al. Inhibition of platelet-mediated, tissue factor-induced thrombin generation by the mouse/human chimeric 7E3 antibody. Potential implications for the effect of c7E3 Fab treatment on acute thrombosis and "clinical restenosis." J Clin Invest 1996;98:863–874.

215. Herault J, et al. Effect of SR121566A, a potent GP IIb-IIIa antagonist on platelet-mediated thrombin generation in vitro and in vivo. Thromb Haemost 1998;79:383–388.

216. van't Meer C, et al. Effect of platelet inhibitors on thrombin generation. Blood 1997;90(Suppl):29a (abstract 114).

217. Moliterno DJ, et al. Effect of platelet glycoprotein IIb/IIIa integrin blockade on activated clotting time during percutaneous transluminal coronary angioplasty or directional atherectomy (the EPIC trial). Evaluation of c7E3 Fab in the Prevention of Ischemic Complications trial. Am J Cardiol 1995;75:559–562.
218. Swords N, Tracy P, Mann K. Intact platelet membranes, not platelet-released microvesicles, support the procoagulant activity of adherent platelets. Arterioscler Thromb 1993;13:1613–1622.
219. Byzova TV, Plow EF. Networking in the hemostatic system. J Biol Chem 1997;272:27,183–27,188.
220. Dicker IB, et al. Both the high affinity thrombin receptor (GPIb-IX-V) and GPIIb/IIIa are implicated in expression of thrombin-induced platelet procoagulant activity. Thromb Haemost 2001;86:1065–1069.
221. Basic-Micic, M, et al. Platelet-induced thrombin generation time: a new sensitive global assay for platelet function and coagulation. Method and first results. Haemostasis 1992;22:309–321.
222. Mach F, et al. Activation of monocyte/macrophage functions related to acute atheroma complication by ligation of CD40: induction of collagenase, stromelysin, and tissue factor. Circulation 1997;96:396–399.
223. Andre P, et al. Pro-coagulant state resulting from high levels of soluble P-selectin in blood. Proc Natl Acad Sci USA 2000;97:13,835–13,840.
224. Ross R, et al. Localization of PDGF-B protein in macrophages in all phases of atherogenesis. Science 1990;248:1009–1012.
225. Kraiss L, et al. Regional expression of the platelet-derived growth factor and its receptors in a primate graft model of vessel wall assembly. J Clin Invest 1993;92:338–348.
226. EPILOG Investigators, Platelet glycoprotein GP IIb/IIIa receptor blockade and low-dose heparin during percutaneous coronary revascularization. The EPILOG Investigators. N Engl J Med 1997;336: 1689–1696.
227. IMPACT-II Investigators. Randomised placebo-controlled trial of eptifibatide on complications of percutaneous coronary intervention: IMPACT-II. Lancet 1997;349:1422–1428.
228. RESTORE Investigators. Effects of platelet glycoprotein IIb/IIIa blockade with tirofiban on adverse cardiac events in patients with unstable angina or acute myocardial infarction undergoing coronary angioplasty. The RESTORE investigators. Randomized Efficacy Study of Tirofiban for Outcomes and REstenosis. Circulation 1997;96:1445–1453.
229. Topol EJ, et al. Randomised trial of coronary intervention with antibody against platelet IIb/IIIa integrin for reduction of clinical restenosis: results at six months. The EPIC Investigators. Lancet 1994;343: 881–886.
230. Strauss B, et al. In vivo collagen turnover following experimental balloon angioplasty injury and the role of matrix metalloproteinases. Circ Res 1996;79:541–550.
231. Bendeck M, et al. Differential expression of α1 type VIII collagen in injured platelet-derived growth factor-BB-stimulated rat carotid arteries. Circ Res 1996;79:524–531.
232. Teirstein P. Overview of glycoprotein IIb/IIIa clinical trials with abciximab and eptifibatide in acute coronary syndromes and percutaneous coronary intervention. J Invasive Cardiol 1999;11(Suppl C): 26C–30C.
233. Lee SP, et al. Elevation and biological activity of CD40 ligand (CD40L): potential mechanism of platelet-mediated inflammation in sickle cell disease. Blood 2001;98:2016.

4

Glycoprotein IIb/IIIa Antagonists
Development of Abciximab and Pharmacology of Abciximab, Tirofiban, and Eptifibatide

Barry S. Coller, MD

CONTENTS

INTRODUCTION
DEVELOPMENT OF ABCIXIMAB AS A GPIIb/IIIa ANTAGONIST
PHARMACOKINETICS OF APPROVED GPIIb/IIIa ANTAGONISTS
ACKNOWLEDGMENTS
REFERENCES

INTRODUCTION

The rationale for developing platelet glycoprotein (GP) IIb/IIIa antagonists as antithrombotic agents for use in ischemic cardiovascular disease emerged from integrating data obtained in the early 1980s by many different investigators working in diverse fields. The data were, however, often controversial or fragmentary, or required extrapolation to human disease from in vitro systems or animals models. Thus, for those who are considering embarking on a similar adventure in drug development, it is important to emphasize that until efficacy and safety was established for these agents in well-controlled, large clinical trials, many individuals remained skeptical about the potential benefits and safety of this approach.

DEVELOPMENT OF ABCIXIMAB AS A GPIIb/IIIa ANTAGONIST

Pathophysiology of Coronary Artery Occlusion

Despite strong evidence from postmortem examinations for a major role of thrombosis in the development of ischemic cardiovascular disease dating back to before 1950 *(1)*, controversies regarding whether the thrombus occurred before or after myocardial infarction *(2)* and the role of coronary spasm *(3)* led to confusion as to the role of thrombosis in the etiology of ischemic damage. Moreover, a plaque hemorrhage model was favored by some investigators in which obstruction was primarily caused by a mechanical flap produced by hemorrhage-induced dissection of the coronary artery *(1)*. It was only with the

From: *Contemporary Cardiology: Platelet Glycoprotein IIb/IIIa
Inhibitors in Cardiovascular Disease, 2nd Edition*
Edited by: A. M. Lincoff © Humana Press Inc., Totowa, NJ

advent of cardiac catheterization of patients with myocardial infarction in the early 1980s that there was general acceptance in the cardiologic community that thrombosis initiated most myocardial infarctions *(4)*. The success of thrombolytic therapy in decreasing mortality from myocardial infarction provided strong support for the importance of thrombosis in the pathogenesis of myocardial infarction *(5,6)*.

Even after it was established that thrombosis is a major contributor to myocardial infarction, however, the relative contributions of platelets and fibrin to this process were unclear. The efficacy of thrombolytic therapy appropriately focused attention on the contribution of fibrin. These data logically led to attempts to develop strategies to decrease fibrin deposition by developing more effective inhibitors of thrombin generation and/or thrombin's action *(7)*. Detailed pathologic studies identified, however, that a white platelet "head" of variable size is usually identifiable at the site of atherosclerotic plaque rupture or erosion, indicating that platelets commonly initiate the thrombotic process *(1,8,9)*. In this formulation, the commonly identified large red fibrin "tail" reflects subsequent activation of the coagulation system (facilitated by thrombin generation on the surface of platelets) and entrapment of erythrocytes in the rapidly forming fibrin meshwork. Biochemical evidence of platelet activation during ischemic vascular events *(10)* provided additional evidence of a role for platelets, although it was not possible to exclude the possibility that platelet activation was an epiphenomenon. Animal models of thrombosis secondary to vascular injury provided compelling evidence that platelets can make a major contribution to thrombus formation *(11–14)*, but all the animal models differ significantly from naturally occurring human cardiovascular disease in the mechanism of injury. Moreover, none of the animal models at that time involved arteries containing the complex types of atherosclerotic lesions on which virtually all human disease occurs.

Perhaps the most compelling evidence supporting an essential role for platelets in myocardial infarction came from the Second International Study of Infarct Survival (ISIS-2), a double-blind, randomized, placebo-controlled study involving more than 17,000 patients with clinically diagnosed myocardial infarction *(6,15)*. This study demonstrated an 18.9% decrease in 35-d vascular mortality from taking aspirin alone (absolute reduction 2.5%), a reduction very similar to the 21.2% achieved with intravenous streptokinase alone *(6)*. Combining aspirin with streptokinase resulted in a 39.4% reduction in mortality, with this additive effect suggesting that the agents operated through different mechanisms of action. Data on the combined use of heparin and aspirin in ISIS-2 were especially important in conceptualizing the roles for antiplatelet and anticoagulant agents. Patients were not randomized with regard to heparin therapy, but the intention of each treating physician to either use or not use heparin was recorded. Aspirin improved the outcome of patients regardless of whether intravaneous, subcutaneous, or no heparin use was planned, providing further evidence that aspirin operates through a mechanism different from that of heparin *(6,15)*. Even the ISIS-2 data supporting an important role for platelets in myocardial infarction could be challenged, however, because it could be argued that aspirin's benefit may have been owing to its effects on nonplatelet proteins or cells, because many such effects have been described *(16)*.

The safety data in ISIS-2 also were extremely important in that they showed that aspirin alone did not increase the risk of hemorrhagic stroke and actually decreased the risk of any stroke by approx 50% *(6,15)*. Aspirin's stroke benefit may result from several mechanisms linked to its antithrombotic action. These include: (1) decreasing the size of mural thrombi, (2) decreasing the size of the myocardial infarctions so that fewer are transmural (the feature most predictive of developing a mural thrombus), (3) decreasing the extent of secondary thrombus formation on emboli that reach the cerebral circulation, and 4) decreasing microvascular thrombus formation that may result from even temporary interruption of the cerebral circulation. The stroke data from ISIS-2, when combined with those of the US Physician's Health Study of primary prophylaxis of myocardial infarction with aspirin *(17)*, which identified an increased risk of hemorrhagic stroke with aspirin treatment, led to the interesting paradox that aspirin decreases the risk of stroke during and immediately after myocardial infarction, a period of high stroke risk, but increases the risk of hemorrhagic stroke in the normal population, in which the risk of stroke is very low. Because the protection from death from myocardial infarction afforded by aspirin, a relatively weak antiplatelet agent, extended to only a minority of patients in ISIS-2 and because aspirin's hemorrhagic toxicity during the first 30 d of treatment was minimal, it seemed logical to conclude that there was a potential role for more powerful antiplatelet agents in the treatment of ischemic cardiovascular events caused by thrombosis.

Theories of the pathogenesis of acute reocclusion after percutaneous coronary interventions (PCIs), including balloon angioplasty, atherectomy, and similar procedures, went through phases similar to those relating to the pathogenesis of myocardial infarction. Thus, in the 1980s, there was considerable controversy as to the relative roles of thrombosis versus mechanical dissection resulting in development of an obstructing intimal flap. Estimates that I obtained at that time from expert interventionalists for a key role for thrombosis ranged from 20 to 80%, with complementary estimates of 80 to 20% for mechanical dissection. Data from at least one relatively small retrospective study indicated that aspirin and dipyridamole decreased the risk of abrupt occlusion *(18)*, but the uncertainty about pathogenesis made it unclear as to whether more potent antiplatelet agents would further decrease the risk of abrupt occlusion after PCI.

Theories about the pathophysiology of unstable angina and acute non-ST segment elevation myocardial infarction (NSTMI) focused on the role of platelet-mediated thrombosis, since there was biochemical evidence of systemic platelet activation and aspirin was demonstrated to be effective in reducing the risk of death or developing a myocardial infarction *(19,20)*. Moreover, adding heparin to aspirin provided additional benefit, but the effect was not dramatic *(20)*. The role of fibrin in these syndromes was uncertain, since thrombolytic therapy did not improve the outcome of patients with unstable angina and NSTMI and may have actually made the outcome worse *(21–23)*. Thus, judging by empiric observations on response to therapy, the pathophysiology of unstable angina and NSTMI appeared to differ from that of acute myocardial infarction. This difference may reflect heterogeneity in the population diagnosed with these disorders, a contention supported by the observation that the group can be divided on the basis of troponin elevation *(24)*, and the variability in angiographic findings *(25)*.

Glanzmann Thrombasthenia

Although first described in 1918, it was not until the 1960s that Glanzmann thrombasthenia was categorized as an autosomal recessive inherited disorder characterized by mucocutaneous hemorrhage, marked prolongation of bleeding time, abnormal clot retraction, and the hallmark failure of platelets to aggregate in response to all the agonists thought to operate in vivo, including ADP, epinephrine, collagen, and thrombin *(26,27)*. Subsequently, it was observed that the platelets of patients with Glanzmann thrombasthenia are deficient in two different glycoproteins, identified as GPIIb and GPIIIa based on their migration in polyacrylamide gels after treatment with sodium dodecyl sulfate *(28,29)*. Soon thereafter, it was established that these proteins exist as a calcium-dependent complex *(30)*.

The nature and severity of the clinical hemorrhagic syndrome caused by Glanzmann thrombasthenia were important factors in the decision to consider GPIIb/IIIa as a target for antithrombotic therapy, since the patients' symptoms could be considered the likely equivalent of maximal GPIIb/IIIa blockade by an antagonist. The spectrum of severity is wide among patients *(26,27,31)*, but easy bruising, menorrhagia, epistaxis, and variable gingival bleeding (depending largely on dental hygiene and tooth repair) are most common. Severe gastrointestinal bleeding and bleeding in other organs occurs, but it is usually episodic and infrequent, unless there is a separate anatomic abnormality. Of particular note is that, unlike the bleeding in hemophilia A and B (factors VIII and IX deficiencies), spontaneous central nervous system bleeding is not common in Glanzmann thrombasthenia *(26)*, highlighting the variability of bleeding syndromes that occur with defects in different components of the hemostatic system. Thus, because it was known that complete absence of GPIIb/IIIa receptors is not incompatible with life, there was reason to hope that even high-grade GPIIb/IIIa blockade could be sustained for at least a short period with acceptable toxicity.

The ability to extrapolate these data to the potential use of GPIIb/IIIa antagonists to treat thrombotic cardiovascular disease was limited, however, by the lack of knowledge about the impact of using a GPIIb/IIIa antagonist in combination with heparin, aspirin, a thrombolytic agent, or perhaps all of them together, since these agents are scrupulously avoided in thrombasthenia patients. Moreover, the invasive instrumentation that is required for PCI and that frequently occurs during the management of myocardial infarction would add a serious hemostatic challenge. Thus, the safety considerations that could be deduced from analysis of patients with Glanzmann thrombasthenia were complex; GPIIb/IIIa antagonists were likely to cause a significant, but perhaps not unacceptable risk of hemorrhage; the use of aspirin, heparin, and thrombolytic agents would probably increase the risk significantly, and there would probably be a need for fastidious attention to the vascular sites of entry of invasive devices.

Observations on patients with Glanzmann thrombasthenia had little to offer with regard to the potential efficacy of GPIIb/IIIa antagonists. Because it is such a rare disorder, few patients who have Glanzmann thrombasthenia are old enough to have thrombotic ischemic vascular disease. Nonetheless, neither we nor Dr. Uri Seligsohn and his colleagues in Israel have identified any patients with Glanzmann thrombasthenia who have had an acute ischemic cardiovascular event *(32)*. Glanzmann thrombasthenia does not, however, appear to afford protection from developing subclinical atherosclerosis, as judged by ultrasound assessment of carotid arteries for intima-media thickness and the presence of atherosclerotic plaques *(33)*.

Platelet Physiology

The development of the platelet aggregometer in the 1960s *(34,35)* opened the modern era of platelet function analysis, with rapid characterization of the aggregation response to ADP, epinephrine, collagen, and thrombin, among others *(36)*. It also allowed for appreciation of the complex interrelation of platelet aggregation and the release reaction *(37)*. It further permitted the characterization of antiplatelet agents, most notably aspirin, which gives a characteristic pattern of inhibition involving the second wave of aggregation *(38, 39)*, the wave that requires thromboxane A_2 production and is associated with the release reaction *(40,41)*.

Platelet aggregation induced by ADP, epinephrine, collagen, and thrombin (the agonists that fail to aggregate platelets from patients with Glanzmann thrombasthenia) was established in the late 1970s to result from the binding of the bivalent adhesive glycoprotein fibrinogen to the platelet surface *(42,43)*, followed by the development of fibrinogen molecule bridges between receptors on two different platelets. Since the GPIIb/IIIa receptor was known to be abnormal in Glanzmann thrombasthenia, it became the logical choice to be the fibrinogen receptor, but even here there was controversy as to whether Glanzmann thrombasthenia patients lacked the receptor or lacked the ability to activate the receptor *(44,45)*. Although several lines of evidence supported the conclusion that the GPIIb/IIIa receptor was, in fact, the receptor that bound fibrinogen *(45,46)*, it was this lingering controversy that led us in the early 1980s to try to develop monoclonal antibodies, which were then coming into general use, to help resolve this issue. We wanted to focus on antibodies that would affect platelet function, and thus our screening assay built on our earlier studies *(45)* demonstrating that platelets could agglutinate fibrinogen-coated beads. In fact, the antibodies we produced that blocked platelet-mediated fibrinogen bead agglutination (10E5 and 7E3) bound to the GPIIb/IIIa complex, providing very strong evidence for GPIIb/IIIa being responsible for the binding of fibrinogen *(47,48)*.

At approximately the same time, additional molecular biologic data from investigators studying adhesion phenomena in many different tissues provided evidence that GPIIb/IIIa was a member of a large family of receptors with similar structures *(49)*. Hynes *(49)* termed these receptors *integrins* to emphasize that they have binding domains on both the exterior of the cell and the cytoplasmic face; the former interact with adhesive ligands, whereas the latter interact with cytoskeletal proteins and proteins involved in both receiving and sending signals. GPIIb/IIIa is a prototypic integrin, being a heterodimer of an α-subunit (GPIIb, αIIb) and a β-subunit (GPIIIa, $\beta3$) *(50,51)*. Monoclonal antibody studies demonstrated that GPIIb/IIIa is essentially specific for platelets and megakaryocytes and is expressed at very high density on platelets [approx 80,000 receptors per platelet *(52)*], making it one of the densest adhesion/aggregation receptors in any biologic system. There is also an internal pool of GPIIb/IIIa receptors associated with α-granule membranes and perhaps other structures *(53,54)*. At least some GPIIb/IIIa receptors probably cycle between the platelet surface and the internal pools *(54)*.

The $\beta3$-subunit of GPIIb/IIIa can also pair with another α-subunit, termed αV, to form the αV$\beta3$ receptor, commonly called the vitronectin receptor *(55)*. This is present on platelets at extremely low levels [approx 50–100 molecules per platelet *(56)*] and is also present on many other cell types, including endothelial cells, osteoclasts, smooth muscle cells, and activated lymphocytes *(57–59)*.

Investigators studying the $\alpha5\beta1$ integrin receptor in the early 1980s made the remarkable discovery that a very small region of the large fibronectin molecule was crucial for the binding *(60)*. Ultimately they localized this to a three-amino acid motif, arginine-glycine-aspartic acid [single-letter code, RGD *(60)*]. They went on to show that small peptides containing this sequence could actually block the binding of ligands to the $\alpha5\beta1$ receptor *(61)*. At approximately the same time, aided by the availability of monoclonal antibodies, it was discovered that the GPIIb/IIIa receptor could bind not only fibrinogen, but also von Willebrand factor (vWf), fibronectin, vitronectin, and other adhesive glycoproteins *(62)*.

With only one exception, as the genes for these proteins were cloned and their amino sequences determined, it became clear that the regions responsible for binding to platelets are the same regions that contain RGD sequences *(63)*. Moreover, the binding of all of these ligands to platelet GPIIb/IIIa could be inhibited by RGD-containing peptides *(64,65)*. The one exception, ironically, is fibrinogen itself, since its binding to GPIIb/IIIa does not appear to be mediated by the RGD-containing domains, but rather by the C-terminal dodecapeptide of the γ-chain *(66,67)*. This peptide contains a glycine-aspartic acid (GD) sequence, as well as a crucial lysine residue (which, like arginine, is positively charged) two amino acids upstream *(68)*. γ-Chain peptides can also inhibit the binding of fibrinogen to platelet GPIIb/IIIa *(69)*. The crystal structure and electron microscopic appearance of fibrinogen demonstrate that the γ-chain dodecapeptides are at the very ends of this highly extended, dimeric molecule *(70,71)*. Thus, even platelets that are almost 500 Å apart can be bridged by a single fibrinogen molecule. It is uncertain whether the RGD and γ-chain peptides bind to the same site on GPIIb/IIIa *(72)*.

The αVβ3 receptor binds many of the same ligands as GPIIb/IIIa, and its ligand binding can also be blocked by RGD peptides *(59,73)*. It appears to have preference for vitronectin *(56)*, however, and, unlike GPIIb/IIIa, it binds to osteopontin when activated *(74,75)*. Moreover, it appears to bind fibrinogen via the latter's C-terminal RGD sequence in the Aα chain *(76)*, and perhaps amino acids 190–202 and 346–358 in the γ-chain *(77)*, but not the γ-chain C-terminal dodecapeptide. A crystal structure of the extracellular segment of the αVβ3 receptor has been reported, which includes points of contact between the αV and β3 (GPIIIa) chains and regions thought to be involved in ligand binding *(78)*. In addition, the crystal structure of αVβ3 in complex with an RGD peptide has been determined, and it was elegantly demonstrated that the binding site is a point of contact between αV and β3, with arginine binding to αV and aspartic acid binding to β3 near the metal ion-dependent adhesion site (MIDAS) domain *(79)*. Based on nuclear magnetic resonance (NMR) data, Beglova et al. *(80)* have proposed that activation of αVβ3 involves a change in struc-ture from a bent form to an upright form by a "switchblade" mechanism, but other models have been suggested *(79)*.

The multiplicity of ligands that can bind to GPIIb/IIIa adds complexity to its biology. Shear conditions may be important in determining the preferred ligand since vWf appears to be the most important ligand under high shear conditions, whereas fibrinogen is favored at low shear *(81)*. One unique feature of the GPIIb/IIIa-fibrinogen interaction is that GPIIb/IIIa activation is required for platelets to bind fibrinogen in the fluid phase *(82)*, but platelet activation is not required for GPIIb/IIIa to mediate adhesion to immobilized fibrinogen *(45,83)*.

The recognition that RGD-containing peptides could inhibit the GPIIb/IIIa receptor opened up exciting new opportunities to synthesize low-molecular-weight peptides, peptidomimetics, and nonpeptides that would have favorable pharmacologic features. This led to the production of literally thousands of compounds, including orally active compounds, that have high affinity for GPIIb/IIIa and high specificity for GPIIb/IIIa, compared to αVβ3 and other integrin receptors (*see* below) *(84–86)*.

Platelet Adhesion and Aggregation

Our current view is that occlusive thrombus formation in coronary arteries probably begins with deposition of platelets on a ruptured or eroded atherosclerotic plaque. The adhesion of platelets to the plaque is primarily mediated by constitutively active receptors on the platelet surface interacting with subendothelial proteins, including but not limited to GPIb/IX (vWf); GPIIb/IIIa (αIIbβ3; immobilized fibrinogen); GPIa/IIa (α2β1) (collagen); GPIc*/IIa (α5β1) (fibronectin); GPIc/IIa (α6β1) (laminin); GPVI (collagen); and perhaps αVβ3 (fibrinogen, vitronectin, vWf, osteopontin) and GPIV (thrombospondin, collagen) *(37)*. The adhesive proteins may be exposed by the initial injury (e.g., collagen and vWf), deposited onto subendothelial proteins either from plasma or from platelet releasates (e.g., binding of vWf to collagen) *(87)*, or deposited from plasma or from platelet releasates onto newly formed fibrin (e.g., vWf) *(88)*. Data demonstrating tissue factor in the lipid-rich core of atherosclerotic plaques, however, raise the possibility that the generation of at least small amounts of thrombin and local fibrin formation may be early events in at least some circumstances *(89)*. The adhesion process is likely to be much more complex after the release or generation of platelet agonists at the site of vascular injury since these agents may be able to cause nearby circulating platelets to expose P-selectin and activate GPIIb/IIIa to a high affinity ligand binding state. Inflammatory cytokines may also affect the process, with platelets rolling or skipping along the surface before settling into stable interactions *(87,90)*. Under the relatively high shear rates found in coronary arteries, the GPIb/IX-vWf interaction appears to play a crucial role *(87)*.

The first layer of adherent platelets probably has little effect on blood flow. It is the recruitment of additional layers of platelets, mediated primarily or exclusively by the GPIIb/IIIa receptor, that poses the greatest risk of platelet thrombus formation and resulting vasoocclusion. Platelet deposition probably also initiates thrombin generation and fibrin deposition, since platelet aggregates have been demonstrated to bind the initiator of the extrinsic pathway of coagulation, tissue factor, which circulates in whole blood *(91–93)*. Moreover, the activated platelets in the thrombus, as well as microparticles released from platelets, furnish highly effective catalytic surfaces on which thrombin can be generated, leading to the initiation of fibrin deposition and further platelet activation and adhesion *(94,95)*. Platelet-rich thrombi resist thrombolysis because platelets facilitate clot retraction and fibrin crosslinking and release inhibitors of fibrinolysis (*see* Mechanisms of Action section below).

Platelets can also contribute to both local and systemic inflammation. Thus, activated platelets can recruit both neutrophils and monocytes via interactions between P-selectin on the surface of activated platelets and P-selectin glycoprotein ligand-1 (PSGL-1) on the surface of the leukocytes (reviewed in ref. *96*). Other platelet receptors, including GPIIb/IIIa, αVβ3, and GPIb/IX may also contribute to strengthening the interactions. Platelets can release cytokines and cytokine precursors, as well as platelet-activating factor, that can activate leukocytes. In addition, activated platelets express CD40 ligand and interleukin-1 (IL-1), potent activators of a number of different inflammatory responses. Finally platelet-neutrophil and platelet-monocyte aggregates circulate in normal blood, and the latter increase when platelets are activated, as occurs after PCI *(97–99)*. Leukocytes that circulate after PCI and those with attached platelets show evidence of activation, as judged by increased expression of αMβ2 *(100,101)*.

Thus, the rationale for targeting the GPIIb/IIIa receptor focused on its pivotal role in mediating the platelet-platelet interactions crucial for vasoocclusive platelet thrombus formation (and the downstream effects of platelet thrombi on coagulation, fibrinolysis, and inflammation), regardless of the agonist responsible for platelet activation. As such, it represents the final common pathway for platelet aggregation. This model predicts that GPIIb/IIIa receptor blockade would have little effect on platelet adhesion, which is largely mediated by other receptors, and this was not considered a disadvantage since the first layer of platelets may contribute to maintaining hemostasis without significantly compromising blood flow.

Animal Models

The goal of the early animal studies was to assess the role of the GPIIb/IIIa receptor in well-established models of thrombosis, in particular models in which aspirin offered less than complete protection *(102)*. We chose antibody 7E3 for these studies because it reacted with human, primate, and dog platelets. The binding characteristics of 7E3 are discussed below in the section on pharmacokinetics. To avoid the possibility that platelets coated with 7E3 would be cleared by dog splenic macrophages containing immunoglobulin Fc receptors, the experiments were conducted with antibodies digested with pepsin to cleave the Fc region from the immunoglobulin, leaving the F(ab')$_2$ fragment *(102)*. To quantify the number of platelet GPIIb/IIIa receptors blocked, we developed an assay using radiolabeled 7E3 *(102)*.

In vivo dose-response experiments with 7E3-F(ab')$_2$ demonstrated that ADP-induced aggregation was not inhibited or minimally inhibited at ≤50% receptor blockade, was partially inhibited by 50–80% receptor blockade, and was essentially eliminated at >80% receptor blockade *(102,103)*. A dose of 7E3-F(ab')$_2$ that just achieves 80% receptor blockade will completely abolish platelet aggregation but will only produce a modest effect on the bleeding time *(103)*. Thus, abolition of platelet aggregation cannot be equated with near 100% receptor blockade, because 80% receptor blockade will achieve this endpoint.

In the dog model developed by Dr. John Folts, a partially occluded and damaged coronary artery undergoes cyclical flow reduction as platelets deposit on the blood vessel wall, aggregate into large platelet thrombi, and then abruptly embolize distally *(11,12)*. Since the thrombi are not occlusive, this model may simulate the events that occur in humans with unstable angina or after PCI. Early studies by Dr. Folts demonstrated that aspirin could preserve patency of the vessel and prevent the cycles, but cycles were restored by epinephrine infusion or increasing the stenosis *(11,104)*. Dr. Willerson and his colleagues *(105,106)* used this same model to define the roles of serotonin, thromboxane A$_2$, and thrombin in platelet thrombus formation. Most importantly, Anderson et al. *(107,108)* demonstrated that a similar phenomenon occurs in some patients after coronary angioplasty, providing support for the relevance of the model for PCI.

7E3-F(ab')$_2$ was the most potent antiplatelet agent Dr. Folts tested in this model, preventing platelet-mediated cyclical flow reductions despite a number of potent prothrombotic provocations, including infusing epinephrine, increasing the vascular stenosis, increasing the vascular damage, and even passing electric current through the cylinder used to create the vascular stenosis *(102,109)*. Similar results were obtained when the model was conducted on the carotid artery of nonhuman primates *(103)*. Dose-response studies demonstrated that the antithrombotic effect could be achieved with approx 60–80% GPIIb/IIIa receptor blockade, which produced only modest effects on the bleeding time *(102,103)*. Later studies by Anderson et al. *(107,108)* demonstrated that derivatives of 7E3 could abolish the cyclical flow reductions that occurred in some patients after coronary artery balloon angioplasty.

Dr. Chip Gold and his colleagues *(14)* had developed a dog model of reocclusion after thrombolysis by producing a severe fixed stenosis of a coronary artery, placing a whole blood thrombus adjacent to the constriction, and then administering tissue plasminogen activation (t-PA) in varying doses and regimens. The coronary arteries of most animals were reperfused by the t-PA, but reocclusion reoccurred nearly always, usually within minutes, and sometimes the reocclusion was followed by cyclical flow reductions similar to those observed in the Folts model *(14)*. Aspirin had only a minimal effect in this model. Pretreating dogs with 7E3-F(ab')$_2$ shortened the time required to achieve reperfusion and completely protected the dogs from reocclusion, even when the dose of t-PA was reduced by as much as 75% *(14,102,110,111)*. In a variation of this model designed to elicit platelet-rich thrombi, t-PA alone did not produce reperfusion, whereas t-PA + 7E3-F(ab')$_2$ was able to achieve reperfusion *(112)*. A minority of animals in Dr. Gold's standard model achieved reperfusion with 7E3-F(ab')$_2$ treatment alone, something virtually never observed in the controls. Later studies by Dr. Gold and his colleagues *(113)* demonstrated similar results in a subset of patients with acute myocardial infarction treated with abciximab. These data were later confirmed in larger studies of myocardial infarction, in which abciximab treatment alone was associated with patency rates similar to those produced by streptokinase and much greater than those associated with aspirin and heparin *(114–116)*.

Independent animal studies conducted by other investigators using 7E3- F(ab')$_2$ produced very similar results in other animal models of thrombosis, including models that lasted as long as 5 d *(111,117–121)*.

Chimeric 7E3 Fab

To minimize the likelihood that humans treated with 7E3 would develop an immune response to the murine antibody, murine 7E3 *(48)* was redesigned as a half-murine, half-human chimeric Fab fragment using recombinant techniques *(122,123)*. The resulting c7E3 Fab (abciximab; ReoPro™) contains the heavy and light chain variable regions from the murine antibody attached to the constant regions of a human IgG$_1$ heavy chain and κ-chain, respectively. c7E3 Fab is prepared by papain digestion of the intact antibody *(123)*.

The antithrombotic effect of abciximab was tested in a primate carotid artery model in which damage was induced by electrolytic injury *(124)*. Abciximab treatment produced dose-response inhibition of thrombus formation; reduced the frequency, or abolished the development, of occlusive thrombi; prolonged the time to occlusion; and decreased thrombus weight. In a baboon femoral artery thrombosis model, abciximab facilitated t-PA-induced thrombolysis, much like murine 7E3-F(ab')$_2$ did in the comparable dog coronary artery model *(111,125)*.

Toxicology studies in nonhuman primates with abciximab, given either as a bolus or as a bolus + continuous infusion for up to 96 h, demonstrated that the drug produced transient mucocutaneous bleeding (gingival bleeding, epistaxis, and bruising) primarily related to sites of blood collection or restraints *(123)*. Similar results were obtained when abciximab was combined with aspirin, heparin, and either t-PA or streptokinase *(123)*.

Abciximab's Mechanisms of Action and Reactivity with αVβ3 and αMβ2

Although the predominant mechanism by which GPIIb/IIIa antagonists prevent ischemic damage is by inhibiting thrombus formation by interfering with platelet aggregation, other potential effects of GPIIb/IIIa receptor blockade may also be important. Since activated platelets can facilitate thrombin generation by releasing factor V(a), binding prothrombin, shedding procoagulant microparticles, and providing a highly efficient catalytic surface for the reactions involved in thrombin generation *(95,126)*, decreasing the number of platelets in a thrombus may decrease thrombin generation. Moreover, in vitro and ex vivo, blockade of GPIIb/IIIa receptors appears to decrease the ability of platelets to undergo the release reaction, shed microparticles, bind prothrombin, and support thrombin generation and fibrin formation in response to tissue factor stimulation and other provocations *(95,126–130)*. In several of these studies *(127–129)*, abciximab inhibited the initiation and/or propagation of thrombin generation more effectively than other GPIIb/IIIa antagonists, perhaps related in part to its ability to also inhibit $\alpha V\beta 3$ *(95)*, which has been demonstrated to bind prothrombin *(131)*, but it is not known whether this results in enhanced clinical efficacy.

Studies of the activated clotting time (ACT) in heparinized patients treated with abciximab and eptifibatide also support the ability of GPIIb/IIIa receptor blockade to decrease thrombin generation in response to contact activation since the ACTs of patients treated with these agents were longer than those of untreated patients *(132,133)*, and adding abciximab to heparin-treated blood prolonged the ACT *(134)*. Studies of in vivo markers of thrombin generation in patients undergoing treatment with GPIIb/IIIa antagonists have provided mixed results. Thus, patients undergoing PCI had lower levels of prothrombin $F_{1.2}$ and fibrinopeptide A when treated with abciximab or tirofiban *(135–137)*. Abciximab treatment did not, however, affect $F_{1.2}$ or thrombin-antithrombin complex levels in patients with acute coronary syndromes without ST segment elevation *(138)*. Only a minority of patients in this study had elevated baseline values, however, and very few patients underwent PCI *(138)*. Abciximab treatment was also unable to prevent increases in $F_{1.2}$ and thrombin-antithrombin complexes in patients treated with a combination of abciximab and reduced-dose alteplase, but there was no control group receiving alteplase alone with which to compare the levels of $F_{1.2}$ and thrombin-antithrombin *(139)*.

The enhanced thrombolysis observed with the combination of GPIIb/IIIa receptor blockade and a thrombolytic agent may be owing to a number of mechanisms, including the following:

1. Inhibition of clot retraction and alterations in fibrin structure *(140–144)*, thus facilitating the diffusion of thrombolytic agents into fibrin thrombi.
2. Inhibition of the release of fibrinolytic inhibitors from platelets, including plasminogen activator inhibitor-1 and α_2-plasmin inhibitor *(145,146)*.
3. Inhibition of factor XIIIa binding to platelets and local release of platelet factor XIII, thus preventing fibrin crosslinking and crosslinking of fibrinolytic inhibitors to fibrin *(147)*.
4. Inhibition of the generation of the thrombin-activatable fibrinolysis inhibitor (TAFI) owing to decreased thrombin generation *(146)*.
5. Inhibition of platelet thrombus formation induced by the platelet-activating activity of thrombolytic agents *(148–150)*, thus allowing the thrombolytic agents to act unopposed by increased deposition of platelets into the thrombus.

Clinical data from the GUSTO V study demonstrated that combination therapy with abciximab and reduced-dose alteplase reduced the rate of reinfarction and other early cardiac events, but did not improve mortality *(151)*.

GPIIb/IIIa receptor blockade may also decrease the release of agents from platelet granules *(95)* that have been implicated in producing intimal hyperplasia, one of the components of the restenosis process. These include platelet-derived growth factor (PDGF), ADP, and serotonin. Moreover, platelet deposition at the site of vascular injury, as judged by the development of cyclical flow reductions, correlates with the subsequent development of intimal hyperplasia in animal models, and antiplatelet therapy can ameliorate the effect *(152)*. However, clinical data on the effect of GPIIb/IIIa antagonists on restenosis, as judged by target vessel revascularization, have been inconsistent (*see* below) (reviewed in refs. *153* and *154*).

Antibody 7E3 and abciximab also react with an activated form of the $\alpha M\beta 2$ receptor found on leukocytes *(155,156)*. Although this receptor plays an important role in leukocyte biology, it is uncertain whether any of abciximab's effect are caused by inhibition of $\alpha M\beta 2$. In human studies, abciximab has been shown to prevent the upregulation of leukocyte $\alpha M\beta 2$ after PCI *(100)*, but this is likely to be the result of preventing large platelet aggregates from binding to leukocytes or inhibiting the release of leukocyte activating agents from platelets rather than a direct effect on $\alpha M\beta 2$ *(99,101)*. Thus, although abciximab reduces monocyte-platelet aggregates in patients undergoing PCI with stenting *(99,101)*, both eptifibatide and tirofiban also produce comparable effects *(157,158)*. Abciximab treatment of patients undergoing PCI also reduces the increases in serum C-reactive protein, IL-6, and tumor necrosis factor-α observed between 24 and 48 h after the procedure, indicating an antiinflammatory effect *(159)*. A reduction in C-reactive protein has also been observed with tirofiban in patients presenting with acute coronary syndromes, however, suggesting that the antiinflammatory effects of these agents may be related to their antiaggregatory effect.

Abciximab reacts not only with GPIIb/IIIa but also with the $\alpha V\beta 3$ receptor *(56,102,160, 161)*; it is unclear, however, whether any of abciximab's clinical effects are caused by this reactivity. There are only a very few $\alpha V\beta 3$ receptors on platelets *(56)*, but they appear to contribute to enhancement of the catalytic efficiency of activated platelets in thrombin generation *(95)*, and activated $\alpha V\beta 3$ receptors appear to uniquely support binding of platelets to osteopontin *(74,75)*. $\alpha V\beta 3$ is present on many different cell types, including endothelial cells, smooth muscle cells, and osteoclasts, and it has been implicated in many different biologic processes, including bone resorption and tumor angiogenesis *(57,162, 163)*. Inhibiting $\alpha V\beta 3$ produces apoptosis of cells that require $\alpha V\beta 3$ for adhesion, most likely as a result of a decrease in the production of "survival" signals from the cytoplasmic protein complexes that are created at focal adhesions where integrin receptors localize and cluster *(57,164,165)*. Thus, it is possible that $\alpha V\beta 3$ blockade can decrease smooth muscle cell proliferation or migration, processes that may be important in intimal hyperplasia. In fact, several animal studies in which $\alpha V\beta 3$ was inhibited with peptides or antibodies support this possibility *(166–172)*, but mice lacking both GPIIb/IIIa and $\alpha V\beta 3$ owing to gene targeting of the GPIIIa ($\beta 3$) subunit are not protected from developing intimal hyperplasia after vascular injury *(173)*.

Although the EPIC study suggested an effect of abciximab treatment on clinical restenosis, no such effect was observed in subsequent studies, including EPILOG, CAPTURE, or ERASER *(153,154,174,175)*. It may be, however, that the duration of abciximab treatment in these studies (12–24 h) was inadequate to truly test the role of $\alpha V\beta 3$ in restenosis since animal data indicate that $\alpha V\beta 3$ upregulation after vascular injury persists for several weeks *(169)*. In the most recently reported study, EPISTENT, there was a >50% reduction in target vessel revascularization in diabetic patients at 6 mo (8.1% vs 16.6%) but no reduction in the nondiabetic population *(176)*. This raises the possibility that restenosis is more dependent on platelet deposition in diabetic patients than in nondiabetics.

GPIIb/IIIa receptor blockade may also decrease damage to the microcirculation distal to the site of vascular injury secondary to embolization of platelet aggregates and platelet-leukocyte aggregates, as well as discharge of thrombin and other vasoactive and proinflammatory agents from platelets and leukocytes *(96,177)*. Several clinical observations support the hypothesis that abciximab treatment may protect the microcirculation, including improved peak blood flow and myocardial contractility 2 wk after stent placement in patients with myocardial infarction *(178)*, more rapid ST-segment resolution after thrombolytic therapy for myocardial infarction *(179)*, and reduction of myocardial perfusion abnormalities after rotational atherectomy *(180)*. Protecting the distal microcirculation might also contribute to the long-term mortality advantage observed with abciximab *(181,182)* if microcirculatory damage ultimately results in fibrosis, electrical instability, and increased risk of sudden death.

PHARMACOKINETICS
OF APPROVED GPIIb/IIIa ANTAGONISTS

The theoretical considerations that led to the current strategy for the dose and duration of therapy for GPIIb/IIIa antagonists are (1) the need for sufficiently high-grade receptor blockade to prevent platelet thrombus formation despite extraordinary provocation, as may exist after vascular injury in the presence of a low flow state; and (2) the need for the high-grade receptor blockade to persist until the blood vessel returns to a state of low platelet reactivity ("passivation"). Animal data in the Gold model *(110)* and a few anecdotal observations *(183)* suggested that ≥80% receptor blockade would be required. Data from patients in the EPIC study who received only a bolus dose of abciximab (instead of a bolus + 12 h infusion) provided additional convincing clinical support for the need for high-grade receptor blockade because as soon as the level of receptor blockade in these patients dropped below approx 80%, there was a marked increase in the onset of new ischemic events *(184)*.

The duration of therapy depends on the passivation process, about which little is known. In animal models of vascular injury of normal blood vessels, it appears to take approx 6–8 h *(185,186)*. Analysis of the time to repeat urgent PCI in the control group in EPIC, however, indicates that the period of high risk after PCI of human vascular lesions is approx 2 d and that a period of lower, but still substantial risk extends from d 2 to 8 *(187)*. Thus, whereas considerable passivation of sites of vascular injury after PCI probably occurs in the first few days, more complete passivation probably takes more than a week. It is possible, however, that subclinical platelet deposition and embolization persists for a longer period. Little is known about the passivation process after stent placement, but with current antiplatelet regimens, clinically significant acute reocclusion is rare. Subclinical platelet deposition and embolization is likely, however, given that abciximab treatment improves microcirculatory function after stenting in patients with myocardial infarction *(178)*.

Abciximab (c7E3 Fab: ReoPro™)

Murine 7E3 and abciximab bind with high affinity to human platelet GPIIb/IIIa (nanomolar K_D) *(48,52,161,188,189)*. Murine 7E3 binds more rapidly to activated than unactivated platelets, probably because activation results in freer access to its binding site *(188)*. Smaller fragments of murine 7E3 [F(ab')$_2$ and Fab'] show less of a differential in initial binding rates to activated vs unactivated platelets, presumably reflecting easier access to the binding site owing to their smaller sizes *(188,189)*. The dissociation (off) rate of abciximab from platelet GPIIb/IIIa was estimated as approx 40–45 min in one study *(189)*, but in two other studies it required approx 120 and approx 180 min to displace 50% of a subsaturating concentration of radiolabeled abciximab from the surface of GPIIb/IIIa-containing HEL cells and platelets, respectively *(52)*. Platelets are able to internalize at least some 7E3 after it binds to the surface *(190)*, an observation consistent with data demonstrating that GPIIb/IIIa receptors cycle from the plasma membrane to α-granule membranes and back *(54)*; the significance of this internalization is unknown.

The precise epitope on GPIIb/IIIa that 7E3 binds to is unknown, but studies in which regions from murine GPIIIa were "swapped" for regions in human GPIIIa have identified two regions that appear either to affect the 7E3 epitope or to actually make up part of the epitope *(191,192)*. The crystal structure reported for the external segment of αVβ3 indicates that these regions are close to each other on the surface of GPIIIa, in close proximity to the RGD bind-ing region *(78,79)*.

After bolus administration of abciximab at the recommended dose of 0.25 mg/kg, approximately 65% of the injected antibody becomes attached within minutes to the GPIIb/IIIa receptors on the platelets in the peripheral circulation and spleen *(123,193)*. In unpublished animal toxicology studies *(194)*, abciximab was also found on bone marrow megakaryocytes. Bone marrow examination of a human patient who developed thrombocytopenia after abciximab treatment also identified abciximab on mature megakaryocytes *(195)*. In most patients, the initial bolus achieves ≥80% GPIIb/IIIa receptor blockade, ≥80% inhibition of ADP-induced platelet aggregation, and marked prolongation of the bleeding time *(123,193,196–199)*. Since the total number of molecules of abciximab that are injected exceeds the number of GPIIb/IIIa receptors normally present by a factor of only 1.5–2.0 *(123)*, the standard dose may not achieve ≥80% receptor blockade in patients with either severe thrombocytosis *(200–202)* or marked splenomegaly with splenic pooling of platelets. The free plasma concentration of abciximab drops very rapidly after injection of a bolus dose or when an infusion is terminated, with an initial half-life of approx 30 min *(123, 193)*. Within an hour or so the level is below the K_D of the antibody. The platelet-inhibiting effects of the bolus injection of abciximab can be sustained by administering a continuous infusion of 10 µg/min or 0.125 µg/kg/min *(123,193,198)*. This produces steady-state levels of approx 100–200 ng/mL (1.9–3.8 nM) *(203)*.

In a study comparing abciximab clearance and inhibition of platelet aggregation in normal controls on aspirin versus patients undergoing elective PCI on aspirin and heparin, it was found that higher concentrations of abciximab were required in the patients than in the normal controls to achieve the same degree of GPIIb/IIIa receptor blockade and inhibition of ADP-induced platelet aggregation *(204)*. The authors estimated the therapeutic plasma range as 100–175 ng/mL. The normal controls in this studies were also studied after discontinuing the abciximab infusion for variable periods of time to assess how much additional abciximab was needed to restore >80% inhibition of platelet aggregation. After 12 h, approx 0.05 mg/kg was required, after 24 h approx 0.1 mg/kg, and after 48 h approx 0.15 mg/kg *(205)*. Very little abciximab can be detected in the urine, making it most likely that its major catabolic route involves digestion by the cells that remove platelets from the circulation *(194)*.

Currently the indicated duration of abciximab treatment is 12 h when the bolus dose is given immediately before PCI *(184,206,207)*. Bleeding time returns to normal within 12 h after the end of the infusion in most patients *(193)*. Platelet aggregation in response to ADP (20 µM) returns to ≥50% of baseline within 1 d in most patients and within 2 d in virtually all patients (Fig. 1). Platelet aggregation in response to a thrombin receptor-activating peptide is less inhibited by bolus abciximab treatment than is platelet aggregation induced by

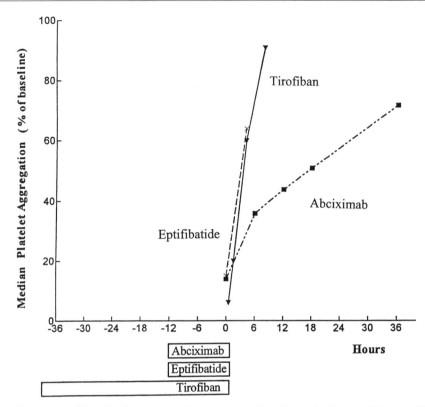

Fig. 1. Recovery of the platelet aggregation response after discontinuing tirofiban, eptifibatide, and abciximab. Aggregation was initiated by 20 μm ADP for the eptifibatide and abciximab studies, and 5 μm ADP for the tirofiban study. Tirofiban was given as a 10 μg/kg bolus + 0.15 μg/kg infusion for 36 h, eptifibatide was given as a 135 μg/kg bolus + 0.5 μg/kg/min infusion for 12 h, and abciximab was given as a 0.25 mg/kg bolus + 10 μg/min for 12 h. Data compiled by Dr. Robert Jordan (Centocor, Malvern, PA).

ADP, most likely because activation of the thrombin receptor induces the release reaction and recruits internal GPIIb/IIIa receptors to the platelet surface *(208)*.

Abciximab can be detected at low levels on the platelets of patients for as long as 14 or more days after the infusion is ended, most likely reflecting the ability of abciximab to redistribute from one platelet to another within minutes to hours *(123,196,197,199,203)*. Thus abciximab binding to platelets is reversible *(123,197,199)*. Platelet transfusions can rapidly reverse the platelet inhibition produced by abciximab in non-human primates and presumably in humans as well *(203,209)*, probably partly because of the ability of the newly transfused platelets to function in hemostasis before they have accumulated a significant amount of abciximab on their surface. Ultimately, however, when abciximab redistribution is complete, the transfer of abciximab from the heavily coated to uncoated platelets results in a decrease in the average GPIIb/IIIa receptor blockade. Decreasing the average blockade to <50% results in considerable return of platelet function.

Combining abciximab with reteplase and/or ticlopidine does not affect the pharmacodynamics of abciximab *(199)*. Pretreating human platelets ex vivo or non-human primate platelets in vivo with tirofiban or eptifibatide does not alter the subsequent binding of abciximab to platelets *(210)*. A pharmacodynamic study of patients with acute coronary syndromes treated with tirofiban or eptifibatide infusions prior to treatment with abciximab at the time of PCI demonstrated that the bolus dose of abciximab caused a further decrease in one or more indices of platelet function, and the platelet inhibition achieved by combination therapy was always equal to, or greater than, that achieved with abciximab alone *(211)*. It is unclear, however, whether abciximab can bind to a GPIIb/IIIa receptor simultaneously with tirofiban and/or eptifibatide, and indirect studies using monoclonal antibodies *(212)* raise the possibility that abciximab binding may actually decrease the binding of the other drugs *(211)*.

In vitro studies using the rapid platelet function assay (*see* Chapter 13) *(213)* to monitor GPIIb/IIIa-dependent platelet function have demonstrated that although most patients achieve ≥80% inhibition of platelet function with the standard bolus dose of abciximab, there is considerable interindividual variability, which increases during the infusion period *(157,214–220)*. In the GOLD study *(214)*, patients undergoing PCI who had the lowest levels of platelet inhibition at 5 min and 8 h after the bolus dose of abciximab had significantly higher rates of major adverse cardiac events (MACE). (At 10 min: <95% inhibition [$n = 125$], 14.4% MACE vs ≥95% inhibition [$n = 344$], 6.4% MACE [$p = 0.006$]; at 8 h: <70% inhibition [$n = 28$], 25% MACE vs ≥70% inhibition [$n = 407$], 8.1% MACE [$p = 0.009$].) This result should be interpreted with caution, however, as the thresholds were established post hoc. Furthermore, although the numbers of patients with <85% inhibition at 10 min in this study were low, patients with 85–95% inhibition at 10 min actually had higher event rates than those with <85% inhibition. Still unknown, however, is whether adjusting the doses in the patients obtaining lesser degrees of platelet function inhibition will result in improved outcomes. Other tests of platelet function have been used to assess the extent of platelet inhibition produced by abciximab, but the data have not been correlated with clinical outcomes *(221)*.

Limited data are available concerning the use of abciximab in patients with renal insufficiency. Pooled data on 39 patients with serum creatinine >2 mg/dL who received abciximab in the EPIC, CAPTURE, EPILOG, and EPISTENT studies did not demonstrate increased bleeding complications *(222)*.

Tirofiban (MK-383; Aggrastat™)

Tirofiban is a nonpeptide derivative of tyrosine (L-tyrosine, *N*-(butlysulfonyl)-*O*-[4 (4-peperidinylbutyl], monohydrochloride) that is highly selective for GPIIb/IIIa compared with αVβ3 *(223–226)*. It inhibits platelet aggregation of gel-filtered platelets induced by ADP (10 μ*M*) with an IC$_{50}$ of 9 n*M*. Infusion of tirofiban at 10 μg/min into dogs produced nearly complete inhibition of ADP-induced platelet aggregation; aggregation returned to approx 70% of normal within 30 min of ending the infusion *(224)*.

In vitro studies demonstrated that 64% of tirofiban is bound to plasma proteins and neither liver microsomes nor liver slices metabolized tirofiban *(227)*. Both renal and biliary excretion contribute to tirofiban clearance, with unchanged tirofiban found in urine and feces *(227,228)*.

In humans, 0.15 μg/kg/min of tirofiban for 4 h produced a 2.5 ± 1.1-fold increase in bleeding time and 97 ± 5% inhibition of ADP (3.4 μ*M*)-induced platelet aggregation *(229, 230)*. Plasma clearance was 329 mL/min, and plasma half-life was 1.6 h. Four hours after stopping tirofiban, the bleeding time returned to normal, and platelet aggregation returned to approx 80% of the pretreatment value (Fig. 1). Aspirin coadministration resulted in enhanced bleeding time prolongation (4.1 ± 1.5-fold increase), which was not owing to an effect on tirofiban plasma levels. The plasma concentration of tirofiban needed to inhibit platelet aggregation by 50% decreased from approx 12 to approx 9 ng/mL when patients also received aspirin. Peak plasma concentration with the 0.15 µg/kg/min infusion was approx 40 ng/mL, and 6 h after stopping the therapy, plasma levels were <3 ng/mL.

A pilot dose-ranging study conducted in patients undergoing coronary artery angioplasty who were simultaneously treated with aspirin and heparin demonstrated that (1) ADP (5 µM)-induced platelet aggregation was inhibited by ≥93% within 5 min of administering a 10 µg/kg bolus dose; (2) bleeding time at 2 h was >30 min when a 10 µg/kg bolus was followed by either a 0.1 or 0.15 µg/kg/min infusion; (3) at the end of the infusions (16–24 h), platelet aggregation was inhibited by 87 and 95%, respectively; and (4) after terminating the infusions, platelet aggregation began to return toward normal in 1.5 h, and by 4 h platelet aggregation was >50% of normal (231).

Studies using the rapid platelet function assay to monitor the response to tirofiban in patients with unstable angina undergoing angioplasty found that at doses of 0.4 µg/kg/min for 30 min, followed by 0.1 µg/kg/min for 20–24 h, there was less inhibition of platelet function than with eptifibatide (180 µ/kg bolus + 2.0 µg/kg/min infusion) or abciximab (0.25 µg/kg bolus + 0.125 µg/kg/min infusion) (219). When tirofiban was given as a 10 µg/kg bolus followed by a 0.1 µg/kg infusion, inhibition of platelet function by tirofiban as measured by the rapid platelet function assay was similar to that produced by abciximab and eptifibatide, but inhibition of platelet function measured by light transmission aggregometry was significantly less (218). In the GOLD study, as with abciximab, there was a trend toward an association between lower levels of platelet function inhibition measured by the rapid platelet function assay and the risk of MACE, but only a small number of patients was studied (214). In the COMPARE study the effects of two doses of tirofiban (0.4 µg/kg/min × 30 min, 0.1 µg/kg/min thereafter, and 10 µg/kg bolus followed by 0.15 µg/kg/min infusion) were evaluated by light transmission aggregometry at 15 min, 30 min, 4 h, and 12 h. Tirofiban achieved less inhibition at the early time points than abciximab or single bolus eptifibatide. At late time points, however, tirofiban achieved high levels of inhibition, comparable to those of eptifibatide, and greater than those of abciximab.

The plasma clearance of tirofiban is reduced in patients with renal insufficiency (creatinine clearance <30 mL/min), and the plasma half-life increases more than threefold (222). The manufacturer recommends 50% dosage reduction in both bolus and infusion doses, but the pharmacokinetic and pharmacodynamic bases for this recommendation have been challenged (222).

In the PRISM-PLUS trial, which studied patients with non-ST-segment elevation acute coronary syndromes, there were 40 patients with creatinine clearance <30 mL/min (232). These patients had more severe coronary artery disease and increased risk of developing ischemic complications. Tirofiban therapy was associated with decreased adverse ischemic outcomes at 48 h and 7 d, but not at 30 d or 6 mo (232). Reduced creatinine clearance was associated with increased risk of bleeding, and tirofiban treatment further increased the risk.

Eptifibatide (Integrilin™)

Eptifibatide is a synthetic disulfide-linked cyclic heptapeptide patterned after the KGD sequence found in the snake venom disintegrin from Sistrurus m. barbouri (233). Based on studies with purified αVβ3, it was originally characterized as being highly specific for

GPIIb/IIIa inhibition compared with $\alpha V\beta 3$ inhibition *(233)*. However, more recent studies indicate that eptifibatide can inhibit $\alpha V\beta 3$-mediated adhesion of human aortic smooth muscle cells and human umbilical vein endothelial cells to $\alpha V\beta 3$ ligands *(225)*.

Early animal studies suggested that eptifibatide produced less prolongation of the bleeding time than other GPIIb/IIIa inhibitors at doses producing comparable inhibition of platelet aggregation. However, it was later discovered that eptifibatide's inhibition of platelet aggregation is significantly augmented when blood is anticoagulated with citrate, the anticoagulant used in the animal studies *(234)*. Thus, the extent of platelet aggregation inhibition was overestimated in those early studies. When the citrate effect is considered, administration of eptifibatide and other GPIIb/IIIa antagonists at doses that produce comparable inhibition of platelet aggregation probably results in comparable levels of bleeding time prolongation.

^{14}C-eptifibatide was administered to eight healthy men as a single 135 µg/kg iv bolus. Peak plasma concentrations were 879 ± 251 ng/mL (mean ± SD) at 5 min, the distribution half-life was 5 ± 2.5 min, and the terminal elimination half-life was 1.1 ± 0.17 h *(235)*. Approximately 73% of administered radioactivity was recovered in 72 h, with renal clearance accounting for 98% of total recovered radioactivity, and approx 40% of total body clearance; unmodified eptifibatide, deamidated eptifibatide, and more polar metabolites were all found in the urine. Only trace amounts of radioactivity were found in the breath and feces.

Since renal clearance is an important component of eptifibatide catabolism, patients with renal impairment can have prolonged inhibition of platelet function after receiving eptifibatide. This is of particular concern in patients with end-stage renal failure since such patients have platelet dysfunction owing to their renal insufficiency. The proper dose of eptifibatide in patients with modest to moderate renal insufficiency (creatinine clearance 2–4 mg/dL) is uncertain *(222)*. Since the steady-state level of eptifibatide is approx 1900 ng/mL when using an infusion rate of 2 µg/kg/min *(236)*, the ratio of eptifibatide molecules to GPIIb/IIIa molecules is >50:1 *(237)*; thus, it is unlikely that platelet transfusions can reverse the effects of the drug, although in vitro data raise some hope in this regard *(238,238)*. As with abciximab, treatment with eptifibatide prolongs the activated clotting time of heparinized patients, suggesting an inhibitory effect on thrombin generation stimulated by contact activation *(132,239)*.

In a pilot study of 21 patients undergoing elective PCI who were also treated with aspirin and heparin (10,000 U bolus + additional doses to maintain activated clotting time at 300–500 s), a bolus dose of 90 µg/kg of eptifibatide, followed by a 1 µg/kg/min infusion for 4 or 12 h, resulted in a decrease in platelet aggregation response using citrated blood to ADP (20 µM) from approx 80% of a full-scale change before eptifibatide treatment to approx 15% at 1 h after the bolus dose and at the end of the infusion *(132)*. There was significant interindividual variability in response, with the 95% confidence limits extending from 0 to 30% and 0 to 40%, respectively, at the two time points. Four hours after stopping the infusion, the average aggregation response was approx 55%, but there was marked interindividual variation (95% confidence limits approx 10% to 90%). Bleeding times were prolonged from approx 6 min before treatment to approx 26 min after 1 h and at the end of the infusion. Bleeding times rapidly returned toward normal after stopping treatment, being approx 9–11 min 1 h after the infusion was stopped.

A subsequent study *(240)* tested four different bolus + 18–24 h infusion regimens in 54 patients undergoing PCI who were also treated with aspirin and heparin (180 µg/kg bolus + 1 µg/kg/min; 135 µg/kg + 0.5 µg/kg/min; 90 µg/kg + 0.75 µg/kg/min; 135 µg/kg + 0.75 µg/kg/min). The 180 µg/kg bolus dose produced high-grade inhibition of ADP-induced platelet aggregation using citrated blood, and this was consistently sustained by the 1 µg/kg/min infusion. There was some return toward normal platelet aggregation in patients treated with the regimens that included the 0.75 µg/kg/min infusion. After stopping treatment for 4 h, platelet aggregation returned to >50% of the pretreatment value (Fig. 1). Bleeding time prolongation was found with all regimens (median values of 22, 12, 12, and 17 min, respectively, compared with control of 7–8 min), and 1 h after stopping the infusion, there was a return toward the control values (9, 10, 9, and 11 min, respectively).

After the citrate effect was discovered, the dose of eptifibatide was increased, and blood was anticoagulated with the direct thrombin inhibitor D-Phe-Pro-Arg chloromethyl ketone (PPACK), which does not chelate calcium *(237)*. Several studies evaluated combinations of different single bolus doses (µg/kg) followed by different infusion doses (µg/kg/min) (135/0.75, 180/2.0, 250/3.0) in patients with acute coronary syndromes *(241)* and during PCI *(219,237,242)*. Although high-level inhibition of ADP-induced aggregation could be achieved soon after the bolus dose, there was an early loss of inhibition of platelet aggregation before steady state was achieved. As a result, regimens employing a second bolus dose 30 min after the first were studied (180/2.0 + second bolus of 90; 250/2.0 + second bolus of 125) *(236)*. From these studies, pharmacokinetic modeling predicted that optimal dosing would involve a bolus dose of 180 µg/kg/min and second bolus dose of 180 µg/kg at 10 min *(236)*. This is the dose used in the ESPRIT trial *(243)*.

Studies of patients with unstable angina undergoing PCI monitored with the rapid platelet function assay and light transmission aggregometry using blood collected into PPACK demonstrated that a bolus dose of 180 µg/kg followed by an infusion of 2.0 µg/kg/min produced more complete and more sustained inhibition of platelet function than abciximab (0.25 mg/kg bolus + 0.125 µg/kg/min infusion) *(219)*. In another, similar study, however, platelet inhibition produced 5 min after the bolus doses by abciximab was greater than that produced by eptifibatide *(218)*. In the GOLD study, among the patients undergoing PCI who were treated with eptifibatide, those with the lowest levels of inhibition of platelet function had the greatest risk of developing MACE. Although only a small number of patients was treated with eptifibatide in this study, the data lend further support to the concept that the extent of platelet function inhibition is an important factor in the efficacy of these agents.

ACKNOWLEDGMENTS

I wish to thank Dr. Robert Jordan for sharing unpublished abciximab data, Drs. Robert Jordan, Marian Nakada, David Phillips, and Robert Gould for reviewing the manuscript and making valuable suggestions, and Suzanne Rivera for outstanding secretarial support. This work was supported in part by grants 19278 and 54469 from the National Heart, Lung, and Blood Institute. Dr. Coller is an inventor of abciximab, and, in compliance with Federal law and the policies of the Research Foundation of the State of University of New York, he has a financial interest in royalties paid to the Foundation for sales of abciximab. Dr. Coller is also an inventor of the rapid platelet function assay (RPFA), and, in compliance with Federal law and the policies of Mount Sinai School of Medicine, he has a financial interest in royalties paid to Mount Sinai for sales of the assay.

REFERENCES

1. Friedberg CK. Diseases of the Heart. WB Saunders, Philadelphia, 1966, pp. 781–785.
2. Roberts WC, Ferrans VJ. The role of thrombosis in the etiology of atherosclerosis (a positive one) and in precipitating fatal ischemic heart disease (a negative one). Semin Thromb Hemost 1976;2:123–135.
3. Maseri A, L'Abbate A, Baroldi G, et al. Coronary vasospasm as a possible cause of myocardial infarction. A conclusion derived from the study of "preinfarction" angina. N Engl J Med 1978;299:1271–1277.
4. DeWood MA, Spores J, Hensley GR, et al. Coronary arteriographic findings in acute transmural myocardial infarction. Circulation 1983;68:I39–I49.
5. Effectiveness of intravenous thrombolytic treatment in acute myocardial infarction. Gruppo Italiano per lo Studio della Streptochinasi nell'Infarto Miocardico (GISSI). Lancet 1986;1:397–402.
6. ISIS-2. (Second International Study of Infarct Survival) Collaborative Group. Randomised trial of intravenous streptokinase, oral aspirin, both, or neither among 17,187 cases of suspected acute myocardial infarction: ISIS-2. Lancet 1988;2:349–360.
7. Markwardt F. The development of hirudin as an antithrombotic drug. Thromb Res 1994;74:1–23.
8. Davies MJ, Thomas A. Thrombosis and acute coronary-artery lesions in sudden cardiac ischemic death. N Engl J Med 1984;310:1147–1140.
9. Falk E. Unstable angina with fatal outcome: dynamic coronary thrombosis leading to infarction and/or sudden death. Circulation 1985;71:699–708.
10. Fitzgerald DJ, Roy L, Catella F, FitzGerald GA. Platelet activation in unstable coronary disease. N Engl J Med 1986;315:983–989.
11. Folts JD, Crowell EB Jr, Rowe GG. Platelet aggregation in partially obstructed vessels and its elimination with aspirin. Circulation 1976;54:365–370.
12. Folts JD, Gallagher K, Rowe GG. Blood flow reductions in stenosed canine coronary arteries: vasospasm or platelet aggregation? Circulation 1982;65:248–255.
13. Ashton JH, Schmitz JM, Campbell NB, et al. Inhibition of cyclic flow variations in stenosed canine coronary arteries by thromboxane A2/prostaglandin H2 receptor antagonists. Circ Res 1986;59:568–578.
14. Yasuda T, Gold HK, Fallon JT, et al. A monoclonal antibody against the platelet GPIIb/IIIa receptor prevents coronary artery reocclusion following reperfusion with recombinant tissue-type plasminogen activator in dogs. J Clin Invest 1988;81:1284–1291.
15. Collins R, Peto R, Baigent C, Sleight P. Aspirin, heparin, and fibrinolytic therapy in suspected acute myocardial infarction. N Engl J Med 1997;336:847–860.
16. Hirsh J, Dalen JE, Fuster V, Harker LB, Patrono C, Roth G. Aspirin and other platelet-active drugs. The relationship among dose, effectiveness, and side effects. Chest 1995;108:247S–257S.
17. Final report on the aspirin component of the ongoing Physicians' Health Study. Steering Committee of the Physicians' Health Study Research Group. N Engl J Med 1989;321:129–135.
18. Barnathan ES, Schwartz JS, Taylor L, et al. Aspirin and dipyridamole in the prevention of acute coronary thrombosis complicating coronary angioplasty. Circulation 1987;76:125–134.
19. Patrono C, Coller B, Dalen JE, et al. Platelet-active drugs: the relationships among dose, effectiveness, and side effects. Chest 2001;119:39S–63S.
20. Cairns JA, Theroux P, Lewis HD Jr, Ezekowitz M, Meade TW. Antithrombotic agents in coronary artery disease. Chest 2001;119:228S–252S.
21. Ambrose JA, Almeida OD, Sharma SK, et al. Adjunctive thrombolytic therapy during angioplasty for ischemic rest angina. Results of the TAUSA Trial. TAUSA Investigators. Thrombolysis and Angioplasty in Unstable Angina trial. Circulation 1994;90:69–77.
22. Effects of tissue plasminogen activator and a comparison of early invasive and conservative strategies in unstable angina and non-Q-wave myocardial infarction. Results of the TIMI IIIB Trial. Thrombolysis in Myocardial Ischemia. Circulation 1994;89:1545–1556.
23. Chen JL. Randomized clinical trial of urokinase versus heparin in unstable angina. J Thromb Thrombolysis 1999;8:223–226.
24. Hamm CW, Heeschen C, Goldmann B, et al. Benefit of abciximab in patients with refractory unstable angina in relation to serum troponin T levels. c7E3 Fab Antiplatelet Therapy in Unstable Refractory Angina (CAPTURE) Study Investigators. N Engl J Med 1999;340:1623–1629.
25. Early effects of tissue-type plasminogen activator added to conventional therapy on the culprit coronary lesion in patients presenting with ischemic cardiac pain at rest. Results of the Thrombolysis in Myocardial Ischemia (TIMI IIIA) Trial. Circulation 1993;87:38–52.

26. Caen JP, Castaldi PA, Leclerc JC, et al. Congenital bleeding disorders with long bleeding time and normal platelet count. I. Glanzmann's thrombasthenia. Am J Med 1966;41:4.

27. Coller BS, Seligsohn U, Peretz H, Newman PJ. Glanzmann thrombasthenia: new insights from an historical perspective. Semin Hematol 1994;31:301–311.

28. Nurden AT, Caen JP. An abnormal platelet glycoprotein pattern in three cases of Glanzmann's thrombasthenia. Br J Haematol 1974;28:253–260.

29. Phillips DR, Agin PP. Platelet membrane defects in Glanzmann's thrombasthenia. Evidence for decreased amounts of two major glycoproteins. J Clin Invest 1977;60:535–545.

30. Kunicki TJ, Pidard D, Rosa JP, Nurden AT. The formation of calcium-dependent complexes of platelet membrane glycoproteins IIb and IIIa in solution as determined by crossed immunoelectrophoresis. Blood 1981;58:268–278.

31. George JN, Caen JP, Nurden AT. Glanzmann's thrombasthenia: the spectrum of clinical disease. Blood 1990;75:1383–1395.

32. Seligsohn U. Personal communication, 2002.

33. Shpilberg O, Rabi I, Schiller K, et al. Patients with Glanzmann thrombasthenia lacking platelet glycoprotein αIIb/β3 (GPIIb/IIIa) and αVβ3 receptors are not protected from atherosclerosis. Circulation 2002;105:1044–1048.

34. Born GV, Hume M. Effects of the numbers and sizes of platelet aggregates on the optical density of plasma. Nature 1967;215:1027–1029.

35. Coller BS. A brief and highly descriptive history of ideas about platelets in health and disease. In: Michelson AD, ed. Platelets. Academic, New York, 2002.

36. Coller BS. Platelet aggregation by ADP, collagen and ristocetin: a critical review of methodology and analysis. In: Schmidt RM, ed. CRC Handbook Series in Clinical Laboratory Science, Section 1: Hematology. CRC, Boca Raton, FL, 1979, pp. 381–396.

37. Ware AJ, Coller BS. Platelet morphology, biochemistry and function. In: Beutler E, Lichtman MA, Coller BS, Kipps TJ, eds. Williams Hematology. McGraw-Hill, New York, 1995, pp. 1161–1201.

38. Weiss HJ, Aledort LM, Kochwa S. The effect of salicylates on the hemostatic properties of platelets in man. J Clin Invest 1968;47:2169–2180.

39. Zucker MB, Peterson J. Inhibition of adenosine diphosphate-induced secondary aggregation and other platelet functions by acetylsalicylic acid ingestion. Proc Soc Exp Biol Med 1968;127:547–551.

40. Needleman P, Minkes M, Raz A. Thromboxanes: selective biosynthesis and distinct biological properties. Science 1976;193:163–165.

41. Samuelsson B. Prostaglandin endoperoxides and thromboxanes: role in platelets and in vascular and respiratory smooth muscle. Acta Biol Med Ger 1976;35:1055–1063.

42. Mustard JF, Kinlough-Rathbone RL, Packham MA, Perry DW, Harfenist EJ, Pai KR. Comparison of fibrinogen association with normal and thrombasthenic platelets on exposure to ADP or chymotrypsin. Blood 1979;54:987–993.

43. Bennett JS, Vilaire G. Exposure of platelet fibrinogen receptors by ADP and epinephrine. J Clin Invest 1979;64:1393–1401.

44. Kornecki E, Niewiarowski S, Morinelli TA, Kloczewiak M. Effects of chymotrypsin and adenosine diphosphate on the exposure of fibrinogen receptors on normal human and Glanzmann's thrombasthenic platelets. J Biol Chem 1981;256:5696–5701.

45. Coller BS. Interaction of normal, thrombasthenic, and Bernard-Soulier platelets with immobilized fibrinogen: defective platelet-fibrinogen interaction in thrombasthenia. Blood 1980;55:169–178.

46. Nachman RL, Leung LL. Complex formation of platelet membrane glycoproteins IIb and IIIa with fibrinogen. J Clin Invest 1982;69:263–269.

47. Coller BS, Peerschke EI, Scudder LE, Sullivan CA. A murine monoclonal antibody that completely blocks the binding of fibrinogen to platelets produces a thrombasthenic-like state in normal platelets and binds to glycoproteins IIb and/or IIIa. J Clin Invest 1983;72:325–338.

48. Coller BS. A new murine monoclonal antibody reports an activation-dependent change in the conformation and/or microenvironment of the platelet GPIIb/IIIa complex. J Clin Invest 1985;76:101–108.

49. Hynes RO. Integrins: a family of cell surface receptors. Cell 1987;48:549–554.

50. Phillips DR, Charo IF, Parise LV, Fitzgerald LA. The platelet membrane glycoprotein IIb-IIIa complex. Blood 1988;71:831–843.

51. Plow EF, D'Souza SE, Ginsberg MH. Ligand binding to GPIIb-IIIa: a status report. Semin Thromb Hemost 1992;18:324–332.

52. Wagner CL, Mascelli MA, Neblock DS, Weisman HF, Coller BS, Jordan RE. Analysis of GPIIb/IIIa receptor number by quantification of 7E3 binding to human platelets. Blood 1996;88:907–914.
53. Niiya K, Hodson E, Bader R, et al. Increased surface expression of the membrane glycoprotein IIb/IIIa complex induced by platelet activation. Relationship to the binding of fibrinogen and platelet aggregation. Blood 1987;70:475–483.
54. Wencel-Drake JD. Plasma membrane GPIIb/IIIa. Evidence for a cycling receptor pool. Am J Clin Pathol 1990;136:61–70.
55. Cheresh DA, Spiro RC. Biosynthetic and functional properties of an Arg-Gly-Asp-directed receptor involved in human melanoma cell attachment to vitronectin, fibrinogen, and von Willebrand factor. J Biol Chem 1987;262:17,703–17,711.
56. Coller BS, Cheresh DA, Asch E, Seligsohn U. Platelet vitronectin receptor expression differentiates Iraqi-Jewish from Arab patients with Glanzmann thrombasthenia in Israel. Blood 1991;77:75–83.
57. Varner JA, Cheresh DA. Integrins and cancer. Curr Opin Cell Biol 1996;8:724–730.
58. Felding-Habermann B, Cheresh DA. Vitronectin and its receptors. Curr Opin Cell Biol 1993;5:864–868.
59. Byzova TV, Rabbani R, D'Souza SE, Plow EF. Role of integrin alpha (v)beta3 in vascular biology. Thromb Haemost 1998;80:726–734.
60. Pierschbacher MD, Ruoslahti E. Cell attachement activity of fibronectin can be duplicated by small synthetic fragments of the molecule. Nature 1984;309:30–33.
61. Pierschbacher MD, Ruoslahti E. Influence of sterochemistry of the sequence Arg-Gly-Asp-Xaa on binding specificity in cell adhesion. J Biol Chem 1987;262:17,294–17,298.
62. Plow EF, McEver RP, Coller BS, Marguerie GA, Ginsburg MH. Related binding mechanisms for fibrinogen, fibronectin, von Willebrand factor and thrombospondin on thrombin-stimulated human platelets. Blood 1985;66:724–727.
63. Ruoslahti E. RGD and other recognition sequences for integrins. Annu Rev Cell Dev Biol 1996;12:697–715.
64. Plow EF, Pierschbacher MD, Ruoslahti E, Marguerie GA, Ginsberg MH. The effect of Arg-Gly-Asp-containing peptides on fibrinogen and von Willebrand factor binding to platelets. Proc Natl Acad Sci USA 1985;82:8057–8061.
65. Haverstick DM, Cowan JF, Yamada KM, Santoro SA. Inhibition of platelet adhesion to fibronectin, fibrinogen, and von Willebrand factor substrates by a synthetic tetrapeptide derived from the cell-binding domain of fibronectin. Blood 1985;66:946–952.
66. Farrell DH, Thiagarajan P. Binding of recombinant fibrinogen mutants to platelets. J Biol Chem 1994;269:226–231.
67. Zaidi T, McIntire LV, Farrell DH, Thiagarajan P. Adhesion of platelets to surface-bound fibrinogen under flow. Blood 1996;88:2967–2972.
68. Kloczewiak M, Timmons S, Bednarek MA, Sakon M, Hawiger J. Platelet receptor recognition domain on the gamma chain of human fibrinogen and its synthetic peptide analogues. Biochemistry 1989;28:2915–2919.
69. Kloczewiak M, Timmons S, Lukas TJ, Hawiger J. Platelet recognition site on human fibrinogen: synthesis and structure-function relationship of peptides corresponding to the carboxy-terminal segment of the gamma chain. Biochemistry 1984;23:1767–1774.
70. Yakovlev S, Litvinovich S, Loukinov D, Medved L. Role of the beta-strand insert in the central domain of the fibrinogen gamma-module. Biochemistry 2000;39:15,721–15,729.
71. Doolittle RF, Yang Z, Mochalkin I. Crystal structure studies on fibrinogen and fibrin. Ann NY Acad Sci 2001;936:31–43.
72. Bennett JS, Shattil SJ, Power JW, Gartner TK. Interaction of fibrinogen with its platelet receptor. Differential effects of alpha and gamma chain fibrinogen peptides on the glycoprotein IIb-IIIa complex. J Biol Chem 1988;263:12,948–12,953.
73. Cheresh DA. Human endothelial cells synthesize and express an Arg-Gly-Asp-directed adhesion receptor involved in attachment to fibrinogen and von Willebrand factor. Proc Natl Acad Sci USA 1987;84:6471–6475.
74. Bennett JS, Chan C, Vilaire G, Mousa SA, DeGrado WF. Agonist-activated alphavbeta3 on platelets and lymphocytes binds to the matrix protein osteopontin. J Biol Chem 1997;272:8137–8140.
75. Helluin O, Chan C, Vilaire G, Mousa S, DeGrado WF, Bennett JS. The activation state of alphavbeta3 regulates platelet and lymphocyte adhesion to intact and thrombin-cleaved osteopontin. J Biol Chem 2000;275:18,337–18,343.

76. Cheresh DA, Berliner SA, Vicente V, Ruggeri ZM. Recognition of distinct adhesive sites on fibrinogen by related integrins on platelets and endothelial cells. Cell 1989;58:945–953.

77. Yokoyama K, Erickson HP, Ikeda Y, Takada Y. Identification of amino acid sequences in fibrinogen gamma-chain and tenascin C C-terminal domains critical for binding to integrin αVβ3. J Biol Chem 2000;275:16,891–16,898.

78. Xiong JP, Stehle T, Diefenbach B, et al. Crystal structure of the extracellular segment of integrin alphaVbeta3. Science 2001;294:339–345.

79. Xiong JP, Stehle T, Zhang R, et al. Crystal structure of the extracellular segment of integrin alphaVbeta3 in complex with an Arg-Gly-Asp ligand. Science 2002;296:151–155.

80. Beglova N, Blacklow SC, Takagi J, Springer TA. Cysteine-rich module structure reveals a fulcrum for integrin rearrangement upon activation. Nat Struct Biol 2002;9:282–287.

81. Weiss HJ, Hawiger J, Ruggeri ZM, Turitto VT, Thiagarajan P, Hoffman T. Fibrinogen-independent platelet adhesion and thrombus formation on subendothelium mediated by glycoprotein IIb-IIIa complex at high shear rate. J Clin Invest 1989;83:288–297.

82. Peerschke EI. The platelet fibrinogen receptor. Semin Hematol 1985;22:241–259.

83. Savage B, Ruggeri ZM. Selective recognition of adhesive sites in surface-bound fibrinogen by glycoprotein IIb-IIIa on nonactivated platelets. J Biol Chem 1991;266:11,227–11,233.

84. Cook NS, Kottirsch G, Zerwes H-G. Platelet glycoprotein IIb/IIIa antagonists. Drugs Future 1994;19: 135–159.

85. Wang W, Borchardt RT, Wang B. Orally active peptidomimetic RGD analogs that are glycoprotein IIb/IIIa antagonists. Curr Med Chem 2000;7:437–453.

86. Cox D, Aoki T, Seki J, Motoyama Y, Yoshida K. The pharmacology of integrins. Med Res Rev 1994; 14:195–228.

87. Ruggeri ZM. von Willebrand factor. J Clin Invest 1997;99:559–564.

88. Loscalzo J, Inbal A, Handin RI. von Willebrand protein facilitates platelet incorporation into polymerizing fibrin. J Clin Invest 1986;78:1112–1119.

89. Fernandez Ortiz A, Badimon JJ, Falk E, et al. Characterization of the relative thrombogenicity of atherosclerotic plaque components: implications for consequences of plaque rupture. J Am Coll Cardiol 1994;23:1562–1569.

90. Frenette PS, Moyna C, Hartwell DW, Lowe JB, Hynes RO, Wagner DD. Platelet-endothelial interactions in inflamed mesenteric venules. Blood 1998;91:1318–1325.

91. Giesen PL, Rauch U, Bohrmann B, et al. Blood-borne tissue factor: another view of thrombosis. Proc Natl Acad Sci USA 1999;96:2311–2315.

92. Rauch U, Bonderman D, Bohrmann B, et al. Transfer of tissue factor from leukocytes to platelets is mediated by CD15 and tissue factor. Blood 2000;96:170–175.

93. Giesen PL, Nemerson Y. Tissue factor on the loose. Semin Thromb Hemost 2000;26:379–384.

94. Siljander P, Carpen O, Lassila R. Platelet-derived microparticles associate with fibrin during thrombosis. Blood 1996;87:4651–4663.

95. Reverter JC, Beguin S, Kessels H, Kumar R, Hemker HC, Coller BS. Inhibition of platelet-mediated, tissue factor-induced thrombin generation by the mouse/human chimeric 7E3 antibody. Potential implications for the effect of c7E3 Fab treatment on acute thrombosis and "clinical restenosis." J Clin Invest 1996;98:863–874.

96. Coller BS. Binding of abciximab to αVβ3 and activated αMβ2 receptors: with a review of platelet-leukocyte interactions. Thromb Haemost 1999;82:326–336.

97. Mickelson JK, Lakkis NM, Villarreal-Levy G, Hughes BJ, Smith CW. Leukocyte activation with platelet adhesion after coronary angioplasty: a mechanism for recurrent disease? J Am Coll Cardiol 1996;28: 345–353.

98. Michelson AD, Barnard MR, Krueger LA, Valeri CR, Furman MI. Circulating monocyte-platelet aggregates are a more sensitive marker of in vivo platelet activation than platelet surface P-selectin: studies in baboons, human coronary intervention, and human acute myocardial infarction. Circulation 2001;104:1533–1537.

99. Furman MI, Kereiakes DJ, Krueger LA, et al. Leukocyte-platelet aggregation, platelet surface P-selectin, and platelet surface glycoprotein IIIa after percutaneous coronary intervention: effects of dalteparin or unfractionated heparin in combination with abciximab. Am Heart J 2001;142:790–798.

100. Mickelson JK, Kleiman NS, Lakkis NM, Chow TW, Hughes BS, Smith CW. Chimeric 7E3 Fab (ReoPro) decreases detectable CD11b on neutrophils from patients undergoing coronary angioplasty. Am J Cardiol 1999;33:97–106.

101. Neumann FJ, Zohlnhofer D, Fakhoury L, Ott I, Gawaz M, Schomig A. Effect of glycoprotein IIb/IIIa receptor blockade on platelet-leukocyte interaction and surface expression of the leukocyte integrin Mac-1 in acute myocardial infarction. J Am Coll Cardiol 1999;34:1420–1426.
102. Coller BS, Scudder LE, Beer J, et al. Monoclonal antibodies to platelet GPIIb/IIIa as antithrombotic agents. Ann NY Acad Sci 1991;614:193–213.
103. Coller BS, Folts JD, Smith SR, Scudder LE, Jordan R. Abolition of in vivo platelet thrombus formation in primates with monoclonal antibodies to the platelet GPIIb/IIIa receptor: correlation with bleeding time, platelet aggregation and blockade of GPIIb/IIIa receptors. Circulation 1989;80:1766–1774.
104. Folts JD, Rowe GG. Epinephrine potentiation of in vivo stimuli reverses aspirin inhibition of platelet thrombus formation in stenosed canine coronary arteries. Thromb Res 1988;50:507–516.
105. Eidt JF, Allison P, Nobel S. Thrombin is an important mediator of platelet aggregation in stenosed canine coronary arteries with endothelial injury. J Clin Invest 1989;84:18–27.
106. Willerson JT, Eidt JF, McNatt J, et al. Role of thromboxane and serotonin as mediators in the development of spontaneous alterations in coronary blood flow and neointimal proliferation in canine models with chronic coronary artery stenoses and endothelial injury. J Am Coll Cardiol 1991;17:101B–110B.
107. Anderson HV, Revana M, Rosales O, et al. Intravenous administration of monoclonal antibody to the platelet GP IIb/IIIa receptor to treat abrupt closure during coronary angioplasty. Am J Cardiol 1992;69:1373–1376.
108. Anderson HV, Kirkeeide RL, Krishnaswami A, et al. Cyclic flow variations after coronary angioplasty in humans: clinical and angiographic characteristics and elimination with 7E3 monoclonal antiplatelet antibody. J Am Coll Cardiol 1994;23:1031–1037.
109. Coller BS, Folts JD, Scudder LE, Smith SR. Antithrombotic effect of a monoclonal antibody to the platelet glycoprotein IIb/IIIa receptor in an experimental animal model. Blood 1986;68:783–786.
110. Gold HK, Coller BS, Yasuda T, et al. Rapid and sustained coronary artery recanalization with combined bolus injection of recombinant tissue-type plasminogen activator and monoclonal anti-platelet GPIIb/IIIa antibody in a dog model. Circulation 1988;77:670–677.
111. Coller BS. Inhibitors of the platelet glycoprotein IIb/IIIa receptor as conjunctive therapy for coronary artery thrombolysis. Coron Art Dis 1992;3:1016–1029.
112. Jang I-K, Gold HK, Ziskind AA, et al. Differential sensitivity of erythrocyte-rich and platelet-rich arterial thrombi to lysis with recombinant tissue-type plasminogen activator. A possible explanation for resistance to coronary thrombolysis. Circulation 1989;79:920–928.
113. Gold HK, Garabedian HD, Dinsmore RL, et al. Restoration of coronary flow in myocardial infarction by intravenous chimeric 7E3 antibody without exogenous plasminogen activators: observations in animals and man. Circulation 1997;95:1755–1759.
114. van den Merkhof LF, Zijlstra F, Olsson H, et al. Abciximab in the treatment of acute myocardial infarction eligible for primary percutaneous transluminal coronary angioplasty. Results of the Glycoprotein Receptor Antagonist Patency Evaluation (GRAPE) pilot study. J Am Coll Cardiol 1999;33:1528–1532.
115. Trial of abciximab with and without low-dose reteplase for acute myocardial infarction. Strategies for Patency Enhancement in the Emergency Department (SPEED) Group. Circulation 2000;101:2788–2794.
116. Antman EM, Giugliano RP, Gibson CM, et al. Abciximab facilitates the rate and extent of thrombolysis: results of the Thrombolysis in Myocardial Infarction (TIMI) 14 trial. The TIMI 14 investigators. Circulation 1999;99:2720–2732.
117. Bates ER, Walsh DG, Mu DX, Abrams GD, Lucchesi BR. Sustained inhibition of the vessel wall-platelet interaction after deep coronary artery injury by temporary inhibition of the platelet glycoprotein IIb/IIIa receptor. Coron Art Dis 1992;3:67–76.
118. Rote WE, Mu DX, Bates ER, Nedelman MA, Lucchesi BR. Prevention of rethrombosis after coronary thrombolysis in a chronic canine model. I. Adjunctive therapy with monoclonal antibody 7E3 F (ab')2 fragment. J Cardiovasc Pharmacol 1994;23:194–202.
119. Fitzgerald DJ, Wright F, FitzGerald GA. Increased thromboxane biosynthesis during coronary thrombolysis: evidence that platelet activation and thromboxane A_2 modulate the response to tissue-type plasminogen activator in vivo. Circ Res 1989;65:83–94.
120. Kiss RG, Stassen JM, Deckmyn H, et al. Contribution of platelets and the vessel wall to the antithrombotic effects of a single bolus injection of Fab fragments of the antiplatelet GPIIb/IIIa antibody 7E3 in a canine arterial eversion graft preparation. Arterioscler Thromb 1994;14:375–380.
121. Kiss RG, Lu HR, Roskams T, et al. Time course of the effects of a single bolus injection of F (ab')2 fragments of the antiplatelet GPIIb/IIIa antibody 7E3 on arterial eversion graft occlusion, platelet aggregation, and bleeding time in dogs. Arterioscler Thromb 1994;14:367–374.

122. Knight DM, Wagner C, Jordan R, et al. The immunogenicity of the 7E3 murine monoclonal Fab antibody fragment variable region is dramatically reduced in humans by substitution of human for murine constant regions. Mol Immunol 1995;32:1271–1281.

123. Jordan RE, Wagner CL, Mascelli M, et al. Preclinical development of c7E3 Fab; a mouse/human chimeric monoclonal antibody fragment that inhibits platelet function by blockade of GPIIb/IIIa receptors with observations on the immunogenicity of c7E3 Fab in humans. In: Horton MD, ed. Adhesion Receptors as Therapeutic Targets. CRC, Boca Raton, FL, 1996, pp. 281–305.

124. Rote WE, Nedelman MA, Mu DX, et al. Chimeric 7E3 prevents carotid artery thrombosis in cynomolgus monkeys. Stroke 1994;25:1223–1232.

125. Kohmura C, Gold HK, Yasuda T, et al. A chimeric murine/human antibody Fab fragment directed against the platelet GPIIb/IIIa receptor enhances and sustains arterial thrombolysis with recombinant tissue-type plasminogen activator in baboons. Arterioscler Thromb 1993;13:1837–1842.

126. Byzova TV, Plow EF. Networking in the hemostatic system. Integrin alphaIIbbeta3 binds prothrombin and influences its activation. J Biol Chem 1997;272:27,183–27,188.

127. Lages B, Weiss HJ. Greater inhibition of platelet procoagulant activity by antibody-derived glycoprotein IIb-IIIa inhibitors than by peptide and peptidomimetic inhibitors. Br J Haematol 2001;113:65–71.

128. Li Y, Spencer FA, Ball S, Becker RC. Inhibition of platelet-dependent prothrombinase activity and thrombin generation by glycoprotein IIb/IIIa receptor-directed antagonists: potential contributing mechanism of benefit in acute coronary syndromes. J Thromb Thrombolysis 2000;10:69–76.

129. Butenas S, Cawthern KM, van't Veer C, DiLorenzo ME, Lock JB, Mann KG. Antiplatelet agents in tissue factor-induced blood coagulation. Blood 2001;97:2314–2322.

130. Dangas G, Badimon JJ, Coller BS, et al. Administration of abciximab during percutaneous coronary intervention reduces both ex vivo platelet thrombus formation and fibrin deposition under dynamic flow conditions. Implications for a potential anticoagulant effect of abciximab. Arterioscler Thromb Vasc Biol 1998;18:1342–1349.

131. Byzova TV, Plow EF. Activation of alphaVbeta3 on vascular cells controls recognition of prothrombin. J Cell Biol 1998;143:2081–2092.

132. Tcheng JE, Harrington RA, Kottke Marchant K, et al. Multicenter, randomized, double-blind, placebo-controlled trial of the platelet integrin glycoprotein IIb/IIIa blocker integrelin in elective coronary intervention. Circulation 1995;91:2151–2157.

133. Moliterno DJ, Califf RM, Aguirre FV, et al. Effect of platelet glycoprotein IIb/IIIa integrin blockade on activated clotting time during percutaneous transluminal coronary angioplasty or directional atherectomy (the EPIC trial). Evaluation of c7E3 Fab in the Prevention of Ischemic Complications trial. Am J Cardiol 1995;75:559–562.

134. Ammar T, Scudder LE, Coller BS. In vitro effects of the platelet GPIIb/IIIa receptor antagonist c7E3 Fab on the activated clotting time. Circulation 1997;95:614–617.

135. Dangas G, Marmur JD, King TE, et al. Effects of platelet glycoprotein IIb/IIIa inhibition with abciximab on thrombin generation and activity during percutaneous coronary intervention. Am Heart J 1999;138:49–54.

136. Ambrose JA, Doss R, Geagea JM, et al. Effects on thrombin generation of the platelet glycoprotein IIb/IIa inhibitors abciximab versus tirofiban during coronary intervention. Am J Cardiol 2001;87:1231–1233.

137. Ambrose JA, Hawkey M, Badimon JJ, et al. In vivo demonstration of an antithrombin effect of abciximab. Am J Cardiol 2000;86:150–152.

138. Merlini PA, Repetto A, Lombardi A, et al. Effect of abciximab on prothrombin activation and thrombin generation in acute coronary syndromes without ST-segment elevation: Global Utilization of Strategies to Open Occluded Coronary Arteries Trial IV in Acute Coronary Syndromes (GUSTO IV ACS) Italian Hematologic Substudy. Circulation 2002;105:928–932.

139. Mak KH, Lee LH, Wong A, et al. Thrombin generation and fibrinolytic activities among patients receiving reduced-dose alteplase plus abciximab or undergoing direct angioplasty plus abciximab for acute myocardial infarction. Am J Cardiol 2002;89:930–936.

140. Cohen I, Burk DL, White JG. The effect of peptides and monoclonal antibodies that bind to platelet glycoprotein IIb-IIIa complex on the development of clot tension. Blood 1989;73:1880–1887.

141. Collet JP, Montalescot G, Lesty C, et al. Effects of abciximab on the architecture of platelet-rich clots in patients with acute myocardial infarction undergoing primary coronary intervention. Circulation 2001;103:2328–2331.

142. Collet JP, Montalescot G, Lesty C, Weisel JW. A structural and dynamic investigation of the facilitating effect of glycoprotein IIb/IIIa inhibitors in dissolving platelet-rich clots. Circ Res 2002;90:428–434.

143. Carr ME Jr, Carr SL, Hantgan RR, Braaten J. Glycoprotein IIb/IIIa blockade inhibits platelet-mediated force development and reduces gel elastic modulus. Thromb Haemost 1995;73:499–505.

144. Collet JP, Montalescot G, Lesty C, et al. Disaggregation of in vitro preformed platelet-rich clots by abciximab increases fibrin exposure and promotes fibrinolysis. Arterioscler Thromb Vasc Biol 2001; 21:142–148.

145. Fay WP, Eitzman DT, Shapiro AD, Madison EL, Ginsburg D. Platelets inhibit fibrinolysis in vitro by both plasminogen activator inhibitor-1 dependent and independent mechanisms. Blood 1994;83: 351–356.

146. Coller BS. Augmentation of thrombolysis with antiplatelet drugs. Overview. Coron Art Dis 1995;6: 911–914.

147. Cox AD, Devine DV. Factor XIIIa binding to activated platelets is mediated through activation of glycoprotein IIb-IIIa. Blood 1994;83:1006–1016.

148. Fitzgerald DJ, Catella F, Roy L, FitzGerald GA. Marked platelet activation in vivo after intravenous streptokinase in patients with acute myocardial infarction. Circulation 1988;77:142–150.

149. Coller BS. Platelets and thrombolytic therapy. N Engl J Med 1990;322:33–42.

150. Rudd MA, George D, Amarante P, Vaughan DE, Loscalzo J. Temporal effects of thrombolytic agents on platelet function in vivo and their modulation by prostaglandins. Circ Res 1990;67:1175–1181.

151. Topol EJ. Reperfusion therapy for acute myocardial infarction with fibrinolytic therapy or combination reduced fibrinolytic therapy and platelet glycoprotein IIb/IIIa inhibition: the GUSTO V randomised trial. Lancet 2001;357:1905–1914.

152. Anderson HV, McNatt J, Clubb FJ, et al. Platelet inhibition reduces cyclic flow variations and neointimal proliferation in normal and hypercholesterolemic-atherosclerotic canine coronary arteries. Circulation 2001;104:2331–2337.

153. Coller BS. Anti-GPIIb/IIIa drugs: current strategies and future directions. Thromb Haemost 2001;86: 437–443.

154. Coller BS. Platelet GPIIb/IIIa antagonists: the first anti-integrin receptor therapeutics. J Clin Invest 1997; 99:1467–1471.

155. Altieri DC, Edgington TS. A monoclonal antibody reacting with distinct adhesion molecules defines a transition in the functional state of the receptor CD11b/CD18 (Mac-1). J Immunol 1988;141:2656–2660.

156. Simon DI, Xu H, Ortlepp S, Rogers C, Rao NK. 7E3 monoclonal antibody directed against the platelet glycoprotein IIb/IIIa cross-reacts with the leukocyte integrin Mac-1 and blocks adhesion to fibrinogen and ICAM-1. Arterioscler Thromb Vasc Biol 1997;17:528–535.

157. Neumann FJ, Hochholzer W, Pogatsa-Murray G, Schomig A, Gawaz M. Antiplatelet effects of abciximab, tirofiban and eptifibatide in patients undergoing coronary stenting. J Am Coll Cardiol 2001;37: 1323–1328.

158. Xiao Z, Theroux P, Frojmovic M. Modulation of platelet-neutrophil interaction with pharmacological inhibition of fibrinogen binding to platelet GPIIb/IIIa receptor. Thromb Haemost 1999;81:281–285.

159. Lincoff AM, Kereiakes DJ, Mascelli MA, et al. Abciximab suppresses the rise in levels of circulating inflammatory markers after percutaneous coronary revascularization. Circulation 2001;104:163–167.

160. Charo IF, Bekeart LS, Phillips DR. Platelet glycoprotein IIb-IIIa-like proteins mediate endothelial cell attachment to adhesive proteins and the extracellular matrix. J Biol Chem 1987;262:9935–9938.

161. Tam SH, Sassoli PM, Jordan RE, Nakada MT. Abciximab (ReoPro, chimeric 7E3 Fab) demonstrates equivalent affinity and functional blockade of glycoprotein IIb/IIIa and alpha (v)beta3 integrins. Circulation 1998;98:1085–1091.

162. Eliceiri BP, Cheresh DA. Adhesion events in angiogenesis. Curr Opin Cell Biol 2001;13:563–568.

163. Feng X, Novack DV, Faccio R, et al. A Glanzmann's mutation in beta 3 integrin specifically impairs osteoclast function. J Clin Invest 2001;107:1137–1144.

164. Brooks PC, Clark RA, Cheresh DA. Requirement of vascular integrin αVβ3 for angiogenesis. Science 1994;264:569–571.

165. Stromblad S, Becker JC, Yebra M, Brooks PC, Cheresh DA. Suppression of p53 activity and p21WAF1/CIP1 expression by vascular cell integrin alphaVbeta3 during angiogenesis. J Clin Invest 1996;98: 426–433.

166. Matsuno H, Stassen JM, Vermylen J, Deckmyn H. Inhibition of integrin function by a cyclic RGD-containing peptide prevents neointima formation. Circulation 1994;90:2203–2206.

167. Choi ET, Engel L, Callow AD, et al. Inhibition of neointimal hyperplasia by blocking $\alpha_v\beta_3$ integrin with a small peptide antagonist G*pen*GRGDSPCA. J Vasc Surg 1994;19:125–134.
168. van der Zee R, Passeri J, Barry JJ, Cheresh DA, Isner JM. A neutralizing antibody to the alpha v beta 3 integrin reduces neointimal thickening in a balloon-injured rabbit iliac artery. Cell Adhes Commun 1998;6:371–379.
169. Srivatsa SS, Fitzpatrick LA, Tsao PW, et al. Selective $\alpha_v\beta_3$ integrin blockade potently limits neointimal hyperplasia and lumen stenosis following deep coronary arterial stent injury: evidence for the functional importance of integrin $\alpha_v\beta_3$ and osteopontin expression during neointima formation. Cardiovasc Res 1997;36:408–428.
170. Slepian MJ, Massia SP, Dehdashti B, Fritz A, Whitesell L. Beta3-integrins rather than beta1-integrins dominate integrin-matrix interactions involved in postinjury smooth muscle cell migration. Circulation 1998;97:1818–1827.
171. Deitch JS, Williams JK, Adams MR, et al. Effects of beta3-integrin blockade (c7E3) on the response to angioplasty and intra-arterial stenting in atherosclerotic nonhuman primates. Arterioscler Thromb Vasc Biol 1998;18:1730–1737.
172. Coleman KR, Braden GA, Willingham MC, Sane DC. Vitaxin, a humanized monoclonal antibody to the vitronectin receptor (alphavbeta3), reduces neointimal hyperplasia and total vessel area after balloon injury in hypercholesterolemic rabbits. Circ Res 1999;84:1268–1276.
173. Smyth SS, Reis ED, Zhang W, Fallon JT, Gordon RE, Coller BS. β3-integrin-deficient mice, but not P-selectin-deficient mice, develop intimal hyperplasia after vascular injury: correlation with leukocyte recruitment to adherent platelets one hour post injury. Circulation 2001;103:2501–2507.
174. The ERASER Investigators. Acute platelet inhibition with abciximab does not reduce in-stent restenosis (ERASER study). Circulation 1999;100:799–806.
175. Neumann FJ, Kastrati A, Schmitt C, et al. Effect of glycoprotein IIb/IIIa receptor blockade with abciximab on clinical and angiographic restenosis rate after the placement of coronary stents following acute myocardial infarction. J Am Coll Cardiol 2000;35:915–921.
176. Marso SP, Lincoff AM, Ellis SG, et al. Optimizing the percutaneous interventional outcomes for patients with diabetes mellitus: results of the EPISTENT (Evaluation of Platelet IIb/IIIa Inhibitor for Stenting Trial) diabetic substudy. Circulation 1999;100:2477–2484.
177. Topol EJ, Yadav JS. Recognition of the importance of embolization in atherosclerotic vascular disease. Circulation 2000;101:570–580.
178. Neumann FJ, Blasini R, Schmitt C, et al. Effect of glycoprotein IIb/IIIa receptor blockade on recovery of coronary flow and left ventricular function after the placement of coronary-artery stents in acute myocardial infarction. Circulation 1998;98:2695–2701.
179. de Lemos JA, Antman EM, Gibson CM, et al. Abciximab improves both epicardial flow and myocardial reperfusion in ST-elevation myocardial infarction. Observations from the TIMI 14 trial. Circulation 2000;101:239–243.
180. Koch KC, Vom DJ, Kleinhans E, et al. Influence of a platelet GPIIb/IIIa receptor antagonist on myocardial hypoperfusion during rotational atherectomy as assessed by myocardial Tc-99m sestamibi scintigraphy. J Am Coll Cardiol 1999;33:998–1004.
181. Anderson KM, Califf RM, Stone GW, et al. Long-term mortality benefit with abciximab in patients undergoing percutaneous coronary intervention. J Am Coll Cardiol 2001;37:2059–2065.
182. Mukherjee D, Reginelli JP, Moliterno DJ, et al. Unexpected mortality reduction with abciximab for in-stent restenosis. J Invasive Cardiol 2000;12:540–544.
183. Gold HK, Gimple L, Yasuda T, et al. Pharmacodynamic study of F (ab')2 fragments of murine monoclonal antibody 7E3 directed against human platelet glycoprotein IIb/IIIa, in patients with unstable angina pectoris. J Clin Invest 1990;86:651–659.
184. EPIC Investigators. Use of a monoclonal antibody directed against the platelet glycoprotein IIb/IIIa receptor in high-risk coronary angioplasty. N Engl J Med 1994;330:956–961.
185. Wilentz JR, Sanborn TA, Haudenschild CC, Valeri CR, Ryan TJ, Faxon DP. Platelet accumulation in experimental angioplasty: time course and relation to vascular injury. Circulation 1987;75:636–642.
186. Groves HM, Kinlough-Rathbone RL, Richardson M, Moore S, Mustard JF. Platelet interaction with damaged rabbit aorta. Lab Invest 1979;40:194–200.
187. Use of a monoclonal antibody directed against the platelet glycoprotein IIb/IIIa receptor in high-risk coronary angioplasty. The EPIC Investigation. N Engl J Med 1994;330:956–961.
188. Coller BS. Activation affects access to the platelet receptor for adhesive glycoproteins. J Cell Biol 1986; 103:451–456.

189. Mousa SA, Forsythe M, Bozarth J, et al. XV454, a novel nonpeptides small-molecule platelet GPIIb/IIIa antagonist with comparable platelet alpha(IIb)beta3-binding kinetics to c7E3. J Cardiovasc Pharmacol 1998;32:736–744.

190. Nurden P, Poujol C, Durrieu-Jais C, et al. Labeling of the internal pool of GP IIb-IIIa in platelets by c7E3 Fab fragments (abciximab): flow and endocytic mechanisms contribute to the transport. Blood 1999;93:1622–1633.

191. Puzon-McLaughlin W, Kamata T, Takada Y. Multiple discontinuous ligand-mimetic antibody binding sites define a ligand binding pocket in integrin alpha (IIb)beta (3). J Biol Chem 2000;275: 7795–7802.

192. Artoni A, Li J, Ruan J, Coller BS, French DL. Studies of the effects of amino acid substitutions in the C177-C184 disulfide loop of human β3 integrin on adhesion to fibrinogen and binding of monoclonal antibody 7E3. Blood 2001;98:517a.

193. Tcheng JE, Ellis SG, George BS, et al. Pharmacodynamics of chimeric glycoprotein IIb/IIIa integrin antiplatelet antibody Fab 7E3 in high-risk coronary angioplasty. Circulation 1994;90:1757–1764.

194. Jordan R. Personal communication, 1998.

195. Poujol C, Durrieu-Jais C, Larrue B, Nurden AT, Nurden P. Accessibility of abciximab to megakaryocytes and endothelial cells in the bone marrow compartment: studies on a patient receiving antithrombotic therapy. Br J Haematol 1999;107:526–531.

196. Mascelli MA, Lance ET, Damaraju L, Wagner CL, Weisman HF, Jordan RE. Pharmacodynamic profile of short-term abciximab treatment demonstrates prolonged platelet inhibition with gradual recovery from GP IIb/IIIa receptor blockade. Circulation 1998;97:1680–1688.

197. Christopoulos C, Mackie I, Lahiri A, Machin S. Flow cytometric observations on the in vivo use of Fab fragments of a chimaeric monoclonal antibody to platelet glycoprotein IIb-IIIa. Blood Coagul Fibrinolysis 1993;4:729–737.

198. Mascelli MA, Worley S, Veriabo NJ, et al. Rapid assessment of platelet function with a modified whole-blood aggregometer in percutaneous transluminal coronary angioplasty patients receiving anti-GP IIb/IIIa therapy. Circulation 1997;96:3860–3866.

199. Peter K, Kohler B, Straub A, et al. Flow cytometric monitoring of glycoprotein IIb/IIIa blockade and platelet function in patients with acute myocardial infarction receiving reteplase, abciximab, and ticlopidine: continuous platelet inhibition by the combination of abciximab and ticlopidine. Circulation 2000;102:1490–1496.

200. Simoons ML, de Boer MJ, van den Brand MJ, et al. Randomized trial of a GPIIb/IIIa platelet receptor blocker in refractory unstable angina. Circulation 1994;89:596–603.

201. Kohl DW, Slavik KJ, Kamath G, Lehr JM, McDonald MJ, Rubio F. High-dose abciximab during coronary angioplasty in a patient with essential thrombocytosis. J Invasive Cardiol 1998;10:173–176.

202. Michaels AD, Whisenant B, MacGregor JS. Multivessel coronary thrombosis treated with abciximab (ReoPro) in a patient with essential thrombocythemia. Clin Cardiol 1998;21:134–138.

203. Jakubowski JA, Jordan RE, Weisman HF. Current antiplatelet therapy. In: Uprichard ACG, Gallagher KP, eds. Handbook of Experimental Pharmacology, vol. 132. Antithrombotics. Springer-Verlag, Heidelberg, 1999, pp. 175–208.

204. Abernethy DR, Pezzullo J, Mascelli MA, Frederick B, Kleiman NS, Freedman J. Pharmacodynamics of abciximab during angioplasty: comparison to healthy subjects. Clin Pharmacol Ther 2002;71: 186–195.

205. Freedman J, Mascelli MA, Pezzullo JC, et al. Pharmacodynamic profile of short-term readministration of abciximab in healthy subjects. Am Heart J 2002;143:87–94.

206. Platelet glycoprotein IIb/IIIa receptor blockade and low-dose heparin during percutaneous coronary revascularization. The EPILOG Investigators. N Engl J Med 1997;336:1689–1696.

207. Randomised placebo-controlled and balloon-angioplasty-controlled trial to assess safety of coronary stenting with use of platelet glycoprotein-IIb/IIIa blockade. The EPISTENT Investigators. Evaluation of Platelet IIb/IIIa Inhibitor for Stenting. Lancet 1998;352:87–92.

208. Kleiman NS, Raizner AE, Jordan R, et al. Differential inhibition of platelet aggregation induced by adenosine diphosphate or a thrombin receptor-activating peptide in patients treated with bolus chimeric 7E3 Fab: implications for inhibition of the internal pool of GPIIb/IIIa receptors. J Am Coll Cardiol 1995;26:1665–1671.

209. Wagner CL, Cunningham MR, Wyand MS, Weisman HF, Coller BS, Jordan RE. Reversal of the antiplatelet effects of chimeric 7E3 Fab treatment by platelet transfusion in cynomolgus monkeys. Thromb Haemostast 1995;73:1313.

210. Nakada MT, Sassoli PM, Tam SH, Nedelman MA, Jordan RE, Kereiakes DJ. Abciximab pharmacodynamics are unaffected by antecedent therapy with other GPIIb/IIIa antagonists in non-human primates. J Cardiovasc Pharmacol, in press.

211. Lev EI, Osende JI, Richard MF, et al. Administration of abciximab to patients receiving tirofiban or eptifibatide: effect on platelet function. J Am Coll Cardiol 2001;37:847–855.

212. Quinn M, Deering A, Stewart M, Cox D, Foley B, Fitzgerald D. Quantifying GPIIb/IIIa receptor binding using 2 monoclonal antibodies: discriminating abciximab and small molecular weight antagonists. Circulation 1999;99:2231–2238.

213. Smith JW, Steinhubl SR, Lincoff AM, et al. Rapid platelet-function assay (RPFA): an automated and quantitative cartridge-based method. Circulation 1999;99:620–625.

214. Steinhubl SR, Talley D, Braden GA, et al. Point-of-care measured platelet inhibition correlates with a reduced risk of an adverse cardiac event following percutaneous coronary intervention. Results of the GOLD (AU-Assessing Ultegra) multicenter study. Circulation 2001;103:2572–2578.

215. Kereiakes DJ, Mueller M, Howard W, et al. Efficacy of abciximab induced platelet blockade using a rapid point of care assay. J Thromb Thrombolysis 1999;7:265–276.

216. Steinhubl SR, Kottke-Marchant K, Moliterno DJ, et al. Attainment and maintenance of platelet inhibition through standard dosing of abciximab in diabetic and nondiabetic patients undergoing percutaneous coronary intervention. Circulation 1999;100:1977–1982.

217. Mukherjee D, Chew DP, Robbins M, Yadav JS, Raymond RE, Moliterno DJ. Clinical application of procedural platelet monitoring during percutaneous coronary intervention among patients at increased bleeding risk. J Thromb Thrombolysis 2001;11:151–154.

218. Simon DI, Liu CB, Ganz P, et al. A comparative study of light transmission aggregometry and automated bedside platelet function assays in patients undergoing percutaneous coronary intervention and receiving abciximab, eptifibatide, or tirofiban. Catheter Cardiovasc Interv 2001;52:425–432.

219. Kereiakes DJ, Broderick TM, Roth EM, et al. Time course, magnitude, and consistency of platelet inhibition by abciximab, tirofiban, or eptifibatide in patients with unstable angina pectoris undergoing percutaneous coronary intervention. Am J Cardiol 1999;84:391–395.

220. Casterella PJ, Kereiakes DJ, Steinhubl SR, et al. The platelet function dose-response to abciximab during percutaneous coronary revascularization is variable. Catheter Cardiovasc Interv 2001;54:497–504.

221. Mukherjee D, Moliterno DJ. Applications of anti-platelet monitoring in catheterization laboratory. J Thromb Thrombolysis 2000;9:293–301.

222. Smith BS, Gandhi PJ. Pharmacokinetics and pharmacodynamics of low-molecular-weight heparins and glycoprotein IIb/IIIa receptor antagonists in renal failure. J Thromb Thrombolysis 2001;11:39–48.

223. Hartman GD, Egbertson MS, Halczenko W, et al. Non-peptide fibrinogen receptor antagonists. 1. Discovery and design of exosite inhibitors. J Med Chem 1992;35:4640–4642.

224. Egbertson MS, Chang CT, Duggan ME, et al. Non-peptide fibrinogen receptor antagonists. 2. Optimization of a tyrosine template as a mimic for Arg-Gly-Asp. J Med Chem 1994;37:2537–2551.

225. Lele M, Sajid M, Wajih N, Stouffer GA. Eptifibatide and 7E3, but not tirofiban, inhibit alpha (v)beta (3) integrin-mediated binding of smooth muscle cells to thrombospondin and prothrombin. Circulation 2001;104:582–587.

226. Kintscher U, Kappert K, Schmidt G, et al. Effects of abciximab and tirofiban on vitronectin receptors in human endothelial and smooth muscle cells. Eur J Pharmacol 2000;390:75–87.

227. Vickers S, Theoharides AD, Arison B, et al. In vitro and in vivo studies on the metabolism of tirofiban. Drug Metab Dispos 1999;27:1360–1366.

228. Tirofiban package insert, 2002.

229. Barrett JS, Murphy G, Peerlinck K, et al. Pharmacokinetics and pharmacodynamics of MK-383, a selective non-peptide platelet glycoprotein-IIb/IIIa receptor antagonist, in healthy men. Clin Pharmacol Ther 1994;56:377–388.

230. Peerlinck K, De Lepeleire I, Goldberg M, et al. MK-383 (L-700,462), a selective nonpeptide platelet glycoprotein IIb/IIIa antagonist, is active in man. Circulation 1993;88:1512–1517.

231. Kereiakes DJ, Kleiman NS, Ambrose J, et al. Randomized, double-blind, placebo-controlled dose-ranging study of tirofiban (MK-383) platelet IIb/IIIa blockade in high risk patients undergoing coronary angioplasty. J Am Coll Cardiol 1996;27:536–542.

232. Januzzi JL Jr, Snapinn SM, DiBattiste PM, Jang IK, Theroux P. Benefits and safety of tirofiban among acute coronary syndrome patients with mild to moderate renal insufficiency: results from the Platelet Receptor Inhibition in Ischemic Syndrome Management in Patients Limited by Unstable Signs and Symptoms (PRISM-PLUS) trial. Circulation 2002;105:2361–2366.

233. Scarborough RM, Naughton MA, Teng W, et al. Design of potent and specific integrin antagonists. Peptide antagonists with high specificity for glycoprotein IIb-IIIa. J Biol Chem 1993;268:1066–1073.

234. Phillips DR, Teng W, Arfsten A, et al. Effect of Ca^{2+} on GPIIb-IIIa interactions with integrilin: enhanced GPIIb-IIIa binding and inhibition of platelet aggregation by reductions in the concentration of ionized calicum in plasma anticoagulated with citrate. Circulation 1997;96:1488–1494.

235. Alton KB, Kosoglou T, Baker S, Affrime MB, Cayen MN, Patrick JE. Disposition of 14C-eptifibatide after intravenous administration to healthy men. Clin Ther 1998;20:307–323.

236. Gilchrist IC, O'Shea JC, Kosoglou T, et al. Pharmacodynamics and pharmacokinetics of higher-dose, double-bolus eptifibatide in percutaneous coronary intervention. Circulation 2001;104:406–411.

237. Phillips DR, Scarborough RM. Clinical pharmacology of eptifibatide. Am J Cardiol 1997;80:11B–20B.

238. Li YF, Spencer FA, Becker RC. Comparative efficacy of fibrinogen and platelet supplementation on the in vitro reversibility of competitive glycoprotein IIb/IIIa (alphaIIb/beta3) receptor-directed platelet inhibition. Am Heart J 2001;142:204–210.

239. The IMPACT-II Investigators. Randomised placebo-controlled trial of effect of eptifibatide on complications of percutaneous coronary intervention: IMPACT-II. Lancet 1997;349:1422–1428.

240. Harrington RA, Kleiman NS, Kottke Marchant K, et al. Immediate and reversible platelet inhibition after intravenous administration of a peptide glycoprotein IIb/IIIa inhibitor during percutaneous coronary intervention. Am J Cardiol 1995;76:1222–1227.

241. Tardiff BE, Jennings LK, Harrington RA, et al. Pharmacodynamics and pharmacokinetics of eptifibatide in patients with acute coronary syndromes: prospective analysis from PURSUIT. Circulation 2001; 104:399–405.

242. Tcheng JE, Talley JD, O'Shea JC, Gilchrist IC, Kleiman NS, Grines CL, et al. Clinical pharmacology of higher dose eptifibatide in percutaneous coronary intervention (the PRIDE study). Am J Cardiol 2001; 88:1097–1102.

243. Novel dosing regimen of eptifibatide in planned coronary stent implantation (ESPRIT): a randomised, placebo-controlled trial. The ESPRIT Investigators. Enhanced Suppression of the Platelet IIb/IIIa Receptor with Integrilin Therapy. Lancet 2000;356:2037–2044.

II

GLYCOPROTEIN IIb/IIIa BLOCKADE DURING CORONARY INTERVENTION

5

Abciximab During Percutaneous Coronary Intervention
EPIC, EPILOG, and EPISTENT Trials

A. Michael Lincoff, MD

CONTENTS

INTRODUCTION
PHARMACOLOGY OF ABCIXIMAB
PIVOTAL TRIALS OF ABCIXIMAB DURING CORONARY INTERVENTION
CONCLUSIONS
REFERENCES

INTRODUCTION

Blockade of the platelet glycoprotein (GP) IIb/IIIa receptor as a therapy for ischemic heart disease was introduced into clinical practice by demonstration that the first of these agents, abciximab, reduces periprocedural complications among patients undergoing high-risk coronary angioplasty. From this initial "proof of concept," subsequent clinical evaluation of this agent progressed through a series of large-scale trials, establishing the broad applicability, marked clinical efficacy, and acceptable safety profile of this therapeutic strategy in the setting of percutaneous coronary revascularization. This chapter reviews the clinical experience with this agent as a pharmacologic adjunct to elective or urgent coronary intervention.

PHARMACOLOGY OF ABCIXIMAB

Preclinical Data

The development and pharmacology of abciximab are reviewed in detail in Chapter 4 by Dr. Coller. In brief, abciximab (ReoPro™, Centocor, Malvern, PA) is a chimeric Fab monoclonal antibody fragment that binds to the platelet GPIIb/IIIa receptor. A murine antibody (7E3) was produced by immunization of mice with human platelets and isolated from hybridoma supernatants by its inhibition of the interaction between platelets and fibrinogen-covered beads. To limit the risk of thrombocytopenia owing to clearance of

From: *Contemporary Cardiology: Platelet Glycoprotein IIb/IIIa
Inhibitors in Cardiovascular Disease, 2nd Edition*
Edited by: A. M. Lincoff © Humana Press Inc., Totowa, NJ

7E3-coated platelets by binding of the Fc region of the IgG molecule to the reticuloendo-thelial system, 7E3 was cleaved with pepsin into $F(ab')_2$ fragments. Animal experiments and initial human studies were carried out using this $F(ab')_2$ form. Because of continued concerns regarding the potential for thrombocytopenia by crosslinking of platelets with the bivalent $F(ab')_2$ antibody, an Fab antibody fragment was produced by papain digestion of m7E3 and subsequently evaluated. Finally, to reduce the risk of immunogenicity to murine protein, genetic reconstruction was used to produce the chimeric c7E3 Fab antibody fragment currently in clinical use (abciximab), which consists of human constant regions and murine variable regions of the IgG antibody.

In preclinical canine and primate animal models (see Chapter 4), 7E3 $F(ab')_2$ or c7E3 Fab were shown to markedly diminish thrombus formation and platelet-mediated cyclic flow reductions in injured and stenosed coronary arteries, to facilitate tissue plasmino-gen activator (t-PA)-induced thrombolysis, and to abolish reocclusion. These antithrom-botic effects were observed at doses that achieved blockade of >60–80% of GPIIb/IIIa receptors.

Clinical Studies

Murine 7E3 and abciximab bind with high affinity to both activated and unactivated platelet GPIIb/IIIa, with inhibition of platelet aggregation observed at levels of receptor blockade >50% and nearly complete abrogation of aggregability at >80% receptor occu-pancy. Although binding is reversible, dissociation of the agent from the receptor is slow, and normalization of platelet aggregation does not occur until 24–36 h following discont-inuation of abciximab infusion (1,2). By flow cytometry, decreasing but measurable levels of platelet-bound abciximab are present for as long as 15 d, beyond the normal circulating platelet lifespan, indicating redistribution of abciximab to new platelets entering the cir-culation (3).

Phase II clinical studies confirmed dose-related inhibition of platelet aggregation and prolongation of bleeding time by 7E3 in the setting of percutaneous coronary interven-tion. In a pilot study of 23 patients undergoing elective angioplasty, escalating bolus doses ranging from 0.15 to 0.35 mg/kg of m7E3 Fab produced levels of receptor blockade ranging from approx 50–90% (4). Doses of ≥0.20 mg/kg led to >70–80% inhibition of platelet aggregation, with partial recovery of platelet function noted by 6 h. Marked pro-longation of bleeding times were observed at all doses, with normalization by 24 h.

Chimeric 7E3 Fab (abciximab) was evaluated in a multicenter, open-label, dose-esca-lation study of 56 patients undergoing elective percutaneous transluminal coronary angio-plasty (PTCA) (2). Levels of receptor blockade and inhibition of platelet aggregation following bolus doses of 0.15, 0.20, and 0.25 mg/kg are detailed in Table 1; although wide variability was observed among patients, particularly at the lowest dose, platelet aggre-gation was consistently suppressed to the theoretical target of ≤20% of baseline by the abciximab bolus dose of 0.25 mg/kg. In the second phase of this study, GPIIb/IIIa recep-tor blockade, platelet aggregation, and bleeding times were measured following a 0.25 mg/kg bolus dose, with and without a subsequent 12-h infusion at a rate of 10 µg/min (Fig. 1). With a bolus only (Fig. 1A), peak receptor blockade and inhibition of platelet aggrega-tion to ≤20% occurred by the first (2-h) measurement, with prolongation of bleeding time to >30 min. Bleeding time returned nearly to normal by 12 h, although recovery of platelet aggregability occurred more gradually, remaining approx 40% and approx 30% inhibited by 12 and 24 h, respectively. Addition of an infusion of abciximab (10 µg/min) following

Table 1
GPIIb/IIIa Receptor Blockade
and Inhibition of Platelet Aggregation after Abciximab Bolus Doses

Bolus dose (mg/kg body weight)	GPIIb/IIIa receptor blockade (% blocked) [median (interquartile range)]	Platelet aggregation to 20 μM ADP (% of baseline) [median (interquartile range)]
0.15	54 (15–94)	46 (34–80)
0.20	80 (67–89)	45 (19–71)
0.25	87 (62–96)	18 (9–25)

Data from ref. 2.

the bolus dose produced consistent levels of receptor occupancy of approx 80%, with inhibition of platelet aggregation to approx 20% and prolongation of bleeding time to >30 min during the 12-h infusion period (Fig. 1B). Following discontinuation of the infusion, recovery of these parameters occurred at rates similar to those following administration of the bolus only. The effectiveness of the 12-h abciximab infusion (10 μg/min or 0.125 μg/ kg min) in maintaining receptor blockade >80% and platelet aggregability <20% in the majority of treated patients was confirmed in a subsequent study of 41 normal volunteers (3).

Kleiman and coworkers (5) evaluated the influence of different agonists on measured inhibition of platelet aggregation by abciximab among 32 patients undergoing coronary angioplasty. Receptor blockade was approx 80% at 2 h following the single abciximab bolus of 0.25 mg/kg, declining to approx 50% by 24 h. This level of receptor occupancy was associated with nearly complete inhibition of platelet aggregation in response to the traditional agonists ADP (20 and 5 μM concentrations) and collagen (mean 76%, 88%, and 85% inhibition at 2 h, respectively). The circulating plasma half-life of abciximab was very short, calculated at <26 min. Inhibition of platelet aggregation at various time points in response to ADP and collagen was significantly correlated with the extent of receptor blockade by abciximab but was not at all related to circulating abciximab plasma concentrations (which were very low by 2 h following the drug bolus). Platelet aggregation in response to stimulation with thrombin receptor-activating peptides (TRAPs), an agonist that mimics platelet activation by thrombin, was significantly less inhibited 2 h following abciximab than was aggregation in response to ADP or collagen. Addition of exogenous abciximab to the platelet-rich plasma, however, led to more complete inhibition of aggregation in response to TRAP.

These investigators postulated that the continued ability of platelets to aggregate in response to TRAP 2 h following the bolus of abciximab may have been related to the "release reaction" induced by thrombin stimulation, in which GPIIb/IIIa receptors in the α-granule membranes and perhaps other sites of the platelet are externalized to the platelet membrane. Given the brief circulating half-life of abciximab, plasma levels of this agent would be insufficient to bind such newly exposed receptors shortly after the bolus is administered. These findings suggested that a continued infusion of abciximab following a bolus would be required to provide complete inhibition of platelet aggregation in the setting of intense stimulation by agonists such as thrombin, in which additional unbound GPIIb/IIIa receptors are externalized to the platelet membrane.

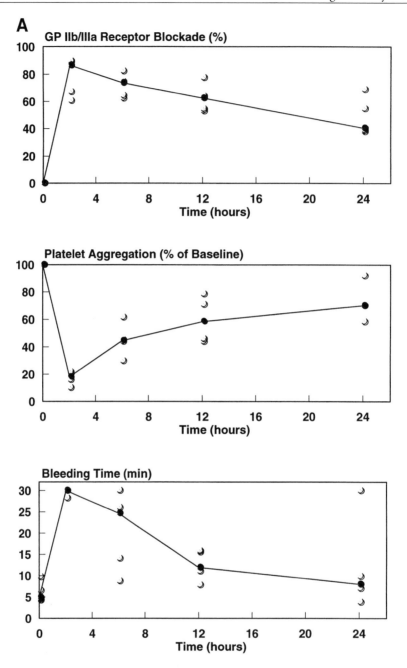

Fig. 1. Pharmacodynamics of a 0.25 mg/kg bolus dose only (**A**) or a 0.25 mg/kg bolus dose followed by a 10 µg/min infusion for 12 h (**B**) of abciximab. The bolus was given at time 0, with the infusion between time 0 and 12 h. Effects were followed for 24 h. Data points for each patient are shown in open circles; median values are in solid squares, and lines join the median values. For each panel: top graph, percentage of GPIIb/IIIa receptors blocked by abciximab; middle graph, inhibition of platelet aggregation, expressed as percentage of baseline aggregation in response to 20 µmol/L ADP; bottom graph, bleeding time. (From ref. 2 with permission.)

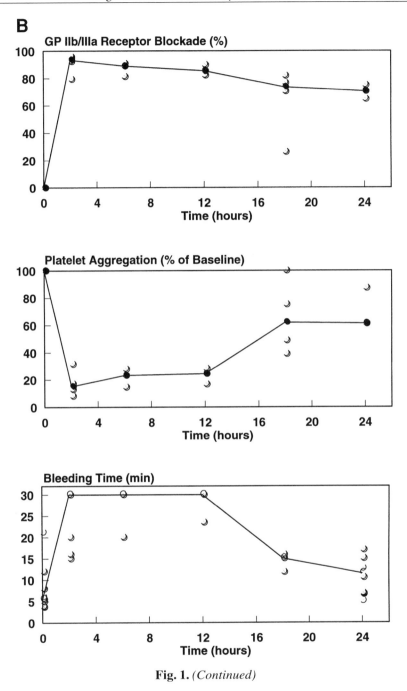

Fig. 1. *(Continued)*

Subsequent studies performed since the availability of point-of-care devices to measure platelet aggregation have documented substantial interpatient variability in the degree of platelet inhibition during abciximab administration. In one study of 100 patients undergoing percutaneous coronary revascularization, all but one achieved >80% inhibition following the bolus of abciximab *(6)*. At 8 h after the bolus, however, during the 12-h abciximab infusion, 13% of patients demonstrated inhibition levels below the 80% target.

Variability in levels of inhibition were even more marked in the hours after discontinuation of infusion, and neither clinical variables nor pretreatment with ticlopidine correlated with response to abciximab.

PIVOTAL TRIALS OF ABCIXIMAB DURING CORONARY INTERVENTION

The role of abciximab during percutaneous coronary revascularization has been assessed in three large-scale, placebo-controlled, randomized trials, enrolling in total over 7000 patients. The first of these trials Evaluation of C7E3 Fab for Prevention of Ischemic Complications (EPIC), focused on patients considered to be at high risk for thrombotic complications. The Evaluation in PTCA to Improve Long-term Outcome with abciximab GP II/IIIa blockade (EPILOG) trial extended the findings of EPIC to the broad spectrum of patients undergoing coronary balloon angioplasty or atherectomy. The Evaluation of Platelet Inhibition in STENTing (EPISTENT) trial investigated the complementarity of abciximab therapy with stenting, the dominant revascularization technique in interventional cardiology.

The three abciximab trials all shared common design and analysis features, which allow for some degree of comparison and contrast among the studies. All trials were blinded, except for the asymmetric balloon angioplasty plus abciximab arm of EPISTENT (*see* the EPISTENT Trial section). All were carried out according to the intention-to-treat principle, wherein patients were randomized before initiation of the interventional procedure and all patients were included in the efficacy analysis, regardless of whether they actually received study drug or underwent revascularization. Endpoints were adjudicated by independent, blinded Clinical Events Committees convened for each trial; these committees utilized data obtained systematically by protocol and identified events that may or may not have been determined by investigators at the individual clinical sites. Endpoint myocardial infarctions were defined by electrocardiographic and enzymatic criteria that were similar in the three trials [in general, infarction was identified by new Q-waves or creative kinase (CK)-MB elevations ≥3 times the control value], with CK-MB values obtained according to a protocolized schedule in all patients, even among those in whom infarction was not clinically suspected.

Similarly, hemoglobin values were obtained prior to hospital discharge for assessment of bleeding complications in all patients, regardless of whether or not bleeding events were observed. Bleeding events were classified according to the criteria of the Thrombolysis in Myocardial Infarction (TIMI) Study Group *(7)*. Major bleeding was defined as intracranial hemorrhage or blood loss resulting in a decrease in hemoglobin by >5 g/dL; minor bleeding was defined by spontaneous gross hematuria or hematemesis, a decrease in hemoglobin by >3 g/dL in association with observed bleeding, or a decrease in hemoglobin by >4 g/dL if a site of blood loss could not be identified. Observed decreases in hemoglobin were adjusted for the influence of red blood cell transfusions *(8)*.

The EPIC Trial

Proof of concept that GPIIb/IIIa inhibition would diminish ischemic complications of percutaneous coronary revascularization was provided by the first Phase III study of this class of agents, the EPIC trial, leading to the marketing approval of abciximab. This trial evaluated the efficacy of two dosing strategies of abciximab versus placebo among patients considered to be at high risk for coronary intervention on the basis of acute ischemic syndromes or clinical and morphologic characteristics (9).

PATIENT POPULATION AND STUDY DESIGN

A total of 2099 patients scheduled to undergo balloon angioplasty or directional atherectomy were enrolled between November, 1991 and November, 1992. Criteria constituting high-risk status for entry into the trial included acute or recent myocardial infarction, unstable angina, complex target lesion angiographic morphology [modified American College of Cardiology/American Heart Association (ACC/AHA) lesion score B2 or C], or a moderately complex target lesion (ACC/AHA score B1) in association with advanced age, female gender, or diabetes mellitus. Patients were excluded from enrollment if they were over 80 yr of age or for known bleeding diatheses, major surgery within 6 wk, or stroke within the prior 2 yr.

The enrolled patient population had a median age of 72 yr, 83% were male, 24% were diabetic, and 57% had a history of prior myocardial infarction. Entry criteria included unstable ischemic syndromes (acute infarction, prior infarction, or unstable angina) in 43% of patients, whereas 57% were enrolled with high-risk morphologic/clinical criteria.

All patients received aspirin and heparin to achieve and maintain an activated clotting time (ACT) of >300–350 s. The initial heparin bolus was 10–12,000 U, followed by additional 3000-U boluses to a maximum of 20,000 U. Randomization was in a double-blind fashion to placebo, abciximab 0.25 mg/kg bolus, or abciximab 0.25 mg/kg bolus followed by abciximab 10 µg/min infusion for 12 h. Heparin infusion was continued, to a target activated partial thromboplastin time (aPTT) of 1.5–2.5 times the control value, and vascular access sheaths remained in place for the 12-h duration of study drug. Balloon angioplasty or directional atherectomy was carried out according to institutional practice, with stent implantation reserved for manifest or threatened vessel closure.

CLINICAL EFFICACY

The primary efficacy endpoint was a composite of death, myocardial infarction, urgent repeat revascularization, or stent or balloon pump placement by 30 d following randomization. This composite event rate was reduced from 12.8% among patients receiving placebo to 11.4% among patients receiving the abciximab bolus (10% relative risk reduction, $p = 0.43$) and to 8.3% among patients receiving the abciximab bolus and 12-h infusion (35% relative risk reduction, $p = 0.008$) (Fig. 2A). The incidences of myocardial infarction and urgent revascularization were significantly reduced by the bolus and infusion of abciximab; the bolus-only regimen resulted in a very modest and statistically insignificant event reduction (Table 2). Mortality rates were not influenced by abciximab according to the intention-to-treat analysis, but three patients who died in the abciximab bolus and infusion arm did so after randomization but before receiving study drug. The treatment effect of abciximab was present in all subgroups analyzed; a trend was observed toward less clinical benefit from abciximab in lighter weight patients, a finding that may have been related to the excess risk of bleeding in this subgroup (see below). Angiographic criteria, including the presence of thrombus, did not predict the extent of clinical benefit derived from abciximab therapy (10).

The clinical efficacy of abciximab in EPIC was maintained at 6-mo and 3-yr clinical follow-up, during which time investigators remained blinded to patient treatment randomization allocation (11,12). By 6 mo, the incidence of death, myocardial infarction, or

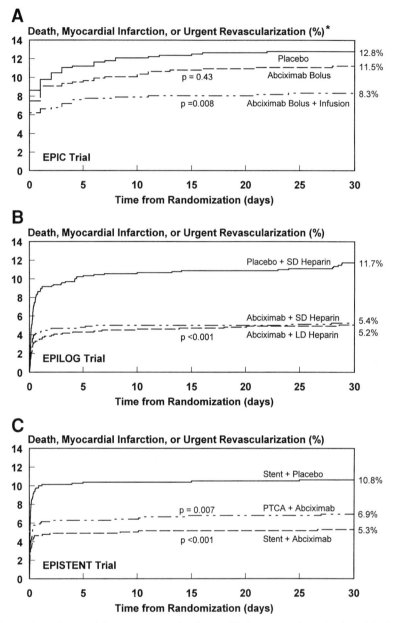

Fig. 2. Kaplan-Meier estimate of the percentage of patients with the composite endpoint of death, myocardial infarction, or urgent repeat revascularization within 30 d of randomization, according to treatment assignment in the EPIC (**A**), EPILOG (**B**), and EPISTENT (**C**) trials. *, The EPIC composite endpoint shown in A also includes stent or intraaortic balloon pump placement. LD = low-dose, weight-adjusted; PTCA = balloon coronary angioplasty; SD = standard-dose, weight-adjusted.

any revascularization (urgent or elective) was 35.1% in the placebo group, 32.6% in the abciximab bolus-only group, and 27.0% in the abciximab bolus and infusion group (23% relative risk reduction, *p* = 0.004) *(11)*. Moreover, use of abciximab was associated with reduction in the need for target vessel revascularization procedures by 6 mo, from 22.3%

Table 2
Components of 30-Day Composite Endpoint in EPIC, EPILOG, and EPISTENT Trials[a]

Endpoint	EPIC			EPILOG			EPISTENT		
	Placebo (n = 696)	Abcix bolus (n = 695)	Abcix bolus + infusion (n = 796)	Placebo (n = 708)	Abcix + LD heparin (n = 939)	Abcix + SD heparin (n = 918)	Stent + placebo (n = 809)	Stent + abcix (n = 794)	PTCA + abcix (n = 796)
Death	1.7	1.3	1.7	0.8	0.3	0.4	0.6	0.3	0.8
MI	8.6	6.2	5.2	8.7	3.7	3.8	9.6	4.5	5.3
Q-wave	2.3	1.0	0.8	0.8	0.4	0.5	1.4	0.9	1.5
Large non-Q wave (CK ≥ 5× control)	4.0	2.7	3.0	5.6	2.0	2.5	5.8	2.0	2.6
Small non-Q wave (CK 3–< 5× control)	2.3	2.4	1.4	1.9	1.2	0.9	2.2	1.5	1.1
Urgent revascularization	7.8	6.4	4.0	5.2	1.6	2.3	2.1	1.3	1.9
Urgent PCI	4.5	3.6	0.8	3.8	1.2	1.5	1.2	0.6	1.3
Urgent CABG	3.6	2.3	2.4	1.7	0.4	0.9	1.1	0.8	0.6

Abbreviations: Abcix, abciximab; CABG, coronary artery bypass graft surgery; CK, creative kinase; LD, low-dose, weight-adjusted; MI, myocardial infarction; PCI, percutaneous coronary intervention; PTCA, coronary balloon angioplasty; SD, standard-dose, weight-adjusted.
[a]Data are percent of patients.

among patients receiving placebo to 16.5% among those receiving the bolus and infusion of abciximab (26% relative risk reduction, $p = 0.007$). Most of the reduction in target vessel revascularization procedures occurred during the first 30 d of follow-up; when only patients who were free of events by 30 d were considered, target vessel revascularization rates were reduced during the period between 1 and 6 mo from 16.9 to 14.4% in the placebo and abciximab bolus and infusion groups, respectively. Although patients did not undergo routine angiographic follow-up in this trial, the finding in EPIC of a reduced need for repeat revascularization procedures over 6 mo led to speculation that this agent may reduce restenosis following coronary intervention.

By 3 yr following randomization, patients treated with abciximab had a sustained reduction in the composite endpoint of death, myocardial infarction, or any revascularization: 47.2% in the placebo group vs 41.1% in the bolus and infusion group ($p = 0.009$) *(12)*. Patients receiving the bolus only of abciximab had no long-term clinical benefit (composite event rate = 47.4% at 3 yr). Survival curves diverged during the first year of follow-up and remained largely parallel from 1 to 3 yr. There was a trend toward decreased mortality by abciximab over 3 yr in the overall cohort, with a more marked 60% reduction by abciximab among the 555 highest risk patients who had been enrolled with unstable angina or acute myocardial infarction (12.7% vs 5.1% in the placebo and abciximab bolus and infusion groups, respectively, $p = 0.01$).

SAFETY

The reduction in ischemic events by abciximab in EPIC was associated with a significant increased risk of bleeding complications, a finding that raised concerns regarding the potential clinical utility of this form of therapy. Compared with placebo, the bolus and infusion of abciximab resulted in a doubling in the rates of major bleeding (7 vs 14%, $p = 0.001$) and red blood cell transfusions (7 vs 15%, $p < 0.001$) *(9)*. Most of the excess bleeding events associated with abciximab occurred at sites of vascular access, although retroperitoneal or spontaneous gastrointestinal bleeding risk was increased as well. No differences among treatment groups in the incidence of intracranial hemorrhage were observed. At least two lines of evidence suggested that concurrent heparin therapy may have played a key role in the pathogenesis of bleeding among patients receiving abciximab in EPIC *(13)*. First, heparin dosages in the trial were not weight-adjusted, and a strong relationship was observed between the risk of bleeding and lighter body weight (and hence, relative "overdosage" of heparin on a per weight basis). Second, major bleeding rates were strongly correlated with total heparin dose and the intensity of anticoagulation (as measured by peak ACT) during the interventional procedure.

Based on the data from EPIC linking bleeding complications to heparin dosing, it was postulated that hemorrhagic risk associated with abciximab might be diminished by reduction in concomitant intraprocedural heparin dose and by removal of vascular access site sheaths during the 12-h abciximab infusion, thus eliminating the need for postprocedural heparin therapy. These strategies were tested in a subsequent pilot study, PROLOG *(14)*. A total of 103 patients undergoing coronary intervention with abciximab were randomized in a 2-by-2 factorial design to receive standard-dose, weight-adjusted heparin (100 U/kg initial bolus) or low-dose, weight-adjusted heparin (70 U/kg bolus) and to undergo late vascular sheath removal (after discontinuation of postprocedural 12-h abciximab and heparin infusion as in the EPIC trial) or early sheath removal (no postprocedural heparin, vascular sheath removal during abciximab infusion).

The efficacy of abciximab in preventing ischemic complications did not appear to be influenced by heparin dose or vascular sheath removal, as ischemic event rates were similar in all treatment groups. Bleeding rates, however, were attenuated independently and in an additive fashion by reduced-dose, weight-adjusted heparin dosing and by early removal of the vascular sheath (during infusion of abciximab). Composite bleeding rates (TIMI major or minor bleeding, blood transfusion, or vascular access site hematoma formation of >5 cm diameter) among patients randomized to standard heparin/late sheath removal, standard heparin/early sheath removal, low-dose heparin/late sheath removal, and low-dose heparin/early sheath removal were 32, 11, 12, and 4%, respectively.

Apart from bleeding, abciximab therapy in EPIC was associated with an increased incidence of thrombocytopenia (platelet count $<100,000/mm^3$ in 3.4 and 5.2% and platelet count $<50,000/mm^3$ in 0.7 and 1.6% of patients in the placebo and bolus plus infusion groups, respectively). Thrombocytopenia owing to abciximab resolved following discontinuation of the agent, with or without platelet transfusions. No patient exhibited an allergic or hypersensitivity response to abciximab, although human antichimeric antibody (HACA) IgG titers were measurable in 6.5% of patients by 30 d after receiving this agent.

The EPILOG Trial

The EPILOG trial was designed to explore the potential role of abciximab therapy in the broad population of patients undergoing coronary intervention and to address the excessive hemorrhagic risk observed in the EPIC trial. The first objective of the trial was therefore to determine whether the clinical benefits of abciximab therapy could be extended to all patients undergoing coronary intervention, regardless of their risk of ischemic complications. Moreover, based on the data from the pilot PROLOG trial, the second key objective was to evaluate whether the incidence of hemorrhagic complications associated with this agent could be reduced without loss of efficacy by weight adjusting or reducing the heparin dose.

Patient Population and Study Design

Patients undergoing elective or urgent percutaneous revascularization with a Food and Drug Administration (FDA)-approved device were enrolled between February and December, 1995 (15). As the EPIC trial suggested that abciximab provided substantial clinical benefit among patients with acute ischemic syndromes (16), patients with unstable angina and associated electrocardiographic changes meeting the EPIC criteria during the previous 24 h were excluded. Patients undergoing primary angioplasty for acute myocardial infarction were under evaluation in a separate dedicated trial at that time (RAPPORT; see Chapter 11) and were therefore also excluded from EPILOG. Other exclusion criteria included planned stent implantation (based on uncertainties regarding the optimal anticoagulation regimen during the time EPILOG was carried out) or rotational atherectomy (owing to the frequent occurrence of CK elevations following this procedure, which may have confounded assessment of the primary endpoint), percutaneous coronary intervention performed within the prior 3 mo, or conditions that would be associated with excessive bleeding risk.

Patients representing a broad spectrum of risk strata and clinical indications for revascularization were enrolled in the trial. Median age was 60 yr, 72% were male, 23% were diabetic, and 49% had a history of prior myocardial infarction. Balloon angioplasty was performed in 95% of cases, directional atherectomy in 5%, and unplanned ("bailout") stenting in 12%. Despite exclusion of patients meeting EPIC criteria for unstable angina, 47% of patients enrolled in EPILOG were considered to have other clinical criteria for unstable angina (without, for example, documented electrocardiographic changes or with symptoms occurring more than 24 hr before randomization). Other indications for revascularization were recent infarction in 21% and stable ischemia in 32%.

Patients were given aspirin and randomized in a double-blind fashion to one of three treatment groups: placebo with standard-dose, weight-adjusted heparin; abciximab with standard- dose, weight-adjusted heparin; or abciximab with low-dose, weight-adjusted heparin. For those receiving abciximab, a 0.25 mg/kg bolus was administered prior to balloon inflation or device activation, followed by a 0.125 µg/kg/min (maximum 10 µg/min) infusion for 12 h. The standard-dose weight-adjusted heparin regimen consisted of an initial heparin bolus prior to the interventional procedure of 100 U/kg (maximum 10,000 U), with additional weight-adjusted boluses according to an algorithm intended to achieve and maintain an ACT of ≥300 seconds. The low-dose weight-adjusted heparin group received an initial bolus of 70 U/kg (maximum 7000 U), with additional boluses as necessary to achieve and maintain an ACT of ≥200 s. Postprocedural heparin was discouraged, and vascular sheaths were to be removed within 2–6 h (during the abciximab infusion). Specific guidelines or algorithms were provided for management of vascular access sites, uncontrolled bleeding, urgent coronary artery bypass surgery, thrombocytopenia, and blood transfusions.

CLINICAL EFFICACY

Planned enrollment was 4800 patients, but the trial was terminated on the recommendation of the independent Data and Safety Monitoring Committee after entry of 2792 patients when an unexpectedly strong clinical benefit was observed at the first interim analysis. This interim analysis revealed that the incidence of death or myocardial infarction at 30 d was reduced from 8.2% among patients in the placebo group to 2.6 or 3.6% among patients treated with abciximab and low-dose or standard-dose heparin, respectively ($p < 0.0001$), meeting the prespecified stopping rule.

The incidence of the primary composite endpoint of death, myocardial infarction, or urgent revascularization at 30 d was 11.7% in the placebo group, 5.2% in the abciximab with low-dose heparin group (56% relative risk reduction, $p < 0.0001$), and 5.4% in the abciximab with standard- dose heparin group (54% relative reduction, $p < 0.0001$; Fig. 2B). The magnitude of risk reduction by abciximab was similar for each of the components of the composite endpoint (Table 2), and the treatment effect of abciximab with either heparin regimen was homogeneous across all patient groups. Proportional hazards regression identified no significant interactions between baseline variables and the efficacy of abciximab therapy.

The early suppression of ischemic events by abciximab in EPILOG was maintained at 6-mo and 1-yr follow-up. In the placebo group, the timing of acute ischemic complications was clustered early in the course following coronary intervention: Of the primary composite end-point events, 72% had accrued during the first 30 d (54% within 24 h), with an additional 19% occurring between 30 d and 6 mo and 9% between 6 mo and 1 yr. Therapy with abciximab resulted in a marked reduction in the risk of complications during the first 30-d period, after which time, incremental event rates were essentially equivalent among the three treatment arms. The composite endpoint (death, myocardial infarction, or urgent revascularization) event rates were 14.7, 8.4, and 8.3% at 6 mo and 16.1, 9.6, and 9.5% at 1 yr in the placebo, abciximab with low-dose heparin, and abciximab with standard-dose heparin groups, respectively.

Thus the treatment effect achieved by abciximab early (at 30 d) was maintained without attenuation throughout the 1-yr follow-up period: the absolute reduction in events (number of events prevented per 100 patients treated) in the combined abciximab groups versus placebo was 6.40 at 30 d, 6.35 at 6 mo, and 6.55 at 1 yr. In contrast to the findings of EPIC, however, rates of repeat target vessel revascularization converged after 30 d. There were no significant differences in rates of target vessel revascularization among the three treatment groups at 6 mo and 1 yr, indicating that abciximab had no effect on the incidence of "clinical restenosis." An angiographic substudy had been planned, in which 900 patients (300 in each treatment group) would return for 6-mo angiographic follow-up to assess the influence of abciximab on angiographic restenosis; because of the early termination of the trial, however, an insufficient number of patients were enrolled in the substudy to allow meaningful analysis of this secondary endpoint to be performed.

SAFETY

Hemorrhagic complications in EPILOG occurred infrequently and were not increased by abciximab therapy. Major bleeding occurred in 3.1, 2.0, and 3.5%, and red cell transfusions were required in 3.9, 1.9, and 3.3% of patients randomized to placebo, abciximab with low-dose heparin, and abciximab with standard-dose heparin, respectively. One patient in each abciximab group, but no patient in the placebo group, suffered a hemorrhagic stroke; two patients receiving abciximab with standard-dose heparin experienced other intracranial bleeding or nonhemorrhagic stroke. Compared with the experience in EPIC, bleeding in EPILOG was reduced in both placebo and abciximab groups, probably as a consequence of weight adjustment, reduction of heparin dosing, and early vascular sheath removal. The treatment effect of abciximab in reducing ischemic complications was enhanced in EPILOG compared with EPIC (56 and 35% relative reductions in the risk of the primary 30-d efficacy endpoint, respectively), suggesting that elimination of excess bleeding may permit the full potential benefit of this form of therapy to be realized.

Thrombocytopenia in association with abciximab appeared to occur less frequently in EPILOG than in EPIC, particularly among patients receiving the low-dose heparin regimen. Severe thrombocytopenia (nadir platelet count <50,000/mm^3) occurred in four (0.4%), four (0.4%), and eight (0.9%, $p = 0.292$) patients in the placebo, abciximab and low-dose heparin, and abciximab and standard-dose heparin groups, respectively.

The EPISTENT Trial

The introduction of GPIIb/IIIa receptor blockade into clinical interventional practice was paralleled by the widespread adoption of elective coronary stenting as the predominant means of percutaneous coronary intervention, based on the efficacy of these devices in reducing repeat revascularization rates (17,18). The initial pivotal studies of GPIIb/IIIa blockade had excluded enrollment of patients undergoing elective stent implantation, reserving the use of stents for "bailout" indications. In the high-risk setting of unplanned coronary stenting, the value of abciximab therapy in reducing ischemic complications had been documented (19), but the question of the role of enhanced antiplatelet therapy with GPIIb/IIIa inhibitors among patients *electively* undergoing revascularization by stents remained to be answered. The EPISTENT trial was designed to evaluate the clinical benefit of abciximab therapy in reducing ischemic complications among patients undergoing elective stent implantation, as well as to assess the clinical efficacy of abciximab (with balloon angioplasty) relative to stenting.

PATIENT POPULATION AND STUDY DESIGN

A total of 2399 patients undergoing elective or urgent percutaneous coronary revascularization were enrolled between July, 1996 and September, 1997 *(20)*. Patients were eligible for inclusion if they had at least one target lesion suitable for allocation to either stenting or balloon angioplasty and were not undergoing primary intervention in the setting of acute myocardial infarction. Exclusions for excessive bleeding risk were similar to those in the EPIC and EPILOG trials; patients were also excluded if a stent had previously been placed in the target lesion, any intervention had been performed in the prior 3 mo, or rotational atherectomy was planned.

EPISTENT enrolled a broad spectrum of patients, representing "real world" coronary stenting rather than the ideal or narrow subgroups assessed in previous stent vs balloon angioplasty trials. Mean age was 59 yr, 75% were male, 20% were diabetic, and 34% had a history of myocardial infarction. Indications for revascularization were (not mutually exclusive) recent infarction (within 7 d) in 16%, unstable angina within the prior 48 h in 36%, unstable ischemic symptoms within the prior 6 mo in 57%, and stable ischemia in 43% of patients.

Patients were treated with aspirin and randomized to one of three treatment groups: stent plus placebo, stent plus abciximab (0.25 mg/kg bolus and 0.125 µg/kg/min infusion for 12 h), or balloon angioplasty (PTCA) plus abciximab. Randomization to abciximab or placebo was blinded in the stented patients. Stenting was to be carried out using the Johnson & Johnson design unless this stent could not be deployed. Stent implantation in the PTCA plus abciximab group was to be reserved for clear "bailout" indications, specified by protocol, rather than suboptimal results. Patients randomized to treatment with abciximab received adjunctive heparin according to the EPILOG low-dose, weight-adjusted regimen (70 U/kg bolus, ACT ≥200 s), whereas those randomized to placebo received the standard-dose, weight-adjusted regimen (100 U/kg bolus, ACT ≥300 s). Vascular sheaths were to be removed early without postprocedural heparin infusion. Ticlopidine was administered following stent placement. As in the EPILOG trial, management guidelines and algorithms were provided for management of bleeding, emergency bypass surgery, blood transfusions, vascular access site care, and thrombocytopenia.

To evaluate the influence of abciximab therapy on restenosis following percutaneous coronary intervention, an angiographic substudy was performed. Approximately 900 patients, 300 in each treatment group, were enrolled consecutively at participating clinical centers to return for systematic angiography and quantitative measurements of target lesion coronary luminal dimensions at 6 months following their index procedure.

CLINICAL EFFICACY

Stents were successfully deployed in 96% of patients for whom they were assigned; 27% of these patients required two or more stents. Crossover to unplanned stenting occurred in only 19.3% of patients in the PTCA plus abciximab group, attesting to the compliance of clinical investigators in reserving stents in this group for clear "bailout" indications. Angiographic complications of abrupt closure, transient closure, or sidebranch closure occurred infrequently but were observed in fewer patients receiving abciximab than placebo.

The primary efficacy composite endpoint of death, myocardial infarction, or urgent repeat revascularization by 30 d following randomization occurred in 10.8% of patients in the stent plus placebo arm, 6.9% of patients in the PTCA plus abciximab arm (36% relative risk reduction, $p = 0.007$), and 5.3% of patients in the stent plus abciximab arm (51% relative risk reduction, $p < 0.001$) (Fig. 2C). Most ischemic events occurred within the first 12 h following the procedure. Compared with stenting alone, adjunctive use of abciximab with stenting reduced rates of death, myocardial infarction, and urgent repeat revascularization, with a similar magnitude of treatment effect for each of the components of the composite endpoint (Table 2). Compared with stenting alone, abciximab with PTCA was associated with equivalent rates of death and urgent repeat revascularization but greater safety with regard to lower rates of myocardial infarction (Table 2). The predominant influence of abciximab on myocardial infarction (86%) was reduction in Q-wave or large non-Q-wave infarction (defined prospectively by CK-MB ≥5 times normal); for the secondary composite endpoint of death or large myocardial infarction (Q-wave or large non-Q-wave infarction), event rates were reduced from 7.8% in the stent plus placebo group to 4.7% in the PTCA plus abciximab group (40% relative risk reduction, $p = 0.009$) and 3.0% in the stent plus abciximab group (62% relative risk reduction, $p < 0.001$). The treatment effect of abciximab was homogeneous across all patient subgroups, as defined by their baseline characteristics or clinical indications for revascularization.

Longer term clinical follow-up was performed at 6 mo *(21)* and 1 yr after randomization *(22)*. Two principal endpoints were assessed at 6 mo: (1) a composite of death or myocardial infarction, and (2) the incidence of repeat target vessel revascularization *(21)*. The rate of death or myocardial infarction was 11.4% in the stent plus placebo group, 5.6% in the stent plus abciximab group ($p < 0.001$), and 7.8% in the PTCA plus abciximab group ($p = 0.013$). The absolute reduction in this composite endpoint (number of events prevented per 100 patients treated) compared with stenting alone was 5.5 at 30 d and 5.8 at 6 mo in the stent plus abciximab group and 4.4 at 30 d and 3.6 at 6 mo in the PTCA plus abciximab group. At 6 mo, mortality was significantly reduced by stenting compared with PTCA among patients receiving abciximab (0.5% vs 1.8%, $p = 0.018$).

By 1 year, the combined treatment resulted in a lower mortality rate than either stenting or abciximab alone (stent + placebo = 2.4%, PTCA + abciximab = 2.1%, stent + abciximab = 1.0%, $p = 0.037$) *(22)*. Cause of death was known to be cardiac in 10 of 19 patients treated with stenting alone, 12 of 17 treated with PTCA + abciximab, and 5 of 8 treated with the combination of stenting + abciximab. Sudden deaths, all presumed to be cardiac, occurred in 7, 3, and 1 patients in the stent + placebo, PTCA + abciximab, and stent + abciximab groups, respectively; sudden deaths all occurred within 180 d of randomization. By multivariate analysis, significant correlates of 1-yr mortality were placebo-stent randomization (compared with abciximab-stent), prior congestive heart failure, diabetes mellitus requiring insulin, age >70 years, less preprocedural stenosis, and postprocedural coronary occlusion.

Rates of repeat target vessel revascularization (percutaneous or surgical) were 10.6% in the stent plus placebo group, 8.7% in the stent plus abciximab group ($p = 0.216$), and 15.4% in the PTCA plus abciximab group ($p = 0.005$) by 6 mo. Among stented patients, treatment with abciximab rather than placebo was associated with a nonsignificant trend toward reduced rates of target vessel revascularization (18% relative risk reduction, $p = 0.215$). Among the subgroup of patients with diabetes, repeat target vessel revascularization rates following stent implantation were significantly reduced by abciximab. Stenting alone (with placebo) did not reduce the incidence of subsequent target vessel revascularization procedures compared with PTCA among diabetics, whereas the rate of this endpoint was halved by the combination of abciximab and stenting.

An angiographic substudy was performed of the first 899 patients in the trial. Minimal luminal diameters (MLDs) post intervention and early gain were significantly better among patients undergoing stenting rather than PTCA. Among stented patients, net gain in MLD was significantly better with abciximab than placebo (0.86 vs 0.73 mm, $p = 0.025$), with a trend toward greater follow-up MLD. Among diabetics, net gain and follow-up MLD were substantially greater among stented patients receiving abciximab than placebo.

SAFETY

Bleeding complications occurred infrequently in EPISTENT and were not increased by abciximab therapy. Major bleeding occurred in 2.2, 1.5, and 1.4%, and transfusions (red cells or platelets, including those related to coronary bypass surgery) were required in 2.2, 2.8, and 3.1% of patients in the stent plus placebo, stent plus abciximab, and PTCA plus abciximab groups, respectively (all p = NS) No patient in the trial suffered an intracranial hemorrhage within 30 d after randomization. Severe thrombocytopenia (platelet count <50,000/mm^3) occurred in 0% of placebo-treated patients and 0.9–1.1% of abciximab-treated patients.

Pooled Trial Findings

Results of analyses of pooled results from the major abciximab interventional trials have demonstrated consistent findings regarding mortality reduction and clinical efficacy in major patient subgroups.

MORTALITY

The trials of GPIIb/IIIa blockade during coronary intervention were not designed with sufficient sample size to detect reductions in short-term mortality, given that the mortality rates at 30 days in this population of patients are expected to be in the range of only 0.5–1.0%. In combination with stenting, however, the magnitude of mortality reduction by abciximab in the EPISTENT trial was of sufficient magnitude (approx 60% risk reduction) to achieve statistical significance by 1 yr, as described in the section above *(22)*. The strength of evidence for reduction in mortality was increased by combining the long-term findings of the different abciximab interventional trials *(23)*. The pooled results of all studies using the bolus and 12-h infusion regimen of abciximab compared with placebo demonstrated mortality rates in the placebo and abciximab groups, respectively, of 1.61% vs 1.14% at 30 d [hazard ratio (HR) = 0.71, 95% confidence interval (CI) 0.50–1.01, $p = 0.056$], 2.86% vs 2.18% at 6 mo (HR = 0.76, 95% CI 0.59–0.99, $p = 0.040$), and 3.33% vs 2.39% at 1 yr (HR = 0.72, 95% CI 0.53–0.97, $p = 0.031$). Similar findings have been reported with longer follow-up, to 7 yr, 4.5 yr, and 3 yr in the EPIC, EPILOG, and EPISTENT trials, respectively *(24)*. The magnitude of long-term reduction in mortality by abciximab is proportional to the mortality risk, as predicted by a clinical risk score, providing further pathophysiologic support for the validity of this finding *(24)*.

SUBGROUPS

Although a treatment effect of abciximab has been observed across the broad spectrum of patients studied in different clinical trials of percutaneous coronary intervention, certain subgroups appeared to derive enhanced benefit. Prominent among these were patients with unstable ischemic syndromes. In the EPIC trial, unstable angina was defined by the presence of early (within 7 d) postinfarction angina, at least two episodes of angina occurring at rest, or angina occurring despite heparin and nitrate therapy; transient electrocardiographic ST-T wave changes accompanying these clinical presentations were required to confirm the diagnosis. Among 470 patients with unstable angina who received study drug and underwent intervention in that trial, the 30-d composite efficacy endpoint rate was decreased by 71% with the abciximab bolus and infusion, from 13.1 to 3.8% ($p = 0.004$) (16). The most serious endpoints of death or myocardial infarction were reduced by 94% at 30 d (11.1% vs 0.6 % in the placebo and abciximab bolus and infusion groups, respectively, $p < 0.001$) and by 88% at 6 mo (16.6% vs 2.0% in the placebo and bolus plus infusion groups, respectively, $p < 0.001$). The magnitude of this reduction by abciximab in the risk of death and myocardial infarction was significantly greater among patients with unstable angina than among those enrolled without unstable angina (interaction: $p = 0.004$ at 30 d, and $p = 0.003$ at 6 months). On 3-yr follow-up of the 555 highest risk patients in EPIC enrolled with unstable angina or acute myocardial infarction, mortality was significantly reduced by abciximab, from 12.7 to 5.1% ($p = 0.01$) (12). Similarly, a pooled analysis of the EPIC, EPILOG, and EPISTENT trials demonstrated a reduction in rates of death or myocardial infarction from 13.2 to 6.7% ($p < 0.001$) by 1 yr among 3478 patients with acute coronary syndromes, compared with a reduction from 13.1 to 9.0% ($p < 0.001$) among 2972 patients with stable ischemia.

Given the greater prevalence, complexity, and complications of atherosclerosis among diabetics, these patients constitute a sizable and important proportion of those for whom coronary revascularization is indicated. However, both percutaneous and surgical coronary revascularization procedures in this patient group are associated with greater risk for complications and worse long-term prognosis than those performed in patients without diabetes. A consistent pattern of benefit with regard to suppression of ischemic complications among diabetic patients has emerged from the abciximab interventional trials, with a magnitude of treatment effect in diabetics equivalent to or greater than that in nondiabetics. In EPILOG, the hazard ratio for the reduction by abciximab in risk of death or myocardial infarction by 6 mo following balloon angioplasty was 0.36 (95% CI = 0.21–0.61) among diabetics vs 0.60 (95% CI = 0.44–0.82) among nondiabetics (25). Similarly, among stented patients in EPISTENT, 6-mo rates of death or myocardial infarction were decreased by abciximab from 12.7 to 6.2% in diabetics ($p = 0.041$) and from 11.0 to 5.4% in nondiabetics ($p > 0.001$) (26).

The pooled results of 1-yr follow-up among patients in the EPIC, EPILOG, and EPISTENT trials provided compelling evidence of an enhanced mortality benefit of abciximab among diabetic patients (27). In the placebo groups, diabetics were at nearly twice the mortality risk at 1 yr as were their nondiabetic counterparts (4.5% vs 2.6% in diabetics and nondiabetics, respectively), but this difference was largely neutralized with abciximab therapy (2.5% vs 1.9%, respectively) (Fig. 3A). Insulin-requiring diabetics had a particularly high mortality rate with placebo, although their risk was halved by treatment with abciximab (8.1% vs 4.2%). Similarly, patients who were classified as insulin resistant on the basis of diabetes, hypertension, and obesity had their mortality reduced from 5.1 to 2.3% with abciximab. The efficacy of abciximab was particularly apparent among diabetic patients who received stents (Fig. 3B), in whom 1-yr mortality was decreased over threefold to levels equivalent to that in patients without diabetes.

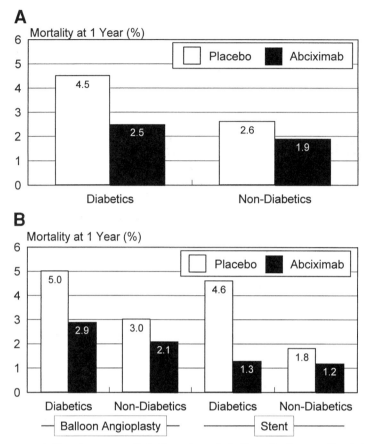

Fig. 3. One-year mortality rates among diabetic and nondiabetic patients according to treatment with placebo or abciximab in a pooled analysis of the EPIC, EPILOG, and EPISTENT trials. (**A**) All diabetic versus nondiabetic patients. (**B**) Outcome separately for patients treated with balloon angioplasty or stents. (Data from ref. *27.*)

The effect of abciximab on target vessel revascularization or restenosis in diabetic patients has been inconsistent. In EPIC and EPILOG, rates of target vessel revascularization were not diminished by abciximab following balloon angioplasty in diabetic patients *(25)*, whereas diabetics in EPISTENT experienced a 50% reduction in the need for target vessel revascularization following stenting (16.6% vs 8.1% in the placebo and abciximab groups, respectively, $p = 0.021$) *(21)*. Abciximab therapy reduced the rate of target vessel revascularization among diabetics in EPISTENT to that of nondiabetics (9.0 and 8.8% in the stent/placebo and stent/abciximab arms, respectively), suggesting that this therapy could neutralize the propensity for restenosis imparted by diabetes mellitus. This apparent effect of abciximab on "clinical restenosis" among diabetics in EPISTENT was supported by findings of the angiographic substudy, in which angiographic indices of in-stent restenosis were improved among diabetics in the abciximab vs placebo arms *(26)*. It is also relevant that diabetic patients in a separate placebo-controlled trial of abciximab during stenting for acute myocardial infarction (ADMIRAL) had significantly lower rates of target vessel revascularization at 6 mo (37.5% vs 13.8%, $p = 0.046$) associated with abciximab therapy *(28)*.

CONCLUSIONS

The EPIC, EPILOG, and EPISTENT randomized, placebo-controlled trials provide a compelling body of evidence among over 7000 patients of the unequivocal and profound efficacy of abciximab in reducing the ischemic complications of death, myocardial infarction, or urgent repeat revascularization associated with percutaneous coronary interventional procedures. This clinical benefit is sustained for at least 3 yr of follow-up and appears to extend to all patients treated, regardless of their underlying risk profile or the modality chosen for percutaneous revascularization. Specific issues regarding optimization of efficacy and safety in the use of this and other agents of its class will be addressed in Chapter 9.

REFERENCES

1. Mascelli MA, Worley S, Veriabo NJ, et al. Rapid assessment of platelet function with a modified whole-blood aggregometer in percutaneous transluminal coronary angioplasty patients receiving anti-GP IIb/IIIa therapy. Circulation 1997;96:3860–3866.
2. Tcheng JE, Ellis SG, George BS, et al. Pharmacodynamics of chimeric glycoprotein IIb/IIIa integrin antiplatelet antibody Fab 7E3 in high-risk coronary angioplasty. Circulation 1994;90:1757–1764.
3. Mascelli MA, Lance ET, Damaraju L, Wagner CL, Weisman HF, Jordan RE. Pharmacodynamic profile of short-term abciximab treatment demonstrates prolonged platelet inhibition with gradual recovery from GP IIb/IIIa receptor blockade. Circulation 1998;97:1680–1688.
4. Ellis SG, Tcheng JE, Navetta FI, et al. Safety and antiplatelet effect of murine monoclonal antibody 7E3 Fab directed against platelet glycoprotein IIb/IIIa in patients undergoing elective coronary angioplasty. Coron Artery Dis 1993;4:167–175.
5. Kleiman NS, Raizner AE, Jordan R, et al. Differential inhibition of platelet aggregation induced by adenosine diphosphate or a thrombin receptor-activating peptide in patients treated with bolus chimeric 7E3 Fab: implications for inhibition of the internal pool of GPIIb/IIIa receptors. J Am Coll Cardiol 1995; 26:1665–1671.
6. Steinhubl S, Kottke-Marchant K, Moliterno D, et al. Attainment and maintenance of platelet inhibition through standard dosing of abciximab in diabetic and nondiabetic patients undergoing percutaneous coronary intervention. Circulation 1999;100:1977–1982.
7. Rao AK, Pratt C, Berke A, et al., for TIMI Investigators. Thrombolysis in myocardial infarction (TIMI) trial—Phase I: hemorrhagic manifestations and changes in plasma fibrinogen and the fibrinolytic system in patients treated with recombinant tissue plasminogen activator and streptokinase. J Am Coll Cardiol 1988;11:1–11.
8. Landefeld LS, Cook EF, Hatley M, Weisberg M, Goldman L. Identification and preliminary validation of predictors of major bleeding in hospitalized patients starting anticoagulant therapy. Am J Med 1987; 82:703–713.
9. EPIC Investigators. Use of a monoclonal antibody directed against the platelet glycoprotein IIb/IIIa receptor in high-risk coronary angioplasty. N Engl J Med 1994;330:956–961.
10. Ellis SG, Lincoff AM, Miller D, et al., for the EPIC and EPILOG Investigators. Reduction in complications of angioplasty with abciximab occurs largely independently of baseline lesion morphology. J Am Coll Cardiol 1998;32:1619–1623.
11. Topol EJ, Califf RM, Weisman HS, et al., for the EPIC Investigators. Reduction of clinical restenosis following coronary intervention with early administration of platelet IIb/IIIa integrin blocking antibody. Lancet 1994;343:881–886.
12. Topol EJ, Ferguson JJ, Weisman HF, et al., for the EPIC Investigator Group. Long-term protection from myocardial ischemic events in a randomized trial of brief integrin β3 blockade with percutaneous coronary intervention. JAMA 1997;278:479–484.
13. Aguirre FV, Topol EJ, Ferguson JJ, et al., for the EPIC Investigators. Bleeding complications with the chimeric antibody to platelet glycoprotein IIb/IIIa integrin in patients undergoing percutaneous coronary intervention. Circulation 1995;91:2882–2890.
14. Lincoff AM, Tcheng JE, Califf RM, et al., for the PROLOG Investigators. Standard versus low dose weight-adjusted heparin in patients treated with the platelet glycoprotein IIb/IIIa receptor antibody fragment abciximab (c7E3 Fab) during percutaneous coronary revascularization. Am J Cardiol 1997;79:286–291.

15. EPILOG Investigators. Platelet glycoprotein IIb/IIIa blockade with abciximab with low-dose heparin during percutaneous coronary revascularization. N Engl J Med 1997;336:1689–1696.

16. Lincoff AM, Califf RM, Anderson KM, et al. Evidence for prevention of death and myocardial infarction with platelet membrane glycoprotein IIb/IIIa receptor blockade by c7E3 Fab (abciximab) among patients with unstable angina undergoing percutaneous coronary revascularization. J Am Coll Cardiol 1997;30:149–156.

17. Serruys PW, de Jaegere P, Kiemeneij F, et al., for the Benestent Study Group. A comparison of balloon-expandable-stent implantation with balloon angioplasty in patients with coronary artery disease. N Engl J Med 1994;331:489–495.

18. Fischman DL, Leon MB, Baim DS, et al., for the Stent Restenosis Study Investigators. A randomized comparison of coronary-stent placement and balloon angioplasty in the treatment of coronary artery disease. N Engl J Med 1994;331:496–501.

19. Kereiakes DJ, Lincoff AM, Miller DP, et al., for the EPILOG Investigators. Abciximab therapy and unplanned coronary stent deployment. Favorable effects on stent use, clinical outcomes, and bleeding complications. Circulation 1998;97:857–864.

20. EPISTENT Investigators. Randomised placebo-controlled and balloon-angioplasty-controlled trial to assess safety of coronary stenting with use of platelet glycoprotein IIb/IIIa blockade. Lancet 1998;352:87–92.

21. Lincoff AM, Califf RM, Moliterno DJ, et al., for the Evaluation of Platelet IIb/IIIa Inhibition in Stenting Investigators. Complementary clinical benefits of coronary-artery stenting and blockade of platelet glycoprotein IIb/IIIa receptors. N Engl J Med 1999;341:319–327.

22. Topol EJ, Mark DB, Lincoff AM, et al., on behalf of the EPISTENT Investigators. Enhanced survival with platelet glycoprotein IIb/IIIa blockade in patients undergoing coronary stenting: one year outcomes and health care economic implications from a multicenter, randomized trial. Lancet 1999;354:2019–2024.

23. Anderson KM, Califf RM, Stone GW, et al. Long-term mortality benefit with abciximab in patients undergoing percutaneous coronary intervention. J Am Coll Cardiol 2001;37:2059–2065.

24. Kereiakes DJ, Lincoff AM, Anderson KM, et al., on behalf of the EPIC E, and EPISTENT Investigators. Abciximab survival advantage following percutaneous coronary intervention is predicted by clinical risk profile. Am J Cardiol 2002;90:628–630.

25. Kleiman NS, Lincoff AM, Kereiakes DJ, et al., for the EPILOG Investigators. Diabetes mellitus, glycoprotein IIb/IIIa blockade, and heparin. Evidence of a complex interaction in a multicenter trial. Circulation 1998;97:1912–1920.

26. Marso S, Lincoff A, Ellis S, et al., EPISTENT Investigators. Optimizing the percutaneous interventional outcomes for patients with diabetes mellitus. Circulation 1999;100:2477–2484.

27. Bhatt D, Marso S, Lincoff A, Wolski K, Ellis S, Topol E. Abciximab reduces mortality in diabetics following percutaneous intervention. J Am Coll Cardiol 2000;35:922–928.

28. Montalescot G, Barragan P, Wittenberg O, et al., for the ADMIRAL Investigators. Platelet glycoprotein IIb/IIIa inhibition with coronary stenting for acute myocardial infarction. N Engl J Med 2001;344:1895–1903.

6

Eptifibatide in Coronary Intervention
The IMPACT and ESPRIT Trials

Jean-Pierre Dery, MD,
J. Conor O'Shea, MD,
and James E. Tcheng, MD

CONTENTS

INTRODUCTION
PLATELET PHYSIOLOGY AND EPTIFIBATIDE
IMPACT
IMPACT HI/LOW
IMPACT II
ESPRIT
REFERENCES

INTRODUCTION

Although percutaneous transluminal coronary intervention has revolutionized the management of patients with coronary artery disease, this technologic advance is neither innocuous nor a panacea. In addition to the technical limitations of the procedure, it is now well recognized that serious vascular injury is caused by the treatment device, which creates an ideal milieu for coronary thrombosis *(1–3)*. Clinical trials of the monoclonal antibody abciximab (c7E3 Fab; ReoPro™, Eli Lilly and Company/Centocor), an agent that blocks the platelet glycoprotein (GP) IIb/IIIa integrin, have clearly documented that inhibition of this receptor during coronary intervention reduces thrombotic complications and improves clinical outcomes *(4–8)*. These positive clinical trial results, coupled with a clearer understanding of platelet physiology, have stimulated the search and encouraged the development of other parenteral inhibitors of the GPIIb/IIIa receptor.

Eptifibatide (Integrilin™, Millenium Pharmaceuticals), a peptide inhibitor of GPIIb/IIIa, is one of a new class of parenteral agents designed and synthesized using the techniques of molecular engineering. This chapter briefly outlines the biopharmacology of

From: *Contemporary Cardiology: Platelet Glycoprotein IIb/IIIa*
Inhibitors in Cardiovascular Disease, 2nd Edition
Edited by: A. M. Lincoff © Humana Press Inc., Totowa, NJ

eptifibatide and then focuses on the experience to date with this novel compound in the setting of coronary intervention.

PLATELET PHYSIOLOGY AND EPTIFIBATIDE

As reviewed in other chapters, the central role of the platelet in vascular thrombosis is now clear. The final act among the processes leading to thrombus formation is mediated by the binding of dimeric adhesion proteins such as fibrinogen and von Willebrand factor to activated GPIIb/IIIa (9,10). The GPIIb/IIIa receptor recognizes an Arg-Gly-Asp (RGD) sequence as well as a Lys-Gln-Ala-Gly-Asp-Val sequence on the fibrinogen molecule (11). These two areas serve as the linkage sites for GPIIb/IIIa receptor binding with fibrinogen (12).

The path leading to the synthesis of eptifibatide has its roots in surveys of naturally occurring proteins. In these surveys, RGD-containing peptides isolated from pit viper venoms were discovered to bind the GPIIb/IIIa receptor and inhibit its function (13). One in particular, barbourin, a protein isolated from the venom of the southeastern pygmy rattlesnake *Sistrurus m. barbouri*, was found to have a higher specificity for GPIIb/IIIa than other molecules. Analysis of the differences in amino acid sequences suggested that the reason for the increased specificity of barbourin was that it differed by a single amino acid substitution of lysine (K) for arginine (14,15).

Eptifibatide was created based on the KGD sequence found in barbourin. It is a cyclic, constrained heptapeptide with a terminal half-life of approx 1.5–2.5 h. In addition to the specificity for GPIIb/IIIa conferred by the KGD sequence, eptifibatide was engineered with a ring structure to impart resistance to proteolysis. Biologic activity is concentration-dependent, and the agent is cleared from the body largely via excretion in the urine as an intact compound (16).

IMPACT

Two Phase II trials of eptifibatide as an adjunct to percutaneous coronary revascularization were conducted in the early 1990s to establish pharmacodynamic and (preliminary) safety profiles of the agent. The first, the Integrelin to Minimize Platelet Aggregation and Coronary Thrombosis (IMPACT) study, was a randomized, placebo-controlled trial of 150 patients undergoing elective percutaneous coronary intervention (17). Patients were allocated to one of three treatment approaches: placebo, a 90 µg/kg bolus before the initiation of the coronary intervention followed by a 1.0 µg/kg/min infusion of eptifibatide for 4 h after the bolus, or the same 90 µg/kg bolus followed by a 1.0 µg/kg/min infusion of eptifibatide for 12 h. Patients were followed for 30 d after the procedure; 101 patients were assigned to eptifibatide, and 49 received placebo. In blood collected in citrate, the 90 µg/kg bolus produced an 86% inhibition of platelet aggregation to stimulation with 20 µM adenosine diphosphate. There was a trend toward lower composite adverse clinical event rates with the longer infusions (12.2% for placebo, 9.6% for the 4-h infusion, and 4.1% for the 12-h infusion, p = NS). Major bleeding event rates were 5% with either eptifibatide treatment compared with 8% with placebo. Minor bleeding, primarily at the vascular access site, occurred in 40% vs 14%, respectively. Although the bleeding profile appeared acceptable, it was suspected that higher dosing of eptifibatide (and potentially better clinical efficacy) might still be possible. This led to the second Phase II study in angioplasty, IMPACT Hi/Low.

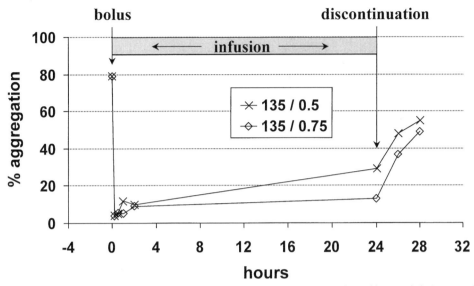

Fig. 1. Inhibition of platelet aggregation with eptifibatide—the IMPACT Hi/Low trial. Among the four different doses of Integrilin evaluated in the IMPACT Hi/Low trial, the 135 μg/kg bolus plus 0.75 μg/kg/min infusion produced a sustained inhibition of platelet aggregation below 20% of baseline, whereas the 135 μg/kg bolus plus 0.5 μg/kg/min infusion permitted some recovery of platelet function by the end of the 24-h infusion. The pharmacodynamic profiles of both regimens were nearly identical in the first 4 h. Data are raw (nonnormalized) results; assays were conducted on blood suspended in citrate. (From ref. *18*.)

IMPACT HI/LOW

The IMPACT Hi/Low study was the second phase II, dose-ranging study of eptifibatide as an adjunct to coronary intervention. The IMPACT Hi/Low study was a placebo-controlled, randomized, dose-escalation trial that measured ex vivo platelet aggregation, bleeding time, and plasma eptifibatide concentration in 73 patients *(18)*. Four different bolus plus infusion combinations were evaluated. A bolus dose of eptifibatide of 180 μg/kg followed by a 1.0 μg/kg/min infusion produced almost complete inhibition (>95%) of platelet aggregation (in whole blood anticoagulated with citrate). Problematically, increasing rates of both minor and major bleeding were observed with increasing doses of eptifibatide. Given the available pharmacodynamic profiles coupled with concerns about bleeding, dosing regimens lower than the maximal doses tested in the IMPACT Hi/Low trial (Fig. 1) were ultimately selected for testing in the phase III study of eptifibatide, the IMPACT II study.

IMPACT II

The IMPACT II study was designed as a pivotal, Phase III study of eptifibatide as an adjunct to coronary intervention. IMPACT II was a multicenter, parallel-group, double-blind, randomized, controlled clinical trial that began patient recruitment in November 1993. It was carried out at 82 centers in the United States, with enrollment closed in November 1994 after 4010 patients had been entered *(19)*. The study specifically included a representative cross-section of all patients undergoing percutaneous revascularization.

Patients were assigned to one of three treatment regimens: a bolus of 135 µg/kg of eptifibatide initiated just before coronary intervention followed by an infusion of 0.5 µg/kg/min of eptifibatide for 20–24 h; a 135 µg/kg bolus followed by a 0.75 µg/kg/min infusion for 20–24 h; or placebo bolus and placebo infusion. All patients received aspirin 325 mg by mouth before (and continued thereafter) the coronary intervention. Heparin was given as a 100 U/kg bolus before the intervention, with additional heparin as needed during the procedure, to attain and maintain an activated clotting time (ACT) between 300 and 350 s.

The primary clinical endpoint was the occurrence within 30 d of the composite of death, myocardial infarction [periprocedural creative kinase (CK) MB ≥3 times the upper limit of normal], urgent or emergency repeat coronary intervention, urgent or emergency coronary artery bypass surgery, or placement of an intracoronary stent during the index procedure for the management of true abrupt closure. The principal safety endpoints were major bleeding, blood transfusion requirements, and stroke. Major bleeding was defined as intracranial hemorrhage or overt bleeding associated with a decrease in hemoglobin of >5 g/dL or a decrease in packed cell volume of ≥15% from baseline.

Primary Composite Clinical Efficacy

In IMPACT II, the clinical efficacy was determined with analyses based on the intention to treat principle. Two different approaches were used. The first, the *treated as randomized* analysis, was of the 3871 (96.5%) patients who received any study drug (whether or not they underwent angioplasty). This approach was used because the delay between randomization allocation (which occurred before arrival of the patient in the catheterization laboratory) and actual treatment administration (which occurred in the catheterization laboratory just before the coronary intervention) resulted in dropout of patients unrelated to either randomization or treatment allocation. Unless otherwise indicated, data presented in this chapter are derived from the treated as randomized analyses. The second approach, the *all randomized* analysis, included all patients enrolled in the study, whether or not the patient received any study drug and/or underwent coronary intervention. All endpoint events were adjudicated by a blinded endpoint committee.

The *treated as randomized* analysis (Table 1) demonstrated a statistically significant 22% reduction in the primary composite clinical endpoint at 30 d with the 135/0.5 treatment approach compared with placebo [9.1% vs 11.6%, $p = 0.035$; odds ratio 0.76 (0.59–0.98)]. A trend toward improved outcomes was observed with the 135/0.75 dosing approach (10.0% vs 11.6%, $p = 0.18$). In absolute terms, treatment with the 135/0.5 regimen prevented 25 events per 1000 patients in the first 30 d. The *all randomized* analysis showed only strong trends favoring a treatment effect. The composite primary endpoint occurred in 151 (11.4%) patients in the placebo group compared with 124 (9.2%) in the 135/0.5 treatment group ($p = 0.063$) and 132 (9.9%) in the 135/0.75 treatment group ($p = 0.22$).

Also included in Table 1 are the primary composite end-point rates as determined by the principal investigators; in other words, events as recorded on the case report forms before adjudication. Several comments can be made about these data. Events documented by the site probably reflect those that were the most clinically apparent (in contrast to those picked up through the meticulous adjudication process). Also, a greater relative difference was reported by the principal investigators than by the adjudication committee; this would suggest that the rigorous adjudication process may produce a conservative underestimate of the actual benefits of drug treatment.

Table 1

Composite Clinical Efficacy Results: Patients Receiving any Study Drug (Treated as Randomized Analyses)

Endpoint	Placebo (n = 1285)	Eptifibatide 35/0.5 (n = 1300)	Eptifibatide 135/0.75 (n = 1286)
24-Hour composite endpoint, n (%; 95% CI)	123 (9.6; 8.0–11.2)	86 (6.6; 5.3–8.0)	89 (6.9; 5.5–8.3)
Significance vs placebo		p = 0.006	p = 0.014
Odds ratio vs placebo (95% CI for OR)	—	0.67 (0.50–0.89)	0.70 (0.53–0.93)
30-Day composite endpoint, n (%; 95% CI)	149 (11.6; 9.8–13.3)	118 (9.1; 7.5–10.6)	128 (10.0; 8.3–11.6)
Significance vs placebo		p = 0.035	p = 0.18
Odds ratio vs placebo (95% CI for OR)	—	0.76 (0.59–0.98)	0.84 (0.66–1.08)
24-Hour composite endpoint as determined by the Principal Investigators, n (%; 95% CI)	82 (6.4; 5.0–7.7)	49 (3.8; 2.7–4.8)	50 (3.9; 2.8–4.9)
Significance vs placebo		p = 0.002	p = 0.004
Odds ratio vs placebo (95% CI for OR)	—	0.57 (0.40–0.83)	0.59 (0.41–0.85)
30-Day composite endpoint as determined by the Principal Investigators, n (%; 95% CI)	103 (8.0; 6.5–9.5)	74 (5.7; 4.4–7.0)	84 (6.5; 5.2–7.9)
Significance vs placebo		p = 0.018	p = 0.142
Odds ratio vs placebo (95% CI for OR)	—	0.69 (0.51–0.94)	0.80 (0.59–1.08)
In-laboratory abrupt closure, n (%; 95% CI)	66 (5.1; 3.9–6.3)	36 (2.8; 1.9–3.7)	48 (3.7; 2.7–4.8)
Significance vs placebo		p = 0.002	p = 0.081
Odds ratio vs placebo (95% CI for OR)	—	0.53 (0.35–0.80)	0.72 (0.49–1.05)

Table 2
30-Day Composite Clinical Efficacy Results by Baseline Characteristics[a]

Characteristic	Eptifibatide 135/0.5 (n = 1300)	Eptifibatide 135/0.75 (n = 1286)
Age		
≤65 yr	0.687 (0.493, 0.958)	0.816 (0.596, 1.117)
>65 yr	0.875 (0.586, 1.306)	0.897 (0.593, 1.356)
Gender		
Male	0.706 (0.523, 0.954)	0.834 (0.626, 1.111)
Female	0.919 (0.565, 1.495)	0.870 (0.524, 1.447)
Tertiles		
Lowest weight (≤77 kg)	0.847 (0.557, 1.288)	0.951 (0.629, 1.439)
Middle weight (77–90 kg)	0.781 (0.507, 1.202)	0.846 (0.549, 1.304)
Highest weight (>90 kg)	0.630 (0.388, 1.025)	0.729 (0.462, 1.153)
Diabetes	0.827 (0.472, 1.450)	0.725 (0.406, 1.295)
No diabetes	0.743 (0.558, 0.989)	0.872 (0.661, 1.151)
Previous intervention	0.979 (0.593, 1.618)	1.108 (0.685, 1.791)
Previous CABG	0.685 (0.373, 1.259)	0.969 (0.553, 1.697)
High-risk stratum	1.005 (0.680, 1.484)	0.885 (0.593, 1.320)
Elective stratum	0.620 (0.442, 0.871)	0.817 (0.593, 1.125)
Balloon angioplasty	0.752 (0.577, 0.980)	0.851 (0.658, 1.100)
Rotablator	0.551 (0.275, 1.104)	0.577 (0.288, 1.158)
Stent implantation	0.377 (0.181, 0.783)	0.473 (0.233, 0.959)

[a]Treated as randomized analyses. Data are point estimates with 95% confidence intervals for the odds ratios.

A consistent, similar degree of benefit was imparted to all patients regardless of risk profile. Efficacy was realized regardless of baseline demographic characteristics, medical history, procedures performed, or angiographic features. Representative data are included in Table 2.

Time to Events

As might be expected of a short-acting parenteral agent, separation and differentiation of the treatment event curves from placebo occurred early, within the first 24 h (the period of drug infusion; Fig. 2). The differences resulted from a reduction in thrombosis, as manifest by a reduction in angiographically apparent true abrupt closure (Table 1). The plots included in Fig. 3, the Kaplan-Meier event curves to 6 mo, illustrate three points. First, the two dosing approaches studied in IMPACT II are indistinguishable in clinical effect; second, the absolute difference achieved during treatment remains constant and durable without degradation over time; and third, the majority of the benefit of eptifibatide treatment was the result of reducing the incidence of myocardial infarction or death. In particular, Fig. 3B points out that eptifibatide treatment had no effect on the need for subsequent (clinically driven) revascularization. With regard to angiographic restenosis, in the 900-patient IMPACT II Angiographic Substudy (in which all patients were required to return for 6-mo follow-up angiography), no differences in rates of angiographic restenosis among the treatment groups were observed (20). Finally, all the plots illustrate that

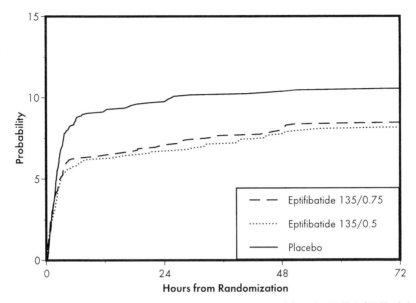

Fig. 2. Kaplan-Meier plot of probability of end-point events to 72 h—the IMPACT II trial. Components of the composite clinical efficacy endpoint were death, myocardial infarction, or urgent revascularization. Most events occurred within 6 h of coronary intervention. Both eptifibatide regimens reduced events to essentially the same degree. (From ref. *19*.)

coronary intervention itself induces adverse clinical events. Of endpoint events to 30 d, >75% of events occurred within the first 24 h of the procedure.

Components of the Composite Endpoint

The event rates for the individual components of the primary efficacy endpoint were reduced with eptifibatide treatment, which was consistent with the overall treatment effect seen in IMPACT II (Table 3). Most of the treatment effect was in reducing the incidence of periprocedural myocardial infarction, with lesser absolute contributions from the other elements tracked. Stents were required for abrupt closure in 18 (1.4%) patients in the placebo group compared with 7 (0.5%) in each of the eptifibatide treatment groups. This finding paralleled the greater overall use of stent implantation in the placebo group at the initial coronary intervention (5.0% vs 2.7% in the 135/0.5 group, $p = 0.002$). Other statistics concerning the individual components of the composite endpoint are listed in Table 3.

Adverse Events

There was no increase in the frequency of major bleeding, blood transfusion, or other morbidity associated with eptifibatide administration. Rates of major bleeding were 4.8% vs 5.1% vs 5.2% for the placebo, 135/0.5, and 135/0.75 groups, respectively. Transfusion rates were likewise comparable. The majority (approx 60%) of all bleeding events were attributable to the vascular access site. Four patients sustained an intracranial hemorrhage, one each in the placebo and 135/0.5 groups and two in the 135/0.75 treatment group. Rates of thrombocytopenia were low overall and indistinguishable among groups, with no patients developing acute profound thrombocytopenia. Finally, no patients developed anti-eptifibatide antibodies.

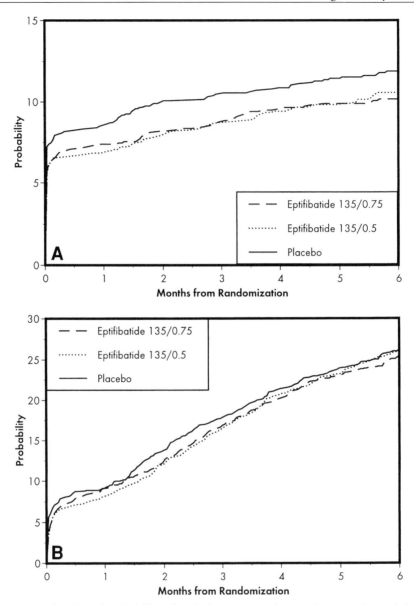

Fig. 3. Kaplan-Meier plots of probability of endpoint events to 6 mo—the IMPACT II trial. (**A**) Plot of death or myocardial infarction. (**B**) Plot of all revascularization (percutaneous coronary intervention or coronary artery bypass surgery). (**A**) Illustrates that the benefit achieved early is maintained for the entire observation period; absolute differences established early remained constant. Almost all the benefit is owing to a reduction in rates of myocardial infarction; no differences in death were realized (data not shown). (**B**) Indicates that eptifibatide treatment did not influence the subsequent need for revascularization. (From ref. *19*.)

IMPACT II: Issues, Questions, and Directions

The IMPACT II study added to the body of evidence focusing on the central role of the platelet in mediating the ischemic complications of coronary intervention. Despite what was accomplished, however, key questions remained after the IMPACT II trial. One

Table 3

Primary Composite Efficacy Outcomes and Components: Patients Receiving Any Study Drug (Treated as Randomized Analyses)

	Placebo (n = 1285)	Eptifibatide 135/0.5 (n = 1300)	Eptifibatide 135/0.75 (n = 1286)
30-Day composite endpoint, n (%; 95% CI)	149 (11.6; 9.8, 13.3)	118 (9.1; 7.5–10.6)	128 (10.0; 8.3–11.6)
Significance vs placebo	—	p = 0.035	p = 0.180
Odds ratio vs placebo (95% CI for OR)	—	0.76 (0.59–0.98)	0.84 (0.66–1.08)
Endpoint components, n (%; 95% CI)			
Death	14 (1.1; 0.5–1.7)	6 (0.5; 0.1–0.8)	11 (0.9; 0.4–1.4)
Myocardial infarction	106 (8.2; 6.7–9.8)	86 (6.6; 5.3–8.0)	90 (7.0; 5.6–8.4)
CK-MB ≥ 3× upper normal limit	72 (5.6; 4.3–6.9)	54 (4.2; 3.1–5.2)	46 (3.6; 2.6–4.6)
CK-MB ≥ 5× upper normal limit	51 (4.0; 2.9–5.0)	38 (2.9; 2.0–3.8)	28 (2.2; 1.4–3.0)
Q waves	20 (1.6; 0.9–2.2)	12 (0.9; 0.4–1.4)	15 (1.2; 0.6–1.8)
Q waves or CK-MB ≥ 5× upper normal limit	59 (4.6; 3.4–5.7)	47 (3.6; 2.6–4.6)	39 (3.0; 2.1–4.0)
Death or CK-MB ≥ 3× upper normal limit	82 (6.4; 5.0–7.7)	57 (4.4; 3.3–5.5)	54 (4.2; 3.1–5.3)
Significance vs placebo	—	p = 0.024	p = 0.013
Odds ratio vs placebo (95% CI for OR)	—	0.67 (0.48, 0.95)	0.64 (0.45, 0.92)
Urgent or emergency bypass surgery	36 (2.8; 1.9–3.7)	19 (1.5; 0.8–2.1)	26 (2.0; 1.3–2.8)
Urgent or emergency repeat percutaneous revascularization	37 (2.9; 2.0–3.8)	35 (2.7; 1.8–3.6)	36 (2.8; 1.9–3.7)
Stent for abrupt closure	18 (1.4; 0.8–2.0)	7 (0.5; 0.1–0.9)	7 (0.5; 0.1–0.9)

Abbreviations: CK, creatine kinase; CI, confidence interval; OR, odds ratio.

issue was the inverse dose-response results at 30 d between the lower dose (135/0.5) and higher dose (135/0.75) regimens in IMPACT II. Curiously, the 30-d (primary endpoint) mark coincided with the greatest separation of effect between the two dosing approaches; as noted above, the 6-mo event curves for the two dosing approaches became virtually identical. These findings appear to be attributable to a number of factors. First, the efficacy of eptifibatide in IMPACT II was largely secondary to the (identical) 135 µg/kg bolus used in both arms, not the continuous infusion. Second, neither of the infusion regimens adequately inhibited platelet function and were more similar than different in biologic activity. Finally, the role of statistical chance cannot be discounted; in fact, the differences between the primary endpoint rates at 30 d are statistically negligible.

Perhaps the critical dilemma was that the treatment effect was less than expected, particularly in the context of the results achieved in the EPIC trial with the monoclonal antibody fragment abciximab (4). Several investigations conducted subsequent to the conclusion of the IMPACT II trial lent support to the notion that higher doses of eptifibatide might provide better clinical efficacy. In a key observation by Phillips and colleagues (21), it was elucidated that the pharmacodynamic effects of eptifibatide were overestimated in the Phase II dose-finding studies. This overestimation was secondary to the use of the anticoagulant sodium citrate to suspend the blood samples; since citrate chelates calcium, and since calcium normally occupies the ligand binding site within GPIIb/IIIa, ex vivo ADP-induced platelet aggregation was artificially enhanced vis à vis the in vivo clinical effect. The best current estimate is that the doses used in IMPACT II achieved only 30–50% of maximal platelet GPIIb/IIIa integrin blockade (22).

Two additional studies have been conducted that have direct relevance to the issue of eptifibatide dosing and the potential for more robust clinical efficacy. The first was the 10,948-patient PURSUIT trial of eptifibatide vs placebo as an adjunct to the management of patients presenting with an acute coronary syndrome (23). In PURSUIT, the dosing of eptifibatide was a bolus of 180 µg/kg followed by an infusion at 2.0 µg/kg-min. Among the 1228 patients in PURSUIT who underwent coronary intervention during study drug infusion, the relative reduction in the composite endpoint of death or myocardial infarction at 30 d was 30% with eptifibatide treatment (16.8% vs 11.8%, $p = 0.01$). This suggested that a higher dose regimen (than that used in IMPACT II) would provide a greater relative risk reduction in end-point events.

In the Platelet Aggregation and Receptor Occupancy with Integrilin—a Dynamic Evaluation (PRIDE) study, the pharmacodynamic effects of three single-bolus and two double-bolus dosing regimens of eptifibatide during coronary intervention were investigated (24). Also incorporated into the PRIDE trial was a lower dose strategy for heparin anticoagulation, using a 70 U/kg heparin bolus to achieve an ACT of 200–300 s. Inhibition of platelet aggregation was determined with blood suspended in a calcium chelator (sodium citrate) and in PPACK (D-Phe-Pro-Arg-CH_2Cl, an anticoagulant that does not chelate calcium) using 20 µM adenosine diphosphate to stimulate platelet aggregation. Representative data from the 135/0.75 and 180/2.0 infusion regimens are depicted in Fig. 4 and show that ex vivo determinations of inhibition of platelet aggregation are dependent on the anticoagulant used to suspend the blood sample. With measurements of platelet aggregation performed on specimens suspended in PPACK, only the 180/2.0 regimen attained >80% platelet inhibition through most of the treatment. Data derived from the PRIDE trial also demonstrated that a concentration of 1650 ng/mL of eptifibatide was necessary to attain 80% of platelet GPIIb/IIIa receptor occupancy (Fig. 5). However, this concentration was

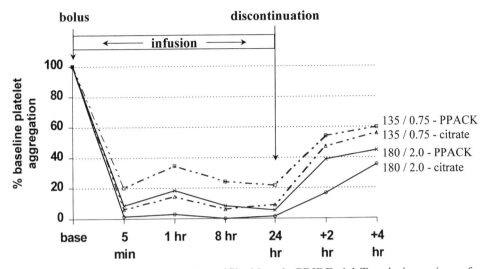

Fig. 4. Inhibition of platelet aggregation by eptifibatide—the PRIDE trial. Two dosing regimens from the PRIDE trial are shown, the 135 μg/kg bolus plus 0.75 μg/kg/min infusion and the 180 μg/kg bolus plus 2.0 μg/kg/min infusion. Blood samples were suspended in either sodium citrate anticoagulant or PPACK anticoagulant. Assays of blood in citrate reported higher degrees of platelet inhibition than blood in PPACK at the same concentration of eptifibatide. The higher dose (180/2.0) regimen suppressed platelet aggregation below 20% of baseline, whereas the lower dose (135/0.75) regimen did not. Data are normalized to 100% aggregation at baseline. PPACK = D-Phe-Pro-Arg-CH$_2$Cl. (From ref. *24.*)

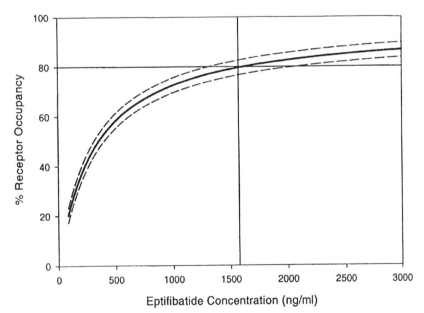

Fig. 5. Relationship of eptifibatide plasma concentration to platelet GPIIb/IIIa receptor occupancy relationship—the PRIDE trial. Ninety-five percent confidence interval (CI) curves are also included. Eighty percent occupancy was achieved when the steady-state concentration exceeded the threshold concentration of 1650 ng/mL (95% CI 1406–1967 ng/mL), as shown. (From ref. *24.*)

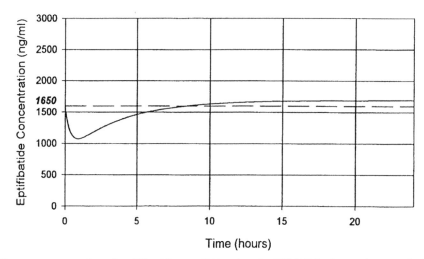

Fig. 6. Plasma concentration of eptifibatide over 24 h using the 180/2.0 dosing regimen—the PRIDE trial. The 1650 ng/mL threshold concentration level is highlighted. (From ref. *24.*)

only reached with the 180/2.0 regimen after 8 h of infusion, once a steady state was achieved (Fig. 6). This led to the hypothesis that a larger bolus (or, alternatively, a second bolus within 10 min of the first) would be necessary to obtain maximal efficacy with the 180/2.0 regimen. Finally, further pharmacodynamic modeling determined that to attain and maintain >80% receptor occupancy (and >80% inhibition of platelet aggregation) throughout the duration of treatment, a 180/2.0/180 double-bolus regimen would be required (Fig. 7) *(25).*

Finally, several other issues remained unresolved after IMPACT-II. First, the PROLOG *(7)* and EPILOG *(6)* trials of abciximab, studies conducted in approximately the same time frame as IMPACT II, reported lower rates of major bleeding with reduced heparin dosing and early sheath removal. Whether the safety profile of eptifibatide could be similarly improved was unknown. More importantly, IMPACT-II did not study the efficacy of eptifibatide in improving outcomes with elective intracoronary stent implantation. Even though extrapolation of the results of the abciximab trials suggested that GPIIb/IIIa inhibition in general would be efficacious in coronary stenting, further studies were still needed after IMPACT-II to evaluate the specific efficacy of eptifibatide.

ESPRIT

The Enhanced Suppression of the Platelet IIb/IIIa Receptor with Integrilin Therapy (ESPRIT) trial was designed as a pivotal, Phase III trial of eptifibatide in patients undergoing stent implantation during percutaneous coronary intervention *(26–28).* The crucial issue was to evaluate a new, novel dosing regimen of eptifibatide developed to attain and maintain >80% platelet GPIIb/IIIa integrin blockade throughout the duration of treatment. The study evaluated the efficacy of treatment in nonurgent PCI in patients receiving second- and third-generation stents using high-pressure stent deployment techniques and concomitant thienopyridine therapy.

ESPRIT was a multicenter, parallel-group, randomized, double-blind, placebo-controlled (with open-label crossover) clinical trial that enrolled 2064 patients in 92 centers in the

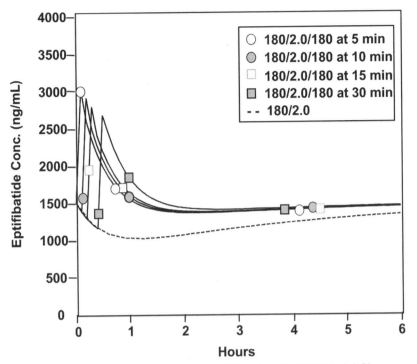

Fig. 7. Pharmacokinetic modeling of double-bolus eptifibatide—the PRIDE trial. Shown are the predicted effects of a 180 µg/kg bolus and 2.0 µg/kg/min infusion alone and after a second 180 µg/kg bolus at 5-, 10-, 15-, or 30-min intervals after the initial bolus. (From ref. *25*.)

United States and Canada. Patient enrollment into ESPRIT took place from June 1999 into February 2000. Figure 8 shows the flow of patients through the trial. Patients with known coronary artery disease scheduled to undergo PCI with stent implantation in a native coronary artery (and who, per the judgment of the operator, did not require pretreatment with a GPIIb/IIIa inhibitor) were considered for inclusion. Patients excluded from the study included those who had sustained a myocardial infarction within 24 h before randomization and patients with continuing chest pain requiring urgent PCI. Other exclusion criteria included PCI within the previous 3 mo, previous stent placement at the target lesion, a target lesion within a saphenous vein graft, treatment with a GPIIb/IIIa inhibitor or a thienopyridine in the previous 30 d, stroke or transient ischemic attack within 30 d, history of hemorrhagic stroke, bleeding diathesis or abnormal bleeding within 30 d of randomization, major surgery in the preceding 6 wk, uncontrolled hypertension (>200/100 mmHg), thrombocytopenia (platelet count < 100×10^9/L), or serum creatinine level > 350 µmol/L (4.0 mg/dL).

Patient were randomized to received either a 180 µg/kg double bolus of eptifibatide administered 10 min apart coupled with a continuous infusion (started immediately after the first bolus) of 2 µg/kg/min for 18–24 h (1 µg/kg/min for patients with serum creatinine >177 µmol/L), or placebo. Concomitant medications included heparin to maintain an ACT between 200 and 300 s, aspirin, and either clopidogrel or ticlopidine (with use of a loading dose).

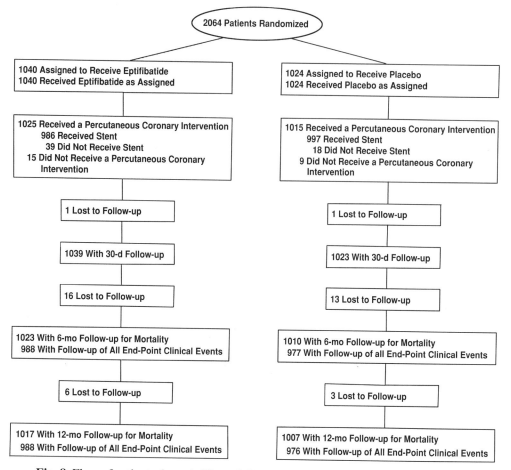

Fig. 8. Flow of patients through 12-mo follow-up—the ESPRIT trial. (From ref. *28.*)

The protocol permitted the use of open-label "bailout" GPIIb/IIIa inhibitor therapy in emergency situations (abrupt closure, no reflow, or coronary thrombosis). Bailout GPIIb/IIIa inhibitor use did not result in unblinding of study drug assignment.

The primary endpoint was a composite of death, myocardial infarction, urgent target vessel revascularization and bailout GPIIb/IIIa inhibitor therapy given for a thrombotic complication within 48 h after randomization. The key secondary efficacy endpoint was the composite of death, myocardial infarction, and urgent target vessel revascularization within 30 d after randomization. Endpoint myocardial infarction was defined by creative kinase (CK)-MB elevation ≥3 times upper limit of normal on two assays in the first 24 h after PCI or a clinical event judged to be compatible with myocardial infarction by the Clinical Events Committee and supported by predetermined electrocardiographic findings and/or cardiac marker elevations. Safety endpoints were bleeding, blood transfusion, and stroke within 48 h or hospital discharge. Bleeding was assessed as major or minor according to the Thrombolysis in Myocardial Infarction (TIMI) criteria.

The sample size was based on a predicted 33% reduction of an expected 11% adverse clinical event rate at 30 d in the placebo arm. With 86% power and an α of 0.05 (two-tailed), the projected sample size for the study was 2400 patients. Because the anticipated recruit-

Table 4
Baseline Characteristics[a]

Characteristic	Eptifibatide (n = 1040)	Placebo (n = 1024)	Total (n = 2064)
Median age (yr) (25–75 quartiles)	62 (54–71)	62 (54–71)	62 (54–71)
Median weight (kg) (25–75 quartiles)	84.0 (73.9–95.3)	84.7 (75.0–97.0)	84.4 (74.0–96.0)
Women	280 (27)	282 (28)	562 (27)
USA/Canada	772 (74)/268 (26)	759 (74)/265 (26)	1531(74)/533 (26)
Previous MI	331 (32)	321 (31)	652 (32)
Previous PCI	237 (23)	246 (24)	483 (23)
Previous CABG	106 (10)	105 (10)	211 (10)
Diabetes	208 (20)	211 (21)	419 (20)
Hypertension	608 (59)	605 (59)	1213 (59)
Hypercholesterolemia	600 (58)	599 (59)	1199 (58)
Smoker	250 (24)	228 (23)	478 (23)
Stable angina	407 (39)	387 (38)	794 (39)
UA/NQMI (2–180 d)	331 (32)	333 (33)	664 (32)
UA/NQMI within 2 d	139 (13)	140 (14)	279 (14)
ST elevation MI within 7 d	44 (4)	49 (5)	93 (5)
Positive functional test only	96 (9)	91 (9)	187 (9)
Other anginal equivalent	23 (2)	24 (2)	47 (2)

Abbreviations: MI, myocardial infarction; PCI, percutaneous coronary intervention; CABG, coronary artery bypass grafting; UA, unstable angina; NQMI, non-Q-wave myocardial infarction.
[a] Data are numbers, with percents in parentheses, except for the first two rows.

ment period was less than 6 mo, no interim analyses were preplanned. However, since the actual recruitment period extended beyond 8 mo, the Data and Safety Monitoring Board independently chose to assess both safety and efficacy. For this analysis, the Data Safety and Monitoring Board prespecified a p value < 0.005 for the rate of death or myocardial infarction at 48 h as criteria warranting termination of the trial. Analyses were by intention to treat. At the interim analysis (conducted with 2007 patients randomized), the Data and Safety Monitoring Board recommended the premature termination of enrollment for efficacy. At the interim analysis, complete data were available of 1758 patients to 48 h and 1384 patients to 30 d. A 43% relative risk reduction in irreversible endpoints of death or myocardial infarction at 48 h (95% CI 19–61; $p = 0.0017$) was the primary determinant of recommendation for termination. Other prerequisite conditions of the board included consistency of reduction in death or myocardial infarction at 30 d, consistency across other components of the endpoint at 48 h and 30 d, absence of safety concerns, and results of other clinical trials of GPIIb/IIIa inhibition in PCI.

The baseline demographic and angiographic characteristics among the 2064 patients enrolled in the study were evenly distributed between treatment groups (Table 4). Patients classified as having an acute coronary syndrome within 48 h or an acute ST-segment elevation myocardial infarction within 7 days before the intervention represented 18% of the study population. Table 5 outlines specific treatment characteristics of the two study groups. A PCI procedure was actually performed in 98.8% of patients, and >96% of the

Table 5
Treatment Indices

Characteristic	Eptifibatide (n = 1040)	Placebo (n = 1024)	Total (n = 2064)
Median infusion duration (h) (25–75 quartiles)	18.3 (18.0–20.1)	18.4 (18.0–20.2)	18.4 (18.0–20.2)
PCI done	1025 (99)	1015 (99)	2040 (99)
Number of stents placed			
Total	986 (95)	997 (97)	1983 (96)
1	676 (65)	650 (64)	1326 (64)
2	234 (23)	242 (24)	476 (23)
3	54 (5)	90 (9)	144 (7)
≥4	22 (2)	15 (2)	37 (2)
Femoral arteriotomy closure device	189 (18)	167 (16)	356 (17)
Median max ACT (s) (25–75 quartiles)	273 (234–316)	263 (230–302)	268 (232–309)
Thienopyridine use	1009 (97)	1006 (98)	2015 (98)

Abbreviations: PCI, percutaneous coronary intervention; Max ACT, maximum procedural activated clotting time.

[a]Data are numbers, with percent in parentheses, except for rows 1 and 9.

patients had one or more stents placed. Almost all subjects (97.7%) received a thienopyridine, mainly clopidogrel.

Early study drug discontinuation occurred at approximately the same rate in both treatment groups. Study drug was discontinued before 12 h in 9.3% (192) and before 16 h in 11.7% (242) of the patients. A total of 35 patients in the eptifibatide group and 43 patients in the placebo group crossed over to open-label eptifibatide therapy.

There was a 37% reduction in the primary composite clinical endpoint of death, myocardial infarction, urgent target vessel revascularization, or crossover bailout therapy for thrombotic complications at 48 h. These events occurred in 108 of the 1024 placebo-treated patients and in 69 of the 1040 eptifibatide-treated patients ($p = 0.0015$). Other event rates for individual components and combinations of components of the endpoint are shown in Fig. 9. All components and combinations of components of the primary endpoint had the same directionality and approximate relative risk reduction as the primary composite endpoint.

Subgroup analysis, depicted in Fig. 10, demonstrated benefit irrespective of baseline characteristics including age, weight, sex, diabetes, and disease presentation. Interestingly, the degree of heparin anticoagulation, as measured by the ACT, did not predict events in any of the treatment groups. In the placebo group, the frequency of the primary composite endpoint was closely similar among patients when they were divided into tertiles of maximum ACT (10.0%, 95% CI 6.9–13.2, in the lowest tertile; 11.5%, 95% CI 8.1–14.8, in the middle tertile; and 10.3%, 95% CI 6.8–13.7, in the highest tertile). The benefit of treatment with eptifibatide was also similar across the tertiles of ACT, with the lowest overall event rate of the primary composite endpoint occurring in patients receiving eptifibatide who were in the lowest tertile. This suggests that, in contradistinction to conventional wisdom, increasing degrees of anticoagulation with heparin do not further reduce adverse clinical event rates in coronary stent PCI.

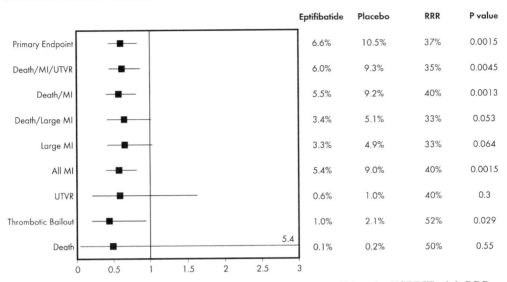

Fig. 9. Risk ratios (95% CI) for major endpoint components at 48 h—the ESPRIT trial. RRR = relative risk ratio; UTVR = urgent target vessel revascularization; MI = myocardial infarction; large MI = CK-MB more than five times upper limit of normal. (From ref. *27*, with permission from Elsevier Science.)

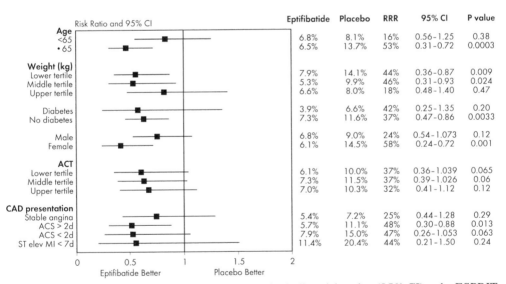

Fig. 10. Subgroup analysis of the primary endpoint including risk ratios (95% CI)—the ESPRIT trial. ACT = activated clotting time; CAD = coronary artery disease; ACS = acute coronary syndrome; RRR = relative risk ratio. The weight tertiles for men were <81 kg, 81–95 kg, and >95 kg, and for women <68 kg, 68–82 kg, and >82 kg. (From ref. *27*, with permission from Elsevier Science.)

The initial benefit found at 48 h was sustained to 30 d (Fig. 11) and at 1 yr (Fig. 12), as shown by the Kaplan-Meier curves. There was a 35% relative risk reduction in the secondary composite endpoint of death, myocardial infarction, and urgent target vessel revascularization at 30 d (10.5% vs 6.8%, $p = 0.0034$). The majority of events occurred in the

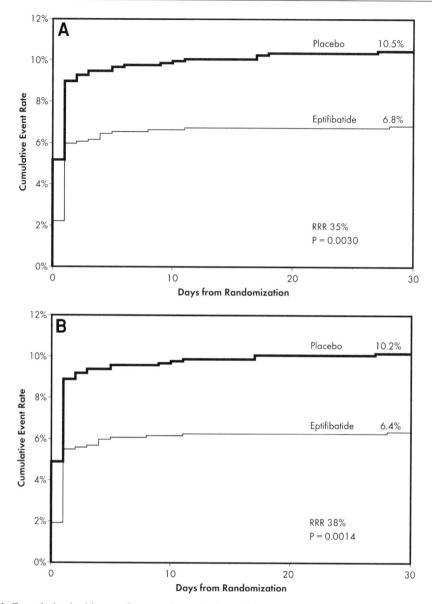

Fig. 11. Cumulative incidence of composite endpoints at 30 d with eptifibatide vs placebo treatment—the ESPRIT trial. (**A**) Composite endpoint of death, myocardial infarction, and urgent TVR. (**B**) Composite endpoint of death and myocardial infarction. TVR = target vessel revascularization; RRR = relative risk ratio. (From ref. *27*, with permission from Elsevier Science.)

first 48 h. Benefits were sustained over time. The absolute difference between the composite of death, myocardial infarction, and all target vessel revascularization was actually larger at 1 yr than at 30 d (3.7% absolute risk reduction at 30 d, 4.6% absolute risk reduction at 1 yr) Although there was a trend favoring mortality reduction, most of the benefit was owing to a reduced rate of myocardial infarction. After 1 yr of follow-up, 20 deaths (2%) occurred in the placebo group compared with 14 deaths (1.4%) with eptifibatide [hazard ratio (HR) 0.69; 95% CI, 0.35–1.36; *p* = 0.28). Over the same period, the

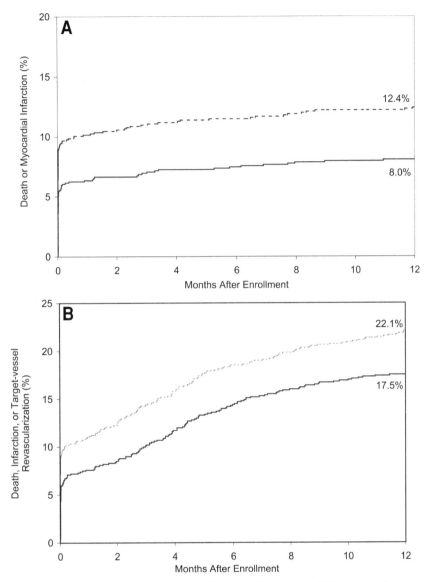

Fig. 12. Cumulative incidence of composite endpoints at 1 yr with eptifibatide vs placebo treatment —the ESPRIT trial. (**A**) Composite endpoint of death and myocardial infarction. Hazard ratio, 0.63; 95% confidence interval, 0.48–0.83; $p = 0.001$. (**B**) Composite endpoint of death, myocardial infarction and urgent TVR. Hazard ratio, 0.76; 95% confidence interval, 0.63–0.93; $p = 0.007$. (From ref. *28*.)

combined endpoint of death and myocardial infarction was reduced from 12.4 to 8.0 with the use of eptifibatide (HR, 0.63; 95% CI, 0.48–0.83; $p = 0.001$; Fig. 12). There was no evidence of an increase in event rate (or rebound) at the time of discontinuation of treatment.

Rates of severe and moderate bleeding as assessed by the site investigator did not differ between groups. However, when measured by the quantitative TIMI bleeding criteria, an increase in bleeding rates with eptifibatide treatment was found. When TIMI bleeding was analyzed by tertiles of the ACT, rates were not increased in the lowest tertile: 0.6%

Table 6
Stroke and Bleeding Complications[a]

Characteristic	Eptifibatide (n = 1040)	Placebo (n = 1024)	Total (n = 2064)
Intracranial bleeding	2 (0.2)	1 (0.1)	3 (0.1)
Nonhemorrhagic stroke	1 (0.1)	0	1 (<0.1)
Severe bleeding	7 (0.7)	5 (0.5)	12 (0.6)
Moderate bleeding	14 (1)	11 (1)	25 (1)
Major bleeding (TIMI)			
Overall*	13 (1)	4 (0.4)	17 (1)
ACT < 244 (n = 661)	2/312 (0.6)	2/349 (0.6)	4/661 (0.6)
ACT 244–292 (n = 678)	6/330 (1.8)	1/348 (0.3)	7/678 (1.0)
ACT > 292 (n = 676)	5/374 (1.3)	1/302 (0.3)	6/676 (0.9)
Minor bleeding (TIMI)	29 (2.8)	18 (1.7)	47 (2.3)
Platelet count < 20,000	2 (0.2)	0	2 (0.1)
RBC transfusion[b]	15 (1)	10 (1)	25 (1)

Abbreviations: RBC, red blood cell; ACT, activated clotting time; TIMI, bleeding classified by TIMI grade as determined by site investigator.

[a]Data are numbers, with percent in parentheses.

[b]Includes CABG-related transfusions of red blood cells.

*p = 0.027.

vs 0.7% for placebo and eptifibatide, respectively. Rates of bleeding increased as the ACT rose, with bleeding being enhanced by treatment with eptifibatide. There were two cases of acute profound thrombocytopenia in the eptifibatide treatment group (a decrease in the platelet count to $<20 \times 10^9$/L within 24 h of start of treatment). No platelet transfusion was necessary as the platelet count rapidly resolved (within hours) after drug discontinuation. No clinical sequelae were reported. Finally, red blood cell transfusion was uncommon (Table 6).

In summary, the ESPRIT trial answered most of the unresolved questions from IMPACT-II. First, whereas IMPACT-II studied patients undergoing balloon angioplasty, the ESPRIT trial proved the benefit of eptifibatide as an adjunct to elective stent implantation in producing significant and clinically relevant reductions in ischemic complications of this procedure. These benefits were achieved despite exclusion of the highest risk patients, the group expected to experience the greatest improvements. Moreover, these results were obtained in the context of high-pressure stent deployment strategies coupled with thienopyridine therapy. Treatment effects were not only robust but were maintained to 1 year and were consistent among all patient subgroups.

Second, the clinical efficacy seen in ESPRIT further solidified the coupling of the degree of platelet GPIIb/IIIa receptor inhibition with clinical efficacy. Pharmacodynamic studies had shown that the eptifibatide dose tested in ESPRIT achieved and maintained blockade of >90% of available GPIIb/IIIa receptors in >90% of patients, corresponding to >90% inhibition of ex vivo platelet aggregation after stimulation by 20 µM ADP in blood suspended in PPACK as the anticoagulant. This was a substantially greater degree of inhibition of platelet aggregation than the 50–60% inhibition achieved in IMPACT-II, and the treatment effect was on a par with that seen in the PCI trials of abciximab. For example, in the Evaluation of IIb/IIIa Platelet Inhibition for Stenting (EPISTENT) trial, the subgroup of patients pretreated with ticlopidine experienced an absolute reduction of the composite endpoint of death, myocardial infarction, and urgent revascularization at 30 d of 3.7% (from 8.9 to 5.2%) with the use of abxicimab compared with placebo *(29)*. This compares favorably with the 3.7% absolute reduction (from 10.5 to 6.8%) for the same endpoint in ESPRIT.

Third, analysis of the bleeding complications and clinical outcomes according to the degree of heparin anticoagulation confirmed the findings first observed in the abxicimab trials that lower doses of heparin (targeting an ACT of 200–250 s) are probably optimal in PCI when adjunctive GPIIb/IIIa blockade is used. In ESPRIT, patients receiving eptifibatide who were in the lowest tertile of heparin anticoagulation had both the lowest rate of the primary composite endpoint and the lowest rate of bleeding complications. Similarly, rates of severe and moderate bleeding per the quantitative TIMI bleeding criteria also did not differ from the rates found in patients randomized to placebo in the lowest tertile. Finally, the low rate of occurrence of thrombocytopenia (0.2%), although still troublesome, compares favorably with the incidence of 0.7% reported with abxicimab *(30)*.

In conclusion, in a population of patients undergoing elective stent implantation, treatment with the 180/2.0/180 double-bolus regimen of eptifibatide lowers the risk of death, myocardial infarction, and target vessel revascularization. The clinical efficacy is consistent and robust across components of the endpoint and across patient subgroups, is durable and long-lasting, and is typical of that seen in other trials of platelet glycoprotein inhibition. When combined with lower degrees of anticoagulation with heparin, these benefits are achieved without increasing the risk of bleeding. In light of these results, all patients (without contraindication for GPIIb/IIIa inhibitors) should be considered for treatment when undergoing percutaneous coronary intervention.

REFERENCES

1. Neuhaus KL, Zeymer U. Prevention and management of thrombotic complications during coronary interventions. Eur Heart J 1995;16(Suppl L):L63–L67.
2. Wilentz JR, Sanborn TA, Haudenschild CC, et al. Platelet accumulation in experimental angioplasty: time-course and relation to vascular injury. Circulation 1987;76:1225–1234.
3. Steele PM, Chesebro JH, Stanson AW, et al. Balloon angioplasty: natural history of the pathophysiological response to injury in a pig model. Circ Res 1985;57:105–112.
4. The EPIC Investigators. Use of a monoclonal antibody directed against the platelet glycoprotein IIb/IIIa receptor in high risk coronary angioplasty. N Engl J Med 1994;330:956–961.
5. Topol EJ, Ferguson JJ, Weisman HF, et al. Long-term protection from myocardial ischemic events in a randomized trial of brief integrin β_3 blockade with percutaneous coronary intervention. JAMA 1997; 278:479–484.
6. The EPILOG Investigators. Platelet glycoprotein IIb/IIIa receptor blockade and low dose heparin during percutaneous coronary revascularisation. N Engl J Med 1997;336:1689–1696.
7. Lincoff AM, Tcheng JE, Califf RM, et al. Standard versus low dose weight adjusted heparin in patients treated with the platelet glycoprotein IIb/IIIa receptor antibody fragment abciximab (c7E3 Fab) during percutaneous coronary revascularisation. The PROLOG investigators. Am J Cardiol 1997;79:286–291.
8. The CAPTURE Investigators. Randomized placebo controlled trial of abciximab before and during coronary intervention in refractory unstable angina: the CAPTURE study. Lancet 1997;349:1429–1435.
9. Lefkovits J, Plow EF, Topol EJ. Platelet glycoprotein IIb/IIIa receptors in cardiovascular medicine. N Engl J Med 1995;332:1553–1559.
10. Phillips DR, Charo IF, Parise LV, Fitzgerald LA. The platelet membrane glycoprotein IIb/IIIa complex. Blood 1988;71:831–843.
11. Pytela R, Pierschbacher MD, Ginsberg MH, Plow EF, Ruoslahti E. Platelet membrane glycoprotein IIb/IIIa: a member of a family of Arg-Gly-Asp-specific adhesion receptors. Science 1986;231:1559–1562.
12. Mustard JF, Kinlough-Rathbone RL, Packham MA. Comparison of fibrinogen association with normal and thrombasthenic platelets on exposure to ADP or chymotrypsin. Blood 1979;54:987–993.

13. Dennis MS, Henzel WJ, Pitti RM, et al. Platelet glycoprotein IIb/IIIa protein antagonists from snake venoms: evidence for a family of platelet aggregation inhibitors. (ArgGlyAsp/fibrinogen receptor/trigramin/echistatin/kistrin). Proc Natl Acad Sci USA 1989;87:2471–2475.

14. Scarborough RM, Naughton MA, Teng W. Design of potent and specific integrin antagonists with high specificity for glycoprotein IIb/IIIa. J Biol Chem 1993;268:1066–1073.

15. Charo IF, Scarborough RM, Du Mee CP, et al. Therapeutics I: pharmacodynamics of the glycoprotein IIb/IIIa antagonist integrelin: phase 1 clinical studies in normal healthy volunteers. Circulation 1992;86 (Suppl I):I–260.

16. Scarborough RM, Rose JW, Hsu MA. Barbourin. A GPIIb/IIIa-specific integrin antagonist from the venom of *Sistrurus m barbouri*. J Biol Chem 1991;266:9359–9362.

17. Tcheng JE, Harrington RA, Kottke-Marchant K, et al. Multicenter, randomized, double-blind, placebo-controlled trial of the platelet integrin glycoprotein IIb/IIIa blocker Integrelin in elective coronary intervention. Circulation 1995;76:2151–2157.

18. Harrington RA, Klieman NS, Kottke-Marchant K, et al. Immediate and reversible platelet inhibition after intravenous administration of a peptide glycoprotein IIb/IIIa inhibitor during percutaneous coronary intervention. Am J Cardiol 1995;76:1222–1227.

19. The IMPACT II Investigators. Randomised placebo-controlled trial of effect of eptifibatide on complications of percutaneous coronary intervention: IMPACT II. Lancet 1997;349:1422–1428.

20. Lincoff AM, Tcheng JE, Ellis SG, et al., for the IMPACT II Investigators. Randomized trial of platelet glycoprotein IIb/IIIa inhibition with Integrelin for prevention of restenosis following coronary intervention: the IMPACT II angiographic substudy. Circ Suppl 1995;92:I–2905.

21. Phillips DR, Teng W, Arfsten A, et al. Effect of calcium on GP IIb/IIIa interactions with Integrelin-enhanced GP IIb/IIIa binding and inhibition of platelet aggregation by reductions in the concentration of ionized calcium in plasma anticoagulated with citrate. Circulation 1997;96:1488–1494.

22. Tcheng JE. Glycoprotein IIb/IIIa inhibitors: putting the EPIC, IMPACT II, RESTORE, and EPILOG trials into perspective. Am J Cardiol 1996;78(Suppl 3A):35–40.

23. The PURSUIT Trial Investigators. Inhibition of platelet glycoprotein IIb/IIIa with eptifibatide in patients with acute coronary syndromes. N Engl J Med 1998;339:436–443.

24. Tcheng JE, Talley JD, O'Shea JC, et al. Clinical pharmacology of higher dose eptifibatide in percutaneous coronary intervention (the PRIDE study). Am J Cardiol 2001;88:1097–1102.

25. Gilchrist IC, O'Shea JC, Kosoglou T, et al. Pharmacodynamics and pharmacokinetics of higher-dose, double-bolus eptifibatide in percutaneous coronary intervention. Circulation 2001;104:406–411.

26. O'Shea JC, Hafley GE, Greenberg S, et al. ESPRIT Investigators (Enhanced Suppression of the Platelet IIb/IIIa Receptor with Integrilin Therapy trial). Platelet glycoprotein IIb/IIIa integrin blockade with eptifibatide in coronary stent intervention: the ESPRIT trial: a randomized controlled trial. JAMA 2001; 285:2468–2473.

27. The ESPRIT Investigators. Enhanced suppression of the platelet iib/iiia receptor with integrilin therapy. Novel dosing regimen of eptifibatide in planned coronary stent implantation (ESPRIT): a randomised, placebo-controlled trial. [erratum appears in Lancet 2001 Apr 28;357:1370]. Lancet 2000;356: 2037–2044.

28. O'Shea JC, Buller CE, Cantor WJ, et al., for the ESPRIT Investigators. Long-term efficacy of platelet glycoprotein IIb/IIIa Integrin blockade with eptifibatide in coronary stent intervention. JAMA 2002; 287:618–621.

29. Steinhubl SR, Ellis SG, Wolski K, Lincoff AM, Topol EJ. Ticlopidine pretreatment before coronary stenting is associated with sustained decrease in adverse cardiac events: data from the evaluation of platelet IIb/IIIa inhibitor for stenting (EPISTENT) trial. Circulation 2001;103:1403–1409.

30. Berkowitz SD, Harrington RA, Rund MM, Tcheng JE. Acute profound thrombocytopenia after c7E3 Fab (abciximab) therapy. Circulation 1997;95:809–813.

7

Tirofiban
in Interventional Cardiology
The RESTORE and TARGET Trials

Nicholas Valettas, MASC, MD
and Howard C. Herrmann, MD

CONTENTS

INTRODUCTION
TIROFIBAN IN PERCUTANEOUS CORONARY INTERVENTION
PCI IN PATIENTS PRETREATED WITH TIROFIBAN
CONCLUSIONS
REFERENCES

INTRODUCTION

The discovery of the pivotal role played by the Arg-Gly-Asp (RGD) tripeptide sequence in the binding of fibrinogen to the glycoprotein IIb/IIIa (GPIIb/IIIa) receptor *(1)*, coupled with the realization that the naturally occurring snake venom disintegrins also exerted their potent antiplatelet effect via the same RGD domain *(2,3)*, led to the development of a series of nonpeptide RGD mimetics with increased specificity for the GPIIb/IIIa integrin *(4,5)*. Subsequent nuclear magnetic resonance studies of one disintegrin, eichistatin, revealed that the key RGD unit resided in a loop segment of the protein with a distinct spatial arrangement *(6)*. A specific search for a similarly structured peptidomimetic led to the discovery of a tyrosine analog inhibitor of GPIIb/IIIa *(7)*. Terminal modification of this compound produced MK-383 (L-700,462; tirofiban), a GPIIb/IIIa inhibitor with substantially increased potency, as evidenced by a >2000-fold decrease in the median inhibitory concentration (IC_{50}) *(8,9)*. Tirofiban (Aggrastat®, Merck & Co., West Point, PA) is indicated for use in patients with acute coronary syndromes including those undergoing percutaneous coronary intervention (PCI). This chapter reviews the clinical use of tirofiban in interventional cardiology with emphasis on its use as primary therapy in PCI and as pretreatment in patients with an acute coronary syndrome prior to PCI. An integral part of this discussion will focus on the key trials, RESTORE and TARGET, that have helped define tirofiban's role in interventional practice.

From: *Contemporary Cardiology: Platelet Glycoprotein IIb/IIIa
Inhibitors in Cardiovascular Disease, 2nd Edition*
Edited by: A. M. Lincoff © Humana Press Inc., Totowa, NJ

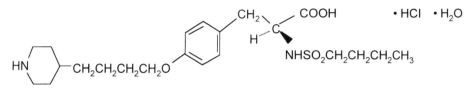

Fig. 1. Structural formula of tirofiban hydrochloride monohydrate.

Pharmacology

Tirofiban HCl (Fig. 1) is a low-molecular-weight (495.08 Daltons) nonpeptide tyrosine derivative that is supplied either as a premixed solution (50 µg/mL) for injection or as a concentrated solution for intravenous infusion after dilution. It selectively binds to the GPIIb/IIIa integrin with greater affinity when the receptor is in the activated state than in the resting state (Fig. 2), with dissociation constants of 1.6 and 15 nM, respectively *(10)*. The hypothetical advantages of this differential affinity, including the possibility of fewer adverse effects, remain to be determined. Unlike abciximab *(11,12)*, tirofiban does not bind to the vitronectin receptor nor to the leukocyte integrin Mac-1 *(13)*. Both these integrins are felt to play putative roles in neointimal hyperplasia and restenosis following coronary angioplasty, vitronectin by stimulating smooth muscle cell proliferation in injured tissue *(14)*, and Mac-1 by recruiting monocytes to the site of vascular injury *(15)*. Although the vitronectin receptor is upregulated shortly after coronary angioplasty *(16)* and antagonism of this integrin by an RGD-peptide inhibitor reduced neointimal proliferation in an animal model of vascular injury *(17)*, subsequent animal *(18)* and human *(19, 20)* studies have failed to confirm any advantage to blockade of this receptor in clinical practice.

The half-life of tirofiban in healthy subjects is approx 2 h, with 65% of the drug cleared from plasma by renal excretion and about 25% excreted unchanged in bile. Patients with a creatinine clearance of <30 mL/min (including patients requiring dialysis) exhibit a >50% decrease in plasma clearance, necessitating a corresponding adjustment in drug dosage. Plasma clearance is also reduced in individuals >65 yr of age by an estimated 20–25% compared with clearance in those <65 yr *(21)*. However, no gender differences in plasma clearance are known to exist *(22)*. Tirofiban binds weakly to plasma proteins, with 35% of an administered dose remaining free in human plasma. Furthermore, hepatic metabolism of the parent compound is limited such that even in patients with moderate hepatic insufficiency, plasma clearance of the drug is not significantly different from its clearance in healthy subjects *(23)*.

Pharmacodynamics

The antiplatelet activity of tirofiban in humans was initially studied in a two-part, double-blind, placebo-controlled, dose-escalation study in healthy male subjects using 1-h and 4-h intravenous infusions *(24)*. Tirofiban inhibited platelet aggregation induced by collagen (2 µg/mL) and ADP (3.4 µM) in a dose-dependent manner, with IC_{50} values of 66 ± 8 nM and 39 ± 4 nM, respectively. The percent inhibition of platelet aggregation as a function of the concentration of tirofiban (Fig. 3) demonstrated a sigmoid relationship between these two variables, with a steep slope and saturation of its antiplatelet effect occurring within a narrow concentration range. These kinetics are consistent with compe-

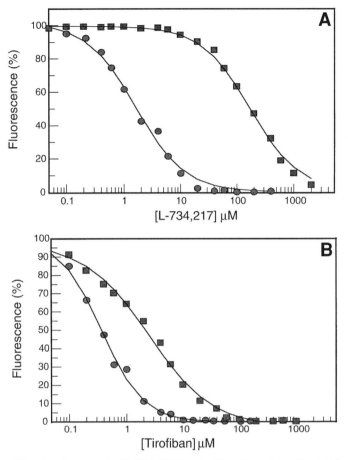

Fig. 2. The competitive displacement of L-736,622 by tirofiban from the activated form (●) and the resting form (■) of purified GPIIb/III yields dissociation constants of 1.6 and 15 n*M*, respectively. (Adapted from ref. *10*, with permission.)

titive inhibition of the GPIIb/IIIa receptor *(25)*. Complete inhibition of both collagen- and ADP-induced platelet aggregation was evident by 30 min following the initiation of an infusion of tirofiban at a rate of 0.40 µg/kg/min. The bleeding time was also prolonged by a mean 4.6-fold and returned to normal 3 h after the end of the 1-h infusion.

The pharmacodynamic activity of tirofiban was further defined in a multicenter, dose-ranging study in high-risk patients undergoing PCI *(26)*. Patients who were randomized to the active treatment arm received one of three dosing regimens initiated the moment the guidewire crossed the lesion: 5, 10, and 10 µg/kg bolus followed by continuous infusions of 0.05, 0.10, and 0.15 µg/kg/min, respectively. The pharmacodynamic effect of tirofiban on ex vivo platelet aggregation in response to 5 µ*M* ADP was then evaluated both before and at several time points during and after drug administration. Rapid inhibition of plate-let aggregation (IPA) was seen with the 10 µg/kg bolus dose, with >90% IPA achieved by 5 min (Fig. 4). IPA was maintained at >90% at 2 h and at the end of the infusion (16–24 h)

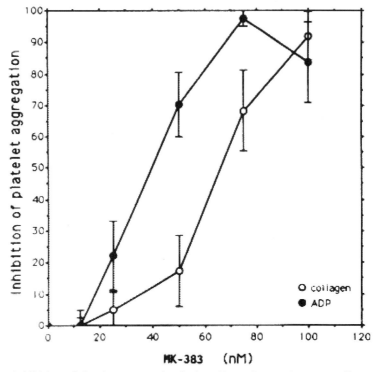

Fig. 3. Percent inhibition of platelet aggregation induced by collagen [2 μg/mL, (O)] and ADP [3.4 μg/mL, (●)] by MK-383. (Adapted from ref. *24*, with permission.)

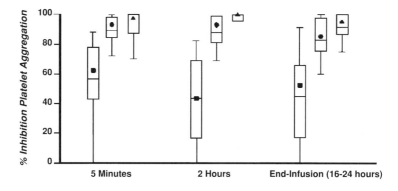

Time Following Initiation of Tirofiban Therapy

Fig. 4. Inhibition of platelet aggregation as a function of time following the initiation of tirofiban therapy (■ = 5 μg/kg bolus + 0.05 μg/kg/min infusion, ● = 10 + 0.10, ▲ = 10 + 0.15). Data depict medians (dose panel symbols), means (horizontal lines), 25th and 75th percentiles (boxes), and 10th and 90th percentiles (whiskers). (Adapted from ref. *26*, with permission.)

with the 0.15 μg/kg/min dose. Four hours after cessation of the infusion, the IPA was <50% for all three dosing regimens (Fig. 5). Heparin alone did not affect the extent of platelet aggregation, although it did double the median bleeding time at the 2-h mark in the placebo group. Median bleeding times in both of the high-dose tirofiban arms at 2 h exceeded 30 min.

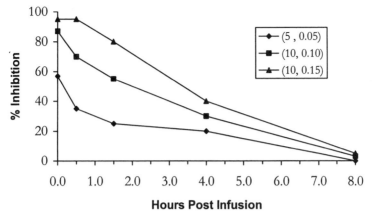

Fig. 5. Recovery of ex vivo platelet aggregation to 5 µM ADP as a function of time from completion of tirofiban infusion for each of the three dosing regimens: (1) 5 µg/kg bolus + 0.05 µg/kg/min infusion, (2) 10 µg/kg bolus + 0.10 µg/kg/min infusion, and (3) 10 µg/kg bolus + 0.15 µg/kg/min infusion. (Adapted from ref. *26,* with permission.)

Although heparin does not affect the antiplatelet activity of tirofiban, there is evidence that administration of tirofiban with heparin results in synergistic antithrombin activity. In a study comparing the effects on thrombin generation of abciximab versus tirofiban during coronary intervention, both agents induced similar elevations in the activated clotting time (ACT) when administered after standard heparinization *(27).* Furthermore, both agents suppressed levels of F1.2, a prothrombin fragment, suggesting that their antithrombin effects are caused by decreased thrombin generation. These data support the concept that the antithrombin activity of GPIIb/IIIa inhibitors is a class effect and that ACT-guided heparin dosing during PCI should be based on an ACT obtained following administration of the GPIIb/IIIa inhibitor.

TIROFIBAN
IN PERCUTANEOUS CORONARY INTERVENTION

Two large-scale trials have been conducted using tirofiban in high-risk patients undergoing PCI: RESTORE *(28)* and TARGET *(29).* Dosing of tirofiban in both studies was based on the dose-ranging study of Kereiakes et al. *(26)* and used the highest dosing regimen (a 10 µg/kg bolus followed by a 0.15 µg/kg/min infusion) to ensure >90% IPA throughout the duration of tirofiban administration.

RESTORE

STUDY DESIGN

The Randomized Efficacy Study of Tirofiban for Outcomes and REstenosis (RESTORE) trial was a randomized, double-blind, placebo-controlled study of tirofiban in patients undergoing percutaneous transluminal coronary angioplasty (PTCA) or directional coronary atherectomy (DCA) within 72 h of presenting with an acute coronary syndrome [unstable angina or myocardial infarction (MI)]. Unstable angina was defined as typical chest pain occurring at rest or with minimal activity and associated with any of the following:

(1) dynamic electrocardiographic (ECG) changes consistent with myocardial ischemia; (2) hemodynamic changes suggestive of ischemia; or (3) angiographic evidence of intra-coronary thrombus. MI was defined as ischemic chest pain lasting >20 min with ST-T changes or pathologic Q waves and creative kinase (CK) elevations greater than twice the upper limit of normal (ULN) or an elevated CK-MB fraction. Notable exclusion criteria included patients who had received thrombolytic therapy within the previous 24 h or who were scheduled for elective coronary stent implantation. Moreover, the protocol instructed investigators to limit the use of coronary stents to "bailout" situations such as actual or threatened abrupt vessel closure.

All patients received 325 mg of aspirin before the procedure and weight-adjusted hep-arin during the procedure to maintain the ACT between 300 and 400 s. Once the guidewire had crossed the lesion, patients were randomized to tirofiban (10 µg/kg bolus over 3 min followed by a 0.15 µg/kg/min infusion for 36 h) or matching placebo. Heparin was dis-continued at the end of the procedure, and the arterial and venous sheaths were removed when the ACT had fallen below 180 s.

The primary endpoint of the study was the 30-d composite of all-cause mortality, MI, coronary artery bypass surgery (CABG), repeat target vessel PCI for recurrent ischemia, or emergent stent implantation for actual or threatened abrupt vessel closure. The criteria required for an MI to qualify as an event depended on the patient's clinical diagnosis upon enrollment in the study. In patients entering the study with unstable angina and normal CK/CK-MB levels, the diagnosis of an MI required: (1) typical chest pain, with new ST-T changes or new pathologic Q waves, in association with an elevated CK-MB, or (2) a CK-MB > 3× ULN in the absence of chest pain or ECG changes. In patients enrolling within 72 h of an MI, the diagnosis of a new MI could be made if (1) the CK-MB was >3× ULN and at least 33% > the previous nadir, or (2) the CK-MB was >3× ULN and at least 100% greater than the previous value if that was <50% of the peak value and <2× ULN. In all patients following hospital discharge, a new MI was defined as (1) typical chest pain with new ST-T changes or new pathologic Q waves and an elevated CK-MB, or (2) a CK-MB level >2× ULN unaccompanied by angina or ECG changes. Although the criteria for an MI to qualify as an event were quite rigorous, routine surveillance for its occurrence was solely limited to a protocol-mandated measurement of CK and CK-MB at the end of the 36-h study drug infusion. Otherwise, cardiac enzymes were drawn only if clinically indicated to eval-uate an episode of myocardial ischemia.

RESULTS

Of the 2212 patients randomized, 71 patients never received the study drug, leaving 2141 patients for inclusion in the efficacy and safety analysis. More than 70% of patients were male, with 20% in each arm being diabetic. Most patients entered the study with a diagnosis of unstable angina and were evenly divided among the two treatment arms. PCI was performed as the primary reperfusion therapy for acute MI in 6% of patients in the placebo group and 7% of patients in the tirofiban group. PTCA was the predominant inter-ventional procedure and was performed in 93 and 92% of patients in the placebo and tirofi-ban groups, respectively. By default, DCA was used in the remainder of patients. Single-vessel intervention was performed in >90% of cases in both groups. Only 2% of treated vessels were bypass grafts. Multiple lesions were treated in 20% of patients in the placebo group and 24% of patients in the tirofiban group.

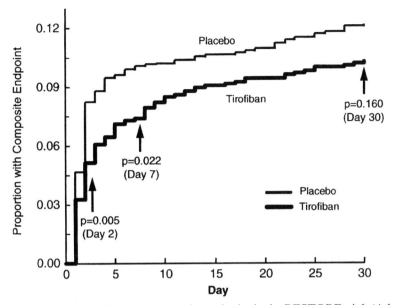

Fig. 6. Kaplan-Meier curves of time to composite endpoint in the RESTORE trial. (Adapted from ref. *28*, with permission.)

Endpoints were evaluated at 2, 7, and 30 d with a clinical and angiographic substudy *(30)* extending the follow-up to 6 mo. At 2 d, the composite endpoint was reduced from 8.7% in the placebo group to 5.4% in the tirofiban group [relative risk reduction (RRR) = 38%, $p < 0.005$], whereas at 7 d, the RRR remained statistically significant at 27% ($p = 0.022$). At both these time points, the benefit of tirofiban was predominantly owing to a reduction in nonfatal MI and the need for repeat angioplasty. At 30 d, however, the reduction in the composite endpoint from 12.2% in the placebo group to 10.3% in the tirofiban group no longer reached statistical significance (Fig. 6). Similarly, 6-mo follow-up also failed to show a statistically significant decrease in the composite endpoint in the tirofiban group, with events occurring in 27.1% of placebo patients and 24.1% of tirofiban patients ($p = 0.11$).

To investigate the effects of tirofiban on the incidence of restenosis, 619 patients were enrolled in a 6-mo angiographic substudy *(30)*. Paired serial angiograms were available in 67% of these patients. Target lesion restenosis was defined as either (1) ≥50% stenosis in those patients who had a <50% stenosis following the initial intervention; (2) late loss in minimal lumen diameter (MLD) of ≥0.72 mm; or (3) late loss ≥50% of the initial gain in MLD. Despite the multitude of definitions for restenosis, the results failed to show a statistically significant difference between the tirofiban and placebo groups. Cumulative distribution curves of MLD before and after PCI and at 6 mo were practically superimposable (Fig. 7).

ANALYSIS

The results of the RESTORE trial confirm that tirofiban is effective in reducing the incidence of acute ischemic complications during PTCA/DCA in patients presenting with an acute coronary syndrome, with extension of these benefits at least into the first week following the intervention. By 30 d, however, the magnitude of the benefit is substantially

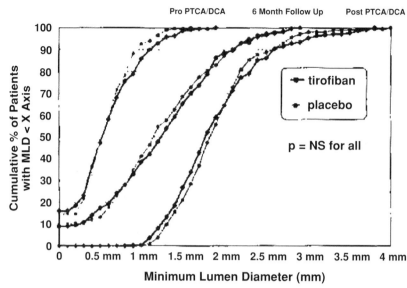

Fig. 7. Cumulative distribution curves of minimum lumen diameter (MLD) before and after intervention and at 6-mo follow-up in patients treated with tirofiban (■) or placebo (●) in the RESTORE trial. (Adapted from ref. *30*, with permission.)

attenuated and no longer statistically significant. Furthermore, treatment with tirofiban does not appear to lower the incidence of restenosis. These results are in contradistinction to those of three contemporary abciximab trials *(19,20,31)* that suggested long-term benefits with abciximab in similar patients. These trials however, included only urgent repeat revascularization as a component of the composite endpoint, whereas the RESTORE trial included any target vessel revascularization in the composite endpoint. In an attempt to account for this difference and allow for comparison of the results between these different trials, the RESTORE investigators performed a *post hoc*, blinded readjudication of the 30-d event rates by including only urgent revascularization (CABG or PCI) in the composite endpoint (Fig. 8). Utilizing this approach, a statistically significant decrease in the 30-d event rate from 10.5% in the placebo arm to 8.0% in the tirofiban arm was observed (RRR = 24%, *p* = 0.052), matching the 8.3% event rate noted in the abciximab arm of the EPIC trial *(31)*.

RESTORE also differed from EPIC and EPILOG in the rate of nonfatal myocardial infarction, reflecting differences in the frequency of serum CK measurements in these trials. In RESTORE, a CK sample was obtained only at the end of the 36-h infusion, whereas in EPIC and EPILOG, CK samples were obtained at multiple time points throughout the first 48 h. Consequently, the nonfatal MI rate in the placebo group of RESTORE was only 5.7%, compared with 8.6 and 8.7% in EPIC and EPILOG, respectively. The lower MI rate in the RESTORE placebo group translated to a smaller absolute risk reduction, even though the absolute MI rates observed in the treatment arms of these trials were similar.

Other important differences between these trials, both in study design and in differing practice patterns present at the time of the respective trials, have prohibited definitive comparisons between the various GPIIb/IIIa inhibitors. For example, in EPIC, drug administration occurred before guidewire placement, as opposed to after guidewire placement,

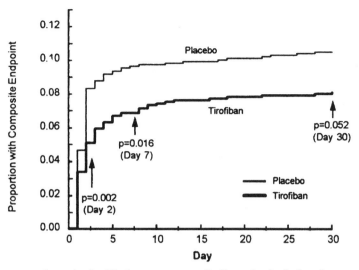

Fig. 8. Time to composite endpoint 30-d event rates readjudicated to include only urgent or emergent revascularizations. (Adapted from ref. *28*, with permission.)

as was the case in RESTORE. Stent usage also differed among these trials. The use of stents for abrupt vessel closure was greater in RESTORE (2.5%) than EPIC (0.6%). As a result, there was a corresponding decrease in the frequency of CABG, from 3.6% in EPIC to 1.3% in RESTORE. In light of these differences and the differing pharmacokinetic and pharmacodynamic properties between tirofiban and abciximab, the TARGET trial was designed to compare these two agents directly.

TARGET

STUDY DESIGN

The Do Tirofiban and ReoPro Give Similar Efficacy Outcomes Trial was a double-blind, double-dummy, multinational study conducted to test whether tirofiban was not inferior to abciximab in patients scheduled to undergo coronary stenting. Eligible patients included those undergoing either an elective or urgent procedure but not those in cardiogenic shock or with ECG evidence of an acute ST-segment elevation myocardial infarction. Patients were randomized to receive either tirofiban (10 μg/kg bolus followed by a 0.15 μg/kg/min infusion for 18–24 h) with abciximab placebo or abciximab (0.25 mg/kg bolus followed by a 0.125 μg/kg/min infusion for 12 h) with tirofiban placebo. Randomization was stratified by the presence or absence of diabetes; all patients received 250–500 mg of aspirin and, when possible, a loading dose of 300 mg of clopidogrel. Heparin was administered at the start of the procedure using a weight-based dosing nomogram to achieve an ACT of 250 s.

The primary endpoint was a composite of death, nonfatal MI, or urgent target vessel revascularization within 30 d of the procedure. A new myocardial infarction was defined biochemically as a CK-MB level > 3× ULN in two successive blood samples, or electrocardiographically by the presence of new pathologic Q waves in two or more contiguous

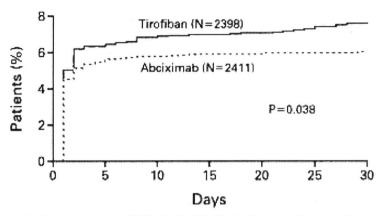

Fig. 9. Incidence of primary endpoint at 30 d in the TARGET trial. (Adapted from ref. *29* with permission.)

leads. Serum chemistry samples were obtained at baseline and every 6 h for 24 h. For patients with a non-ST-elevation MI who were enrolled in the study, the CK-MB value also had to be 50% greater than the last preprocedural level for an event to qualify as an MI. Pre-specified secondary endpoints included the occurrence of a primary endpoint in specific subgroups: diabetics, females, patients >65 yr of age, patients pretreated with clopidogrel, and patients enrolled in participating U.S. sites.

RESULTS

A total of 5308 patients were enrolled in the trial; 4809 of these patients actually received study drug (2398 in the tirofiban group and 2411 in the abciximab group) and were included in the analysis. Approximately 75% in each group were men, and 23% in each group were diabetics. Most patients (63%) were enrolled with a diagnosis of an acute coronary syndrome, and almost all (95%) patients in both groups received a coronary stent. A native coronary artery was the target vessel in 95% of cases. Restenotic lesions were treated in 5% of cases in each group. Most patients (81%) were treated in the United States.

The primary endpoint occurred in 7.6% of patients in the tirofiban group compared to 6.0% in the abciximab group. To meet prespecified criteria for noninferiority, the upper bound of the 95% confidence interval (CI) of the hazard ratio (HR) had to be <1.47. In fact, the upper bound of the one-sided 95% CI was 1.51, failing to meet the criteria necessary to confirm the noninferiority of tirofiban to abciximab. Once the noninferiority of tirofiban could not be established, the researchers were then able to assess whether abciximab was superior to tirofiban. The HR comparing tirofiban with abciximab showed a statistically significant difference at 1.26 (95% CI = 1.01–1.57, $p = 0.038$) (Fig. 9). Most of the benefit was derived from the difference in the nonfatal MI rates between the two drugs (6.9% vs 5.4%, $p = 0.04$) (Fig. 10). Stratification of the MI rates by the magnitude of the CK-MB level showed that the protective effect of abciximab was more prominent with larger infarctions. For example, whereas the risk ratio comparing tirofiban with abciximab was 0.86 ($p = NS$) for CK-MB elevations of 3–5× ULN, at CK-MB levels of >10× ULN, it increased to 1.47 ($p = NS$). Furthermore, the risk ratio for the development of new abnormal Q waves was 1.66 ($p = NS$). Although underpowered to detect statistically significant differences, these results suggest that the main benefit of abciximab over

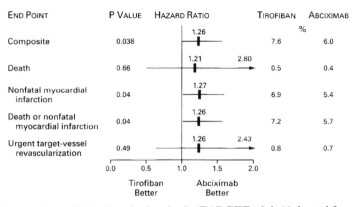

Fig. 10. Hazard ratios for individual endpoints in the TARGET trial. (Adapted from ref. *29*, with permission.)

tirofiban may well be in the prevention of Q-wave or sizable non-Q-wave MIs. The benefit of abciximab was obtained without any increase in risk of major bleeding, which was <1.0% in both groups. There was, however, a significantly higher incidence of minor bleeding attributable to abciximab (4.3% vs 2.8%, $p < 0.001$). There also was a significantly greater incidence of thrombocytopenia in the abciximab group, although this did not result in a higher incidence of either red cell or platelet transfusions.

Prespecified subgroup analyses revealed that patients who received a stent for the treatment of an acute coronary syndrome obtained greater benefit from abciximab than those patients who received a stent for other reasons. Patients <65 yr of age obtained greater benefit with abciximab than with tirofiban, whereas both agents were equally effective in patients >65 yr of age. The presence of diabetes did not result in any difference in efficacy between the two agents. Stratification of outcome by treatment center revealed a significant benefit of abciximab over tirofiban in patients treated at non-US centers, with an event rate of 2.9% with abciximab and 6.9% with tirofiban. In fact, in the 3910 patients treated at US centers, the HR was only 1.14, with the lower boundary of the 95% CI falling below unity. The most likely explanation for this difference can be found in the unexpectedly low event rate (2.9%) in the abciximab group of non-US patients. In EPISTENT (*32*), for comparison, the 30-d composite endpoint of death, MI, or urgent target vessel revascularization occurred in 5.3% of patients randomized to receive a stent and abciximab. Furthermore, most patients enrolled in EPISTENT did not have an acute coronary syndrome and thus would be expected to have a lower event rate than those in TARGET, in which 63% of patients were enrolled with a diagnosis of an acute coronary syndrome.

At 6 mo the difference between the two agents in the composite endpoint (14.4 vs 13.8, $p =$ NS) was attenuated and, although still favoring abciximab, was no longer statistically significant (*33*). Once again, it was the nonfatal-MI event rates that predominantly influenced the composite endpoint. A small decrease in the absolute risk reduction from 1.5% at 30 d to 1.4% at 6 mo was sufficient to prevent the composite endpoint from reaching statistical significance. Target vessel revascularization also failed to show a statistically significant difference, not only at 30 d but, more importantly, also at 6 mo, confirming that the nonspecificity of abciximab for the GPIIb/IIIa integrin does not affect the clinical restenosis rate.

ANALYSIS

The TARGET trial is the only trial to date that has directly compared two different GPIIb/IIIa inhibitors. Based on the results of this trial, several conclusions can be drawn that can help guide clinical practice. It is safe to say that in patients <65 yr of age and particularly in those presenting with an acute coronary syndrome and who have a culprit lesion that is amenable to PCI with stenting, abciximab is the preferred agent. Not only is it associated with an improved clinical outcome, but it also provides this benefit without an increase in clinically significant bleeding. Vigilance must be exercised, however, since abciximab is more likely than tirofiban to cause a profound thrombocytopenia (<20,000/mm^3). One recent study cited an incidence of profound thrombocytopenia of approx 0.5% *(34)*, which correlates well with the 0.3% incidence observed in the TARGET trial. Consequently, early (e.g., 4 h post bolus) and sequential complete blood counts should be performed in all patients treated with abciximab.

The TARGET trial failed to show any difference between the two agents in elderly patients (>65 yr) or those with chronic stable angina who are referred for elective PCI. Multivariate modeling is necessary to understand these subgroup comparisons fully and to identify patients who might derive equal benefit from both agents. The data do not support the theory that the nonplatelet effects of abciximab influence the clinical restenosis rate. More significant, and most likely reflecting the evolutionary improvements in the procedural aspects of PCI in general, was the observation that the clinical restenosis rate, reflected by the 6-mo target vessel revascularization rate, was only approx 8% in both treatment arms *(33)*.

It must be kept in mind that the main benefit of abciximab is in lowering the incidence of periprocedural myocardial infarctions, as manifested by an asymptomatic elevation in the CK-MB. Although the protective effect of abciximab is greater with larger infarctions, in absolute numbers most of the periprocedural myocardial enzyme elevations are of small magnitude, and their clinical significance remains a subject of significant debate *(35)*. The lack of a significant mortality difference at 6-mo and 1 yr *(33a)* follow-up suggests that the increase in the periprocedural MI event rate is not associated with an increase in cardiac death. Longer follow-up will be required to determine whether these infarctions result in progressive LV dysfunction or late sudden cardiac death.

Several theories have been advanced to explain the superiority of abciximab over tirofiban that was observed in the TARGET trial *(29)*. Preferential blockade of the vitronectin and Mac-1 receptors by abciximab leads to inhibition of platelet-endothelial cell, platelet-smooth muscle cell, and monocyte-platelet aggregates and, as a result, interferes with the recruitment of inflammatory cells to sites of vessel injury *(36)*. It is plausible that attenuation of this inflammatory response may help stabilize a ruptured plaque or dampen the magnitude of the periprocedural platelet activation that has been shown to predict the risk of acute ischemic events after PCI *(37)*. Though GUSTO-IV *(38)* failed to show any benefit of abciximab as adjunctive therapy in the medical treatment of patients with unstable angina or non-ST-elevation myocardial infarction, differences in the timing of the event relative to drug administration or differences in the characteristics between spontaneous or mechanical plaque disruption may explain abciximab's demonstrated benefit in PCI.

Dosing Considerations

An alternative explanation for the observed differences between abciximab and tirofiban is that the dose of tirofiban used was suboptimal and did not provide an equivalent degree of platelet inhibition to that provided by abciximab. In a pharmacodynamic dose-escalation trial of abciximab *(39)* that served as the basis for the dose used in the EPIC trial, a threshold of >80% inhibition of platelet aggregation to 20 µM ADP was selected as the target for pharmacological efficacy. This degree of platelet inhibition correlated to >80% receptor occupancy which, in animal models of coronary stenosis, has been shown to prevent platelet thrombosis during coronary angioplasty *(40)*. Consequently, studies with the small-molecule agents adopted this threshold as the minimum degree of platelet inhibition required to ensure efficacious dosing. However, in the only dose-ranging study of tirofiban in patients undergoing PCI *(26)*, the concentration of ADP used as agonist for the light aggregometry assays was only 5 µM as opposed to the 20 µM ADP used in the pharmacodynamic study for abciximab described above. So, despite the fact that the dose of tirofiban that was eventually used both in the RESTORE and TARGET trials, was shown to provide >90% inhibition of platelet activation, it remains uncertain that the degree of platelet inhibition between the two agents in the TARGET trial was truly equivalent given this difference in the potency of the agonist. In fact, in a study that did use 20 µM ADP as the agonist, 30 patients with unstable angina were randomly assigned to receive either standard-dose abciximab, PURSUIT-dose eptifibatide *(41)*, or PRISM-PLUS-dose tirofiban *(42)*. The IPA was then assessed in PPACK-anticoagulated blood at baseline, at 10 and 40 min after the bolus, and at 4–6, 12, and 18–20 h. The median IPA was found to exceed 80% at all time points for abciximab and eptifibatide, whereas with tirofiban, only at the 18-h sample was the median IPA > 80% *(43)*. Unfortunately, the generalizability of these results to other acute coronary syndrome patients undergoing PCI is limited by the difference in the dose of tirofiban used in this study (acute coronary syndrome dose) and that used in the TARGET trial (PCI dose).

In another comparative trial investigating the extent of platelet inhibition produced by the three agents, Simon et al. *(44)* used a hybrid dose of tirofiban [RESTORE bolus (10 µg/kg) + PRISM-PLUS infusion (0.10 µg/kg/min)] and measured 20 µM ADP-induced platelet aggregation at 10 min following the bolus. Once again, tirofiban exhibited a significantly lower degree of platelet inhibition than did either abciximab or eptifibatide. Given the timing of the blood sample, the suggestion is that the bolus dose of tirofiban may be inadequate. Several limitations of the study, including differences in the patients' baseline characteristics, differences in dosing regimens, and the lack of information regarding the use of clopidogrel preclude definitive conclusions *(45)*.

In an attempt to investigate further the issue of inadequate dosing of tirofiban, especially since patients with an acute coronary syndrome have been shown to exhibit a greater degree of platelet activation *(46)* than in patients without, we *(47)* randomly assigned 20 acute coronary syndrome patients who were undergoing planned coronary stenting to tirofiban (10 µg/kg bolus, 0.15 µg/kg/min × 18 h) or abciximab (0.25 mg/kg bolus, 0.125 µg/kg/min × 12 h) and measured the IPA to 20 µM ADP at baseline, 5, 15, 30, 45, and 60 min after drug administration. All patients were pretreated with ASA (325 mg) and clopidogrel (300 mg) and received heparin to maintain an ACT of at least 250 s. At all time points, the IPA with tirofiban was less than that with abciximab (Fig. 11). This difference was statistically significant only at the 15-min time interval, consistent with the suggestion that the bolus dose of tirofiban may be suboptimal. Furthermore, the mean time to balloon inflation (13 ± 2 min) coincided with the timing of the maximal difference in the IPA between the two drugs, suggesting that at the crucial moment of initial balloon inflation, tirofiban less effectively inhibits platelet activation than does abciximab.

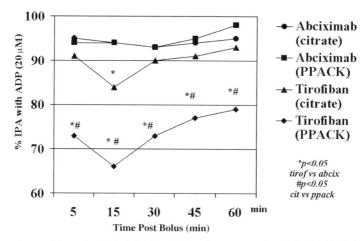

Fig. 11. Comparison of the extent of inhibition of platelet aggregation (20 μ*M* ADP) by tirofiban and abciximab as a function of time post bolus and anticoagulant. With citrate as anticoagulant, the inhibition of platelet aggregation at 15 min is significantly lower with tirofiban than abciximab. (Adapted from ref. *47*, with permission.)

Additional, although circumstantial, evidence to support the theory that it is the bolus dose of tirofiban that may be inadequate can be found in a German study *(48)* that measured the IPA in 60 patients undergoing coronary stenting for symptomatic coronary artery disease who were randomized to abciximab, eptifibatide, or tirofiban. The dose of tirofiban was the same as that used in the TARGET trial. Platelet aggregometry using 20 μ*M* ADP was performed on serial blood samples obtained starting at 2 h following initial drug administration. At the 2-h time interval, there were no significant differences in the mean inhibition or in the percentage of patients achieving >80% inhibition with either drug. This degree of platelet inhibition was subsequently maintained for the duration of the infusion. The results of these two studies suggest that following a bolus of 10 μg/kg, tirofiban less effectively inhibits platelet aggregation than does the corresponding abciximab bolus but by 1–2 h into the infusion the degree of platelet inhibition is equivalent. These observations may also help explain the efficacy of tirofiban in the medical management of patients presenting with an acute coronary syndrome who are pretreated with tirofiban prior to undergoing PCI.

PCI IN PATIENTS PRETREATED WITH TIROFIBAN

Two large-scale trials, PRISM-PLUS *(42)* and TACTICS-TIMI 18 *(49)*, have involved patients presenting with unstable angina or non-ST-elevation MI who were initially treated with tirofiban and subsequently underwent PCI. A review of these trials will help to define further the role of tirofiban in the cardiac catheterization laboratory, especially since many patients are referred for coronary angiography and intervention only after having failed aggressive medical therapy with aspirin, heparin, and a GPIIb/IIIa inhibitor such as tirofiban.

PRISM-PLUS

STUDY DESIGN

The Platelet Receptor Inhibition in Ischemic Syndrome Management in Patients Limited by Unstable Signs and Symptoms (PRISM-PLUS) trial was a randomized, double-blind, multicenter study of 1915 patients with Canadian Cardiovascular Society class III or IV angina and either ischemic ECG changes or elevated levels of cardiac enzymes who were randomized to one of three dosing regimens: (1) tirofiban (0.6 µg/kg/min for 30 min, followed by an infusion of 0.15 µg/kg/min) plus placebo heparin; (2) tirofiban (0.4 µg/kg/min bolus over 30 min, followed by an infusion of 0.1 µg/kg/min) plus dose-adjusted heparin; or (3) dose-adjusted heparin plus placebo tirofiban. Study medications were infused for a minimum of 48 h, and all patients also received 325 mg of aspirin daily. Between 48 and 96 h, all patients were encouraged to proceed with coronary angiography and coronary intervention if indicated. In patients undergoing PCI, tirofiban (or tirofiban placebo) was continued for 12–24 h following the procedure, whereas the heparin was discontinued at the end of the procedure and the sheaths removed at least 2 h later. After the first interim efficacy analysis, the tirofiban-only arm was discontinued because of an excess mortality (4.6% vs 1.1%, tirofiban vs heparin, respectively).

The primary endpoint of the trial was the 7-d composite of all-cause mortality, new MI, refractory ischemia, or rehospitalization for unstable angina. A prospectively defined analysis examined the occurrence of the composite endpoint at 30 d in the subgroup of 475 patients who underwent PTCA.

RESULTS

The addition of tirofiban to heparin therapy significantly decreased the occurrence of the composite endpoint at 7 d from 17.9% in the heparin-only arm to 12.9% in the tirofiban plus heparin arm (RR = 0.68, 95% CI = 0.53-0.88, p = 0.004). Although the absolute difference decreased over time, the reduction in the composite endpoint remained statistically significant at 30 d and 6 mo. This reduction was primarily driven by a 47% reduction in the incidence of MI and a 50% reduction in the incidence of refractory ischemia. The mortality rate at all time points was similar in both groups. The beneficial effect of tirofiban on the incidence of MI was apparent as early as 48 h into therapy, coincident with the duration of the medical stabilization phase of the trial.

During the initial hospitalization 90% of patients underwent coronary angiography, and angioplasty was subsequently performed on 30.5% of all patients, at the discretion of the attending physician. In this subgroup, the 30-d composite endpoint occurred in 8.8% of patients in the tirofiban plus heparin group and in 15.3% of patients in the heparin-only group, suggesting that patients with an acute coronary syndrome who undergo PCI derive particular benefit from pretreatment with tirofiban in addition to aspirin and heparin.

The mechanism of this benefit is most likely a reduction in intracoronary thrombus burden and improved coronary flow. In an angiographic substudy of PRISM-PLUS, 1491 angiograms were analyzed at the core angiographic laboratory for the extent of intracoronary thrombus, Thrombolysis in Myocardial Infarction (TIMI) flow grade, and lesion severity (50). The clot burden was classified using the TIMI thrombus grading system, in which grade 1 is defined as a possible thrombus, grade 2 a small thrombus [<0.5× normal lumen diameter (NLD)], grade 3 a medium-sized thrombus (0.5–1.5× NLD), grade 4 a large thrombus (>1.5× NLD), grade 5 a recent thrombotic occlusion, and grade 6 a chronic occlusion. The primary angiographic endpoint was the proportion of patients with each grade of TIMI thrombus excluding grade 6, since chronic occlusions were unlikely to be the cause of the presenting acute coronary syndrome. Predefined secondary endpoints included TIMI flow grade and lesion severity. Compared with heparin alone, tirofiban plus heparin significantly reduced intracoronary thrombus burden by 23% (OR = 0.77,

$p = 0.022$) and significantly increased the proportion of patients with TIMI 3 flow (OR = 0.65 for TIMI 2 or less vs TIMI 3, $p = 0.002$). Persistence of thrombus was associated with a twofold increase in the composite endpoint at 30 d.

ANALYSIS

The results of the PRISM-PLUS study suggest that significant clinical benefit can be anticipated from the early initiation of tirofiban in patients with acute coronary syndrome. This benefit was evident as early as 48 h into therapy, implying that tirofiban is effective in patients who are treated medically. These results are consistent with a recent metaanalysis of trials of GPIIb/IIIa inhibitors in acute coronary syndrome: an overall 34% reduction in the incidence of death or nonfatal MI was noted during the initial period of medical stabilization prior to PCI *(51)*.

A reduction in the composite endpoint in PRISM-PLUS was also present at 7 d, 30 d, and 6 mo in the combination therapy group. Most of the benefit at these time points was conferred on the subset of patients who underwent PCI. In fact, the incidence of the composite endpoint at 30 d in the group of patients treated with medical management alone, although favoring combination therapy, was not significantly different from that in the heparin-only group (RR = 0.87, 95% CI = 0.6-1.25).

Based on the results of the angiographic substudy, it is evident that the mechanism responsible for the observed clinical benefit is a reduction in the thrombus burden and an improvement in coronary flow. Mechanistically, this may also explain why some of the initial comparative trials of early invasive or conservative therapy for patients with acute coronary syndrome, which did not include GPIIb/IIIa inhibitor therapy, demonstrated a worse outcome in the invasive arms *(52)*. In light of this apparent paradox, the TACTICS-TIMI 18 trial was designed to compare directly an early invasive or conservative treatment strategy in acute coronary syndrome patients treated with tirofiban combination therapy.

TACTICS-TIMI 18

STUDY DESIGN

The Treat Angina with Aggrastat and Determine Cost of Therapy with an Invasive or Conservative Strategy (TACTICS-TIMI 18) trial randomized 2220 patients with unstable angina or non-ST-elevation MI to early invasive or conservative therapy. All patients were treated with aspirin and unfractionated heparin (5000 U bolus followed by a 1000 U/h infusion for 48 h), and tirofiban was administered as a 0.4 µg/kg/min bolus over 30 min followed by a maintenance infusion of 0.1 µg/kg/min for 48 h or until revascularization. For patients undergoing percutaneous revascularization, the tirofiban infusion was continued for at least 12 h after the procedure. Patients were eligible for inclusion if they had experienced either a prolonged episode of angina or recurrent episodes at rest or with minimal exertion within the previous 24 h that were associated with ischemic ECG changes, abnormal cardiac enzymes, or prior evidence of documented coronary artery disease. Patients were excluded if they presented with persistent ST-segment elevation, had undergone a PCI or CABG within the previous 6 mo, had evidence of severe congestive heart failure or cardiogenic shock, or were felt to be at increased risk of bleeding.

Patients randomized to an early invasive strategy were to undergo diagnostic catheterization between 4 and 48 h after randomization, followed by PCI or CABG as appropriate. Patients randomized to early conservative therapy underwent invasive procedures only if they failed medical therapy, as defined by the occurrence of any of the following: refractory angina, hemodynamic instability, documented ischemia on routine or nuclear stress testing, rehospitalization for recurrent angina, or new MI. The primary endpoint was the 6-mo composite of death, nonfatal MI, and rehospitalization for an acute coronary syndrome.

RESULTS

In the group of patients randomized to an early invasive therapy, diagnostic catheterization was performed in 97%, a median (25th, 75th percentiles) of 22 (18, 39) h after randomization. Subsequent revascularization with PCI or CABG was performed in 60% of patients, a median of 25 (19, 46) and 89 (48, 142) h after randomization, respectively. Coronary stents were used in 83% of coronary interventions in the invasive group. Tirofiban therapy was administered in 94% of cases.

At 6 mo, the primary endpoint had occurred in 15.9% of patients in the invasive group as opposed to 19.4% of patients in the conservative group (OR = 0.78, 95% CI = 0.62–0.97, $p = 0.025$). This reduction was evident as early as 30 d after randomization (7.4% vs 10.5%, $p = 0.009$). The predominant benefit was seen in the reduction of nonfatal MI and rehospitalization for recurrent angina and not in a reduction in mortality.

ANALYSIS

The many similarities between the patients in the TACTICS trial and those in the TARGET trial allow for several important comparisons. The difference in the incidence of death or nonfatal MI (an endpoint chosen for comparison given the different definitions of the primary endpoint in each study) between abciximab and tirofiban at 30 d in TARGET is no longer evident when the event rate in the abciximab arm in TARGET (5.7%) is compared with the event rate in the invasive arm of TACTICS (4.7%). The fact that the patients in the invasive arm of TACTICS underwent PCI later than those in TARGET suggests several hypotheses that may explain the above observation. It is possible that suboptimal bolus dosing of tirofiban contributed to its reduced efficacy in TARGET, or that a longer tirofiban infusion is required prior to PCI in order to passivate the lesion and reduce complications. The preponderance of evidence to date clearly shows that several hours into an infusion of tirofiban the inhibition of platelet aggregation is similar to that provided by abciximab and well above the accepted cutoff of 80% (see TARGET section). Additionally, pretreatment with tirofiban, which, in PRISM-PLUS, was shown to decrease the thrombus burden and improve coronary flow, may prevent the occurrence of distal microembolization that often results in small myocardial infarctions. Prevention of these periprocedural infarcts is consistent with the observation that the main benefit observed in these trials was in a lower incidence of nonfatal MI.

In light of the increased use of tirofiban in the initial treatment of patients with acute coronary syndrome, the results of the TARGET trial raise the question of whether to switch to abciximab in patients on tirofiban who are referred for PCI. Although a small, single-center study of 50 patients did document a further reduction in platelet function without a higher incidence of bleeding or thrombocytopenia when abciximab was substituted for tirofiban in acute coronary syndrome patients undergoing PCI (53), our practice is to continue the tirofiban during the intervention. This strategy is supported by the low incidence of adverse outcomes in the patients randomized to the early invasive arm of the TACTICS trial and by the pharmacodynamic studies showing equivalent degrees of platelet inhibition between abciximab and tirofiban after the first 2 h of drug infusion.

CONCLUSIONS

Tirofiban is a specific antagonist of the GPIIb/IIIa receptor with unique pharmacologic properties that distinguish it from the other agents in its class that have been approved by the Food and Drug Administration. A wealth of evidence from well-designed, large-scale trials now exists confirming that therapy with tirofiban reduces the incidence of adverse cardiac events in acute coronary syndrome patients treated medically as well as in patients undergoing PCI directly. In both groups, the observed benefits include a reduction in the combined incidence of death or MI as well as a reduction in the incidence of refractory ischemia or need for urgent repeat revascularization. Furthermore, it is evident that in patients with acute coronary syndrome who are initially treated medically, the ones who derive the greatest benefit are those who subsequently proceed to cardiac catheterization and coronary intervention.

Inevitable comparisons with abciximab suggest that for younger acute coronary syndrome patients, abciximab is the superior agent, resulting in a reduced incidence of nonfatal MI within 30 d after intervention. However, for nonacute coronary syndrome patients undergoing elective stenting, there appears to be no discernable difference in outcomes between the two agents, and the shorter half-life, lower incidence of profound thrombocytopenia, and lower cost of tirofiban make it an attractive alternative to abciximab. Moreover, multiple small-scale studies have suggested that the difference in efficacy between the two agents may be a result of an inadequate bolus dose of tirofiban, resulting in suboptimal platelet inhibition at the time of coronary intervention. A multicenter, dose-escalation study of the bolus dose of tirofiban is currently under way to address this issue.

REFERENCES

1. Pytela R, Pierschbacher MD, Ginsberg MH, Plow EF, Ruoslahti E. Platelet membrane glycoprotein IIb/IIIa: member of a family of Arg-Gly-Asp-specific adhesion receptors. Science 1986;231:1559–1562.
2. Gould RJ, Polokoff MA, Friedman PA, et al. Disintegrins: a family of integrin inhibitory proteins from viper venoms. Proc Soc Exp Biol Med 1990;195:168–171.
3. Musial J, Niewiarowski S, Rucinski B, et al. Inhibition of platelet adhesion to surfaces of extracorporeal circuits by disintegrins. RGD-containing peptides from viper venoms. Circulation 1990;82:261–273.
4. Hartman GD, Egbertson MS, Halczenko W, et al. Non-peptide fibrinogen receptor antagonists: 1. Discovery and design of exosite inhibitors. J Med Chem 1992;35:4640–4642.
5. Thibault G, Tardif P, Lapalme G. Comparative specificity of platelet $\alpha_{IIb}\beta_3$ integrin antagonists. J Pharmacol Exp Ther 2001;296:690–696.
6. Chen Y, Pitzenberger SM, Garsky VM, Lumma PK, Sanval G, Baum J. Proton NMR assignments and secondary structure of the snake venom protein eichistatin. Biochemistry 1991;30:11,625–11,636.
7. Egbertson MS, Chang CTC, Duggan ME, et al. Non-peptide fibrinogen receptor antagonists: 2. Optimization of a tyrosine template as a mimic for Arg-Gly-Asp. J Med Chem 1994;37:2537–2551.
8. Deckelbaum LI, Sax Fl, Grossman W. Tirofiban, a nonpeptide inhibitor of the platelet glycoprotein IIb/IIIa receptor. In: Sasahara AA, Loscalzo J, eds. New Therapeutic Agents in Thrombosis and Thrombolysis. Marcel Dekker, New York, 1997, pp. 355–365.
9. Hartman GD. Tirofiban hydrochloride platelet antiaggregatory GP IIb/IIIa receptor antagonist. Drugs Future 1995;20:897–901.
10. Bednar RA, Gaul SL, Hamill TG, et al. Identification of low molecular weight GP IIb/IIIa antagonists that bind preferentially to activated platelets. J Pharmacol Exp Ther 1998;285:1317–1326.
11. Tam SH, Sassoli PM, Jordan RE, Nakada MT. Abciximab (ReoPro, chimeric 7E3 Fab) demonstrates equivalent affinity and functional blockade of glycoprotein IIb/IIIa and alpha(v)beta3 integrins. Circulation 1998;98:1085–1091.
12. Simon DI, Xu H, Ortlepp S, Rogers C, Rao NK. 7E3 monoclonal antibody directed against the platelet glycoprotein IIb/IIIa cross-reacts with the leukocyte integrin Mac-1 and blocks adhesion to fibrinogen and ICAM-1. Arterioscler Thromb Vasc Biol 1997;17:528–535.

13. Gould RJ, Chang CTC, Lynch RJ, et al. MK-383 is a potent non-peptide mimic of RGD that inhibits glycoprotein IIb/IIIa (Abstract). Thromb Haemost 1993;69:976.

14. The EPIC Investigator Group. Long-term protection from myocardial ischemic events in a randomized trial of brief integrin β_3 blockade with percutaneous coronary intervention. JAMA 1997;278:479–484.

15. Chandrasekar B, Tanguay J-F. Platelets and restenosis. J Am Coll Cardiol 2000;35:555–562.

16. Scarborough RM, Kleiman NS, Phillips DR. Platelet glycoprotein IIb/IIIa antagonists: what are the relevant issues concerning their pharmacology and clinical use? Circulation 1999;100:437–444.

17. Matsuno H, Stassen JM, Varmylen J, Deckmyn H. Inhibition of integrin function by a cyclic RGD-containing peptide prevents neointima formation. Circulation 1994;90:2203–2206.

18. Deitch JS, Williams JK, Adams MR, et al. Effects of β-3 integrin blockade (c7E3) on the response to angioplasty and intra-arterial stenting in atherosclerotic nonhuman primates. Arterioscler Thromb Vasc Biol 1998;18:1730–1737.

19. The CAPTURE Investigators. Randomised placebo-controlled trial of abciximab before and during coronary intervention in refractory unstable angina: the CAPTURE study. Lancet 1997;349:1429–1435.

20. The EPILOG Investigators. Platelet glycoprotein IIb/IIIa receptor blockade and low-dose heparin during percutaneous coronary revascularization. N Engl J Med 1997;336:1689–1696.

21. Aggrastat Product Monograph, Merck & Co., 1998.

22. Cook JJ, Bednar B, Lynch JR, et al. Tirofiban(Aggrastat®). Cardiovasc Drug Rev 1999;17:199–224.

23. Talley JD. Pharmacology of GP IIb-IIIa platelet inhibitors, Part IV. J Intervent Cardiol 2000;13:243–254.

24. Peerlink K, De Lepeleire I, Goldberg M, et al. MK-383 (L-700,462), a selective nonpeptide platelet glycoprotein IIb/IIIa antagonist is active in man. Circulation 1993;88:1512–1517.

25. Kumar A, Herrmann HC. Tirofiban: an investigational platelet glycoprotein IIb/IIIa receptor antagonist. Exp Opin Invest Drugs 1996;6:1257–1267.

26. Kereiakes DJ, Kleiman NS, Ambrose J, et al. Randomized, double-blind, placebo-controlled dose-ranging study of tirofiban (MK-383) platelet IIb/IIIa blockade in high risk patients undergoing coronary angioplasty. J Am Coll Cardiol 1996;27:536–542.

27. Ambrose JA, Doss R, Geagea J-PM, et al. Effects on thrombin generation of the platelet glycoprotein IIb/IIIa inhibitors abciximab versus tirofiban during coronary intervention. Am J Cardiol 2001;87:1231–1233.

28. The RESTORE Investigators. Effects of platelet glycoprotein IIb/IIIa blockade with tirofiban on adverse cardiac events in patients with unstable angina or acute myocardial infarction undergoing coronary angioplasty. Circulation 1997;96:1445–1453.

29. The TARGET Investigators. Comparison of two platelet glycoprotein IIb/IIIa inhibitors, tirofiban and abciximab, for the prevention of ischemic events with percutaneous coronary revascularization. N Engl J Med 2001;344:1888–1894.

30. Gibson CM, Goel M, Cohen DJ, et al., for the RESTORE investigators. Six-month angiographic and clinical follow-up of patients prospectively randomized to receive either tirofiban or placebo during angioplasty in the RESTORE trial. J Am Coll Cardiol 1998;32:28–34.

31. The EPIC Investigators. Use of a monoclonal antibody directed against the platelet glycoprotein IIb/IIIa receptor in high risk angioplasty. N Engl J Med 1994;330:956–961.

32. The EPISTENT Investigators. Randomised placebo-controlled and balloon-angioplasty controlled trial to assess safety of coronary stenting with use of platelet glycoprotein-IIb/IIIa blockade. Lancet 1998;352:87–92.

33. Moliterno DJ, Yakubov SJ, DiBattiste PM, et al. Outcomes at 6 months for the direct comparison of tirofiban and abciximab during percutaneous coronary revascularization with stent placement: the TARGET follow-up study. Lancet 2002;360:355–360.

33a. Roffi M, Moliterno DJ, Meier B, et al. Impact of different platelet glycoprotein IIb/IIIa receptor inhibitors among diabetic patients undergoing percutaneous coronary intervention: TARGET 1-year follow-up. Circulation 2002;105:2730–2736.

34. Berkowitz SD, Harrington RA, Rund MM, Tcheng JE. Acute profound thrombocytopenia after c7E3 Fab (abciximab) therapy. Circulation 1997;96:809–813.

35. Stone GW, Mehran R, Dangas G, Lansky AJ, Kornowski R, Leon MB. Differential impact on survival of electrocardiographic Q-wave versus enzymatic myocardial infarction after percutaneous intervention: a device specific analysis of 7147 patients. Circulation 2001;104:642–647.

36. Nurden AT, Poujol C, Durrieu-Jais C, Nurden P. Platelet glycoprotein IIb/IIIa inhibitors: basic and clinical aspects. Arterioscler Thromb Vasc Biol 1999;19:2835–2840.

37. Tschoepe D, Schultheiss HP, Kolarov P, et al. Platelet membrane activation markers are predictive for increased risk of acute ischemic events after PTCA. Circulation 1993;88:37–42.

38. GUSTO IV-ACS Investigators. Effect of glycoprotein IIb/IIIa receptor blocker abciximab on outcome in patients with acute coronary syndromes without early revascularisation: the GUSTO IV-ACS randomised trial. Lancet 2001;357:1915–1924.

39. Tcheng JE, Ellis SG, George BS, et al. Pharmacodynamics of chimeric glycoprotein IIb/IIIa integrin antiplatelet antibody Fab 7E3 in high-risk coronary angioplasty. Circulation 1994;90:1757–1764.

40. Bates ER, McGillem MJ, Mickelson JK, Pitt B, Mancini GB. A monoclonal antibody against the platelet glycoprotein IIb/IIIa receptor complex prevents platelet aggregation and thrombosis in a canine model of coronary angioplasty. Circulation 1991;84:2463–2469.

41. The PURSUIT Trial Investigators. Inhibition of platelet glycoprotein IIb/IIIa with eptifibatide in patients with acute coronary syndromes. N Engl J Med 1998;339:436–443.

42. The PRISM-PLUS Investigators. Inhibition of the platelet glycoprotein IIb/IIIa receptor with tirofiban in unstable angina and non-Q-wave myocardial infarction. N Engl J Med 1998;338:1488–1497.

43. Kereiakes DJ, Broderick TM, Roth EM, et al. Time course, magnitude, and consistency of platelet inhibition by abciximab, tirofiban, or eptifibatide in patients with unstable angina pectoris undergoing percutaneous coronary intervention. Am J Cardiol 1999;84:391–395.

44. Simon DI, Liu CB, Ganz P, et al. A comparative study of light transmission aggregometry and automated bedside platelet function assays in patients undergoing percutaneous coronary intervention and receiving abciximab, eptifibatide, or tirofiban. Cathet Cardiovasc Intervent 2001;52:425–432.

45. Swierkosz TA, Valettas N, Herrmann HC. IIb or not IIb: when, how, and which GP IIb/IIIa inhibitor? Editorial comment. Cathet Cardiovasc Intervent 2001;52:433–434.

46. Ault KA, Cannon CP, Mitchell J, McCahan J, et al. Platelet activation in patients after an acute coronary syndrome: results from the TIMI-12 trial. J Am Coll Cardiol 1999;33:634–639.

47. Herrmann HC, Swierkosz TA, Kapoor S, et al. Comparison of degree of platelet inhibition by abciximab-vs-tirofiban in patients with unstable angina and non-Q-wave myocardial infarction undergoing percutaneous coronary interventions. Am J Cardiol 2002;89:1293–1297.

48. Neumann F-J, Hochholzer W, Pogatsa-Murray G, Schomig A, Gawaz M. Antiplatelet effects of abciximab, tirofiban and epifibatide in patients undergoing coronary stenting. J Am Coll Cardiol 2001;37:1323–1328.

49. The TACTICS-TIMI18 Investigators. Comparison of early invasive and conservative strategies in patients with unstable coronary syndromes treated with the glycoprotein IIb/IIIa inhibitor tirofiban. N Engl J Med 2001;344:1879–1887.

50. Zhao X-Q, Theroux P, Snapinn SM, Sax FL, for the PRISM-PLUS Investigators. Intracoronary thrombus and platelet glycoprotein IIb/IIIa receptor blockade with tirofiban in unstable angina or non-Q-wave myocardial infarction: angiographic results from the PRISM-PLUS trial. Circulation 1999;100:1609–1615.

51. Boersma E, Akkerhuis KM, Theroux P, Califf RM, Topol EJ, Simoon ML. Platelet glycoprotein IIb/IIIa receptor inhibition in non-ST-elevation acute coronary syndromes: early benefit during medical treatment only, with additional protection during percutaneous coronary intervention. Circulation 1999;100:2045–2048.

52. Lefkovits J, Topol EJ. Intravenous glycoprotein IIb/IIIa receptor inhibitor agents in ischemic heart disease. In: Topol EJ, ed. Acute Coronary Syndromes. Marcel Decker, New York, 2001, pp. 419–452.

53. Lev EI, Osende JI, Richard MF, et al. Administration of abciximab to patients receiving tirofiban or eptifibatide: effect on platelet function. J Am Coll Cardiol 2001;37:847–855.

8

Overview of the Glycoprotein IIb/IIIa Interventional Trials

A. Michael Lincoff, MD and Eric J. Topol, MD

CONTENTS

INTRODUCTION
THE AGENTS
THE RANDOMIZED TRIALS
SYNTHESIS OF THE RANDOMIZED TRIALS
RECOMMENDATIONS
SUMMARY
REFERENCES

INTRODUCTION

Plaque rupture and vascular thrombosis are key initiating factors in the pathogenesis of ischemic complications of percutaneous coronary revascularization *(1,2)*. The central role of platelet activity in this setting is highlighted by the unequivocal benefit of aspirin in preventing death or myocardial infarction among patients undergoing coronary intervention *(3)*. Newer strategies for more potent inhibition of platelet activity at the injured coronary plaque focus on the integrin glycoprotein (GP) IIb/IIIa receptor on the platelet surface membrane, which binds circulating fibrinogen or von Willebrand factor and cross-links adjacent platelets as the final common pathway to platelet aggregation *(4)*. Pharmacologic compounds directed against GPIIb/IIIa block this receptor, prevent binding of circulating adhesion molecules, and potently inhibit platelet aggregation.

The studies and trials evaluating the roles of specific GPIIb/IIIa inhibitors in the setting of percutaneous coronary intervention (PCI) have been described in detail in Chapters 5–7. Trials evaluating the efficacy of GPIIb/IIIa blockade during primary angioplasty for acute myocardial infarction are discussed in Chapter 12. The present chapter reviews the body of clinical data regarding this class of agents during coronary revascularization and provides a perspective on the efficacy, safety, patient selection, and optimal use of this new therapeutic strategy.

From: *Contemporary Cardiology: Platelet Glycoprotein IIb/IIIa*
Inhibitors in Cardiovascular Disease, 2nd Edition
Edited by: A. M. Lincoff © Humana Press Inc., Totowa, NJ

THE AGENTS

Three intravenous GPIIb/IIIa antagonists have undergone large-scale Phase III and Phase IV trial evaluation in the setting of percutaneous coronary revascularization, and all are currently approved for clinical use by the United States Food and Drug Administration. *Abciximab* (c7E3 Fab, ReoPro™, Centocor, Malvern, PA), the first agent of this class, is a human-murine chimeric monoclonal Fab antibody fragment that binds with high affinity and a slow dissociation rate to the GPIIb/IIIa receptor *(5,6)*. Abciximab is cleared rapidly from the plasma (half-life of approx 25 min) *(7)* but remains bound to circulating platelets for as long as 21 d *(8)*. Binding of abciximab is not specific for the platelet GPIIb/IIIa receptor; this agent has equal affinity for the vitronectin receptor ($\alpha_v\beta_3$), which appears to play a role in cell adhesion, migration, and proliferation. *Eptifibatide* (Integrilin™, COR Therapeutics, South San Francisco, CA), a cyclic heptapeptide based on the Lys-Gly-Asp (KGD) amino acid sequence, is a highly specific, competitive inhibitor of the GPIIb/IIIa complex. Blockade of the receptor by eptifibatide is rapidly reversible, with a plasma half-life in humans of about 2.5 h *(9)*. *Tirofiban* (Aggrastat™, Merck, White House Station, NJ) is a tyrosine-derivative nonpeptide mimetic inhibitor of GPIIb/IIIa, which also specifically and competitively binds to the receptor in a rapidly reversible fashion *(10)* and has a short (approx 1.6 h) serum half-life. Platelet aggregation is inhibited by all these agents in a dose-related manner, with nearly complete abolition of platelet thrombosis at levels of receptor occupancy >80% *(6)*. After discontinuation of abciximab, platelet aggregation returns toward baseline over the subsequent 12–36 h *(6)*, whereas normalization of platelet function occurs much more quickly (over 30 min to 4 h) following discontinuation of the reversible eptifibatide or tirofiban *(9,10)*.

THE RANDOMIZED TRIALS

The role of GPIIb/IIIa inhibitors administered as periprocedural intravenous therapy in the setting of PCI has been tested in 12 large-scale, randomized, controlled trials enrolling in total over 25,000 patients. Six of these trials were placebo-controlled evaluations during elective or urgent PCI: EPIC of abciximab among patients considered to be at high risk, EPILOG of abciximab in a broad spectrum of patients undergoing elective or urgent revascularization, EPISTENT of abciximab among patients suitable for stent implantation, IMPACT-II of lower dose eptifibatide in a broad patient population undergoing balloon angioplasty, ESPRIT of a high-dose, double-bolus eptifibatide regimen during elective or urgent stenting, and RESTORE of tirofiban during balloon angioplasty for unstable ischemic syndromes. Four trials have tested abciximab vs placebo or "conventional care" among patients with acute myocardial infarction undergoing balloon angioplasty (RAPPORT) or stenting (ISAR-2, ADMIRAL) or in a 2-by-2 factorial design randomized to angioplasty or stenting (CADILLAC). CAPTURE tested the role of abciximab as treatment *prior to* angioplasty among patients with refractory unstable angina. TARGET is the only direct comparative trial carried out thus far, testing the relative efficacy of abciximab and tirofiban during PCI among patients outside the setting of acute myocardial infarction.

Trial Designs

Study algorithms are summarized in Fig. 1, enrollment details provided in Table 1, and details regarding heparin dosing listed in Table 2. Individual trial protocols are described, and efficacy and safety findings are detailed in subsequent sections.

Trial Protocols

THE EPIC TRIAL

EPIC is described in detail in Chapter 5. This trial provided the "proof of concept" of the efficacy of GPIIb/IIIa blockade in improving clinical outcome among patients undergoing coronary balloon angioplasty or directional atherectomy. A total of 2099 patients deemed to be at high risk for ischemic complications on the basis of acute ischemic syndromes (myocardial infarction or unstable angina) or adverse clinical and lesion morphologic characteristics were enrolled between 1992 and 1993 *(11)*. Given the prolonged duration of abciximab's binding to the GPIIb/IIIa receptor, this trial assessed whether a single bolus of the agent would be effective or if a more prolonged period of administration would be required. Patients were therefore randomized to treatment with placebo, an abciximab 0.25 mg/kg bolus administered immediately prior to initiation of the interventional procedure, or an abciximab bolus followed by a 10 µg/min infusion for 12 h. All patients received aspirin; concomitant heparin was administered as a preprocedural bolus of 10–12,000 U [with additional boluses as necessary to achieve and maintain an activated clotting time (ACT) of 300–350 s], followed by a postprocedural infusion for at least the 12-h duration of the abciximab study drug. Vascular access sheaths were left in place during the heparin and study drug infusions and were removed 6 h after the heparin was discontinued. The primary efficacy endpoint was death, myocardial infarction, urgent repeat revascularization, or stent or intraaortic balloon pump placement; double blinding was maintained and clinical assessments were also performed at 6 mo and 3 yr following randomization.

THE EPILOG TRIAL

EPILOG is described in detail in Chapter 5. This study was designed to extend the findings of the EPIC trial in two ways. First, to determine whether the clinical benefits of abciximab therapy observed among high-risk patients in EPIC could be extrapolated to all patients treated by percutaneous coronary revascularization, regardless of their perceived risk for ischemic complications, a broad spectrum of patients undergoing elective or urgent intervention was enrolled. The second objective was to determine whether the substantial increase in bleeding complications associated with abciximab therapy in EPIC (see below) could be attenuated by modification of conjunctive heparin dosing. The EPILOG trial design was based on the findings of the pilot PROLOG study *(12)*, which suggested that hemorrhagic complications of abciximab could be reduced without loss of clinical efficacy by weight adjustment and reduction of heparin dose and by early sheath removal during the abciximab infusion (with no postprocedural heparin). Patients were randomized to placebo with standard-dose, weight-adjusted heparin; abciximab with standard-dose, weight-adjusted heparin; or abciximab with low-dose, weight-adjusted heparin (Table 2) *(13)*. Abciximab was administered as a bolus of 0.25 mg/kg, followed by an infusion of 0.125 µg/kg/min (maximum 10 µg/min) for 12 h. Postprocedural heparin was not given, and vascular sheaths were removed 2–6 h after the procedure. Planned sample size was 4800 patients, but the trial was terminated early after the first interim analysis demonstrated an unexpectedly marked treatment efficacy of abciximab therapy; at that point, a total of 2792 patients had been enrolled between February and December, 1995. The primary efficacy endpoint was death, myocardial infarction, or urgent repeat revascularization by 30 d; patients were also followed in a double-blinded fashion to 6 mo and 1 yr.

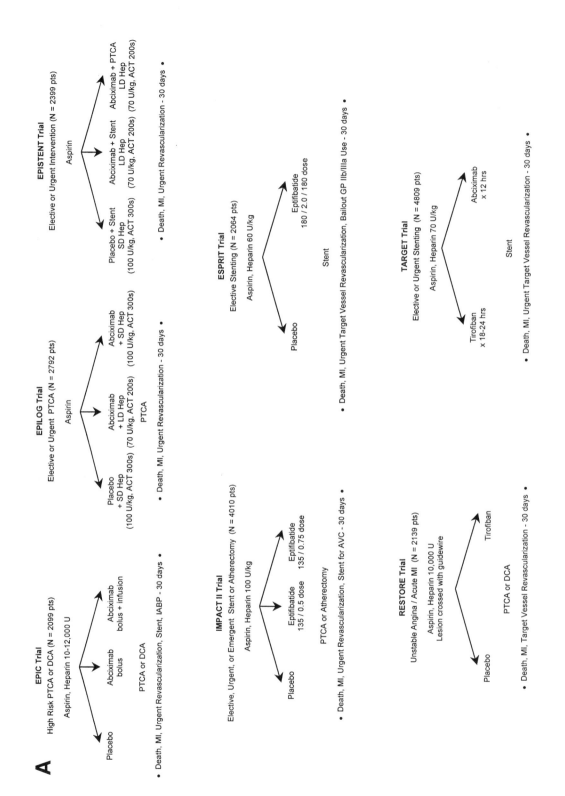

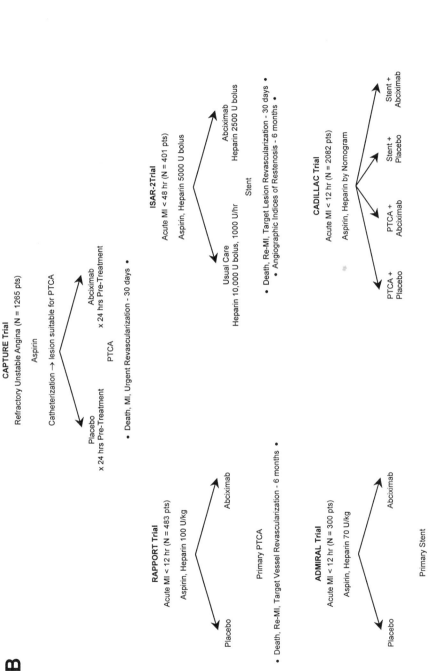

Fig. 1. Protocol outlines for the 11 large-scale trials of glycoprotein (GP)IIb/IIIa blockade in interventional cardiology. (**A**) Trials during elective or urgent PCI. (**B**) Trials during refractory unstable angina or acute myocardial infarction. ACT, activated clotting time; AVC, abrupt vessel closure; DCA, directional coronary atherectomy; IABP, intraaortic balloon pump; LD Hep, low-dose, weight-adjusted heparin; MI, myocardial infarction; PTCA, balloon angioplasty; SD Hep, standard-dose, weight-adjusted heparin; 135/0.5, 135/0.75, and 180/2.0/180 = eptifibatide doses (*see* text); pts, patients.

Table 1

Randomized Interventional Trials: Patient Populations

Trial	Agent tested	No. of patients	Enrollment period	Entry criteria
EPIC	Abciximab	2099	11/91–11/92	High-risk PTCA or DCA Acute MI—within 12 h (direct or rescue PTCA) Recent MI—within prior 7 d Unstable angina—within 24 h of chest pain (rest or postinfarction angina with ischemic ECG changes) Clinical-morphologic criteria (ACC/AHA lesion score B2 or C, ACC/AHA score B1 with DM or with women age > 65 yr)
EPILOG	Abciximab	2792	2/95—12/95	Urgent or elective PTCA, DCA, TEC, or laser Excluding unstable angina or acute MI (EPIC criteria) within prior 24 h, elective stents, rotational atherectomy
EPISTENT	Abciximab	2399	7/96–9/97	Coronary intervention suitable for PTCA or elective stent Excluding acute MI within 24 h, rotational atherectomy
IMPACT II	Eptifibatide	4010	11/93–11/94	All clinical indications, all approved interventions
ESPRIT	Eptifibatide	2064	6/99–2/00	Elective stent for which GPIIb/IIIa inhibitor would not be routinely used Excluding acute MI within 24 h or unstable ischemia with ongoing chest pain or prior thienopyridine use
RESTORE	Tirofiban	2139	1/95–12/95	High-risk PTCA or DCA Acute MI—within 72 h (Q-wave or non-Q-wave) Unstable angina—within 72 h (chest pain at rest or on minimal effort with ECG changes, hemodynamic changes, or angiographic thrombus)
CAPTURE	Abciximab	1265	5/93–12/95	Refractory unstable angina Unstable angina—within 48 h (chest pain with ECG changes) despite iv heparin and nitroglycerin
RAPPORT	Abciximab	483	11/95–2/97	Primary PTCA for acute ST elevation MI—within 12 h
ISAR-2	Abciximab	401	N/A	Primary stent for acute ST elevation MI—within 48 h
ADMIRAL	Abciximab	300	7/97–12/98	Primary PCI for acute ST elevation MI—within 12 h
CADILLAC	Abciximab	2681	11/97–9/99	Primary PCI for acute ST elevation MI—within 12 h
TARGET	Abciximab vs tirofiban	4809	12/99–8/00	Coronary intervention suitable for stent Excluding acute MI or cardiogenic shock

Abbreviations: ACC/AHA, American College of Cardiology/American Heart Association modified lesion complexity score (61); DCA, directional coronary atherectomy; DM, diabetes mellitus; ECG, electrocardiographic; MI, myocardial infarction; N/A, not available; PCI, percutaneous coronary intervention (balloon angioplasty, stent, or other device); PTCA, coronary balloon angioplasty; TEC, transluminal extraction catheter atherectomy.

Table 2
Randomized Interventional Trials: Heparin Regimens and Vascular Sheath Removal

Trial	Bolus[a]	Heparin target ACT[a] (s)	Postprocedural infusion[b]	Sheath removal[b] (time after interventional procedure)
EPIC	10–12,000 U initial 3000 U additional to maximum total 20,000 U	300–350 s	>12 h Target aPTT 1.5–2.5 × control	>6 h after 12-h study drug infusion (>18 h total)
EPILOG	"Standard-dose": 100 U/kg "Low-dose": 70 U/kg	"Standard-dose" > 300 s "Low-dose" > 200 s	None None	When ACT < 175 s (approx 2–6 h)
EPISTENT	Placebo: 100 U/kg Abciximab: 70 U/kg	Placebo > 300 s Abciximab > 200 s	None	When ACT < 175 s (approx 2–6 h)
IMPACT II	100 U/kg	300–350 s	None	When aPTT < 45 s (4–6 h)
ESPRIT RESTORE	60 U/kg 10,000 U	200–300 s 300–400 s	None None	3–4 postprocedure When ACT < 180 s
CAPTURE	150 U/kg for weight < 70 kg 10,000 U	>300 s	1 h after PTCA (all patients received infusion for 24 h before PTCA: target aPTT 2.0–2.5 × control)	4–6 h (>24–30 h total, including during preprocedural study drug infusion)
RAPPORT	100 U/kg	>300 s	None	When ACT < 175 s (4–6 h)
ISAR-2	(5000 U before catheterization) Control: 10,000 U Abciximab: 2500 U	None	Control: 1000 U/h for 12 h after sheath Abciximab: none	N/A
ADMIRAL	70 U/kg	>200 s	7 U/kg/h for 24 h	4–6 h after heparin infusion stopped
CADILLAC	(5000 U before catheterization) by nomogram	Control > 350 s Abciximab 200–300 s	None	N/A
TARGET	70 U/kg	>250 s	None	When ACT < 175 s (approx 2–6 h)

Abbreviations: ACT, activated clotting time; N/A, information not available; aPTT, activated partial thromboplastin time.
[a] Prior to first balloon inflation or device activation of interventional procedure.
[b] Recommended by protocol.

THE **EPISTENT** TRIAL

EPISTENT is described in detail in Chapter 5. Previous trials of GPIIb/IIIa receptor blockade during PCI had excluded patients undergoing elective stent implantation, because of rapid changes in the "optimal stenting" technique during the time periods that these trials were under way as well as uncertainties regarding the best conjunctive anticoagulation regimen. EPISTENT was therefore designed to evaluate the complementary and comparative roles of GPIIb/IIIa blockade with abciximab and stenting. A total of 2399 patients undergoing urgent or elective percutaneous revascularization of lesions suitable for balloon angioplasty (PTCA) or stenting were enrolled between 1996 and 1997 and randomized to stent plus placebo, stent plus abciximab (bolus and 12-h infusion), or PTCA plus abciximab *(14)*. "Bailout" or unplanned stents were utilized in only 19% of patients in the PTCA group. The primary efficacy endpoint of death, myocardial infarction, or urgent revascularization was assessed at 30 d, with clinical follow-up to 6 mo and 1 yr. Additionally, an angiographic substudy of 900 patients (300 in each treatment group) was carried out to evaluate the influence of abciximab on restenosis.

THE **IMPACT II** TRIAL

IMPACT II is described in detail in Chapter 6. This "all comers" trial tested the clinical efficacy of eptifibatide among 4010 patients undergoing percutaneous intervention for any clinical indication between 1993 to 1994 *(15)*. Patients received aspirin and weight-adjusted heparin and were randomized to placebo, eptifibatide 135 µg/kg bolus followed by an infusion of 0.5 µg/kg/min for 20–24 h ("135/0.5 group"), or eptifibatide 135 µg/kg bolus followed by an infusion of 0.75 µg/kg/min for 20–24 h ("135/0.75 group"). Clinical outcome was assessed at 30 d and 6 mo. An angiographic substudy, enrolling approx 900 patients, was performed to assess the influence of eptifibatide on angiographic restenosis.

THE **ESPRIT** TRIAL

The ESPRIT trial is described in Chapter 6. The disappointing treatment effect of eptifibatide observed in the IMPACT-II trial (*see* the 30-Day Efficacy section) was thought to be at least partly caused by the dose employed, which was subsequently observed to result in blockade of only 30–50% of GPIIb/IIIa receptors *(16)*. Further dosing studies *(17)* and pharmacodynamic modeling demonstrated that a double bolus of 180 µg/kg given 10 min apart with a 2.0 µg/kg/min infusion of eptifibatide uniformly produced and maintained >80% blockade of GPIIb/IIIa receptors. This high-dose eptifibatide regimen was tested among patients in the setting of coronary stenting in the ESPRIT trial. Because of ethical concerns regarding randomization of patients to placebo during 1999–2000, a time when the efficacy of GPIIb/IIIa blockade had already been well documented, patients were eligible for inclusion in ESPRIT only if they "...in the opinion of the treating physician would not routinely be treated with a glycoprotein IIb/IIIa inhibitor during PCI..." *(18)*. Patients within 24 h of acute myocardial infarction or with unstable myocardial ischemia and "continuing chest pain precipitating urgent PCI" were excluded, as were those who were pretreated with a thienopyridine platelet inhibitor (ticlopidine or clopidogrel).

The patients were randomized in a double-blind fashion to receive either placebo or eptifibatide immediately prior to stent implantation, with infusions for 18–24 h; heparin doses in both the placebo and eptifibatide arms were reduced, with 60 U/kg bolus and target ACT >250 s. The planned sample size was 2400 patients, but the trial was terminated on the basis of an interim review demonstrating efficacy after 2064 patients had been enrolled. The primary endpoint was the composite of death, myocardial infarction, urgent target vessel revascularization, or bailout GPIIb/IIIa inhibitor therapy within 48 h, with follow-up to 30 d, 6 mo, and 1 yr.

THE RESTORE TRIAL

RESTORE is described in detail in Chapter 7. The clinical efficacy of tirofiban was tested during 1995 among a total of 2139 patients considered to be at high risk for coronary balloon angioplasty owing to unstable angina or myocardial infarction *(19)*. Patients were randomized after passage of a guidewire across a target lesion to placebo or tirofiban, administered as a 10 µg/kg bolus followed by a 0.15 µg/kg/min infusion for 36 h. The predefined primary endpoint of the study was the occurrence of death, myocardial infarction, or *any* target vessel repeat revascularization by 30 d; clinical outcome was also assessed at 6 mo. A *post hoc* reclassification of revascularization events was performed to produce a composite endpoint comparable to that of other interventional trials by including only *urgent* revascularization procedures. An angiographic substudy of approx 600 patients (300 in each group) evaluated the effect of tirofiban on restenosis.

THE CAPTURE TRIAL

CAPTURE is described in detail in Chapter 9. This trial differed from the other interventional GPIIb/IIIa trials in that CAPTURE evaluated a strategy of *pretreatment* with abciximab prior to balloon angioplasty among patients with refractory unstable angina. Patients qualified for enrollment if they had unstable angina with episodes of chest pain and ischemic electrocardiographic changes, despite therapy with intravenous heparin and nitroglycerin, and had been demonstrated on angiography to have a lesion suitable for coronary angioplasty *(20)*. All patients received aspirin and were randomized to placebo or abciximab for 18–24 h prior to angioplasty and continued for 1 h after completion of the procedure. Heparin was administered and vascular sheaths remained in place from enrollment throughout the pretreatment phase and until at least 1 h after angioplasty. Planned sample size was 1400 patients, but the trial was stopped on the basis of efficacy at the third interim analysis with 1265 patients enrolled between 1993 and 1995. The primary endpoint of death, myocardial infarction, or urgent revascularization was assessed at 30 d, with continued clinical follow-up through 6 mo.

THE RAPPORT TRIAL

RAPPORT is described in detail in Chapter 12. A total of 483 patients treated by primary balloon angioplasty within 12 h of symptoms of acute myocardial infarction were randomized to receive placebo or abciximab (bolus and 12 h infusion) in addition to aspirin and heparin *(21)*. The primary endpoint was death, recurrent myocardial infarction, or any (elective or urgent) repeat target vessel revascularization by 6 mo. A composite endpoint of the acute ischemic events of death, reinfarction, or urgent repeat target vessel revascularization (comparable to the primary endpoints used in the other trials) was also assessed at 7 d, 30 d, and 6 mo.

THE ISAR-2 TRIAL

ISAR-2 is described in detail in Chapter 12. This was a nonblinded study intended primarily to assess the impact of abciximab on restenosis following primary PCI for acute myocardial infarction. A total of 401 patients were randomized to either "conventional care" or adjunctive abciximab (bolus plus infusion) during stent implantation performed within 48 h of onset of chest pain *(22)*. Heparin doses were reduced in the abciximab arm. The primary endpoint was late loss of angiographic luminal dimensions by 6-mo follow-up; clinical events (death, myocardial reinfarction, or target vessel revascularization) were assessed at 30 d and 6 mo.

THE ADMIRAL TRIAL

ADMIRAL is described in Chapter 12. This trial was designed to determine the influence of abciximab therapy among a broad unselected population of patients with acute myocardial infarction in the context of a management strategy of primary stent implantation. Patients within 12 h of acute infarction in whom stenting was planned were enrolled and randomized in a double-blind fashion to placebo or abciximab bolus plus infusion *(23)*. The initial heparin bolus was 70 U/kg in both arms. Of the 300 patients enrolled, 26% were randomized and administered study drug in the ambulance or emergency department, with the remainder receiving study agent in the intensive care unit or catheterization laboratory. Percutaneous coronary revascularization was attempted in 92–95% of patients after angiography. The primary composite endpoint of death, myocardial reinfarction, or urgent target vessel revascularization was assessed at 30 d and 6 mo.

THE CADILLAC TRIAL

CADILLAC is described in detail in Chapter 12. This large-scale trial assessed the effectiveness of stenting and abciximab among 2082 patients undergoing primary PCI within 12 h of acute myocardial infarction *(24)*. Excluded from enrollment were those with bypass graft stenoses, coronary lesions requiring multivessel intervention, or "pre-specified anatomical conditions...that would reduce the likelihood of successful stenting." Using a 2-by-2 factorial design, patients were randomized to PTCA alone, PTCA plus abciximab, stent alone, or stent plus abciximab. Heparin doses were adjusted by nomogram to provide a lower ACT target range for patients receiving abciximab. The primary endpoint was the composite of death, reinfarction, repeat target vessel revascularization, or disabling stroke *by 6 mo* after randomization; clinical endpoints were also assessed at 30 d. An angiographic substudy of 900 patients was performed to determine the impact of therapy on the risk of restenosis at 6 mo.

THE TARGET TRIAL

TARGET is described in Chapter 7. This is was the first (and to date only) comparative trial of two different GPIIb/IIIa antagonists, performed to determine whether or not tirofiban was inferior to abciximab during coronary stenting. As all patients received a GPIIb/IIIa inhibitor, those undergoing urgent or elective procedures were eligible for enrollment *(25)*. Patients were randomized on a double-blind, double-dummy basis to receive either abciximab 0.25 mg/kg bolus and 0.125 µg/kg/min (maximum 10 µg/min) infusion for12-h or tirofiban 10 µg/kg bolus and 0.15 µg/kg/min infusion for 18–24 h. Pretreatment with clopidogrel and aspirin was encouraged, and a reduced-dose, weight-adjusted heparin regimen (70 U/kg, target ACT > 250 s) was used in both arms. Of the total 5308 patients enrolled, 4809 received study drug and formed the study population. The primary endpoint was the composite of death, myocardial infarction, or urgent target vessel revascularization at 30 d, with clinical follow-up at 6 mo and 1 yr.

Intertrial Comparisons

Pooled analyses of these 12 large-scale trials of GPIIb/IIIa blockade allow general principles regarding the efficacy and safety of this treatment strategy to be evaluated. Important differences among the trials must be recognized, however, with regard to patient populations, study drug regimens, adjunctive medical therapies, and endpoint assessment.

ENTRY CRITERIA

As a general rule, therapies that are effective will often exhibit the most clinical efficacy among patients who are at heightened risk for the events to be prevented. For this reason, initial trials of GPIIb/IIIa blockade during coronary intervention often focused on patients deemed to be at high risk for periprocedural ischemic complications. The first trial, EPIC, designated high-risk status by either the unequivocal unstable ischemic syndromes or complex angiographic target lesion morphology in combination with clinical criteria. The RESTORE entry criteria were even narrower than those of EPIC, including only patients with unstable ischemic syndromes, the subgroup that had been found in EPIC to have experienced the most clinical benefit from GPIIb/IIIa blockade (*see* below) *(26)*. CAPTURE was a trial focused on the particular application of GPIIb/IIIa blockade as pretreatment among patients with refractory unstable angina, defined by ongoing ischemic symptoms and electrocardiographic changes despite optimal medical management. RAPPORT, ISAR-2, ADMIRAL, and CADILLAC specifically evaluated patients undergoing primary angioplasty or stenting for ST elevation acute myocardial infarction.

In contrast, one of the primary objectives of the EPILOG trial was to assess whether the clinical efficacy of abciximab therapy could be extended to the low- as well as high-risk patients undergoing coronary intervention; all patients were therefore to be included, except those with severe unstable angina (with symptoms and electrocardiographic changes within the previous 24 h) for whom the profound benefit of abciximab had already been demonstrated in EPIC *(26)*, or those with acute myocardial infarction, a setting under evaluation in dedicated trials. Similarly, the philosophy behind design of IMPACT-II was one of broad applicability, and patients representing various risk profiles were enrolled. More recently, the EPISTENT and ESPRIT trials sought to evaluate the role of GPIIb/IIIa blockade with abciximab and eptifibatide, respectively, during the current interventional era of widespread stenting with adjunctive thienopyridine therapy.

STUDY DRUG REGIMENS

Aside from CAPTURE, all trials evaluated a strategy whereby study drug (GPIIb/IIIa inhibitor or placebo) was administered as a bolus immediately prior to coronary intervention, followed by infusions of varying durations. The EPIC trial was the only study to test a bolus-only regimen of a GPIIb/IIIa antagonist. Given that abciximab has the longest duration of GPIIb/IIIa blockade of all the agents under evaluation, and that the group in EPIC receiving the bolus of abciximab experienced only a small and statistically insignificant reduction in endpoints compared with placebo (*see* below), it was concluded that post-bolus infusions would be required with all these compounds in subsequent trials for optimal passivation of the arterial plaque and reduction in clinical ischemic events. The durations of study drug infusion were based on pharmacodynamic differences among the agents: 24-h or 36-h infusions of eptifibatide and tirofiban were chosen for the IMPACT-II and RESTORE trials, respectively, given the rapidly reversible pharmacodynamics of these drugs, compared with the 12-h infusion of abciximab. With the greater postprocedural stability imparted by stenting compared with balloon angioplasty (particularly with thieno-pyridine therapy), the more contemporary trials of eptifibatide (ESPRIT) and tirofiban (TARGET) used infusions of only 18–24 h (or less) to enhance compatibility with shortened hospital length-of-stays.

As previously described, CAPTURE utilized a 24-h pretreatment regimen of study drug. Abciximab was administered for only 1 h after the interventional procedure, partly because this trial was designed and initiated before the findings of EPIC regarding the importance of a postprocedural abciximab infusion were fully appreciated. The short post-procedural drug infusion may have adversely influenced the magnitude of treatment effect observed in the CAPTURE trial.

Conjunctive Heparin and Vascular Access Site Management

Protocol guidelines for conjunctive heparin dosing and vascular sheath removal are summarized in Table 2. As described below, a major limitation of abciximab therapy in EPIC was a marked increase in the incidence of bleeding complications. This hemorrhagic risk appeared to be linked to excessive intraprocedural heparin dosing as well as the prac-tice of leaving vascular access sheaths in place with ongoing heparin infusion for the entire 12-h study drug infusion period. A pilot study demonstrated that vascular sheaths could be removed and hemostasis achieved during abciximab infusion, if heparin had been dis-continued, and that bleeding rates actually tended to be less with this strategy than with prolonged sheath dwell times (12). Moreover, the risk of hemorrhagic complications was further diminished by reduction and weight adjustment of the procedural heparin doses.

Based on these findings, the EPILOG trial explicitly tested low-dose vs standard-dose weight-adjusted heparin regimens with abciximab, and the other trials incorporated some form of protocol-directed limitation or weight adjustment of heparin dosing. Trials per-formed after EPIC recommended that little or no heparin infusion be administered after the procedure and that vascular access sheaths be removed early (usually during study drug infusion). Notably, however, postprocedural heparin infusions were often used during the trials of primary PCI for acute myocardial infarction; in RAPPORT, for example, median dwell times for vascular access sheaths were 17–19 h. Similarly, vascular sheaths remained in place with ongoing heparin infusion for the entire 24-h pretreatment period between qualifying angiography and percutaneous revascularization in CAPTURE.

Other Medications

All patients in these interventional trials of intravenous GPIIb/IIIa blockade were treated with aspirin before the procedure and indefinitely thereafter. Although it is unlikely that aspirin adds significant platelet antiaggregatory effect during ongoing administration of a GPIIb/IIIa antagonist, there may well be an incremental benefit of its inhibition of plate-let activation or antiinflammatory properties. Moreover, long-term ischemic event rates are suppressed by chronic aspirin therapy but would not be expected to be influenced by a brief periprocedural administration of a GPIIb/IIIa agent. Other anticoagulant drugs were generally restricted by protocol to the extent that they could exacerbate bleeding com-plications of the study agent. Patients on therapeutic warfarin therapy were excluded, as were those in whom administration of dextran was planned. Thrombolytic therapy as an adjunct to angioplasty was discouraged, with reduced doses suggested if administration of these drugs was considered imperative. Antianginal and other medical therapies were not protocol-directed and were utilized at the discretion of physicians at the clinical sites.

The protocol-specified use of thienopyridines in these trials varied in parallel with the evolution of enhanced antiplatelet regimens for coronary stenting. Trials performed early in the stent era specified that ticlopidine or clopidogrel be administered for 4 wk after stenting. Data derived from EPISTENT as well as other studies, however, suggested that periprocedural ischemic events were reduced by pretreatment with thienopyridines (27). As a result, the TARGET trial strongly encouraged administration of a loading dose of clopidogrel (300 mg) 2–6 h prior to PCI as "background" therapy to enhance the efficacy of tirofiban relative to abciximab. Conversely, the exclusion of patients pretreated with clopidogrel from enrollment in the ESPRIT trial could be seen as a means of enhancing the apparent differences between placebo and eptifibatide.

TRIAL CONDUCT AND ENDPOINTS

The interventional trials shared many common design and analysis features. Most trials were blinded, with the exception of ISAR-2, CADILLAC, and the asymmetric balloon angioplasty plus abciximab arm of EPISTENT. Endpoints were adjudicated by review of primary data by independent, blinded Clinical Events Committees for all studies except ISAR-2. Myocardial infarction was in general identified by new Q-waves or creatine kinase-MB fraction (CK-MB) elevations ≥3 times the control value. Urgent repeat revascularization was defined by evidence of precipitating myocardial ischemia and rapid (within 24 h) performance of the revascularization procedure. Bleeding events were classified as "major" or "minor" based on observed hemorrhage and changes in hemoglobin according to the criteria of the Thrombolysis in Myocardial Infarction (TIMI) Study Group (28).

Important differences existed, however, with regard to assessment of periprocedural myocardial infarctions. In all but two of the trials, Clinical Events Committees reviewed CK-MB enzyme values that had been obtained systematically by a protocol-driven schedule (every 6–8 h for the first 24 h) and thereby identified myocardial infarctions that may or may not have been noted by site investigators. In contrast, myocardial enzyme values were not routinely obtained in the RESTORE or CADILLAC trials, but were instead drawn only when ischemic events were suspected to have occurred; Clinical Events Committee reviews were thus confined to adjudication of events that had been identified by the site investigators. As a consequence, endpoint (re-)infarction rates in RESTORE and CADILLAC were substantially lower than in the other trials discussed here, thereby substantially reducing the ability of those trials to identify the therapeutic effect of GPIIb/IIIa blockade.

30-Day Efficacy

Event rates for the composite 30-d endpoint of death, myocardial infarction, or urgent repeat revascularization in the various treatment groups of the 11 interventional trials without active controls (i.e., excluding TARGET) are summarized in Fig. 2. Ischemic endpoint event rates were consistently diminished by GPIIb/IIIa blockade in all the trials, although the magnitude of treatment effect was variable. In EPIC (11), this composite event rate was reduced from 12.8% among patients receiving placebo to 11.4% among patients randomized to the abciximab bolus (10% relative risk reduction, $p = 0.43$) and to 8.3% among patients randomized to the abciximab bolus and 12-h infusion (35% relative risk reduction, $p = 0.008$). The treatment effect of abciximab appeared to be amplified (up to

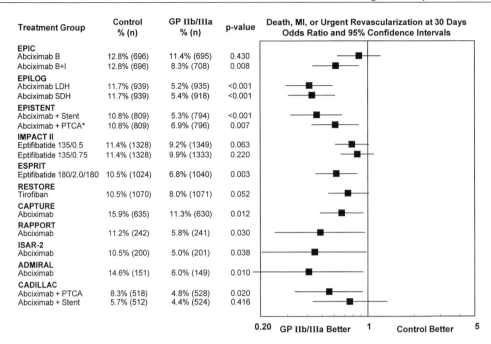

Treatment Group	Control % (n)	GP IIb/IIIa % (n)	p-value	Death, MI, or Urgent Revascularization at 30 Days Odds Ratio and 95% Confidence Intervals
EPIC				
Abciximab B	12.8% (696)	11.4% (695)	0.430	
Abciximab B+I	12.8% (696)	8.3% (708)	0.008	
EPILOG				
Abciximab LDH	11.7% (939)	5.2% (935)	<0.001	
Abciximab SDH	11.7% (939)	5.4% (918)	<0.001	
EPISTENT				
Abciximab + Stent	10.8% (809)	5.3% (794)	<0.001	
Abciximab + PTCA*	10.8% (809)	6.9% (796)	0.007	
IMPACT II				
Eptifibatide 135/0.5	11.4% (1328)	9.2% (1349)	0.063	
Eptifibatide 135/0.75	11.4% (1328)	9.9% (1333)	0.220	
ESPRIT				
Eptifibatide 180/2.0/180	10.5% (1024)	6.8% (1040)	0.003	
RESTORE				
Tirofiban	10.5% (1070)	8.0% (1071)	0.052	
CAPTURE				
Abciximab	15.9% (635)	11.3% (630)	0.012	
RAPPORT				
Abciximab	11.2% (242)	5.8% (241)	0.030	
ISAR-2				
Abciximab	10.5% (200)	5.0% (201)	0.038	
ADMIRAL				
Abciximab	14.6% (151)	6.0% (149)	0.010	
CADILLAC				
Abciximab + PTCA	8.3% (518)	4.8% (528)	0.020	
Abciximab + Stent	5.7% (512)	4.4% (524)	0.416	

0.20   GP IIb/IIIa Better   1   Control Better   5

Fig. 2. Composite 30-d endpoint (death, myocardial infarction, or urgent repeat revascularization) event rates for the 11 GPIIb/IIIa interventional trials without active controls (i.e., TARGET excluded). RESTORE trial endpoints listed here are for the published *post hoc* analysis including only *urgent* repeat revascularization for consistency with the other trials. The reported composite endpoint at 30 d in CADILLAC was death, myocardial reinfarction, urgent target vessel revascularization, or disabling stroke. The reported composite endpoint at 30 d in RAPPORT, ISAR-2, and ADMIRAL was death, myocardial reinfarction, or urgent target vessel revascularization. *EPISTENT trial groups compared with reference group of Placebo + Stent; thus, the "placebo control" for the Abciximab + PTCA group underwent stenting rather than PTCA. B, bolus; B+I, bolus plus infusion; LDH, low-dose, weight-adjusted heparin; MI, myocardial infarction; PTCA, percutaneous transluminal coronary angioplasty; SDH, standard-dose, weight-adjusted heparin; 135/0.5, 135/0.75, and 180/2.0/180 = eptifibatide doses (*see* text).

a 56% risk reduction) in the subsequent EPILOG trial *(13)*: the composite endpoint event rate was 11.7% in the placebo group, 5.2% in the abciximab with low-dose heparin group (56% relative risk reduction, $p < 0.0001$), and 5.4% in the abciximab with standard-dose heparin group (54% relative reduction, $p < 0.0001$). A treatment effect of similar proportion was observed among patients receiving abciximab compared with placebo in EPISTENT *(14)*; the primary efficacy composite endpoint occurred in 10.8% of patients in the stent plus placebo arm, 6.9% of patients in the balloon plus abciximab arm (36% relative risk reduction, $p = 0.007$), and 5.3% of patients in the stent plus abciximab arm (51% relative risk reduction, $p < 0.001$).

In contrast, although the IMPACT-II trial provided evidence that eptifibatide diminished periprocedural ischemic events, the magnitude of treatment effect was less marked than in the abciximab trials and did not quite reach statistical significance *(15)*. The composite endpoint in IMPACT-II occurred in 11.4% of patients in the placebo group, 9.2% of patients in the eptifibatide 135/0.5 group (19% relative risk reduction, $p = 0.063$), and

9.9% of patients in the eptifibatide 135/0.75 group (16% relative risk reduction, $p = 0.22$). No dose response was observed among the eptifibatide doses evaluated in this study. Subsequent to IMPACT-II, it was observed that the binding of eptifibatide to the GPIIb/IIIa receptor was exaggerated in blood anticoagulated by the calcium-chelating anticoagulant citrate (which had been used in the GPIIb/IIIa dose-finding studies) relative to that which would occur at physiologic calcium concentrations *(16)*. A higher dose of eptifibatide, with a double bolus to ensure adequate platelet receptor blockade during the early period immediately after plaque injury, led to a substantially greater treatment effect in the ESPRIT trial *(18)*, in which the 30-d composite endpoint was reduced from 10.5 to 6.8% (35% risk reduction, $p = 0.0034$).

In the RESTORE trial *(19)*, the efficacy of tirofiban during high-risk balloon angioplasty was also less than had been anticipated based on the results of the EPIC trial. The predefined primary endpoint of death, myocardial infarction, or repeat target lesion revascularization in RESTORE occurred in 12.2% of patients in the placebo group and 10.3% of patients in the tirofiban group (16% relative risk reduction, $p = 0.16$). With the *post hoc* reclassification of revascularization events to allow comparison with the other trials, the 30-d composite of death, myocardial infarction, or urgent revascularization was 10.5% in the placebo group and 8.0% in the tirofiban group (24% relative risk reduction, $p = 0.052$).

In CAPTURE *(20)*, a 24-h period of pretreatment with abciximab among patients with refractory unstable angina prior to angioplasty reduced the primary composite endpoint from 15.9% in the placebo group to 11.3% in the abciximab group (29% relative risk reduction, $p = 0.012$). Clinical benefit of abciximab began to accrue during the pretreatment phase before the angioplasty procedure, with the preprocedural myocardial infarction rate reduced from 2.1% among control patients to 0.6% among those treated with abciximab ($p = 0.029$).

Among patients undergoing primary PCI for acute myocardial infarction, the treatment effect of abciximab was generally concordant with that observed in the elective PCI trials. In RAPPORT *(21)*, the composite endpoint of death, recurrent myocardial infarction, or urgent target vessel revascularization at 30 d was significantly reduced by abciximab from 11.2 to 5.8% (48% relative risk reduction, $p = 0.038$). Similarly, the 30-d composite endpoint was reduced from 10.5 to 5.0% (52% relative risk reduction, $p = 0.038$) in ISAR-2 *(22)* and from 14.6 to 6.0% (59% relative risk reduction, $p = 0.01$) in ADMIRAL *(23)*. Notably, among the subset of patients in ADMIRAL who had been randomized and received their study drug before arriving in the catheterization laboratory, event rates were markedly reduced, from 21.1 to 2.5%.

In contrast, the CADILLAC trial did not show a significant benefit of abciximab in reducing 30-d complication rates among patients receiving stents (5.7% vs 4.4%, $p = NS$), although there was a treatment effect of abciximab in patients treated with balloon angioplasty (8.3% vs 4.8%, $p = 0.02$) *(24)*. Importantly, however, end-point event rates overall in CADILLAC were much lower than in the other acute MI abciximab trials, particularly for the endpoint of reinfarction (which was *not* systematically adjudicated), raising important concerns regarding whether CADILLAC was appropriately designed to evaluate the treatment effect of GPIIb/IIIa inhibition on acute ischemic complications. It was notable, for example, that although subacute thrombosis rates were reduced by abciximab from 1.4 to 0.4% ($p < 0.001$), no differences in reinfarction rates were detected (0.9 vs 0.8%).

When directly compared with abciximab among patients undergoing stenting in the TARGET trial *(29)*, tirofiban was found to provide inferior protection from acute ischemic events. The 30-d composite endpoint occurred in 7.6% of patients receiving tirofiban, compared with 6.0% of patients randomized to abciximab (hazard ratio for tirofiban 1.26, 95% confidence interval 1.01–1.57, $p = 0.038$). Differences in outcome between the two agents emerged within 2 d of the PCI procedure.

COMPONENTS OF THE 30-DAY ENDPOINT

The breakdown of individual 30-d endpoints is detailed in Table 3. In general, the treatment effect of GPIIb/IIIa blockade was similar for each of the components of the composite endpoints used in this trial. Point estimates of event rates for infrequent complications such as death were imprecise, and although a trend toward diminished mortality was observed in most of the studies, these differences did not reach statistical significance. Myocardial infarction rates were consistently diminished by treatment with GPIIb/IIIa inhibitors compared with placebo; rates of urgent repeat revascularization were usually reduced as well. The EPISTENT trial requires particular explanation owing to the asymmetry of the treatment groups (abciximab plus stent or abciximab plus PTCA compared with the reference arm of placebo plus stent). Compared with stenting alone, adjunctive use of abciximab with stenting reduced the rates of death, myocardial infarction, and repeat revascularization. Compared with stenting alone, abciximab with balloon angioplasty was associated with equivalent rates of death and revascularization but lower rates of myocardial infarction.

The most frequent ischemic event prevented in these GPIIb/IIIa interventional trials was myocardial infarction, predominantly non-Q-wave infarction. Although the clinical importance of such periprocedural non-Q-wave infarctions following percutaneous coronary revascularization was initially controversial, virtually every contemporary study that has examined the impact of periprocedural enzyme release over an adequate follow-up period has demonstrated that patients who experience myocardial infarction during or after coronary intervention are at significantly greater risk for late cardiac death than those who do not *(30–36)*. Although an increased risk of late events has been observed in these studies even among patients with "small" CK-MB elevations (>1–1.5 times control) *(33–35)*, the extent of mortality risk appears to be proportional to the degree of enzyme elevation. It is therefore relevant that the effect of the GPIIb/IIIa inhibitors on reducing periprocedural myocardial infarction in these trials was primarily observed for large non-Q-wave infarctions (CK-MB >5 times control), confirming that the ischemic events prevented were clinically relevant, not merely laboratory abnormalities.

EFFICACY IN PATIENT SUBGROUPS

Although it might be anticipated that intense platelet inhibition with a GPIIb/IIIa inhibitor would provide substantial clinical benefit only among patients at high risk for thrombotic complications, a consistent treatment effect has been observed among all subgroups of patients enrolled in the trials. No clinical or angiographic *(37)* parameter has been found to identify patients reliably who do not benefit from GPIIb/IIIa blockade. This finding was most apparent in EPILOG and EPISTENT, as well as ESPRIT, in which the reduction in acute 30-d ischemic endpoints was of similar magnitude among patients defined by ischemic syndrome or a number of demographic or clinical characteristics.

Long-Term Efficacy

Patients were followed for at least 6 mo after randomization in all the interventional trials for assessment of clinical endpoints, and routine follow-up for 1 yr was obtained

Table 3
Randomized Interventional Trials—30-Day Efficacy Endpoint Events

Trial	Death (%)	MI (%)	Urgent revasc. (%)
EPIC			
Placebo	1.7	8.6	4.5, PCI, 3.6, CABG
Abciximab bolus	1.3	6.2	3.6, PCI, 2.3, CABG
Abciximab bolus + infusion	1.7	5.2	0.8, PCI, 2.4, CABG
EPILOG			
Placebo	0.8	8.7	5.2
Abciximab + reduced-dose heparin	0.3	3.7	1.6
Abciximab + standard-dose heparin	0.4	3.8	2.3
EPISTENT			
Placebo + stent	0.6	9.6	2.1
Abciximab + stent	0.3	4.5	1.3
Abciximab + PTCA	0.8	5.3	2.1
IMPACT II			
Placebo	1.1	8.1	2.8, PCI, 2.8, CABG
Eptifibatide 135/0.5 dose	0.5	6.6	2.6, PCI, 1.6, CABG
Eptifibatide 135/0.75 dose	0.8	6.9	2.9, PCI, 2.0, CABG
ESPRIT			
Placebo	0.6	9.7	1.7[a]
Eptifibatide 180/2.0/180 dose	0.4	6.2	1.1[a]
RESTORE			
Placebo	0.7	5.7	4.0, PCI[b], 1.4, CABG[b]
Tirofiban	0.8	4.2	2.3, PCI[b], 1.1, CABG[b]
CAPTURE			
Placebo	1.3	8.2	10.9
Abciximab	1.0	4.1	7.8
RAPPORT			
Placebo	2.1	4.1	6.6[a]
Abciximab	2.5	3.3	1.7[a]
ISAR-2			
Control	4.5	1.5	5.0[a]
Abciximab	2.0	0.5	3.0[a]
ADMIRAL			
Placebo	6.6	2.6	6.6
Abciximab	3.4	1.3	1.3
CADILLAC			
PTCA + Control	2.5	0.8	5.6
PTCA + Abciximab	1.1	0.8	3.4
Stent + Control	2.2	1.0	3.2
Stent + Abciximab	2.7	0.8	1.6
TARGET			
Tirofiban	0.5	6.9	0.8[a]
Abciximab	0.4	5.4	0.7[a]

Abbreviations: CABG, coronary artery bypass graft surgery; MI, myocardial infarction; PCI, percutaneous coronary intervention; PTCA, percutaneous transluminal coronary angioplasty; 135/0.5, 135/0/75, and 180/2.0/180 = eptifibatide doses (*see* text).

[a] Revascularization endpoint is Urgent Target Vessel revascularization, compared with Urgent Revascularization for other trials.

[b] The RESTORE endpoints listed here are for the published *post hoc* analysis including only *urgent* repeat revascularization, for consistency with the other trials.

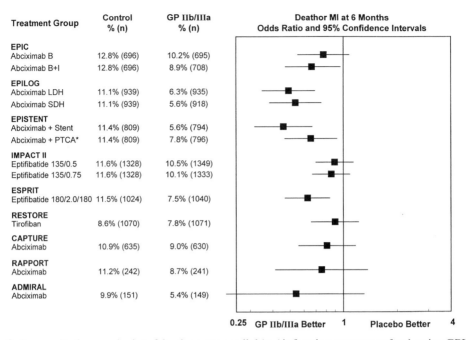

Treatment Group	Control % (n)	GP IIb/IIIa % (n)	Deathor MI at 6 Months Odds Ratio and 95% Confidence Intervals
EPIC			
Abciximab B	12.8% (696)	10.2% (695)	
Abciximab B+I	12.8% (696)	8.9% (708)	
EPILOG			
Abciximab LDH	11.1% (939)	6.3% (935)	
Abciximab SDH	11.1% (939)	5.6% (918)	
EPISTENT			
Abciximab + Stent	11.4% (809)	5.6% (794)	
Abciximab + PTCA*	11.4% (809)	7.8% (796)	
IMPACT II			
Eptifibatide 135/0.5	11.6% (1328)	10.5% (1349)	
Eptifibatide 135/0.75	11.6% (1328)	10.1% (1333)	
ESPRIT			
Eptifibatide 180/2.0/180	11.5% (1024)	7.5% (1040)	
RESTORE			
Tirofiban	8.6% (1070)	7.8% (1071)	
CAPTURE			
Abciximab	10.9% (635)	9.0% (630)	
RAPPORT			
Abciximab	11.2% (242)	8.7% (241)	
ADMIRAL			
Abciximab	9.9% (151)	5.4% (149)	

0.25   GP IIb/IIIa Better   1   Placebo Better   4

Fig. 3. Composite 6-mo endpoint of death or myocardial (re-)infarction event rates for the nine GPIIb/IIIa interventional trials without active controls (i.e., TARGET excluded) for which data were available. EPISTENT trial groups compared with reference group of Placebo + Stent. Abbreviations as for Fig. 2.

in many of the studies. In EPIC, the earliest of these studies, double blinding was maintained and clinical data for all endpoints were obtained for up to 3 yr. Recently, an analysis of long-term mortality outcome of the three major abciximab studies has been reported, with EPIC data to 7 yr, EPILOG data to 4.5 yr, and EPISTENT data to 3 yr.

ACUTE ISCHEMIC ENDPOINTS

Rates of the composite endpoint of death or myocardial infarction at 6 mo in the nine trials without active controls (i.e., excluding TARGET) for which data are available are summarized in Fig. 3. In general, the treatment effect in reducing these acute ischemic events that was achieved early (by 30 d) with GPIIb/IIIa blockade was maintained without attenuation over the long term. The same observation held true for the suppression of urgent revascularization events in those trials in which the urgency of revascularization procedures was adjudicated over long-term follow-up. In EPILOG, for example, the composite endpoint of death, myocardial infarction, or urgent repeat revascularization was reduced in the combined abciximab groups compared with placebo from 11.7 to 5.3% at 30 d, from 14.7 to 8.4% at 6 mo, and from 16.1 to 9.6% at 1 yr; thus, the absolute reduction by abciximab in the composite endpoint (number of events prevented per 100 patients treated) was remarkably constant, 6.3–6.5, at each of these time points. In the TARGET trial, rates of death or myocardial infarction at 6 mo were 8.7% vs 7.4% in the tirofiban and abciximab arms, respectively ($p = 0.108$). Although the difference in rates of myocardial infarction between abciximab and tirofiban treatment groups was no longer statistically significant by 6 mo, the absolute number of events prevented was unchanged at these two time points, demonstrating no diminution of the difference between therapies:

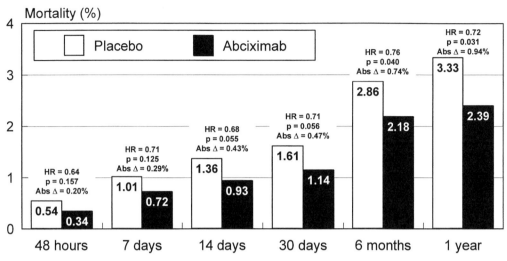

Fig. 4. Pooled results of mortality reduction over time by abciximab relative to control for all interventional trials using the bolus and 12-h infusion regimen of abciximab during percutaneous coronary intervention. Abs Δ, absolute % reduction in mortality; HR, hazard ratio. (Data from ref. *38*.)

6.9% vs 5.4% (*p* = 0.04), absolute difference 1.5% at 30 d; 8.0% vs 6.6% (*p* = 0.07), absolute difference 1.4% at 6 mo.

In the CAPTURE trial, the incidences of death or revascularization over 6 mo were not different among placebo- and abciximab-treated patients. The treatment effect of abciximab on myocardial infarction rates persisted by 6 mo, but was somewhat attenuated (8.2% vs 4.1%, absolute 4.1% difference at 30 d; 9.3% vs 6.6%, absolute 2.7% difference at 6 mo). Such attenuation over long-term follow-up is in contradistinction to the experience in the other GP IIb/IIIa trials during coronary intervention and may be related to the severity of the acute ischemic syndrome or to inadequacy of the 1-h postprocedural abciximab infusion in CAPTURE.

MORTALITY

The long-term follow-up at 1 yr after randomization in the EPISTENT trial provided compelling evidence of a complementary clinical benefit of GPIIb/IIIa blockade and stenting. The combination of stenting and abciximab resulted in a significantly lower mortality rate than either therapy alone (placebo plus stent, 2.4%; abciximab plus angioplasty, 2.1%; abciximab plus stent, 1.0%; hazard ratio = 0.43 for the comparison of abciximab plus stent vs placebo plus stent, *p* = 0.037). Further evidence for this finding of a mortality reduction by abciximab during PCI was obtained by pooling the long-term findings of the different abciximab interventional trials *(38)*. Among all studies using the bolus and 12-h infusion regimen of abciximab, mortality rates compared with placebo were significantly diminished by 25–30% for as long as 3 yr (Fig. 4). The mechanism of mortality reduction with abciximab in these studies remains to be defined. Although the occurrence of a periprocedural myocardial infarction or urgent revascularization clearly increased the risk of subsequent death over the ensuing year, 70–75% of the observed mortality by 1 yr occurred in patients who had *not* suffered an ischemic event within the early

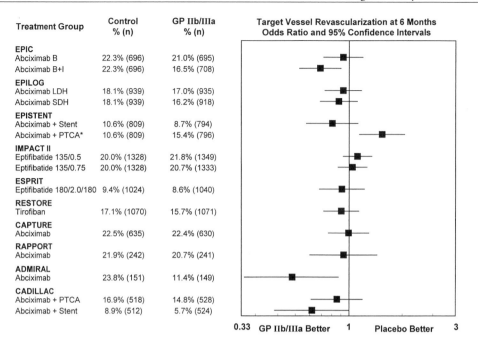

Treatment Group	Control % (n)	GP IIb/IIIa % (n)
EPIC		
Abciximab B	22.3% (696)	21.0% (695)
Abciximab B+I	22.3% (696)	16.5% (708)
EPILOG		
Abciximab LDH	18.1% (939)	17.0% (935)
Abciximab SDH	18.1% (939)	16.2% (918)
EPISTENT		
Abciximab + Stent	10.6% (809)	8.7% (794)
Abciximab + PTCA*	10.6% (809)	15.4% (796)
IMPACT II		
Eptifibatide 135/0.5	20.0% (1328)	21.8% (1349)
Eptifibatide 135/0.75	20.0% (1328)	20.7% (1333)
ESPRIT		
Eptifibatide 180/2.0/180	9.4% (1024)	8.6% (1040)
RESTORE		
Tirofiban	17.1% (1070)	15.7% (1071)
CAPTURE		
Abciximab	22.5% (635)	22.4% (630)
RAPPORT		
Abciximab	21.9% (242)	20.7% (241)
ADMIRAL		
Abciximab	23.8% (151)	11.4% (149)
CADILLAC		
Abciximab + PTCA	16.9% (518)	14.8% (528)
Abciximab + Stent	8.9% (512)	5.7% (524)

Target Vessel Revascularization at 6 Months
Odds Ratio and 95% Confidence Intervals

0.33   GP IIb/IIIa Better   1   Placebo Better   3

Fig. 5. Rates of 6-mo target vessel revascularization for the GPIIb/IIIa interventional trials. EPISTENT trial groups compared with reference group of Placebo + Stent. Abbreviations as for Fig. 3.

period after their index intervention *(38)*. Thus, abciximab did not appear to exert its mortality benefit exclusively through prevention of early ischemic complications.

A significant reduction in long-term mortality by the small-molecule GPIIb/IIIa inhibitors has not been demonstrated; no effects of eptifibatide or tirofiban on death rates were observed in the IMPACT-II or RESTORE trials. There was, however, a nonsignificant trend toward mortality reduction at 1 yr with the high-dose eptifibatide regimen in the ESPRIT trial (placebo 2.0% vs eptifibatide 1.4%; hazard ratio = 0.69; $p = 0.28$) *(39)*. Moreover, there were no differences between the tirofiban and abciximab treatment arms with with regard to 1-yr mortality rates in the TARGET trial (1.92% vs 1.74%, respectively), although TARGET was not statistically powered to assess for equivalence with regard to the infrequent mortality endpoint.

TARGET VESSEL REVASCULARIZATION

The 6-mo results of the EPIC trial demonstrated that therapy with abciximab was associated with a significant reduction in the need for target vessel revascularization procedures (elective or urgent) at 6 mo, from 22.3% among patients receiving placebo to 16.5% among those receiving the bolus and infusion of abciximab (26% relative risk reduction, $p = 0.007$), a finding that led to speculation that this agent may reduce restenosis following coronary intervention. Routine angiographic follow-up was not performed in EPIC; thus, the influence of abciximab on angiographic restenosis could not be confirmed. A significant reduction in the need for late target vessel revascularization procedures by abciximab was not observed at 6 mo or 1 yr in the subsequent EPILOG trial; with the exception of ADMIRAL, neither have any of the other interventional trials with GPIIb/IIIa blockade during balloon angioplasty or stenting demonstrated a significant decrease in "clinical restenosis" (Fig. 5). In the only trial directly comparing two agents, TARGET, differences between the GPIIb/IIIa inhibitors were not observed: at 6 mo, rates of target vessel revascularization were 7.5 and 8.0% (p = NS) in the tirofiban and abciximab groups, respectively. Angiographic substudies within the EPISTENT, IMPACT II, RESTORE, ISAR-2, and CADILLAC trials showed no differences among control or abciximab treatment groups in angiographic measurements of luminal dimensions or restenosis. Moreover, the influence of 12-h or 24-h infusions of abciximab on in-stent restenosis was assessed among 225 patients in the mechanistic ERASER study utilizing intravascular ultrasound (IVUS) measurements of in-stent neointimal tissue volume *(40)*. No effect of either abciximab regimen on neointimal hyperplasia following stenting was observed by IVUS, a finding confirmed by quantitative coronary angiography.

The only intriguing exception to the apparent lack of effect of GPIIb/IIIa blockade on restenosis has been suggested in the EPISTENT and ADMIRAL trials among patients with diabetes mellitus. Rates of target vessel revascularization by 6 mo after stenting were reduced in diabetic patients from 16.6 to 8.1% (p = 0.021) in EPISTENT and from 37.5 to 13.8% (p = 0.046) in ADMIRAL. The angiographic substudy within EPISTENT confirmed a reduction in in-stent neointimal hyperplasia by abciximab in the diabetic subgroup. Notably, rates of target vessel revascularization at 6 mo were the same (although relatively low) among diabetics in the abciximab and tirofiban treatment arms of TARGET (10.8 and 8.8%, respectively, p = 0.257), suggesting that if an anti-restenotic effect of abciximab exists in diabetics, it is probably shared by tirofiban as well.

Safety

The major limitation of abciximab therapy in the first interventional trial, EPIC, was a substantially increased risk of bleeding: the bolus and infusion regimen of abciximab was associated with a doubling in the incidence of major bleeding events and the need for red blood cell transfusions. A high rate of bleeding was also observed in RAPPORT, probably related to the relatively high heparin dose and long vascular sheath dwell times. During subsequent trials, in which heparin doses were limited and vascular sheaths removed early, bleeding rates were diminished in all treatment groups, and appreciable increases in major hemorrhagic risk were no longer associated with GPIIb/IIIa therapy (Table 4) Minor bleeding events (defined as gastrointestinal or genitourinary bleeding or hemoglobin drop of 3–5 gm/dL) tended to occur more frequently in these trials among patients receiving GPIIb/IIIa agents compared with placebo, even with reduced-dose heparin regimens. In the two recent major stent trials, for example, rates of minor bleeding were 1.7% vs 2.9% in the placebo and abciximab groups of EPISTENT and 1.7% vs 2.8% in the placebo and eptifibatide groups of ESPRIT. Similarly, although there were no differences between tirofiban and abciximab treatment groups in rates of major bleeding (0.9 and 0.7%, respectively), abciximab therapy was associated with more minor bleeding in that trial (2.8% vs 4.3%, p < 0.001).

Thrombocytopenia occurred infrequently but was somewhat increased among patients receiving GPIIb/IIIa antagonists, particularly abciximab (Table 5). An increased risk of severe thrombocytopenia (platelet count < 50,000 mm^{-3}) occurred almost exclusively with abciximab therapy, with rates as high as 1.0–1.8%. In the TARGET trial, severe thrombocytopenia occurred in 0.1 and 0.9% of patients randomized to tirofiban and abciximab, respectively (p < 0.001).

Table 4
Rates of In-Hospital of 30-Day TIMI Major Bleeding and Transfusions

Trial	Major bleeding[a] (%)	Transfusions (%)
EPIC		
Placebo	6.6	7.0
Abciximab bolus	10.9	13.2
Abciximab bolus + infusion	14.0	15.4
EPILOG		
Placebo	3.1	3.9
Abciximab + reduced-dose heparin	2.0	1.9
Abciximab + standard-dose heparin	3.5	3.3
EPISTENT		
Placebo + stent	2.2	2.2
Abciximab + stent	1.5	2.8
Abciximab + PTCA	1.4	3.1
IMPACT II		
Placebo	4.8	5.2
Eptifibatide 135/0.5 dose	5.1	5.6
Eptifibatide 135/0.75 dose	5.2	5.9
ESPRIT		
Placebo	0.4	1.0
Eptifibatide 180/2.0/180 dose	1.0	1.4
RESTORE		
Placebo	2.1	2.2[b]
Tirofiban	2.4	3.5[b]
CAPTURE		
Placebo	2.5	3.4
Abciximab	4.1	7.1
RAPPORT		
Placebo	9.5	7.9
Abciximab	16.6	13.7
ISAR-2		
Control	N/A	4.5
Abciximab	N/A	3.5
ADMIRAL		
Placebo	0	N/A
Abciximab	0.7	N/A
CADILLAC		
PTCA + Control	0.6	3.7
PTCA + Abciximab	0.4	5.1
Stent + Control	0.2	4.1
Stent + Abciximab	0.8	5.0
TARGET		
Tirofiban	0.9	1.2
Abciximab	0.7	1.5

Abbreviations: 135/0.5, 135/0/75, and 180/2.0/180 = eptifibatide doses (*see* text); N/A, not available.
[a] Major Bleeding defined by the Thrombolysis in Myocardial Infarction (TIMI) criteria *(28)* as intracranial hemorrhage or bleeding associated with a decrease in hemoglobin of ≥ 5 g/dL.
[b] Transfusion rates in RESTORE reported only for >2 U.

Table 5
Rates of Thrombocytopenia

Trial	Agent	Control (%)	GPIIb/IIIa inhibitor (%)
Moderate thrombocytopenia (platelet count < 100,000 mm^{-3})			
EPIC	Abciximab	3.4	3.6 (bolus)
			5.2 (bolus + infusion)
EPILOG	Abciximab	1.5	2.6 (std. dose heparin)
			2.5 (low-dose heparin)
EPISTENT	Abciximab	0.6	3.1 (plus stent)
			2.9 (plus PTCA)
CAPTURE	Abciximab	1.3	5.6
RAPPORT	Abciximab	2.9	5.0
ADMIRAL	Abciximab	1.3	4.7
CADILLAC	Abciximab	2.0	4.0
IMPACT II	Eptifibatide	2.7	3.2 (135/0.5 dose)
			2.8 (135/0.75 dose)
RESTORE[a]	Tirofiban	0.9	1.1
Severe thrombocytopenia (platelet count < 50,000 mm^{-3})[b]			
EPIC	Abciximab	0.7	0.4 (bolus)
			1.6 (bolus + infusion)
EPILOG	Abciximab	0.4	0.9 (std. dose heparin)
			0.4 (low-dose heparin)
EPISTENT	Abciximab	0	1.1 (plus stent)
			0.9 (plus PTCA)
CAPTURE	Abciximab	0.3	1.8
ADMIRAL	Abciximab	1.3	1.3
IMPACT II	Eptifibatide	0.6	0.2 (135/0.5 dose)
			0.4 (135/0.75 dose)
ESPRIT	Eptifibatide	0	0.2
RESTORE	Tirofiban	0.1	0.2

[a]Reported in RESTORE for platelet count < 90,000 mm^{-3}.
[b]Reported in ESPRIT trial for platelet count < 20,000 mm^{-3}.

Coronary Intervention in Trials of Unstable Angina

Six large-scale trials have assessed GPIIb/IIIa inhibition among patients with unstable angina or non-Q-wave myocardial infarction in whom percutaneous revascularization was not mandated. In three of these trials, PURSUIT *(41)* and PRISM PLUS *(42)*, and PARAGON B *(43)*, a substantial number of patients underwent early coronary intervention while on study drug infusion, providing important information regarding the efficacy of these agents as preprocedural and postprocedural therapy. In PURSUIT, 9461 patients were randomized to receive placebo or eptifibatide (180 µg/kg bolus, then 2.0 µg/kg/min infusion for 72–96 h) in addition to heparin or aspirin; of these, 1228 underwent percutaneous revascularization within the first 72 h (while receiving study drug) *(41)*. Eptifibatide was associated with a significant reduction in the risk of myocardial infarction prior to the revascularization procedure (5.5% vs 1.8%, $p < 0.001$), as well as a significant reduction in the composite endpoint of death or myocardial infarction by 30 d (16.8 vs 11.8%, 30% relative risk reduction, $p = 0.01$).

In PRISM PLUS, 1570 patients were treated with placebo or tirofiban (0.4 µg/kg/min for 30 min and then 0.1 µg/kg/min infusion for 48–96 h in addition to aspirin and heparin) *(42)*. Catheterization and percutaneous revascularization were encouraged, but to be deferred for 48 h, and 475 patients underwent coronary intervention while receiving study drug. During the first 48 h (before intervention), death or myocardial infarction rates were reduced from 2.6 to 0.9% by tirofiban in the overall 1570 patient cohort ($p = 0.01$); among the 475 patients undergoing intervention, 30-d rates of death or myocardial infarction were 10.2 and 5.9% in the placebo and tirofiban groups, respectively (42% relative risk reduction, $p = 0.12$). In PARAGON B, 5225 patients were randomized to receive placebo or lamifiban, a non-peptide small molecule GPIIb/IIIa inhibitor similar to tirofiban, for 72 h *(43)*. Catheterization and revascularization were performed at the physician's discretion. Among the 678 patients undergoing PCI while on study drug, the composite endpoint of death or myocardial infarction was reduced from 0.85 to 0.31% prior to PCI and from 12.8 to 8.9% following PCI.

SYNTHESIS OF THE RANDOMIZED TRIALS

Efficacy

The consistent finding among over 25,000 patients enrolled in the trials of GPIIb/IIIa receptor blockade during coronary intervention has been that of reduction in the risk of important acute ischemic events by as much as 50–60%, unequivocally establishing the clinical efficacy of this class of therapy in this setting. This treatment effect extends to each of the components of the composite clinical endpoint (death, myocardial infarction, and emergency revascularization), attesting to the common platelet/thrombus-mediated pathophysiology of these events. The inhibition of acute ischemic events is achieved early, primarily in the first 12–48 h after the revascularization procedure, and is almost invariably maintained without attenuation thereafter. Over long-term (3-yr or more) follow-up, a 20–25% relative reduction in mortality has been convincingly demonstrated with abciximab; it is unknown whether a similar benefit is associated with eptifibatide or tirofiban.

Improved outcome with this therapy has been apparent in every subgroup of patients tested, and no demographic, clinical, angiographic, or procedural characteristic has been observed that will identify patients who do *not* benefit from GPIIb/IIIa blockade. Patients with acute ischemic syndromes such as unstable angina, however, may derive exceptional treatment effect from this class of therapy. Other subsets of patients who are at increased risk for acute ischemic events, such as those requiring bailout stenting *(44)* or with diabetes *(45,46)*, also tended to experience a enhanced absolute treatment effect from GPIIb/IIIa inhibition.

Clinical benefit is derived from GPIIb/IIIa blockade irrespective of the technique or modality used for percutaneous coronary revascularization. The EPISTENT trial clearly demonstrated a magnitude of treatment effect with abciximab during elective stenting (absolute risk reduction 5.5%, relative risk reduction 51%) that was essentially identical to that obtained with abciximab during balloon angioplasty in EPILOG (absolute risk reduction 6.4%, relative risk reduction 56%). Similarly, subgroup analysis of patients in EPIC and EPILOG undergoing directional atherectomy confirmed previous findings that atherectomy patients are at substantially greater risk for ischemic complications than their counterparts treated with angioplasty and that the treatment effect of abciximab during atherectomy tended, if anything, to be greater than that during balloon angioplasty *(47)*. The decision to utilize these agents during a revascularization procedure thus should not be made contingent on whether balloon angioplasty, stent implantation, or atherectomy is planned.

An important influence of GPIIb/IIIa blockade on restenosis following PCI is unlikely. Although a significant reduction by abciximab in long-term target vessel revascularization rates was observed in the EPIC trial, this treatment effect has not been definitively confirmed in any subsequent study of a GPIIb/IIIa inhibitor. In-stent restenosis among diabetic patients may be somewhat favorably influenced by abciximab or tirofiban, but this finding cannot be definitively confirmed.

DIFFERENCES IN EFFICACY AMONG THE AGENTS

Although all three of the GPIIb/IIIa inhibitors reduce ischemic risk, there has been apparent heterogeneity among the drugs since the earliest trials with regard to the magnitude of treatment effect. The bolus and 12-h infusion regimen of abciximab reduced 30-d endpoints by as much as 50–60% in the EPILOG and EPISTENT trials, whereas more modest risk reductions on the order of 15–25% were seen with eptifibatide and tirofiban in IMPACT-II and RESTORE, respectively. It has been hypothesized that variability in efficacy among agents, if it exists, may relate to the pharmacodynamics of receptor binding. Abciximab dissociates slowly from the GPIIb/IIIa receptor, thus providing gradually diminished inhibition of platelet aggregation for 12–24 h or more after termination of drug infusion *(6,8)*; in contrast, platelet aggregation following discontinuation of the rapidly reversible agents (eptifibatide and tirofiban) is normalized within 2–4 h *(9,10)*. Additionally, the nonspecific blockade by abciximab of the $\alpha_v\beta_3$ (vitronectin) and $\alpha_m\beta_2$ (Mac-1) receptors in addition to platelet GPIIb/IIIa ($\alpha_{IIb}\beta_3$) theoretically may provide advantages over the specific agents (which bind exclusively to GPIIb/IIIa). Ex vivo experimental studies, for example, have suggested that blockade of GPIIb/IIIa and the vitronectin receptors more completely suppresses platelet-mediated thrombin generation than does inhibition of either receptor alone *(48)*. Inhibition of Mac-1 may have additional salutary effects related to suppression of inflammation or vascular smooth muscle cell death *(49)*.

More contemporary trials of the small-molecule GPIIb/IIIa inhibitors have provided conflicting evidence regarding the effectiveness of eptifibatide and tirofiban relative to abciximab. The ESPRIT trial showed a substantial clinical benefit of high-dose eptifibatide compared with placebo, convincingly demonstrating the importance of adequate platelet inhibition with these agents. The treatment effect of eptifibatide in ESPRIT can be compared only indirectly with that of abciximab in EPISTENT, with all the limitations inherent to intertrial comparisons. Nevertheless, three general observations can be made.

First, ESPRIT enrolled a lower risk group of patients than did EPISTENT, by virtue of its exclusion of those with severe unstable angina, recent myocardial infarction, or bypass graft disease. Second, the use of a low-dose heparin regimen (60 U/kg) in *both* treatment arms raises the question of whether insufficient anticoagulation was provided for those randomized to placebo; the median ACT was only 263 s in the placebo arm of ESPRIT, whereas retrospective studies have suggested that an optimal ACT level for PCI performed without GPIIb/IIIa blockade is in the range of 350–375 s *(50)*. In contrast, the heparin dose in EPISTENT was higher in the placebo arm (100 U/kg) than in the abciximab arms (70 U/kg), and the median ACT among patients randomized to placebo in EPISTENT

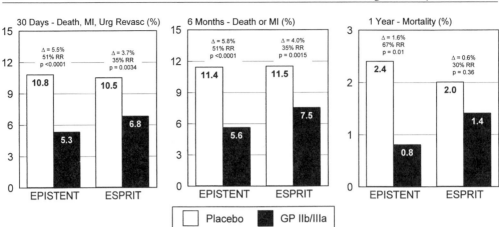

Fig. 6. Comparison of EPISTENT (abciximab vs placebo) and ESPRIT (eptifibatide vs placebo) trial endpoints at 30 d, 6 mo, and 1 yr. MI, myocardial infarction; RR, risk reduction; Urg Revasc, urgent revascularization. One-year mortality endpoint is treated patient analysis.

was 346 s. Concerns regarding the adequacy of anticoagulation in ESPRIT are compounded by the prohibition of thienopyridine pretreatment. These factors could have increased the ischemic event rate in the placebo group of that trial, thereby exaggerating the apparent treatment effect of eptifibatide. Third, the magnitude of short-term and long-term treatment effect with eptifibatide in ESPRIT was numerically less than that of abciximab in EPISTENT at each time point (Fig. 6); although there is clearly no statistical basis to conclude that the results of these trials are dissimilar, the trends are noteworthy.

In contrast to eptifibatide, tirofiban has been compared directly with abciximab in the TARGET trial. Although this study was intended to show noninferiority of tirofiban, short-term ischemic event rates were significantly lower with abciximab, reinforcing the evidence for a differential treatment effect among the agents. Notably, this early difference in ischemic complications did not translate to a significant difference between tirofiban and abciximab treatment groups with regard to mortality at 1 yr, although TARGET was not designed with an adequate sample size to have statistical power to assess this infrequent mortality endpoint.

Safety

BLEEDING

The major potential safety issue with this as well as other classes of agents directed against platelet function or coagulation is that of bleeding. The findings of the first trial of this class of therapy, EPIC, highlighted the potential for hemorrhagic risk with these agents. Most bleeding with GPIIb/IIIa antagonists in this and subsequent trials was at sites of vascular access, although spontaneous gastrointestinal and genitourinary bleeding also occurred; long-term sequelae were infrequent. Importantly, pooled analysis of the trials indicates that rates of intracranial hemorrhage do *not* appear to be increased *(51)*. The improvement in the safety profile of these agents subsequent to the EPIC experience shows that modification of conjunctive anticoagulant therapy with heparin by weight adjustment and dose reduction is a key intervention in abrogating excess bleeding risk.

Early removal of vascular sheaths and meticulous care of the access site are probably also important means of avoiding hemorrhage. Bleeding may nevertheless be a concern in certain groups of patients, such as those who receive GPIIb/IIIa blockade as an unplanned or bailout intervention in the setting of full-dose heparinization or those undergoing rescue angioplasty for failed reperfusion after full-dose thrombolysis. Partial reversal of heparinization with protamine in the former situation and very careful heparin dose reduction and ACT monitoring in the latter will probably improve the balance between risk and benefit in these patients.

For patients who develop refractory or life-threatening bleeding, the antiplatelet effect of abciximab may be reversed by discontinuation of drug infusion and by platelet transfusion after the approx 10–30 min required for clearance of circulating drug. After introduction of new platelets into the circulation, abciximab redistributes from old to new platelets, reducing the mean level of receptor blockade. In experimental studies, transfusion of the equivalent of 10 U of platelets in primates treated with abciximab led to prompt reduction in mean receptor blockade from 80–90% to <70%, near normalization of bleeding times, and partial (approx 30%) recovery of platelet aggregation *(52)*. Platelet transfusions should rarely be necessary with the rapidly reversible agents eptifibatide and tirofiban, but theoretically they would not be effective during the approx 2 h required for elimination of high concentrations of these agents from the circulating plasma phase.

EMERGENCY CORONARY BYPASS SURGERY

There has been concern about the risk of excessive perioperative bleeding if patients require urgent coronary artery bypass surgery for failed angioplasty after administration of a GPIIb/IIIa inhibitor. The rapidly reversible agents eptifibatide and tirofiban should present little in the way of perioperative bleeding risk in this regard; platelet aggregation and bleeding times return to normal following discontinuation of both of these agents within a few hours, the time period required for coronary artery bypass to be performed. Despite its more prolonged duration of action, however, antecedent treatment with abciximab should not be considered a contraindication to necessary emergency surgical revascularization.

In a detailed study of surgical outcomes among 85 patients requiring urgent coronary surgery in the EPILOG and EPISTENT trials, abciximab therapy was not associated with a major increase in perioperative blood loss *(53)*. Platelet transfusions were administered more frequently (in part prophylactically) to patients who had received abciximab, but the need for other blood products was the same in the abciximab and placebo groups. Although surgical reexploration for bleeding tended to be more frequent in patients who had received abciximab, surgical cross-clamp, cardiopulmonary bypass, and closure times were not prolonged, and the utilization of optimal mammary artery conduits was not impaired. Moreover, ischemic events tended to be less frequent in abciximab-treated patients. Thus, hemorrhagic risk may be modestly increased by abciximab in the event of urgent coronary bypass surgery, but it is unlikely to be associated with excess mortality or important morbidity. Conventional procedures for intraoperative ACT-guided heparin dosing and selective application of platelet transfusions appear to be appropriate for the management of these patients.

THROMBOCYTOPENIA

Thrombocytopenia occurs infrequently following GPIIb/IIIa inhibition, but it may be precipitous and profound (platelet count $<20,000$ mm^{-3}); the excess risk of profound thrombocytopenia associated with abciximab (0.4–1.1%) appears to be higher than with eptifibatide (0–0.2%) or tirofiban (0.1–0.3%). Thrombocytopenia in this setting is not a benign event. In a pooled analysis of 7290 patients in the EPIC, EPILOG, and EPISTENT trials, 178 (2.4%) developed thrombocytopenia, with an independent association observed with abciximab therapy (odds ratio 1.75) *(54)*. Even with the analysis confined to the 126 patients without antecedent coronary bypass surgery, those with thrombocytopenia had significantly higher rates of major and minor hemorrhage (33% vs 9%, $p < 0.001$), red cell transfusions (21% vs 5%, $p < 0.001$), and 30-d mortality (4.8% vs 0.6%, $p < 0.001$) than did patients without thrombocytopenia. Perhaps somewhat surprisingly, however, bleeding complications and mortality were *less* frequent if thrombocytopenia occurred in patients who had been randomized to abciximab than if thrombocytopenia was in the context of placebo administration.

The mechanism of thrombocytopenia associated with GPIIb/IIIa inhibitors is unknown. Thrombocytopenia occurring after administration of a GPIIb/IIIa agent can usually be differentiated from that caused by the heparin-induced thrombocytopenia syndrome by the early and precipitous onset, generally within 1–24 h after administration of the GPIIb/IIIa inhibitor *(55)*, as well as by the absence of thrombotic complications. There is little evidence of ongoing platelet clearance following discontinuation of the GPIIb/IIIa antagonist, and most patients experience an increase in platelet count of about 20–30,000 mm^{-3}/d (the rate of bone marrow production). Unlike heparin-induced thrombocytopenia, platelet transfusions are a safe and protective therapy for profound thrombocytopenia with or without serious bleeding induced by GPIIb/IIIa inhibitors. Platelet counts should be measured within the first 2–4 h after administration of these agents and followed for the duration of therapy.

READMINISTRATION

Approximately 5–6% of patients will develop a human antichimeric antibody (HACA) response to abciximab; no antibody response has been observed with eptifibatide, tirofiban, or lamifiban. A prospective registry found no instances of hypersensitivity or anaphylactic reactions following abciximab readministration in 500 patients, and efficacy of the agent in reducing ischemic complications appeared to be similar with readministration as with first-time use *(56)*. The rates of profound thrombocytopenia (platelet count <20,000 mm^{-3}) following readministration were somewhat higher, however, than expected with first-time administration. Moreover, in contrast to the typically rapid resolution of thrombocytopenia seen with first-time administration, a protracted time course of thrombocytopenia for up to 1 wk was observed in these patients following readministration. The presence or absence of a positive HACA titer did not appear to be predictive of a lack of clinical effectiveness, development of thrombocytopenia, or other sequelae in patients undergoing readministration.

RECOMMENDATIONS

Whom to Treat

Although trial data support the use of GPIIb/IIIa inhibitors in virtually all patients undergoing percutaneous coronary revascularization, these agents are not universally employed in clinical practice, primarily because of economic considerations. Economic aspects of GPIIb/IIIa blockade are discussed in detail in Chapter 14; it is important to recognize that cost savings derived from reduction in ischemic events offset much of the acquisition cost of these agents. Moreover, the cost effectiveness of abciximab in reducing mortality during coronary stenting appears quite favorable, approx $6200 per life-year saved, well within the range of other accepted medical therapies *(57)*. Economic considerations aside, the benefits of this therapy should certainly be provided to patients at elevated risk for periprocedural complications, such as those with unstable angina or acute myocardial infarction, diabetes mellitus, complex lesion morphology, extensive myocardium at jeopardy, or multivessel or multilesion interventions. Although anecdotal data suggest that abciximab may be useful in an unplanned or bailout fashion to reverse thrombotic complications of coronary intervention *(58,59)*, this approach has never been tested in a randomized fashion and must be regarded as suboptimal relative to planned use.

Which Agent to Use

Aside from the economic considerations, the available data suggest that the current efficacy standard during and after percutaneous coronary intervention remains abciximab administered as a bolus followed by a 12-h infusion. Aspirin, heparin, and ticlopidine or clopidogrel (in patients receiving stents) should also be administered *(60)*. A pretreatment regimen of abciximab, as was used in CAPTURE, may be effective in stabilizing patients prior to coronary revascularization, but it offers no clear advantage in stable patients or even in unstable patients for whom revascularization can be immediately performed. Regardless of whether or not a period of pretreatment with abciximab is used, the 12-h postprocedural infusion appears to be necessary for optimal clinical benefit.

Even for situations in which broad use of abciximab is precluded because of economic considerations, there is little justification for withholding the less expensive agents eptifibatide or tirofiban. The treatment effects of these GPIIb/IIIa inhibitors are considerable, if not clearly equivalent to that of abciximab, and certainly justify their relatively modest costs. A reasonable compromise between efficacy and cost might be to utilize abciximab for those settings in which enhanced benefit has been observed with this agent relative to the reversible inhibitors. In particular, patients with severe unstable ischemic syndromes were excluded from inclusion in the ESPRIT trial and had a particularly inferior outcome with tirofiban in TARGET. Abciximab is the only agent that has been tested during primary PCI for acute myocardial infarction. The robust mortality benefit of abciximab in diabetics has also not been duplicated with the reversible agents.

For patients presenting with unstable angina or non-Q-wave myocardial infarction in whom revascularization is not immediately planned, both eptifibatide and tirofiban have been unequivocally shown to improve clinical outcome prior to intervention, following intervention, or in patients treated conservatively without early intervention (*see* Chapter 10). Once a course of empiric therapy with eptifibatide or tirofiban has been initiated, there are no data to suggest that patients would experience incremental benefit by conversion to abciximab during subsequent percutaneous coronary revascularization, as the treatment effects of eptifibatide and tirofiban in PURSUIT and PRISM PLUS were considerable in these patients.

Conjunctive Heparin and Vascular Access Site Management

A low-dose, weight-adjusted heparin regimen, using an initial bolus of 60–70 U/kg (maximum 6000–7000 U) adjusted to attain and maintain an ACT of ≥200 s, has clearly been shown to be a safe and effective means of administering heparin when GPIIb/IIIa inhibitor therapy is planned. There are no data to suggest that postprocedural heparin provides additional benefit in this setting, even in patients treated for acute ischemic syndromes; vascular access sheaths can typically be removed 2–6 h after the procedure, during the GPIIb/IIIa inhibitor infusion, once the ACT is <175 s or the aPTT is <50 s. Manual or mechanical groin compression should be maintained for at least 30 min, followed by strict bed rest with leg immobilization for 6–8 h after sheath removal. Alternatively, vascular closure devices may be used immediately and appear to be effective in patients who have received GPIIb/IIIa antagonists. Other measures to help reduce bleeding risk at the vascular access site include anterior arterial puncture only (rather than the traditional Seldinger "through-and-through" technique), avoidance of routine venous sheath placement, and adequate patient sedation and immobilization during periods of strict bed rest.

SUMMARY

Platelet GPIIb/IIIa receptor blockade represents one of the most significant advances in the practice of interventional cardiology. Large-scale randomized controlled trials have unequivocally demonstrated that these agents reduce the risk of periprocedural ischemic complications by up to 50–60% and are efficacious in a broad spectrum of patients undergoing revascularization irrespective of risk profile, clinical indication for revascularization, or interventional technique. This clinical benefit may be achieved without excess major bleeding risk by modification of conjunctive heparin dosing. Issues for future study include critical evaluation of the medicoeconomic aspects of this therapy, the effectiveness of these agents when used in an unplanned or bailout fashion, and the potential for combining GPIIb/IIIa antagonists with novel inhibitors of thrombin or other components of the coagulation cascade.

REFERENCES

1. Steele PM, Chesebro JH, Stanson AW, et al. Balloon angioplasty. Natural history of the pathophysiological response to injury in a pig model. Circ Res 1985;57:105–112.
2. Uchida Y, Hasegawa K, Kawamura K, Shibuya I. Angioscopic observation of the coronary luminal changes induced by percutaneous transluminal coronary angioplasty. Am Heart J 1989;117:769–776.
3. Schwartz L, Bourassa MG, Lesperance J, et al. Aspirin and dipyridamole in the prevention of restenosis after percutaneous transluminal coronary angioplasty. N Engl J Med 1988;318:1714–1719.
4. Phillips DR, Charo IF, Parise LV, Fitzgerald LA. The platelet membrane glycoprotein IIb/IIIa complex. Blood 1988;71:831–843.
5. Coller BS. Blockade of platelet GPIIb/IIIa receptors as an antithrombotic strategy. Circulation 1995;92: 2373–2380.
6. Tcheng JE, Ellis SG, George BS, et al. Pharmacodynamics of chimeric glycoprotein IIb/IIIa integrin antiplatelet antibody Fab 7E3 in high-risk coronary angioplasty. Circulation 1994;90:1757–1764.
7. Kleiman NS, Raizner AE, Jordan R, et al. Differential inhibition of platelet aggregation induced by adenosine diphosphate or a thrombin receptor-activating peptide in patients treated with bolus chimeric 7E3 Fab: implications for inhibition of the internal pool of GPIIb/IIIa receptors. J Am Coll Cardiol 1995;26: 1665–1671.
8. Mascelli MA, Lance ET, Damaraju L, Wagner CL, Weisman HF, Jordan RE. Pharmacodynamic profile of short-term abciximab treatment demonstrates prolonged platelet inhibition with gradual recovery from GP IIb/IIIa receptor blockade. Circulation 1998;97:1680–1688.
9. Harrington RA, Kleiman NS, Kottke-Marchant K, et al. Immediate and reversible platelet inhibition after intravenous administration of a peptide glycoprotein IIb/IIIa inhibitor during percutaneous coronary intervention. Am J Cardiol 1995;76:1222–1227.
10. Kereiakes DJ, Kleiman NS, Ambrose J, et al. Randomized, double-blind, placebo-controlled dose-ranging study of tirofiban (MK-383) platelet IIb/IIIa blockade in high risk patients undergoing coronary angioplasty. J Am Coll Cardiol 1996;27:536–542.

11. EPIC Investigators. Use of a monoclonal antibody directed against the platelet glycoprotein IIb/IIIa receptor in high-risk coronary angioplasty. N Engl J Med 1994;330:956–961.

12. Lincoff AM, Tcheng JH, Bass TA, et al. A multicenter, randomized, double-blind pilot trial of standard versus low dose weight-adjusted heparin in patients treated with the platelet glycoprotein IIb/IIIa receptor antibody 7E3 during percutaneous coronary revascularization (abstr). J Am Coll Cardiol 1995;25: 80A.

13. EPILOG Investigators. Platelet glycoprotein IIb/IIIa blockade with abciximab with low-dose heparin during percutaneous coronary revascularization. N Engl J Med 1997;336:1689–1696.

14. EPISTENT Investigators. Randomised placebo-controlled and balloon-angioplasty-controlled trial to assess safety of coronary stenting with use of platelet glycoprotein IIb/IIIa blockade. Lancet 1998;352: 87–92.

15. IMPACT II Investigators. Randomized placebo-controlled trial of effect of eptifibatide on complications of percutaneous coronary intervention: IMPACT II. Lancet 1997;349:1422–1428.

16. Phillips DR, Teng W, Arfstent A, et al. Effect of Ca^{2+} on GP IIb-IIIa interactions with Integrilin. Enhanced GP IIb-IIIa binding and inhibition of platelet aggregation by reductions in the concentration of ionized calcium in plasma anticoagulated with citrate. Circulation 1997;96:1488–1494.

17. Tcheng JE, Talley JD, O'Shea JC, et al. Clinical pharmacology of higher-dose eptifibatide in percutaneous coronary intervention: results of the PRIDE study. Am J Cardiol 2001;88:1097–1102.

18. ESPRIT Investigators. Novel dosing regimen of eptifibatide in planned coronary stent implantation (ESPRIT): a randomised, placebo-controlled trial. Lancet 2000;356:2037–2044.

19. RESTORE Investigators. Effects of platelet glycoprotein IIb/IIIa blockade with tirofiban on adverse cardiac events in patients with unstable angina or acute myocardial infarction undergoing coronary angioplasty. Circulation 1997;96:1445–1453.

20. CAPTURE Investigators. Randomised placebo-controlled trial of abciximab before and during coronary intervention in refractory unstable angina: the CAPTURE Study. Lancet 1997;349:1429–1435.

21. Brener SJ, Barr LA, Burchenal JEB, et al., on behalf of the ReoPro and Primary PTCA Organization and Randomized Trial (RAPPORT) Investigators. A randomized, placebo-controlled trial of platelet glycoprotein IIb/IIIa blockade with primary angioplasty for acute myocardial infarction. Circulation 1998;98: 734–741.

22. Neumann F, Kastrati A, Schmitt C, et al. Effect of glycoprotein IIb/IIIa receptor blockade with abciximab on clinical and angiographic restenosis rate after the placement of coronary stents following acute myocardial infarction. J Am Coll Cardiol 2000;35:915–921.

23. Montalescot G, Barragan P, Wittenberg O, et al., for the ADMIRAL Investigators. Platelet glycoprotein IIb/IIIa inhibition with coronary stenting for acute myocardial infarction. N Engl J Med 2001;344: 1895–1903.

24. Stone GW, Grines CL, Cox DA, et al., CADILLAC Investigators. Comparison of angioplasty with stenting, with or without abciximab, in acute myocardial infarction. N Engl J Med 2002;346:957–966.

25. Topol EJ, Moliterno DJ, Herrmann HC, et al., for the TARGET Investigators. Comparison of two platelet glycoprotein IIb/IIIa inhibitors, tirofiban and abciximab, for the prevention of ischemic events with percutaneous coronary revascularization. N Engl J Med 2001;344:1888–1894.

26. Lincoff AM, Califf RM, Anderson KM, et al. Evidence for prevention of death and myocardial infarction with platelet membrane glycoprotein IIb/IIIa receptor blockade by c7E3 Fab (abciximab) among patients with unstable angina undergoing percutaneous coronary revascularization. J Am Coll Cardiol 1997;30: 149–156.

27. Steinhubl SR, Lauer MD, Mukherjee DP, et al. The duration of pretreatment with ticlopidine prior to stenting is associated with the risk of procedure-related non-Q-wave myocardial infarctions. J Am Coll Cardiol 1998;32:1366–1370.

28. Rao AK, Pratt C, Berke A, et al., for TIMI Investigators. Thrombolysis in Myocardial Infarction (TIMI) trial—Phase I: hemorrhagic manifestations and changes in plasma fibrinogen and the fibrinolytic system in patients treated with recombinant tissue plasminogen activator and streptokinase. J Am Coll Cardiol 1988;11:1–11.

29. TARGET Investigators. Comparison of two platelet glycoprotein IIb/IIIa inhibitors, tirofiban and abciximab, for the prevention of ischemic events with percutaneous coronary revascularization. N Engl J Med 2001;344:1888–1894.

30. Abdelmeguid AE, Topol EJ, Whitlow PL, Sapp SK, Ellis SG. Significance of mild transient release of creatine kinase-MB fraction after percutaneous coronary intervention. Circulation 1996;94:1528–1536.

31. Kugelmass AD, Cohen CJ, Moscucci M, et al. Elevation in creatine kinase myocardial isoform following otherwise successful directional coronary atherectomy and stenting. Am J Cardiol 1994;74:748–754.

32. Harrington RA, Lincoff AM, Califf RM, et al., for the CAVEAT investigators. Characteristics and consequences of myocardial infarction after percutaneous coronary intervention: insights from the coronary angioplasty versus excisional atherectomy trial (CAVEAT). J Am Coll Cardiol 1995;25:1693–1699.

33. Kong TQ, Davidson CJ, Meyers SN, Tauke JT, Parker MA, Bonow RO. Prognostic implication of creatine kinase elevation following elective coronary artery interventions. JAMA 1997;277:461–466.

34. Tardiff BE, Califf RM, Tcheng JE, et al., for the IMPACT-II Investigators. Post-intervention cardiac enzyme elevations: prognostic significance in IMPACT II (abstr). J Am Coll Cardiol 1996;27:83A.

35. Redwood SR, Popma JJ, Kent KK, et al. Predictors of late mortality following ablative new-device angioplasty in native coronary arteries (abstr). J Am Coll Cardiol 1996;27:167A.

36. Topol EJ, Ferguson JJ, Weisman HF, et al., for the EPIC Investigator Group. Long-term protection from myocardial ischemic events in a randomized trial of brief integrin β3 blockade with percutaneous coronary intervention. JAMA 1997;278:479–484.

37. Ellis SG, Lincoff AM, Miller D, et al., for the EPIC and EPILOG Investigators. Reduction in complications of angioplasty with abciximab occurs largely independently of baseline lesion morphology. J Am Coll Cardiol 1998;32:1619–1623.

38. Anderson KM, Califf RM, Stone GW, et al. Long-term mortality benefit with abciximab in patients undergoing percutaneous coronary intervention. J Am Coll Cardiol 2001;37:2059–2065.

39. O'Shea JC, Buller CE, Cantor WJ, et al., for the EsPRIT Investigators. Long-term efficacy of platelet glycoprotein IIb/IIIa integrin blockade with eptifibatide in coronary stent intervention. JAMA 2002;287: 618–621.

40. ERASER Investigators. Acute platelet inhibition with abciixmab does not reduce in-stent restenosis (ERASER Study). Circulation 1999;100:799–806.

41. PURSUIT Trial Investigators. Inhibition of platelet glycoprotein IIb/IIIa with eptifibatide in patients with acute coronary syndromes. N Engl J Med 1998;339:436–443.

42. PRISM PLUS Study Investigators. Inhibition of the platelet glycoprotein IIb/IIIa receptor with tirofiban in unstable angina and non-Q-wave myocardial infarction. N Engl J Med 1998;338:1488–1497.

43. PARAGON-B Investigators. Randomized, placebo-controlled trial of titrated intravenous lamifiban for acute coronary syndromes. Circulation 2002;105:316–321.

44. Kereiakes DJ, Lincoff AM, Miller DP, et al., for the EPILOG Investigators. Abciximab therapy and unplanned coronary stent deployment. Favorable effects on stent use, clinical outcomes, and bleeding complications. Circulation 1998;97:857–864.

45. Marso S, Lincoff A, Ellis S, et al., EPISTENT Investigators. Optimizing the percutaneous interventional outcomes for patients with diabetes mellitus. Circulation 1999;100:2477–2484.

46. Bhatt D, Marso S, Lincoff A, Wolski K, Ellis S, Topol E. Abciximab reduces mortality in diabetics following percutaneous intervention. JACC 2000;35:922–928.

47. Ghaffari S, Kereiakes DJ, Lincoff AM, et al., for the EPILOG Investigators. Platelet glycoprotein IIb/IIIa receptor blockade with abciximab reduces ischemic complications in patients undergoing directional coronary atherectomy. Am J Cardiol 1998;82:7–12.

48. Reverter JC, Beguin S, Kessels H, Kumar R, Hemker HC, Coller BS. Inhibition of platelet-mediated, tissue factor-induced thrombin generation by the mouse/human chimeric 7E3 antibody. J Clin Invest 1996; 98:863–874.

49. Seshiah PN, Kereiakes DJ, Vasudevan SS, et al. Activated monocytes induce smooth muscle cell death. Role of macrophage colony stimulating factor and cell contact. Circulation 2002;105:174–180.

50. Chew DP, Bhatt DL, Lincoff AM, et al. Defining the optimal activated clotting time during percutaneous coronary intervention. Circulation 2001;103:961–966.

51. Akkerhuis KM, Deckers JW, Lincoff AM, et al. Risk of stroke associated with abciximab among patients undergoing percutaneous coronary intervention. JAMA 2001;286:78–82.

52. Wagner CL, Cunningham MR, Wyand MS, Weisman HF, Coller BS, Jordan RE. Reversal of the antiplatelet effects of chimeric 7E3 Fab treatment by platelet transfusion in cynomolgous monkeys (abstr). Thromb Haemost 1995;73:1313.

53. Lincoff AM, LeNarz RA, Despotis GJ, et al., for the EPILOG and EPISTENT Investigators. Abciximab and bleeding complications during coronary surgery: results from the EPILOG and EPISTENT trials. Ann Thorac Surg 2000;70:516–526.

54. Kereiakes DJ, Berkowitz SD, Lincoff AM, et al. Clinical correlates and course of thrombocytopenia during percutaneous coronary intervention in the era of abciximab glycoprotein IIb/IIIa blockade. Am H J 2000;140:74–80.

55. Berkowitz SD, Harrington RA, Rund MM, Tcheng JE. Acute profound thrombocytopenia after c7E3 Fab (abciximab) therapy. Circulation 1997;95:809–813.

56. Tcheng JE, Kereiakes DJ, Lincoff AM, et al., for the ReoPro Readminstration Registry Investigators. Abciximab readministration. Results of the ReoPro Readministration Registry. Circulation 2001;104: 870–875.

57. Topol EJ, Mark DB, Lincoff AM, et al., on behalf of the EPISTENT Investigators. Enhanced survival with platelet glycoprotein IIb/IIIa blockade in patients undergoing coronary stenting: one year outcomes and health care economic implications from a multicenter, randomized trial. Lancet 1999;354:2019–2024.

58. Garbarz E, Farah B, Vuillemenot A, et al. "Rescue" abciximab for complicated percutaneous transluminal coronary angioplasty. Am J Cardiol 1998;82:800–803.

59. Muhlestein JB, Karagounis LA, Treehan S, Anderson JL. "Rescue" utilization of abciximab for the dissolution of coronary thrombus developing as a complication of coronary angioplasty. J Am Coll Cardiol 1997;30:1729–1734.

60. Popma JJ, Weitz J, Bittl JA, et al. Antithrombotic therapy in patients undergoing coronary angioplasty. Chest 1998;114:7288–7418.

61. Ellis SG, Vandormael MG, Cowley MJ, et al. Coronary morphologic and clinical determinants of procedural outcome with angioplasty for multivessel coronary disease. Implications for patient selection. Circulation 1990;82:1193–1202.

III

GLYCOPROTEIN IIb/IIIa BLOCKADE FOR ACUTE ISCHEMIC SYNDROMES

9

The Use of Abciximab in Therapy-Resistant Unstable Angina

Clinical and Angiographic Results of the CAPTURE Pilot Trial and the CAPTURE Study

Marcel J. B. M. van den Brand, MD
and Maarten L. Simoons, MD

CONTENTS

INTRODUCTION
PATIENTS AND METHODS
RESULTS
DISCUSSION
ACKNOWLEDGMENTS
REFERENCES

INTRODUCTION

In 1989 Braunwald *(1)* provided a classification for patients with unstable angina, based on the clinical circumstances under which the syndrome occurred and the severity of the symptoms. A further subdivision took the intensity of medical treatment and the presence or absence of reversible electrocardiographic changes during anginal attacks into consideration. Outcome of patients with unstable angina could be predicted using this classification *(2)*.

The underlying cause of unstable angina is thought to be rupture and ulceration of a preexistent atherosclerotic plaque, leading to platelet adhesion and aggregation, and thrombus formation *(3)*. In most patients the syndrome can be stabilized with bed rest and antiischemic and antithrombotic therapy *(4)*. However, in a minority of patients, ischemic symptoms continue in spite of intensive medical therapy. Such patients with unstable angina refractory to medical treatment are usually referred for urgent angioplasty or bypass operation *(2)*, even though interventions are associated with a higher complication rate compared with stable or stabilized unstable angina patients *(5,6)*. Prevention and or resolution of platelet aggregates and thrombi may help to diminish ongoing ischemic attacks as well as angioplasty complications.

From: *Contemporary Cardiology: Platelet Glycoprotein IIb/IIIa
Inhibitors in Cardiovascular Disease, 2nd Edition*
Edited by: A. M. Lincoff © Humana Press Inc., Totowa, NJ

The chimeric 7E3 (c7E3) monoclonal antibody Fab fragment (abciximab) is a potent inhibitor of platelet aggregation. It blocks the glycoprotein IIb/IIIa fibrinogen receptor on the platelet surface, and, by preventing the binding of fibrinogen to the platelet surface, platelet aggregation and, platelet thrombus formation are thus inhibited *(7)*.

In a double-blind, randomized, placebo-controlled pilot study, the safety and preliminary efficacy of c7E3 Fab treatment were studied in patients with refractory unstable angina undergoing percutaneous coronary angioplasty (PTCA) *(7a)*. It was hypothesized that c7E3 Fab in combination with nitrates, heparin, and aspirin would facilitate stabilization of the culprit lesion and thus reduce recurrent ischemia prior to PTCA and reduce the complication rate during and after the PTCA procedure. The effect of c7E3 Fab on the severity of the culprit lesion was assessed by qualitative and quantitative angiographic analysis.

After this pilot study, yielding favorable results, a larger trial was designed in patients presenting with the same refractory unstable angina syndrome *(7b)*. The doses of abciximab and concomitant medication, as well as the duration of administration in relation to the angioplasty procedure, were identical to the study outline of the CAPTURE pilot trial.

All angiograms were revised centrally by the Angiographic Committee, to assess qualitative lesional aspects, and the outcome of the angioplasty procedure. The CAPTURE (c7E3 Fab Antiplatelet Therapy in Refractory Unstable Angina) study was discontinued on the recommendation of the Safety and Efficay Monitoring Committee after interim analysis of 1050 patients (1400 patients planned).

PATIENTS AND METHODS

Sixty patients were enrolled in the pilot CAPTURE trial from September 1991 to July 1992 in seven hospitals in the Netherlands, Belgium, Germany, and United Kingdom *(7a)*. The CAPTURE trial recruited 1265 patients from 69 hospitals in 12 countries between May 1993 and December 1995 *(7b)*. Patients were eligible for the pilot study as well as for the main study if they had refractory unstable angina defined as chest pain at rest with concomitant electrocardiographic (ECG) abnormalities compatible with myocardial ischemia (ST-segment depression, ST-segment elevation, or abnormal T waves), and one or more episodes of typical chest pain, ECG abnormalities, or both, compatible with myocardial ischemia during therapy with intravenous heparin and glyceryl trinitrate, started at least 2 h previously. The latest episode of ischemia should have occurred within 48 h before enrollment, corresponding to Braunwald class III "acute"unstable angina *(1,2)*.

All patients had undergone angiography and had significant coronary artery disease, with a culprit lesion suitable for angioplasty. Patients were enrolled within 24 h of angiography, and angioplasty was scheduled 18–24 h after the start of study medication. In the pilot trial, diagnostic angiography was performed within 12 h of the most recent episode of coronary ischemia. After this angiogram, enrollment and start of the trial medication had to be accomplished within 4 h. If necessary because of recurrent ischemia, angioplasty could be done earlier, at the discretion of the investigator. Reasons for exclusion from both studies were as follows:

1. Recent myocardial infarction, unless creatine kinase values had returned to below two times the upper limit of normal (in the pilot CAPTURE trial, patients were excluded if they experienced a Q-wave myocardial infarction within 7 d in the region subtended by the culprit artery).
2. Features of persisting ischemia that would require immediate intervention.
3. A >50% occlusion of the left main coronary artery or a culprit lesion located in a bypass graft.

Total occluded vessels were only acceptable in the pretrial if the occlusion was suspected to be of recent origin by the presence of thrombi or contrast staining at the site of the total occlusion. In CAPTURE, all total occluded vessels could be included, if these were considered culprit arteries. Re-PTCA of the same segment was excluded in the pilot trial, but not in the CAPTURE trial. Other exclusions included bleeding risk factors such as surgery, gastrointestinal or genitourinary bleeding during the 6 wk before enrollment, or a cerebrovascular accident within the previous 2 yr; planned administration of oral anticoagulants, intravenous dextran, or a thrombolytic agent before or during PTCA; underlying medical conditions such as persistent hypertension despite treatment; history of hemorrhagic diathesis; history of autoimmune disease, or a platelet count $<100 \times 10^9$/L.

After enrollment, patients received aspirin at a daily dose of 50 mg. In patients not previously on aspirin, the first dose was at least 250 mg. Heparin was administered from before randomization until at least 1 h after the PTCA procedure and was adjusted to achieve an activated partial thromboplastin time between 2–0 and 2–5 times normal. The protocol recommended that the initial bolus dose before PTCA should not exceed 100 U/kg or 10,000 U, whichever was lower. Subsequent heparin boluses were given during PTCA after the clotting time had been checked. The recommended anticoagulation target was an activated clotting time of 300 s or an activated partial thromboplastin time of 70 s.

Heparin was administered until at least 1 h after PTCA. All patients received intravenous glyceryl trinitrate. β-Blockers, calcium-channel blockers, and other cardiovascular drugs were allowed. In addition, patients were randomly assigned abciximab (0.25 mg/kg bolus followed by a continuous infusion of 10 µg/min) or matching placebo. Randomization was obtained by telephone call to an independent service organized by the Department of Clinical Epidemiology of the University of Amsterdam. The randomization treatment was started within 2 h of allocation and given during the 18–24 h before angioplasty and for 1 h after completion of the procedure.

Arterial sheaths were kept in place after the diagnostic angiogram, during administration of study drug, and were exchanged before angioplasty. Balloon angioplasty was done by standard techniques. The use of stents was not encouraged, unless it was required to maintain immediate patency of the dilated segment. Sheaths remained in place from the time of the qualifying angiogram until 4–6 h after discontinuation of heparin and study drug. Special care was taken to obtain complete hemostasis at the site of arterial access. During the hospital stay in the pilot trial and also during 30-d follow-up in the CAPTURE trial, all events and medications were recorded, with special attention to bleeding complications and recurrent ischemic symptoms.

The primary endpoint in the trials was the occurrence of death (from any cause), myocardial infarction, or an urgent intervention for treatment of recurrent ischemia (angioplasty, coronary artery bypass surgery, intracoronary stent placement, intraaortic balloon pump) during the initial hospital stay for the pilot trial, and within 30 d in the CAPTURE trial.

Serum samples drawn at the time of randomisation were available for determination of troponin T and C-reactive protein (CRP). Troponin T was measured using a one-step enzyme immunoassay based on electrochemiluminescence technology (Elecsys 2010, Boehringer Mannheim, Germany). The lower detection limit of this assay was 0.01 mg/L, and the diagnostic threshold level was 0.10 mg/L. Patients with postinfarction angina were not included in the troponin T analysis. CRP was measured by N Latex CRP Mono tests, performed on a Behring BN ll Nephelometer (Dade Behring, Deerfield, IL) using polystyrene microbeads coated with monoclonal mouse antibodies. The detection limit of the assay was 0.2 mg/L. For clinical practice, a threshold level of 5.0 mg/L is recommended.

Electrocardiography

ECGs were obtained before enrollment and both during and after episodes of chest pain. Additional ECGs were recorded at enrollment; 6, 12, and 18 h after enrollment; just before PTCA; 1, 6, and 24 h after PTCA; at discharge; and whenever patients experienced recurrent chest pain. Myocardial infarction during the index hospital stay was defined as values of creatine kinase or its MB isoenzyme more than three times the upper limit of normal in at least two samples and increased by 50% over the previous value, or an ECG with new significant Q-waves in two or more contiguous leads. Myocardial infarction after discharge was defined as concentrations of creatinine kinase or its MB isoenzyme above two times the upper limit of normal, or new significant Q waves in two or more contiguous ECG leads.

Additional Measures

For the CAPTURE trial, the following additional measures were taken to ensure independent reporting of data.

A Clinical Endpoint Committee reviewed all case report forms, ECGs, and supporting documents for confirmation that patients met the study entry criteria for refractory unstable angina; the occurrence of endpoints; the frequency of recurrent ischemia; and important adverse events (bleeding, thrombocytopenia, and stroke).

Bleeding was classified as major, minor, or insignificant, by previously published criteria *(8)*. Major bleeding was defined as intracranial bleeding or episodes associated with a decrease in haemoglobin of >3.5 mmol/L (5 g/L). Bleeding was defined as minor if it was spontaneous and observed as gross hematuria or hematemesis, or if blood loss (spontaneous or not) was observed with a decrease in hemoglobin of >2.1 mmol/L, or if there was a decrease in hemoglobin of >2.8 mmol/L with no significant bleeding site identified.

Blood loss insufficient to meet criteria for minor bleeding was classified as insignificant. To account for transfusion, packed cell volume and hemoglobin measurements were adjusted for any transfusion of packed red blood cells or whole blood within the 48 h before measurement by the method of Landefeld and colleagues *(9)*. Thrombocytopenia was defined as an acute fall in platelet count during or after administration of the study agent to $<100 \times 10^9$/L or a decrease of $\geq 25\%$ from baseline.

The protocol recommended that blood transfusion should be given according to the guidelines of the American College of Physicians *(10)*. These guidelines state that normovolemic anemia is acceptable for patients without symptoms and that those with symptoms should receive transfusions on a unit-by-unit basis to relieve symptoms.

Analytic Methods

A Safety and Efficacy Monitoring Committee was established to monitor safety data continuously and to carry out interim analyses after enrollment of 350 and 700 patients. After the second interim analysis, the Committee recommended a third interim analysis after 1050 patients.

The protocol specified that the trial would be stopped if the difference in the rate of the primary endpoint between the abciximab and placebo groups was significant with a

p value of 0.0001, 0.001, or 0.0072 at the first (350 patients), second (700 patients), or third interim analysis, respectively. The study design was group sequential, with plans for accrual of up to 1400 patients. This sample would allow detection of a reduction in the primary endpoint from 15 to 10% with $\alpha = 0.05$ and power = 0.80. The Lan-DeMets method was used to assign p values for interim analysis (11).

A log-rank test was done at interim and final analysis to test for differences in the rates of occurrence of the primary endpoint in the abciximab and placebo groups.

Event rates were calculated for patients in each treatment group by the Kaplan-Meier method. Fisher's exact test was used to make pairwise comparisons among the groups for binary measurements. Logistic regression analysis was used to verify the association among bleeding complications, body weight, and heparin dose. Analyses were by intention to treat.

Coronary Arteriography and Angioplasty

Coronary arteriography and left ventricular angiography were performed as soon as possible after the qualifying anginal attack using the Judkins technique. Heparin 2500–5000 IU was administered at the beginning of the procedure. A second angiogram was performed within 24 h after the start of study medication followed by angioplasty. The coronary artery responsible for the ischemia was identified through lesion characteristics, ECG location of reversible ST-T segment changes, and left ventricular wall contraction abnormalities. For quantitative analysis of angiograms, the following additional measures were taken in the pilot trial. At least two orthogonal projections were made of the culprit coronary segment, after injection of 1–3 mg of isosorbide dinitrate. During the first and second angiogram, the same projections and X-ray gantry settings were employed to compare lesion severity. Low osmolar contrast medium was used for all angiograms.

Qualitative and Quantitative Assessment of Coronary Angiograms

In the pilot trial both a qualitative and quantitative assessment of all angiograms was performed by the Core Laboratory at Cardialysis, Rotterdam.

The following items were visually scored after the first contrast injection: Thrombolysis in Myocardial Infarction (TIMI) flow grade (12) of the culprit artery; stenosis severity, as visually assessed in multiple projections, and presence of intracorornary thrombus, defined as an intraluminal filling defect, visible during at least one complete cine-run, and surrounded on three sides by contrast medium (13). A totally occluded coronary artery could contain a filling defect but was not automatically scored as containing such a defect. In addition, all angiograms were analyzed quantitatively, using the computer-assisted cardiovascular angiography analysis system (14,15). Any area sized 6.9×6.9 mm in a selected cineframe (overall dimensions 18×24 mm) encompassing the desired arterial segment was digitized by a high-resolution CCD camera with a resolution of 512×512 pixels and 8 bits of gray level. Vessel contours were determined automatically, based on the weighted sum of the first and second derivative functions applied to the digitized information along scanlines perpendicular to the local centerline directions of an arterial segment. A computer-derived estimation of the original arterial dimensions at the site of the obstruction was used to define the interpolated reference diameter. This technique is based on a computer-derived estimation of the original diameter values over the analyzed region (assuming there was no disease present) according to the diameter function. The absolute diameter of the stenosis and the reference diameter were measured, using the known guiding catheter diameter as a calibration factor. All contour positions of the catheter and arterial segments were corrected for pincushion distortion. *Plaque area* is the difference in area in mm^2 between the reference and the detected contours over the length of the lesion *(16)*.

In the CAPTURE trial no quantitative measurements were performed on the coronary arteriograms. The qualitative assessment was more extensive than in the pilot trial and was carried out by an Angiographic Committee, consisting of six experienced interventional cardiologists.

From the angiograms at baseline and before angioplasty the ischemia-related artery (IRA), severity of all lesions present, collateral flow to the IRA, and TIMI flow *(12)* in the IRA, as well as all AHA/ACC lesion characteristics *(17)*, were scored individually from multiple projections.

These lesion characteristics included length (<10 mm; 10–20 mm; >20 mm), eccentricity or concentricity, ostial or nonostial location, smoothness or irregularity, angulated or nonangulated, easy or difficult accessibility, presence or absence of thrombus, none, moderate, or heavy calcification, and involvement or noninvolvement of a side branch at the lesion site. *TIMI flow* was scored visually as TIMI 0 if no contrast penetrated distal to the entire IRA for the duration of the filming sequence, TIMI 1 if contrast penetrated the site of the lesion without complete filling of the distal IRA for the duration of the cine-run, TIMI 2 if contrast medium filled the IRA completely, but rate of inflow or clearing of contrast was slower than in comparable areas, TIMI 3 if both inflow and clearance of contrast were at the same speed in the IRA compared with other vessels.

Thrombus was scored as present if a filling defect without calcification could be visualized near the lesion, or an embolus in the distal territory of the IRA. A lesion was classified as *angulated* if the artery at the site of the lesion exhibited an angle of ≥45 degrees. *Lesion length* was estimated by taking the length of the inflated balloon as a reference and was defined as that segment of the artery with a narrowing of ≥50% of the reference diameter. A *bifurcation* was scored as being present at the lesion site, when the inflated balloon covered the ostium of a side branch with a minimal estimated diameter of 1.5 mm. A lesion was scored as *ostial* if the inception of the lesion started within 10 mm of the origin of the left anterior descending or right coronary artery. *Eccentricity* was scored if the remaining connection between the proximal and distal part of the IRA at the site of the lesion was not situated in the middle of the artery. The stenotic site was judged to be *irregular* if its luminal edge was irregular or had a sawtooth component. *Accessibility* was scored as easy if the lesion was distal to maximal one bend of ≥45 degrees, as moderately tortuous if the stenosis was distal to two bends of ≥45 degrees, and as excessive tortuous if the lesion was distal to three or more bends of ≥45 degrees. *Calcification* was scored if moderate or heavy radiodensities were noted with fluoroscopy or cinearteriography at the site of the target lesion.

If one of the characteristics could only be verified in one angiographic projection, this was considered enough evidence for the existence of the pertinent item.

The definitions of TIMI flow, lesion severity, and AHA/ACC characteristics were discussed with the members of the Angiographic Committee before angiograms were reviewed. The actual viewing was performed by one cardiologist and an angiographic technician from Cardialysis and agreement reached after deliberation. In case of disagreement, consensus was reached by a verdict of a second cardiologist.

After angioplasty, the procedure was scored as angiographically successful if the TIMI flow in the IRA was 3 (normal) and the remaining stenosis occupied less than half the diameter of the vessel, compared with the adjacent segment.

The use of a stent(s) if visible on the angiogram was also noted, as were side branch occlusions if the side branch was at least 1.5 mm in diameter. Dissections after the procedure were categorized according to modified National Heart, Lung, and Blood Institute criteria as A–F *(18)*.

Dilation of other significant stenoses outside the IRA during the same procedure was discouraged, but if deemed necessary by the investigator, the result of dilation of the additional lesions was also evaluated.

Statistical Analysis

Differences between groups were analyzed by intention to treat. Categorical variables were summarized by count and/or percentages. Continuous variables were summarized by means and standard deviations. Fisher's exact test was used to assess differences in categorical variables with respect to treatment.

Multivariable logistics modeling was used to examine relationships between primary endpoint and individual lesion characteristics, age, gender, and treatment and between bleeding complications, body weight, and heparin dose. Variable selection was done in a stepwise fashion. The selected variables were tested for interactions with all other variables. For the modeling, the continuous variable age was dichotomized. Odds ratios with their 95% confidence intervals were calculated from the logistic model. When an odds ratio needed to be calculated from more than one regression coefficient, the relevant variance and covariance components from the variance-covariance matrix were used for calculation of the 95% confidence intervals for the subgroup odds ratios.

RESULTS

CAPTURE Pilot Trial

BASELINE CHARACTERISTICS

Between September 1991 and July 1992, 60 patients were enrolled in six different hospitals. Baseline characteristics are summarized in Table 1. The groups were balanced, although more patients in the placebo group had sustained a previous infarct compared with the treatment group (p = NS), and more patients in the placebo group demonstrated multivessel disease, defined as a >50% diameter stenosis in one of the three main epicardial vessels. Medication at the time of the qualifying ischemic attack was intense and similar in both groups.

RECURRENT ISCHEMIA

During infusion of the study drug, ischemia occurred in nine patients treated with c7E3 Fab and in 16 placebo patients (p = 0.06), whereas nine and six patients, respectively, developed ischemia after PTCA (Table 2). Most patients had multiple episodes. The total number of patients with different types of ischemia did not differ between the two treatment groups (p = 0.15), and the total number of episodes was not significantly different between patients receiving c7E3 Fab (33 episodes) or placebo (56 episodes, p = 0.17). In one placebo patient, an urgent intervention was performed because of recurrent ischemia before the scheduled PTCA.

Table 1
Baseline Clinical, Electrocardiographic,
and Angiographic Characteristics of Patient Groups

Group	c7E3Fab	Placebo
Male/female	20/10	24/6
Age (yr); (median, range)	61, 38–73	60, 38–73
Previous infarct	9	16
Within 7 d	6	5
Previous CABG	0	2
Previous PTCA	4	5
Medication prior to qualifying ischemic attack		
Heparin	25	27
Aspirin	21	24
Nitrates		
Intravenous	24	27
Oral	4	2
β-Blocker	22	24
Calcium channel blocker	15	22
Ischemia-related vessel		
Left anterior descending artery	16	14
Left circumflex	8	6
Right coronary artery	6	10
Multivessel disease	6*	15*

Abbreviations: CABG, coronary artery bypass grafting; PTCA, percutaneous transluminal coronary angioplasty.

    *$p = < 0.05$.

Table 2
Recurrent Ischemia

Ischemia	c7E3	Placebo
No. of patients	30	30
Pain + ST-T changes	2	5
Pain − ST-T changes	1	2
Pain, no ECG available	1	0
Silent ST-T changes	5	12
Patients with pain or ST-T changes	9	16

    Patients with recurrent ischemia between diagnostic and second angiography. Multiple episodes and different types of ischemia could occur in one patient. Episodes of ischemia during angiography or PTCA were not included.

While the patients were in hospital, a total of 12 major ischemic events occurred in seven placebo patients: death ($n = 1$), myocardial infarction ($n = 4$), and urgent intervention because of severe recurrent ischaemia ($n = 7$). One event (a myocardial infarction) occurred in a patient treated with c7E3 Fab (Table 3; 1 vs 7 patients, $p = 0.03$) . Three placebo patients experienced more than one major event. Multivessel disease was present in five of the seven placebo patients who developed an event, whereas the c7E3 Fab-treated patient with an event had single-vessel disease. After correction for the imbalance in baseline characteristics, the difference between the two groups was not statistically significant

Table 3
Major Events

Events	c7E3 Fab (n = 30)	Placebo (n = 30)
Death	0	1
Myocardial infarction	1	4
Before PTCA	0	1
After PTCA	1	3
Urgent procedure	0	7
PTCA	0	3
CABG	0	3
Stent	0	1
Total events	1	12
Total number of patients with one or more major events	1	7

Abbreviations: CABG, coronary artery bypass grafting; PTCA, percutaneous transluminal coronary angioplasty.

Table 4
Qualitative Angiographic Data[a]

Angiography	c7E3 Fab (n = 30)		Placebo (n = 30)	
	B	A	B	A
TIMI flow				
0	1	1	4	3
1	2	1	0	1
2	10	5	7	6
3	17	23	19	20
Improved		6		4
Worsened		0		3
Intracoronary filling defect	5	2	1	1

[a]B, before study drug infusion; A, after study drug infusion.

in this pilot study ($p = 0.16$). One patient from the placebo group died 26 d after allocation after a complicated clinical course, including two urgent PTCA procedures, myocardial infarction, heart failure, intraaortic balloon pump, and severe bleeding.

QUALITATIVE EVALUATION OF CORONARY ANGIOGRAMS

TIMI flow grade 3 in culprit arteries, assessed centrally by the Core Laboratory, was present in 57% and 63% of patients at the first angiogram in the placebo and treatment groups, respectively. A substantial improvement in coronary blood flow occurred after treatment in the c7E3 Fab patient group. In the placebo group, a mix of either improvement or deterioration was observed in TIMI flow score (Table 4). Extensive filling defects in the coronary arteries were rare. Most filling defects were small, although they were visible in more than one projection and located distally from the culprit lesion. The numbers of intracoronary filling defects and total occlusions in the pre- and posttreatment

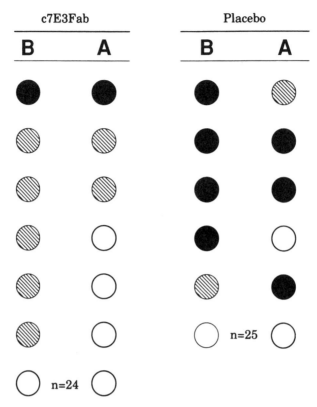

Fig. 1. Qualitative coronary angiographic data of the ischemia-related coronary artery before (**B**) and after (**A**) study drug infusion. ● = totally occluded coronary artery; ◐ = intracoronary filling defect; ○= patent coronary artery, without filling defect. The number of patent vessels with no filling defect in either angiogram is depicted in the bottom line.

angiograms are presented in Fig. 1. In the placebo group, one new occlusion was observed, in two cases patency was restored, with thrombotic remnants in one of these two cases. Three of five coronary clots resolved in the c7E3 group.

QUANTITATIVE CORONARY ANGIOGRAPHIC ANALYSIS

Quantitative coronary angiographic data are summarized in Table 5. In one patient with a very proximal left anterior descending coronary artery lesion, calculation of percentage diameter stenosis was not possible because the reference diameter could not be ascertained. Plaque area and extent of obstruction could only be calculated in patent coronary arteries. A significant decrease in percentage diameter stenosis, extent of obstruction, and plaque area was observed in the c7E3 patients. In the placebo group, similar changes were observed to a lesser extent, except for the extent of obstruction, which increased in the placebo group patients. Differences between groups were not significant.

ANGIOPLASTY PROCEDURE

Angioplasty was performed in all 60 patients. In one patient who received c7E3 Fab, PTCA was deferred because of a total occlusion owing to a large intracoronary clot at the second angiogram. He was treated with intracoronary alteplase 50 mg infused over 30 min,

Table 5
Quantitative Angiographic Data From the First Angiogram (I) and After Study
Drug Infusion (II) and the Difference Between Both Measurements (II–I)

	No.	c7E3 Fab (n = 30)	No.	Placebo (n = 30)
DS (%)				
I	30	65.7 (8.6)	29	67.7 (16.1)
II	30	62.3 (10.5)	29	65.6 (15.8)
II–I	30	–3.4 (6.7)*	29	–2.1 (12.4)
MLD (mm)				
I	30	0.9 (0.3)	30	0.9 (0.4)
II	30	1.0 (0.3)	30	0.9 (0.4)
II–I	30	0.1 (0.2)	30	0.0 (0.3)
Ext Ob (mm)				
I	29	7.3 (2.2)	26	7.2 (3.4)
II	29	6.9 (2.1)	26	7.3 (2.9)
II–I	29	–0.5 (1.2)*	26	0.3 (1.8)
Plq area (mm^2)				
I	29	8.2 (3.4)	26	9.1 (6.8)
II	29	7.1 (2.5)	27	8.6 (4.8)
II–I	29	–1.1 (1.9)*	25	–0.5 (3.3)
AS (%)				
I	20	89.2 (6.7)	21	90.7 (7.9)
II	23	88.3 (8.4)	22	89.6 (10.2)
II–I	19	–1.8 (8.1)	19	–1.3 (6.4)

Abbreviations: DS, diameter stenosis; MLD, minimal lumen diameter; Ext Ob, extent
of the obstruction; Plq area, plaque area; AS, area stenosis.
*$p \leq 0.05$ for paired comparison of angiogram I vs II in each patient group. The changes
between patient groups (c7E3 fab vs placebo) did not reach statistical significance. Numbers
in third and fifth columns represent means (SD).

followed by 50 mg intravenously over 2 h. The next day, the clots were partly resolved, and PTCA was performed successfully. One other c7E3 Fab patient with a thrombocytosis of unknown origin received alteplase during PTCA because of persistent thrombus formation. PTCA was completed with success, and the subsequent clinical course was uncomplicated. The total success rate of the angioplasty procedure was 83% in the c7E3 Fab group and 70% in the placebo group (Table 6).

Capture Trial

The CAPTURE trial was discontinued after the third interim analysis of 1050 patients. Complete data, fully reviewed by the Clinical Endpoint Committee, were available for 976 patients, and 74 patients were partially reviewed. By that point, 87 (16.4%) of 532 patients in the placebo group and 56 (10.8%) of 518 in the abciximab group had a primary endpoint (death, myocardial infarction, or urgent intervention within 30 d). Since the p value for the difference ($p = 0.0064$) was below the prespecified stopping criterion ($p = 0.0072$), and since the data were consistent among all subgroups analyzed, the Safety and Efficacy Monitoring Committee recommended that recruitment should cease. This recommendation was followed by the Steering Committee, after consultation with regulatory authorities.

Table 6
Complications and Untoward Events
During and After Coronary Angioplasty

	C7E3Fab (n = 30)	Placebo (n = 30)
Mortality	0	1
Myocardial necrosis	1	3
Urgent CABG	0	3
Re-PTCA	0	2
Residual stenosis > 50%	4	6
Number of patients with one or more untoward events	5	9
Procedural success (%)	83	70

Abbreviations: CABG, coronary artery bypass grafting; PTCA, percutaneous transluminal coronary angioplasty.

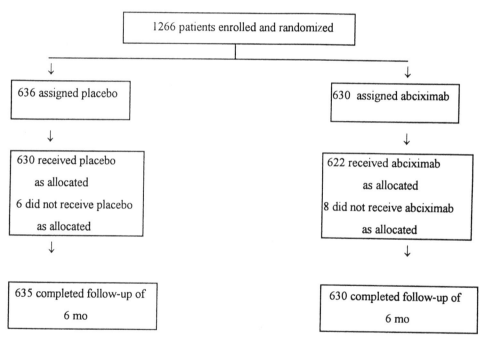

Fig. 2. Trial profile.

Figure 2 shows the flow of patients through the trial; 1266 patients were enrolled, of
1400 scheduled. Follow-up data were complete for all but one patient (placebo), who
withdrew consent after randomization.

Five other patients in the placebo group did not receive placebo (two refused but
allowed follow-up and three for logistic reasons). Eight patients did not receive abciximab
(one received other therapy, five withdrew consent but allowed follow-up, two for logistic
reasons).

Table 7
Baseline Data and Concomitant Medication

	Placebo (n = 635)	Abciximab (n = 630)
M/F	459/176	461/169
Mean (SD) age in years	61 (10)	61 (10)
Anthropometry: mean (SD)		
Weight (kg)	76 (12)	76 (12)
Height (cm)	170 (9)	170 (9)
Number of patients with [no. (%)]		
Angina > 7 d previously[a]	322 (51.4)	300 (48.6)
Infarction within previous 7 d	78 (12.3)	88 (14.0)
Infarction 8–30 d	43 (6.8)	53 (8.4)
Infarction > 30 d previously	116 (18.3)	116 (18.4)
Infarction, date not reported	6 (0.9)	7 (1.1)
PTCA	86 (13.5)	84 (13.3)
CABG	21 (3.3)	11 (1.7)
Risk factors [no. (%)]		
Diabetes[a]	82 (13.0)	95 (15.1)
Hypertension[a]	261 (41.4)	271 (43.4)
Current smokers[a]	255 (40.8)	235 (37.5)
Medication within 7 d before enrollment [no. (%)]		
Aspirin	582 (91.7)	586 (93.0)
Intravenous heparin	634 (99.8)	627 (99.5)
Nitrates	633 (99.7)	627 (99.5)
β-Blockers	392 (61.7)	400 (63.5)
Calcium antagonists	297 (46.8)	286 (45.4)
Medication after enrollment [no. (%)]		
Aspirin	608 (95.7)	604 (95.9)
Ticlopidin	25 (3.9)	25 (4.0)
Intravenous heparin	616 (97.0)	613 (97.3)
β-Blockers	395 (62.2)	412 (65.4)
Nitrates	616 (97.0)	613 (97.3)
Calcium antagonists	314 (49.4)	289 (45.9)

[a] In a few patients no data were available for these items; percentages calculated for patients in whom these data were reported.

The two treatment groups were similar in terms of baseline characteristics (Table 7): 73% were male, 50% had a history of angina, and 41% had had a previous myocardial infarction. Seventy-two percent of patients were enrolled within 6 h of the first (diagnostic) angiogram, 60% had experienced myocardial ischemia within the 12 h before treatment, and 95% had an ischemic episode after a minimum of 2-h treatment with nitrates and intravenous heparin. Study drug was started in 1253 patients. It was discontinued early (before 30 min after PTCA) in 86 patients (45 placebo, 41 abciximab) for various reasons, including bleeding (1, 9), bypass surgery (5, 1), and stent placement (8, 3). Angioplasty was attempted in 1241 patients (98%). The procedure was done earlier than planned in 23 patients (1.8%), 14 of whom were in the placebo group (Table 8). According to the investigators, the procedure was not successful, with a residual stenosis >50%, in 70 patients

Table 8
Angiography and PTCA Results[a]

	Placebo (n = 635)	Abciximab (n = 630)
Artery with culprit lesion		
Left anterior descending	383 (60.3)	385 (61.1)
Left circumflex	104 (16.4)	105 (16.7)
Right coronary	144 (22.7)	138 (21.9)
PTCA timing		
Urgent (before planned)	14 (2.2)	9 (1.4)
18–26 h[b]	613 (96.5)	597 (94.8)
Delayed (>26 h)	8 (1.3)	15 (2.4)
No PTCA	11 (1.7)	13 (2.1)
PTCA result		
Attempted	624	617
Succeeded[c]	554 (88.8)	580 (94.0)
Failed[c]	70 (11.2)	37 (6.0)

[a]Data are numbers, with percent in parentheses.
[b]Prespecified time window was 18–24 h after enrollment; in 70 patients procedure was done between 24 and 26 h for logistic reasons.
[c]Percentages of those attempted.

receiving placebo and in 37 receiving abciximab (11.2 vs 6.0%, $p = 0.001$). Treatment with abciximab also resulted in lower rates of urgent repeat PTCA, urgent stent placement, and bypass surgery (Table 9); however, these differences were not statistically significant.

The primary endpoint (death, myocardial infarction, or urgent intervention within 30 d of enrollment) occurred in 101 (15.9%) patients in the placebo group and 71 (11.3%) in the abciximab group ($p = 0.012$; Table 9, Fig. 3). This difference was owing mainly to a difference in the proportion with myocardial infarction [52 (8.2%) vs 26 (4.1%), $p = 0.002$; Table 9].

The findings were consistent in all subgroups studied and were independent of age, sex, ECG findings at enrollment, and the presence of diabetes, peripheral vascular disease, or renal dysfunction. Progression to myocardial infarction during the first 18–24 h after enrollment was rare, despite the inclusion of patients with acute, refractory, unstable angina. Even so, the frequency of myocardial infarction before PTCA was significantly lower in patients receiving abciximab than in those receiving placebo (Table 9, $p = 0.029$). Most infarcts occurred during or within 24 h of PTCA ($p = 0.021$, Fig. 4), whereas infarction rates were low in both groups 2–30 d after PTCA (Table 9). The lower rate of myocardial infarction in patients receiving abciximab than in those receiving placebo was found for both Q-wave and non-Q-wave infarcts, and independently of the creatine kinase threshold used to define an infarct (Table 9).

Major bleeding complications occurred in only 3.8% of patients, although both major and minor bleeding events were more common during treatment with abciximab than during placebo treatment (Table 9).

Table 9
Clinical Events at 30-day Follow-Up[a]

	Placebo (n = 635)	Abciximab (n = 630)	p value[b]
Death, infarction, or urgent intervention	101 (15.9)	71 (11.3)	0.012
Death	8 (1.3)	6 (1.0)	>0.1
Myocardial infarction			
Before PTCA	13 (2.1)	4 (0.6)	0.029
During PTCA (<24 h)	34 (5.5)	16 (2.6)	0.009
After PTCA (2–30 d)	5 (0.9)	6 (1.0)	>0.1
Non-Q-wave	36 (5.5)[c]	19 (3.0)	0.036
Q-wave	17 (2.7)[c]	7 (1.1)	0.067
Peak CK > 5× normal	21 (3.3)	10 (1.6)	0.067
Peak CK > 10× normal	15 (2.6)	5 (0.8)	0.040
All myocardial infarction	52 (8.2)	26 (4.1)	0.002
Myocardial infarction/death	57 (9.0)	30 (4.8)	0.003
Urgent intervention			
Urgent PTCA			
Before planned time	14 (2.2)	9 (1.4)	>0.1
Repeat PTCA	28 (4.4)	19 (3.1)	>0.1
Urgent CABG	11 (1.7)	6 (1.0)	>0.1
Urgent stent	42 (6.6)	35 (5.6)	>0.1
All urgent interventions	69 (10.9)	49 (7.8)	0.054
Nonurgent interventions			
Repeat PTCA	16 (2.6)	21 (3.4)	>0.1
CABG	9 (1.4)	4 (0.6)	>0.1
Stent	47 (7.4)	49 (7.8)	>0.1
Stroke	3 (0.5)	1 (0.2)	>0.1
Major bleeding[d]			
Puncture site	9	19	>0.1
Retroperitoneal	0	2	>0.1
Pulmonary	0	1	>0.1
Gastrointestinal	0	3	>0.1
Urogenital	1	0	>0.1
All major bleeding	12 (19)	24 (3.8)	0.043
Minor bleeding[d]	13 (2.0)	30 (4.8)	0.008
Transfusion[d]	21 (3.4)	44 (7.1)	0.005

Abbreviations: CK, creatine kinase; CABG, coronary artery bypass graft; PTCA, percutaneous transluminal coronary angioplasty.
[a]Data are numbers, with percent in parentheses.
[b]p values (two-sided) < 0.1 are reported.
[c]One patient had both.
[d]Excluding those in patients who underwent CABG.

No excess strokes were observed with abciximab. In the placebo group, two patients had nonhemorrhagic stroke, and one had an intracranial hemorrhage (1, 5, and 7 d after enrollment, respectively). Stroke occurred in a single patient treated with abciximab (15 d after enrollment), but the type of stroke could not be determined. Most bleeding complications occurred at arterial puncture sites. In both treatment groups, bleeding was more

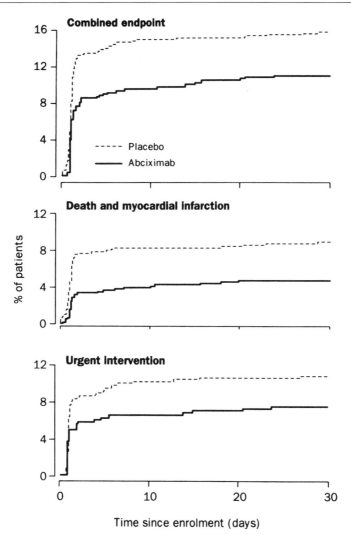

Fig. 3. Time course of combined primary endpoint and its major components.

common in patients who received a high dose of heparin during PTCA, and in patients with low body weight. For patients receiving <100 IU/kg heparin, the bleeding rates were 1.2 and 4.4% in the placebo and abciximab groups, respectively. The corresponding rates were 2.7 and 6.6% in those receiving 100–149 IU/kg and 7.9 and 14.8% in patients receiving ≥150 IU/kg heparin. In logistic regression analysis, both heparin dose per kg ($p = 0.0001$) and use of abciximab ($p = 0.0008$) were significantly related to bleeding risk. By contrast, the reduction in primary endpoint was related only to use of abciximab ($p = 0.016$) and not to heparin dose ($p = 0.70$).

Thrombocytopenia (platelets $<100 \times 10^9/L$) occurred in 5.6% of the abciximab group and 1.3% of the placebo group. Ten patients receiving abciximab had platelet counts <50 × 10/L within 24 h; no placebo recipient had this complication. None of these patients had bleeding complications. Two patients had platelet counts $<20 \times 10/L$. Treatment with study drug (abciximab) was discontinued in five patients, who all received platelet transfusions.

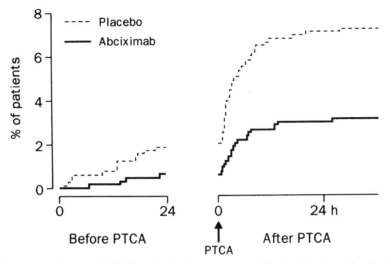

Fig. 4. Development of myocardial infarction during treatment with abciximab or placebo, before and in association with PTCA.

Full recovery of platelet counts (to >100×10^9/L) occurred within 24 h in three patients, within 48 h in three, and within 5 d in three. Follow-up measurements were not available in one patient.

At follow-up 6 mo later, death or myocardial infarction had occurred in 56 (8.9%) abciximab-treated patients and 69 (10.9%) placebo recipients ($p = 0.19$, Fig. 5). Bypass surgery had been required by 33 (5.2%) and 44 (6.9%), respectively ($p = 0.20$). PTCA was needed for similar proportions of patients in both groups, mainly because of restenosis (Table 10). Also, medication up to 6 mo of follow-up was similar in the two groups (Table 11). At 6 mo, 242 events had occurred in 193 abciximab-treated patients compared with 274 events in 193 placebo recipients. Thus, the number of events per patient was lower after abciximab ($p = 0.067$).

Four years postrandomization, follow-up data were obtained in 1157 patients (94% of all patients alive at 6 mo). Death and myocardial infarction rates were continuously (non-significantly) lower over a 4-yr period in patients randomized to abciximab (Table 11).

The initial large and significant difference in death or myocardial infarction favoring abciximab among patients with a positive troponin-T test at randomization ($\geq$0.1 ng/L) was maintained throughout the 4-yr follow-up period (*18a*) (Fig. 6). Death or myocardial infarction at 4 yr occurred in 16.9 and 24.8% of troponin-T-positive patients receiving abciximab or placebo ($p = 0.015$). The incidence of these events in troponin-T positive patients was comparable with that of troponin-T-negative patients receiving abciximab or placebo.

A high CRP (>10 mg/L) at randomization was predictive of a higher incidence of death or myocardial infarction at 6 mo (*18b*). The same difference in outcome related to initial CRP level was found at 4-yr follow-up (Fig. 7). The mortality at 4 yr was 9.2% for patients with high CRP values and 3.9% for patients with low values at entrance ($p = 0.001$). In contrast to the risk reduction of abciximab in patients with elevated troponin-T levels, the risk reduction of abciximab was not dependent on CRP levels at randomization.

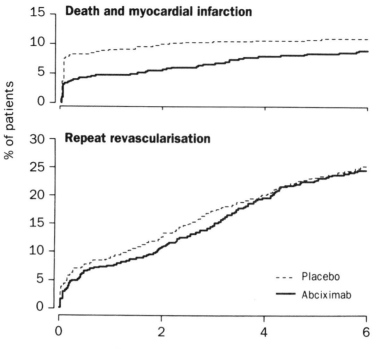

Fig. 5. Time-course of death and myocardial infarction and repeat revascularization during 6-mo follow-up.

Table 10
Clinical Events During 4-Year Follow-Up[a]

Event	Placebo (n = 635)	Abciximab (n = 630)
At 6 mo postrandomization		
Death	14 (2.2)	17 (2.8)
Myocardial infarction	59 (9.3)	41 (6.6)
Death or myocardial infarction	69 (10.9)	56 (8.9)
Repeat PTCA	127 (20.0)	131 (20.8)
CABG	44 (6.9)	33 (5.2)
Any of the above	193 (30.4)	193 (30.6)
At 4 yr postrandomization		
Death	38 (6.0)	40 (6.4)
Myocardial infarction	79 (12.4)	68 (10.8)
Death or myocardial infarction	107 (16.9)	99 (15.7)
Repeat PTCA	175 (27.6)	194 (30.8)
CABG	71 (11.2)	54 (8.6)
Any of the above	271 (42.7)	288 (45.7)

Abbreviations: CABG, coronary artery bypass grafting; PTCA, percutaneous transluminal coronary angioplasty.

[a]None of the differences were significant at $p < 0.05$. Data are as absolute numbers, with percents in parentheses.

Table 11
Clinical Events During 4-Year Follow-Up[a]

Event	Placebo (n = 635)	Abciximab (n = 630)
At 6 mo postrandomization		
Death	14 (2.2)	17 (2.7)
Myocardial infarction	59 (9.3)	41 (6.5)
Death or myocardial infarction	69 (10.9)	56 (8.9)
Repeat PTCA	127 (20.0)	131 (20.8)
CABG	44 (6.9)	33 (5.2)
Any of the above	193 (30.4)	193 (30.6)
At 4 yr postrandomization		
Death	38 (6.0)	40 (6.4)
Myocardial infarction	79 (12.4)	68 (10.8)
Death or myocardial infarction	107 (16.9)	99 (15.7)
Repeat PTCA	175 (27.6)	194 (30.8)
CABG	71 (11.2)	54 (8.6)
Any of the above	271 (42.7)	288 (45.7)

Abbreviations: CABG, coronary artery bypass grafting; PTCA, percutaneous transluminal coronary angioplasty.

[a]None of the differences were significant at $p < 0.05$. Data are absolute numbers, with percents in parentheses.

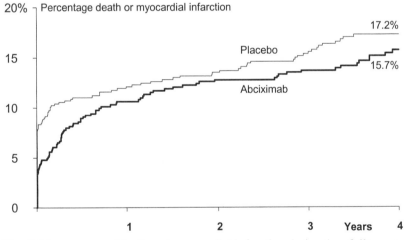

Fig. 6. Time-course of death and myocardial infarction during 4-yr follow-up.

Troponin-T and CRP had independent prognostic values (Fig. 8). Patients with both elevated troponin-T and CRP had the highest 4-yr event rate (death or myocardial infarction: 16.8%), whereas patients with low CRP and negative troponin had the lowest event rate (3.9%; $p < 0.001$). CRP and troponin T both remained independent significant determinants of long-term cardiac outcome after correction by multivariable analysis for the established risk factors [age, sex, diabetes, hypertension, smoking, hypercholesterolemia, previous cardiovascular disease (i.e., myocardial infarction, heart failure, PTCA, CABG

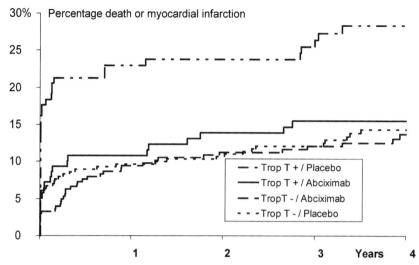

Fig. 7. Kaplan-Meier curves of death and/or myocardial infarction according to troponin T (Trop T) status and treatment received. Significantly ($p = 0.015$) more events occurred in patients with positive troponin T and receiving placebo.

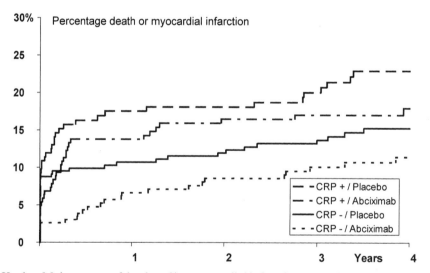

Fig. 8. Kaplan-Meier curves of death and/or myocardial infarction according to C-reactive protein (CRP) status and treatment received. There was no significant difference between the groups.

or stroke and peripheral vascular disease)]. The long-term risk reduction with abciximab was most pronounced in troponin-T-positive patients regardless of CRP value (hazard ratio 0.44 vs 0.92, abciximab vs placebo, respectively; $p = 0.073$).

ANGIOGRAPHIC RESULTS OF THE CAPTURE TRIAL

Of 1265 patients enrolled in the CAPTURE trial, 1233 underwent angioplasty after treatment with abciximab or placebo. Of these 1233 patients, two angiograms were available

Table 12
Baseline and Demographic Data from the Total Study Population
and the Angio-Available and Angio-Not-Available Group

	Total population[a]	Angio available	Angio not available
No. of patients	1233	1197	36
Males (%)	73.2	72.8	86.1
Age [mean (SD)]	61 (10)	61 (10)	60 (11)
Weight [kg (SD)]	76 (12)	76 (12)	79 (10.0)
Height [cm (SD)]	170 (9)	170 (9)	171 (6)
Previous angina (%)	50	50	58*
Previous infarct (%)	39	39	50*

[a]Patients undergoing PTCA.
*$p < 0.05$, angio available vs not available.

for central review in 1197 patients and one angiogram in another 6 patients. So of 97.1% of all treated patients, both angiograms were available for review. Patients without angio review had more previous angina and previous infarction than those with review of the angiograms (Table 12). A primary composite endpoint (death, MI, and urgent reintervention) was reached in 13.1% of the angio-available patients, 19.4% in the angio-not-available group ($p = $ NS), and 13.3% of all study patients. The incidence in reaching a primary composite endpoint at 30 d of the angio-available patients treated with placebo or abciximab was 15.5 and 10.8%, ($p = 0.017$) respectively, with a significant reduction in death and nonfatal myocardial infarction in the abciximab-treated patients from 8.5 to 4.5% ($p = 0.007$) and a marginally significant reduction in urgent reinterventions from 10.8 to 7.2% ($p = 0.034$). In the angio-not-available patients, the primary endpoint was also lower after abciximab (26.3% vs 11.8%, $p = 0.408$), although this was not statistically significant in this small group of patients.

TIMI flow could be assessed in 1168 pairs of baseline and pre-PTCA angiograms. No significant differences were present at baseline (Fig. 9). After infusion 88, abciximab patients improved the TIMI flow rate of the IRA by at least one class vs 81 placebo group patients ($p = $ NS). Worsening of TIMI flow by at least one class was seen in 27 placebo- and 16 abciximab-treated patients ($p = $ NS). Thrombus in any coronary segment was present in the first angiogram in 50 and 49 patients from the placebo- and abciximab-treated patients and resolved prior to angioplasty in 11 and 21 patients, respectively (22% vs 43% $p = 0.033$) (Fig. 10).

Lesion type according to the AHA/ACC criteria assessed in the first angiogram was not different between the two groups (Table 13). Missing data are owing to total occluded vessels. In the placebo group more complications occurred and endpoints were reached in patients with more severe lesions (Table 13). Treatment with abciximab did not affect endpoints in patients with type A or B_1 lesions but reduced events in patients with complex lesions.

By univariate analysis, endpoints (death, myocardial infarction, or urgent reinterventions) were more frequent in patients with long lesions or angulated or bifurcation lesions (Table 14). By multivariable analysis, only lesions at bifurcation were associated with an increased endpoint risk, particularly in younger patients.

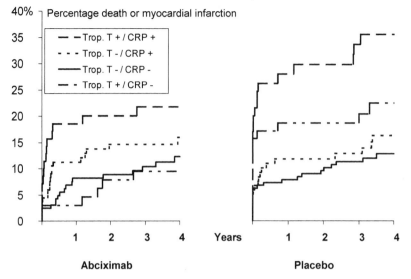

Fig. 9. Kaplan-Meier curves of death and/or myocardial infarction according to C-reactive protein (CRP) and troponin T (Trop T) status and treatment received.

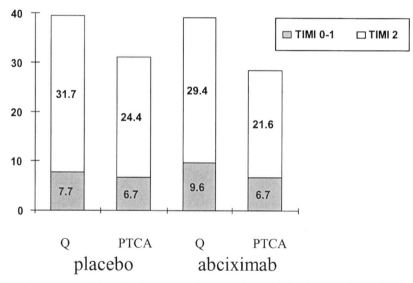

Fig. 10. TIMI flow grade of the infarct-related artery (IRA) in abciximab-treated and placebo patients at the time of diagnostic angiography before treatment (Q) and 18–24 h later during treatment (PTCA). Neither differences between groups nor changes are statistically significant.

The angioplasty procedure was angiographically successful in 88.0% of placebo patients and 94.1% of abciximab patients ($p < 0.001$). Placebo patients showed a higher incidence of both failure to cross (11 vs 2, $p = 0.02$) and failure to dilate (66 vs 34, $p = 0.001$) the lesion successfully. Of all patients with a failed procedure, 33.3% of placebo-treated patients reached a primary endpoint, whereas this occurred in only 11.4% of abciximab-treated patients with a failed procedure ($p = 0,019$). If the procedure was successful, the respective numbers were 13.0 and 10.7%. Stents were implanted in 56 placebo and 60

Table 13
Lesion Type According to AHA/ACC Criteria
as Scored in the Baseline Angiogram, and Primary Composite Endpoint[a]

Lesion type	Placebo (n = 584)	Endpoint	Abciximab (n = 569)	Endpoint	p value
A	48 (8.2)	21 (9.6)	50 (8.8)	22 (9.6)	NS
B$_1$	170 (29.1)		179 (31.5)		
B$_2$	188 (32.2)	32 (17.0)	166 (29.2)	20 (12.0)	NS
>B$_2$	166 (28.4)		167 (29.3)		
C	12 (2.1)	34 (19.1)	7 (1.2)	20 (11.5)	0.055

[a]Data are numbers, with percent in parentheses.

Table 14
Individual IRS Lesion Characteristics
and Outcome in Patients Treated with Abciximab or Placebo

Lesion characteristic	No.	Abciximab primary endpoint [no. (%)]	No.	Placebo primary endpoint [no. (%)]
Length				
<10 mm	418	46 (11.0)	442	57 (12.9)
≥10 mm, <20 mm	143	16 (11.2)	128	26 (20.3)*
≥20 mm	0	0 (0.0)	12	3 (25.0)
Eccentricity				
Concentric	97	7 (7.2)	93	15 (16.1)
Eccentric	470	54 (11.5)	486	71 (14.6)
Angulation				
<45 degrees	528	57 (10.8)	532	74 (13.9)
>45 degrees	40	4 (10.0)	44	11 (25.0)*
Contour				
Smooth	451	46 (10.2)	457	69 (15.1)
Irregular	115	16 (13.9)	123	17 (13.8)
Calcification				
Yes	86	11 (12.8)	89	15 (16.9)
No	481	50 (10.4)	486	69 (14.2)
Bifurcation				
Yes	129	13 (10.1)	153	36 (23.5)*
No	437	49 (11.2)	427	50 (11.7)
Thrombus				
Yes	41	5 (12.2)	40	9 (22.5)
No	551	54 (10.6)	558	76 (14.4)
Ostial				
Yes	23	1 (4.3)	25	4 (16.0)
No	545	61 (11.2)	558	82 (14.7)
Accessibility				
Readily accessible	554	62 (11.2)	564	84 (14.9)
Moderate tortuosity	0	0 (0)	14	2 (14.3)

*p < 0.05 placebo vs abciximab.

abciximab patients. All implants in the abciximab patients were successful, but implantation was not successful in nine placebo patients ($p = 0.003$).

After the procedure, more abciximab patients showed a type A–C dissection of the dilated vessel than placebo-treated patients (31.5% vs 25.1%, $p = 0.014$). Higher grade dissections were equal in both groups (2.2% in abciximab vs 2.0% in placebo patients). Occlusion of a side branch of ≥1.5 mm diameter, originating from the dilation site, occurred in 2.8% of placebo patients and 1.0% of abciximab patients ($p = 0.03$). No vessel perforation was visible on any angiogram. A single additional non-IRA lesion was dilated in 113 patients. Two or more additional lesions were treated in another 17 patients.

The results of these dilations were similar to those of the IRA dilation, with success rates in the abciximab-treated patients of 92.5% and in the placebo-treated patients of 83.7%.

DISCUSSION

Both the pre-CAPTURE and the CAPTURE trial showed a significant reduction in the primary endpoint of death, myocardial infarction, or urgent repeat intervention when patients were pretreated with abciximab, compared with placebo. The corresponding reduction in the rate of myocardial infarction was 50%. These findings accord with those of other clinical studies of abciximab *(19–21)* and studies with other inhibitors of the platelet glycoprotein IIb/IIIa receptor *(22,23)*. In the EPIC (Evaluation of c7e3 for the Prevention of Ischemic Complications) trial *(19)*, administration of a bolus abciximab followed by 12 h infusion at the same dose as in our study reduced the rate of death or myocardial infarction from 9.6% (placebo) to 6.1% ($p = 0.015$) and reduced the need for urgent reintervention. A bolus-only regimen was less effective *(19)*. In our study, pretreatment with abciximab reduced the rates of these events before, during, and immediately after the interventions. In the EPILOG (Evaluation of PTCA to Improve Long-term Outcome by ReoPro GPIIb/IIIa receptor blockade) study *(21)*, which was also stopped early by the Safety and Efficacy Monitoring Committee, similar results were obtained in patients undergoing elective PTCA.

In all three studies with abciximab, the initial treatment effects were maintained for at least 30 d. Modest reductions in the same events, although not statistically significant, were observed in patients undergoing PTCA and treated with tirofiban ($p = 0.16$) *(22)* or eptifibatide ($p = 0.06$) *(23)*. These two agents differ from abciximab in that they are small molecules with short half-lives and with more reversible binding to the IIb/IIIa receptor. Nevertheless, these studies consistently support the efficacy of platelet glycoprotein IIb/IIIa receptor blockers in preventing thrombotic complications before and during coronary intervention.

In contrast to other studies, patients in CAPTURE with more severe, refractory, unstable angina were treated during the 18–24 h before planned PTCA. Abciximab resulted in a reduction of events during this period as well as of procedure-related events (Fig. 4). Apparently, some stabilization of the unstable plaque was achieved during this treatment period. Since most infarctions occurred during or after the intervention, further event reduction might have been achieved by a longer treatment period before PTCA. PTCA might even have been avoided in some of these patients after stabilization of the plaque had been achieved. Thus, further studies can be justified to investigate the efficacy of abciximab and related drugs in patients with unstable angina but no planned coronary revascularization procedure. As in the EPIC trial *(19,20)*, patients treated with abciximab in CAPTURE

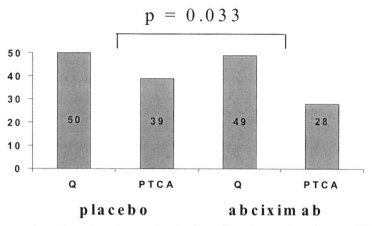

Fig. 11. Presence of any thrombus observed at the first (Q) and second angiogram (PTCA). There is a significant difference in thrombus resolution between patients treated with placebo or abciximab.

had higher bleeding rates than those in the placebo group. However, the rate of major bleeding complications was much lower in CAPTURE than in the previous study (3.8 vs 10.6%), by the same definitions. Minor bleeding rates were also lower in our study (4.8 vs 18.8% in EPIC).

This reduction was achieved by reduction of the heparin dose and greater attention to the site for vascular access. However, we also observed a significant relation between heparin use and bleeding risk. A further reduction of heparin doses and early sheath removal in the EPILOG study *(21)* avoided excess bleeding episodes in patients receiving abciximab. Heparin dose should be monitored closely in patients treated with abciximab. During PTCA, heparin dose should be restricted to 70 IU/kg.

Complications during coronary angioplasty are of either mechanical or thrombotic origin. Balloon angioplasty results in a disruption or dissection of the arterial wall, which lead to exposure of plaque contents, collagen, and other components of the vascular wall to the blood, resulting in platelet activation and thrombosis. Mechanical complications from large dissection flaps can now be treated by stents *(24,25)*. Stents may also reduce the area of exposure of thrombogenic components of the vascular wall. Many of the thrombotic complications and associated myocardial infarctions can be avoided when abciximab is given, whether for 18–24 h before the procedure as in CAPTURE, or for 10–30 min before and 12 h after intervention, as in the other studies *(19–21)*.

Review of the angiograms of patients participating in the CAPTURE trial showed that more thrombi were resolved in the patients treated with abciximab, underscoring the thrombolytic potential of the drug *(26)* (Fig. 11). This finding is in agreement with the qualitative angiographic data from the CAPTURE pilot trial, in which three of six vessels being occluded or showing thrombi at the first angiogram contained no intracoronary filling defects after treatment with abciximab, whereas this occurred in only one of five patients pretreated with placebo. Similar results were obtained in a study with tirofiban (PRISM PLUS) in which angiograms were analyzed in 1168 patients who had been treated with this IIb/IIIa receptor blocker or placebo during 65 ± 17 h. In these patients, medium or large thrombi were reported in 20% of placebo patients and in 14% of patients receiving tirofiban *(27)*.

The angiographic success rate of the procedure was higher if patients were pretreated with abciximab (94.1 vs 88.0%; $p < 0.001$). Most of the failures of angioplasty were caused by inability to dilate the culprit lesion successfully. This is also true if a stent was implanted. Stent implantation resulted in a 100% angiographically successful procedure in abciximab-treated patients, whereas success after stent implantation was only achieved in 86% of placebo-treated patients ($p = 0.003$). Abciximab thus improves the angiographic outcome both with and without stent implantation. Again, these data have recently been confirmed in other trials comparing patients receiving stents with or without abciximab (28).

Apparently heparin and aspirin are unable to control for ongoing thrombus formation at the dilation site, whereas abciximab is able to control this process, thus resulting in a successful procedure. Angiography might not be the most sensitive diagnostic tool to detect thrombi in coronary arteries (18), but it is tempting to ascribe the better angiographic outcome after abciximab to less thrombus formation at the site of the dilation. In keeping with this finding is our observation of significantly fewer occurrences of side-branch occlusion after dilation when patients are pretreated with abciximab. Although this finding was rather rare in both groups, the absolute difference of 1.8% of side-branch occlusion between both groups might have contributed to the absolute difference of 3.6% in the number of infarctions between both groups, since most of these infarctions occurred in conjunction with the angioplasty procedure (Fig. 4).

It is remarkable that in this trial patients pretreated with abciximab and a failed angioplasty procedure did not exhibit a higher incidence of the primary endpoint at 30 d (11.4%) than the total group of patients treated with abciximab (10.8%). However, 33% of patients in the placebo group with a failed angioplasty procedure reached a primary endpoint vs 13% of placebo patients with a successful angioplasty procedure.

This raises the question of whether treatment with abciximab during a longer waiting period before angioplasty could further reduce the number of events, and even reduce the total number of revascularization procedures.

An improvement in TIMI flow of at least one grade between the first and the second angiogram was observed in equal numbers in both patient groups in the CAPTURE trial, as was already noted in the pilot CAPTURE trial.

Grading lesions according to the system devised by the AHA/ACC task force has led to the recognition of lesions more susceptible to angioplasty complications. In the group of patients treated with placebo or abciximab, the number of primary endpoints for A or B_1 lesions was 9.6% vs 9.6%; for B_2 lesions 17.0% vs 12.0%; and for $>B_2$ or C lesions 19.1% vs 11.5%. When looking at individual lesion characteristics only a lesion at the site of a bifurcation led to a significant higher incidence of complications when patients were not pretreated with abciximab.

The short course of abciximab treatment did not affect the rate of recurrent myocardial infarction after the first few days; such infarctions are probably caused by new plaque rupture at the same or at another coronary segment. Furthermore, there was no indication that abciximab influenced the restenosis process, since rates of repeat PTCA were the same in abciximab and placebo groups.

These results contrast with those of the EPIC study, in which a consistently lower rate of target lesion revascularization was observed with abciximab up to 6 mo and 3 yr after enrollment (20). This difference between CAPTURE and EPIC follow-up results may be a chance finding, or it may be owing to the difference in treatment regimen. In CAPTURE, abciximab infusion was discontinued 1 h after PTCA, whereas the infusion continued for

12 h in EPIC. Higher plasma concentrations of abciximab after PTCA might result in binding of abciximab to the $\alpha_v\beta_3$ (vitronectin) receptor, which is exposed on vascular smooth muscle cells after vessel injury. This receptor, to which abciximab binds with the same affinity as to the glycoprotein platelet IIb/IIIa receptor, is thought to be involved in migration and proliferation of smooth muscle cells (29).

This hypothesis has been studied in more detail in the ERASER trial. Instent restenosis rates did not differ at 6 mo after angioplasty, when patients were treated with placebo or 12- or 24-h abciximab infusion (30).

Follow-up data from EPILOG (21) show results intermediate between those of CAPTURE and EPIC; there was sustained benefit of treatment with abciximab, with similar low event rates between 1 mo and 6 mo in the two treatment groups.

The collective experience in large trials with more than 6000 patients has shown unequivocally that treatment with abciximab greatly reduces the rate of thrombotic complications in association with PTCA. Treatment with abciximab during and after the intervention can be recommended in all patients undergoing PTCA, if the drug costs are not prohibitive (4,31). Patients with elevated troponin-T levels are at particular risk of myocardial infarction and will benefit most from pretreatment with abciximab. A longer pretreatment period, for example 2 or 3 d, may be even more beneficial, although there is not yet sufficient evidence. Continuation of treatment for at least 12 h after PTCA seems prudent in view of the long-term efficacy observed with that regimen (20). Additional long-term benefit might be obtained by long-term treatment with related agents that can be taken orally.

In view of the costs of abciximab, some physicians may decide to use this drug only or mainly to treat thrombotic complications when these occur during an intervention. Such use may be effective, but it has not been tested rigorously in randomized trials. Currently available data indicate that pretreatment with abciximab is warranted in all patients undergoing PTCA, particularly in patients with refractory unstable angina with more complex lesions as determined by angiography.

ACKNOWLEDGMENTS

Parts of this chapter were reprinted with permission from refs. 7a and 7b.

REFERENCES

1. Braunwald A. Unstable angina. A classification. Circulation 1989;80:410–414.
2. Van Miltenburg-van Zijl A, Simoons ML, Veerhoek RJ, Bossuyt PM. Incidence and follow-up of Braunwald subgroups in unstable angina pectoris. J Am Coll Cardiol 1995;25:1286–1292.
3. Falk E. Morphologic features of unstable atherothrombotic plaques underlying acute coronary syndromes. Am J Cardiol 1989;63:114E–120E.
4. Theroux P, Quimet H, McCans J, et al. Aspirin, heparin, or both to treat acute unstable angina. N Engl J Med 1988;319:1105–1111.
5. Goldman BS, Katz A, Christakis G, Weisel R. Determinants of risk for coronary artery bypass grafting in stable and unstable angina pectoris. Can J Surg 1985;28:505–508.
6. de Feyter PJ, Suryapranata H, Serruys PW, et al. Coronary angioplasty for unstable angina: immediate and late results in 200 consecutive patients with identification of risk factors for unfavorable early and late outcome. J Am Coll Cardiol 1988;12:324–333.
7. Gold HK, Gimple LW, Yasuda T, et al. Pharmacodynamic study of F(ab')$_2$ fragments of murine monoclonal antibody 7E3 directed against human platelet glycoprotein IIb/IIIa in patients with unstable angina pectoris. J Clin Invest 1990;86:651–659.

7a. van den Braud MJBM, Simoons ML, De Boer MJ, et al. Antiplatelet therapy in therapy-resistant unstable angina. A pilot study with ReoPro (c7E3). Eur Heart J 1995;16(Suppl L):36–42.

7b. The CAPTURE Investigators. Randomized placebo controlled trial of abciximab before and during coronary intervention in refractory unstable angina: the CAPTURE trial. Lancet 1997;349:1429–1435.

8. Rao AK, Pratt C, Berke A, et al. Thrombolysis in myocardial infarction trial—Phase I: Hemorrhagic manifestations and changes in plasma fibrinogen and the fibrinolytic system in patients treated with recombinant tissue plasminogen activator and streptokinase. J Am Coll Cardiol 1988;12:1–11.

9. Landefeld LS, Cook EF, Hatley M. Identifications and preliminary validation of predictors of major bleeding in hospitalised patients starting anticoagulant therapy. Am J Med 1987;82:703–713.

10. American College of Physicians Clinical Guideline: practice strategies for elective red blood cell transfusion. Ann Intern Med 1992;116:403–406.

11. Lan KK, de Mets DL. Discrete sequential boundaries for clinical trials. Biometrika 1983;70:659–663.

12. Chesebro JH, Knatterud G, Roberts R, et al. Thrombolysis in myocardial infarction (TIMI) trial, Phase I: A comparison between intravenous tissue plasminogen activator and intravenous streptokinase. Clinical findings through hospital discharge. Circulation 1987;76:142–154.

13. Capone G, Wolf NM, Meyer B, Meister SG. Frequency of intracoronary filling defects by angiography in angina pectoris at rest. Am J Cardiol 1985;56:403–406.

14. Reiber JH, Serruys PW, Kooijman CJ, et al. Assessment of short-, medium-, and long-term variations in arterial dimensions from computer assisted quantification of coronary cineangiograms. Circulation 1985;71:280–288.

15. Strauss BH, Juilliere Y, Rensing BJ, Reiber JH, Serruys PW. Edge detection versus densitometry for assessing coronary stenting quantatively. Am J Cardiol 1991;67:484–490.

16. Crawford DW, Brooks SH, Selzer RH, Brandt R, Beckenbach ES, Blankenhorn DH. Computer densitometry for angiographic assessment of arterial cholesterol contents and gross pathology in human atherosclerosis. J Lab Clin Med 1977;89:378–392.

17. Ryan TJ, Faxon DP, Gunnar RM, et al. Guidelines for percutaneous transluminal coronary angioplasty: a report of the American College of Cardiology/American Heart Association Task Force on assessment of diagnostic and therapeutic cardiovascular procedures (Subcommittee on Percutaneous Transluminal Coronary Angioplasty). J Am Coll Cardiol 1988;12:529–549.

18. den Heyer P, Foley DP, Escaned J, et al. Angioscopic versus angiographic detection of intimal dissection and intracoronary thrombus. J Am Coll Cardiol 1994;24:649–654.

18a. Hamm CW, Heeschen C, Goldmann B, et al., for the CAPTURE study investigators. Benefit of abciximab in patients with refractory unstable angina in relation to serum troponin-T levels. N Engl J Med 1999;340:1623–1629.

18b. Heeschen C, Hamm CW, Bruemmer J, et al., for the CAPTURE investigators. Predictive value of C-reactive protein and troponin T in patients with unstable angina: a comparative analysis. J Am Coll Cardiol 2000;35:1535–1542.

19. EPIC investigators. Use of a monoclonal antibody directed against the platelet glycoprotein IIb/IIIa receptor in high risk coronary angioplasty. N Engl J Med 1994;330:956–961.

20. Topol EJ, Califf RM, Weisman HF, et al. Randomised trial of coronary intervention with antibody against platelet IIb/IIIa integrin for reduction of clinical restenosis: results at six months. Lancet 1994;343:881–886.

21. The EPILOG investigators. Platelet glycoprotein IIb/IIIa receptor blockade and low-dose heparin during percutaneous coronary revascularization. N Engl J Med 1997;336:1689–1696.

22. The RESTORE Investigators. Effects of platelet glycoprotein IIb/IIIa blockade with tirofiban on adverse cardiac events in patients with unstable angina or acute myocardial infarction undergoing coronary angioplasty. Circulation 1997;96:1445–1453.

23. The IMPACT II investigators. Randomised placebo-controlled trial of effect of eptifibatide on complications of percutaneous coronary intervention: IMPACT II. Lancet 1997;349:1422–1428.

24. Serruys PW, Jaegere P de, Kiemeneij F, et al. A comparison of balloon-expandable-stent implantation with balloon angioplasty in patients with coronary artery disease. N Engl J Med 1994;331:489–495.

25. Fischman DL, Leon MB, Baim DS, et al. A randomised comparison of coronary-stent placement and balloon angioplasty in the treatment of coronary artery-disease. N Engl J Med 1994;331:496–501.

26. Muhlestein JB, Karagounis LA, Treehan S, Anderson JL. "Rescue" utilization of abciximab for the dissolution of coronary thrombus developing as a complication of coronary angioplasty. J Am Coll Cardiol 1997;30:1729–1734.

27. Xue-Qiao Zhao, Snapinn S, Sax FL, et al. Angiographic results from platelet receptor inhibition for ischemic syndrome management in patients with documented unstable angina or non Q wave MI (PRISM-plus). Circulation 1997;96:I–474 (abstract).
28. Kereiakes D, Lincoff AM, Miller DP, et al., for the EPILOG trial investigators. Abciximab therapy and unplanned coronary stent deployment. Favourable effects on stent use, clinical outcomes, and bleeding complications. Circulation 1998;97:857–864.
29. Choi ET, Engel L, Callow AD, et al. Inhibition of neointimal hyperplasia by blocking $\alpha_v\beta_3$ integrin with a small peptide antagonist G*penGRGDSPC*A. J Vasc Surg 1994;19:125–134.
30. The ERASER investigators. Acute platelet inhibition with abciximab does not reduce in-stent restenosis (ERASER study). Circulation 1999;100:799–806.
31. Mark DB, Talley JD, Topol EJ, et al. Economic assessment of platelet glycoprotein IIb/IIIa inhibition for prevention of ischemic complications of high-risk coronary angioplasty. Circulation 1996;94:629–635.

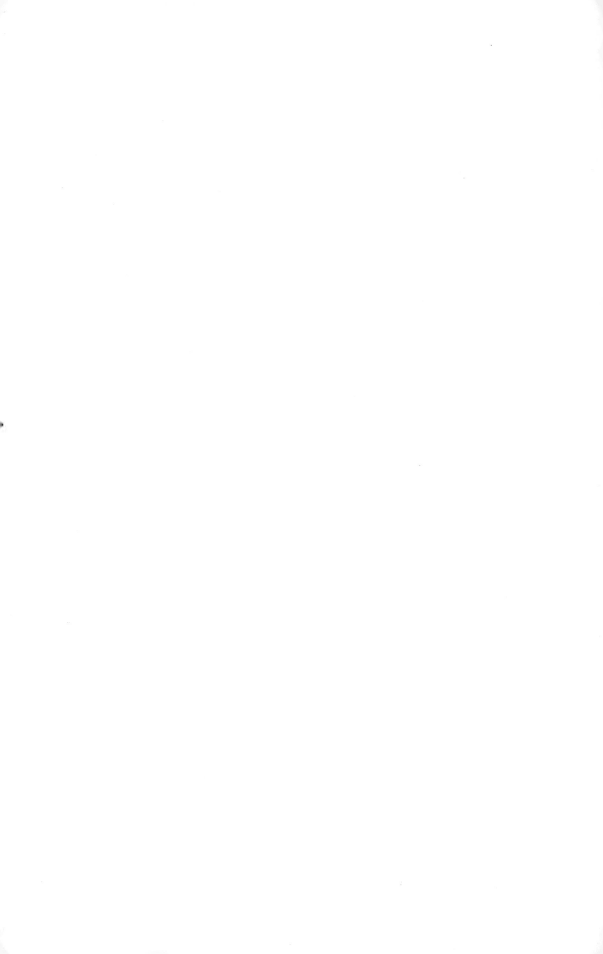

10

Unstable Angina Trials
PARAGON, PURSUIT, PRISM, PRISM-PLUS, and GUSTO-IV

David J. Moliterno, MD

CONTENTS

INTRODUCTION
ANTIPLATELET THERAPIES
GPIIb/IIIa RECEPTOR ANTAGONISTS
CLINICAL OUTCOME: PARAGON A AND B, PRISM, PRISM-PLUS,
   PURSUIT (5 Ps), AND GUSTO-IV
CURRENT ISSUES
SUMMARY AND FUTURE DIRECTIONS
REFERENCES

INTRODUCTION

Unstable angina is part of the acute coronary syndrome (ACS) spectrum; it is related to non-Q-wave myocardial infarction and slightly more distantly related to Q-wave myocardial infarction. The diversity of conditions leading to unstable angina as well as the varying symptoms upon presentation have made the definition and classification of unstable angina difficult *(1)*. The Global Unstable Angina Registry and Treatment Evaluation (GUARANTEE) study reported that one-third of hospitalized patients with cardiac chest pain had new or accelerated symptoms associated with exertion, whereas two-thirds had rest angina *(2)*. This distinction is important, since patients with exertional angina may have a gradual worsening of an underlying atherosclerotic coronary arterial narrowing, as opposed to those with rest angina, who have an abrupt reduction in myocardial perfusion owing to a ruptured plaque (*see* Chapter 1). Angina at rest is often associated with electrocardiographic changes of ischemia and shares a similar underlying mechanism with threatened vessel closure following percutaneous coronary angioplasty, i.e., plaque disruption. Whether spontaneous or as a result of angioplasty, plaque rupture leads to exposure of the coronary arterial subendothelial components, platelet activation, and thrombus formation.

From: *Contemporary Cardiology: Platelet Glycoprotein IIb/IIIa*
Inhibitors in Cardiovascular Disease, 2nd Edition
Edited by: A. M. Lincoff © Humana Press Inc., Totowa, NJ

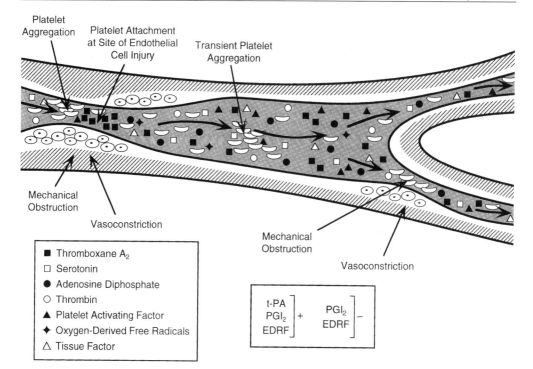

Fig. 1. Schematic diagram of mechanism underlying primary acute coronary syndromes. At the site of the atherosclerotic plaque (anatomic obstruction), endothelial injury is present. In combination with the release of vasoactive and platelet-activating substances such as thromboxane A_2, serotonin, thrombin, and adenosine diphosphate (ADP), this causes a physiologic obstruction superimposed on the anatomic obstruction. Platelet activation and aggregation can occur as a result of these substances or in response to exposure of the subendothelial matrix following plaque fissuring or rupture. Platelets release additional vasoactive factors and fibrinogen, which, in turn, leads to further vasoconstriction, platelet activation, thrombin formation, and potentially vessel obstruction. EDRF, endothelium-derived relaxing factor; PGI_2, prostacyclin; t-PA; tissue plasminogen activator. (Adapted with permission from ref. *3.*)

The subendothelial constituents exposed following plaque rupture (e.g., collagen, von Willebrand factor, and fibronectin) are recognized by platelet surface receptors [primarily glycoprotein (GP)Ib], and platelet adhesion and activation occurs. During activation, platelets secrete a host of substances from their α-granules, which leads to vasoconstriction, chemotaxis, mitogenesis, and activation of neighboring platelets *(3,4)* (Fig. 1). Platelet activation leads to the recruitment and "functionalization" of GPIIb/IIIa integrins or specialized surface receptors that mediate aggregation (platelet-platelet binding). Aggregated platelets accelerate the production of thrombin by providing the surface for the binding of cofactors required for the conversion of prothrombin to thrombin. In a reciprocating fashion, thrombin is a potent agonist for further platelet activation, and it stabilizes the thrombus by converting fibrinogen to fibrin. Because the final common pathway leading to platelet aggregation is via fibrinogen binding between adjacent platelet GPIIb/IIIa receptors, blocking these receptors is a strategically ideal means of limiting ischemic events associated with unstable angina.

Despite the increased use of aspirin, an effective although weak antiplatelet agent, unstable angina remains among the leading causes of adult hospitalizations in industrialized countries. In fact, the incidence of unstable angina continues to increase, and reportedly approx 1 million hospitalizations each year in the United States are with a primary diagnosis of unstable angina. Thus, the testing of platelet GPIIb/IIIa inhibitors and their institution into the medical armamentarium of the acute coronary syndromes is as necessary and clinically relevant as ever. This chapter reviews the use of antiplatelets and GPIIb/IIIa inhibitors in unstable angina and non-Q-wave myocardial infarction, with particular emphasis on the Phase III trials of intravenous GPIIb/IIIa inhibitors.

ANTIPLATELET THERAPIES

Aspirin

The benefit of aspirin therapy alone or in combination with heparin in the treatment of unstable angina has been proved in several randomized trials (5–9). Aspirin, a cyclooxygenase and hydroperoxidase inhibitor, blocks synthesis of thromboxane A_2 and hinders platelet aggregation from some, but not all stimuli. In the study by Théroux and colleagues (5) entitled "Aspirin, Heparin, or Both to Treat Acute Unstable Angina," there was a significant reduction in cardiac death or myocardial infarction (MI) from 11.9% in the placebo group, to 3.3% with aspirin alone, to 1.6% with the combination of aspirin and heparin ($p = 0.0042$). The Research Group on Instability in Coronary Artery Disease in Southeast Sweden (RISC) (6) demonstrated a 57% ($p = 0.033$) reduction in MI and death with aspirin therapy compared with placebo, whereas intermittent intravenous heparin showed no significant influence on these endpoints. One-year follow-up of these patients continued to show nearly a 50% reduction ($p < 0.0001$) in death and MI in aspirin-treated patients compared with placebo (7). Although the dose of aspirin and the duration of follow-up varied in each of these studies, a substantial reduction in relative risk of adverse cardiac events was consistently seen. Pooled data from over 2000 patients (5,7–9) (Table 1) showed that the occurrence of infarction or death was reduced from 11.8% (control) to 6.0% (aspirin). Similar results were reported by the Antiplatelet Trialists' Collaboration study for aspirin-treated patients with infarction (10) (Table 1). Based on pooled data from the most recent report from the Antiplatelet Trialists' Collaboration (11), a dose of 75–150 mg of aspirin provides optimal reduction of ischemic events (Fig. 2).

Ticlopidine

Ticlopidine, an antiplatelet agent commonly used after intracoronary stent implantation, inhibits ADP-mediated platelet aggregation (12) and antagonizes the interaction of fibrinogen with the GPIIb/IIIa receptors of platelets (13). Although these mechanisms are distinctly different from the actions of aspirin and require 48–72 h to become clinically manifest (14), available data suggest that ticlopidine is as effective as aspirin in reducing adverse cardiac events in unstable angina. Balsano et al. (15) reported the use of ticlopidine in a randomized study of 652 patients with unstable angina. Nonfatal infarction and vascular death were reported in 13.6% of control subjects and 7.3% of patients receiving ticlopidine, or a 46% risk reduction ($p = 0.009$). Considering available trial data with aspirin or ticlopidine compared with placebo, the Antiplatelet Trialists' Collaboration reported on seven trials including 4018 patients: the occurrence of adverse vascular events

Table 1
Randomized Trials of Aspirin in Patients with Acute Coronary Syndromes

Study	No. of patients	ASA duration (mo)	Daily dose (mg)	Death or MI		Δ Relative risk (%)	P-Value
				Control (%)	Aspirin (%)		
Unstable angina							
Lewis et al. *(9)*	1266	3	324	10.1	5.0	−51	<0.001
Cairns et al. *(8)*	278	24	1300	14.1	11.5	−20	0.008
Théroux et al. *(5)*	239	<1	650	11.9	3.3	−72	0.012
Wallentin et al. *(7)*	288	3	75	17.6	7.4	−58	0.004
Pooled	2071	~6		11.8	6.0	−49	<0.001
Acute MI trials							
Antiplatelet Trialists' Collaboration *(10)*	20,543	~1	~150–325	14.4	10.6	−26	<0.001

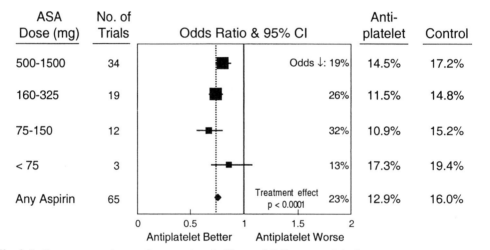

Fig. 2. Indirect comparisons of proportional effects of different aspirin doses on vascular events in high-risk patients. Considering over 60 trials and nearly 60,000 patients, aspirin in the range of 75–150 mg daily appears to provide as much protection from ischemic vascular events as any other studied dose. (Adapted with permission from ref. *11*.)

(MI, stroke, or vascular death) was reduced by 35% with antiplatelet therapy (14.1% vs 9.1%, $p < 0.001$) *(10)*.

Clopidogrel

Clopidogrel, an analog of ticlopidine, also antagonizes the ADP-dependent activation of the platelet GPIIb/IIIa receptor by irreversibly and selectively blocking the binding of ADP to the P2Y$_{12}$ receptor on the platelet surface. The largest comparative antiplatelet trial was a secondary prevention study testing aspirin versus clopidogrel among 19,185 patients with prior MI, ischemic stroke, or symptomatic peripheral arterial disease. The Clopidogrel versus Aspirin in Patients at Risk for further Ischemic Events (CAPRIE) trial enrolled patients between 1992 and 1995 in 16 countries *(16)*. At a mean follow-up of approximately 2 yr, there was a 9% relative reduction in the composite of ischemic stroke, myocardial (re)infarction, or vascular death with the use of clopidogrel. The annual occurrence of the primary endpoint was 5.83% of those treated with aspirin and 5.32% ($p = 0.043$) of those treated with clopidogrel. Among the subgroup enrolled following myocardial infarction ($n = 6302$), no reduction in the primary endpoint was observed with clopidogrel, but rather a nonsignificant ($p = 0.66$) 4% relative increase in events compared with aspirin therapy. In the setting of ACS, the Clopidogrel in Unstable Angina to Prevent Recurrent Ischemic Events trial (CURE) randomized 12,562 inpatients to aspirin or aspirin plus clopidogrel. After a mean follow-up of 9 mo, the combination of clopidogrel plus aspirin was seen to reduce the composite of cardiovascular death, nonfatal MI, and stroke by 20% compared with aspirin treatment alone (9.3 vs 11.4; $p < 0.001$) *(17)*. Of note, <7% of patients in CURE were managed with a platelet GPIIb/IIIa antagonist.

GPIIb/IIIa RECEPTOR ANTAGONISTS

The most potent family of antiplatelet agents are the GPIIb/IIIa receptor inhibitors. As mentioned, platelet aggregation can be initiated by a number of pathways. However, the final common pathway—irrespective of how it is initiated—involves the binding of the GPIIb/IIIa receptors of adjacent platelets by an interposing fibrinogen molecule. By blocking GPIIb/IIIa receptors, platelet aggregation can be effectively prevented. Many intravenous antagonists to the GPIIb/IIIa receptor have been developed, and three are commercially available. Platelet GPIIb/IIIa receptor antagonists are approved for the primary treatment of unstable angina and non-Q-wave MI. Results from six such large clinical trials, the so-called 5 Ps and the fourth GUSTO trial, were recently published: the Platelet IIb/IIIa Antagonism for the Reduction of Acute Coronary Syndrome Events in A Global Organization Network (PARAGON A and B) trials *(18,19)*; the Platelet Receptor Inhibition in Ischemic Syndrome Management (PRISM) study *(20)*; the Platelet Receptor Inhibition in Ischemic Syndrome Management in Patients Limited by Unstable Signs and Symptoms (PRISM-PLUS) study *(21)*; the Platelet IIb/IIIa in Unstable Angina: Receptor Suppression Using Integrilin Therapy (PURSUIT) trial *(22)*; and the fourth Global Use of Strategies to Open Occluded Arteries (GUSTO-IV) trial *(23)*.

Abciximab

The first large-scale study with platelet GPIIb/IIIa inhibitors was with abciximab in the setting of percutaneous coronary revascularization *(24)* (*see* Chapter 5). Subsequently, several large studies have been completed with this monoclonal antibody to the GPIIb/IIIa receptor. The Evaluation of c7E3 for the Prevention of Ischemic Events (EPIC) *(24)* trial enrolled high-risk angioplasty patients; the Evaluation of PTCA to Improve Long-term Outcomes by c7E3 Glycoprotein Receptor Blockade (EPILOG) *(25)* trial enrolled "all comers" and excluded only those having an acute infarction or unstable angina with electrocardiographic changes at rest. Likewise, the Evaluation of IIb/IIIa Platelet Inhibitor for Stenting (EPISTENT) included a large number of patients with unstable angina *(26–28)*. The Coronary Angioplasty for Refractory Unstable Angina (CAPTURE) enrolled only those angioplasty patients with medically refractory unstable angina *(29)* (*see* Chapter 9). Although the overall cohort receiving abciximab (c7E3, ReoPro™) in these four trials had a dramatic reduction in the composite occurrence of death, MI, or need for urgent revascularization following angioplasty or atherectomy, an even greater benefit was extended to those with unstable angina. Compared with placebo, those with unstable angina who

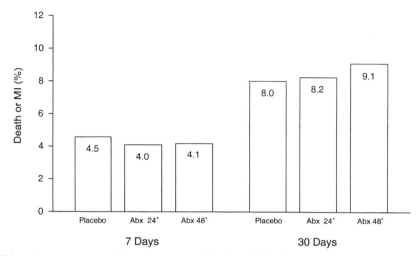

Fig. 3. Thirty-day occurrence of the composite of death or MI in GUSTO-IV. This primary endpoint occurred 14% more often in the group receiving abciximab for 48 h (abx 48°) compared with placebo. On the other hand, when considering this endpoint at 7 d, the same treatment group actually had 10% fewer events compared with placebo. Therefore, when indirectly comparing different clinical trials, it is best to refer to a similar endpoint and at a similar time of follow-up. (Data from ref. *23*.)

received abciximab as bolus plus infusion had a 62–70% reduction in death, MI, or urgent revascularization in the first 30 d of follow-up *(26)*. The EPIC investigators reported a 60% reduction in death at 3-yr follow-up among patients with unstable angina or evolving infarction receiving bolus plus infusion of abciximab during angioplasty *(27)*. Interestingly, this benefit became most evident after the first year of follow-up.

The indications for abciximab for patients with unstable angina have become more clearly focused following the completion of the Do Tirofiban and ReoPro Give Similar Efficacy Outcome Trial (TARGET) *(30)* and GUSTO-IV trials. These two studies are discussed in detail elsewhere. In brief, GUSTO-IV tested abciximab as primary medical therapy (i.e., without angioplasty) vs placebo among 7800 patients. No reduction in ischemic events was seen with abciximab use among these medically treated patients. In fact, a tendency for worse outcome was seen among those receiving a 48-h infusion of abciximab (Fig. 3). In contrast, in the TARGET trial, 4809 patients undergoing intracoronary stent placement were equally randomized to abciximab or tirofiban, and abciximab was found to be superior to tirofiban in reducing ischemic events. The 30-d composite of death, MI, and urgent target vessel revascularization was 26% lower with abciximab (7.6% vs 6.0%; $p = 0.038$) *(30)*. Moreover, the cohort of patients receiving the highest benefit at early and late follow-up was that with unstable angina. Compared with tirofiban, abciximab reduced MI at 30 d and 6 mo by 32% and 27%, respectively among ACS patients ($p \leq 0.01$) *(31)*.

Lamifiban

Lamifiban (Hofmann-LaRoche, Basel, Switzerland) is a low-molecular-weight, synthetic, nonpeptide, highly-specific GPIIb/IIIa receptor antagonist. Lamifiban (Ro 44-9883) was first studied in unstable angina patients in The Canadian Lamifiban study *(32)*,

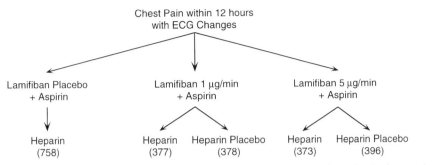

Fig. 4. Flow diagram summarizing the PARAGON study protocol, partial factorial design, and number of patients randomized. (From ref. *19*, with permission.)

a Phase II dose-exploring study of 365 patients. Aspirin was given to all patients, and heparin was given to a minority (26%) of patients (at the discretion of the primary physician). Lamifiban was used as bolus plus infusion, with the bolus ranging from 150 to 750 µg and infusion doses ranging from 1 to 5 µg/min for 72 h. In a dose-dependent fashion, platelet aggregation to 10 µmol ADP was inhibited by 60% to >95%, and bleeding time was prolonged. At 30-d follow-up, compared with placebo, those assigned to low-dose lamifiban (1 or 2 µg/min) had a 23% reduction, and those assigned to high-dose lamifiban (4 or 5 µg/min) had a 70% reduction in the composite of death and MI.

A Phase IIIa study of lamifiban in unstable angina, the Platelet IIb/IIIa Antagonism for the Reduction of Acute Coronary Syndrome Events in a Global Organization Network (PARAGON A) trial, with 2282 patients, was subsequently completed *(19)*. The objective of this trial was to assess several treatment strategies of GPIIb/IIIa inhibition (lamifiban), with the optimal strategy to be further tested versus standard therapy *(33)*. Therefore, a partial factorial design was implemented with patients randomized to low-dose vs high-dose lamifiban and to heparin or no heparin therapy. The fifth possible group to be randomized to was the control group, which received placebo and heparin. Thus, each patient received lamifiban, unfractionated heparin, or both in addition to aspirin (Fig. 4). Patients assigned to low-dose lamifiban received a 300 µg bolus followed by a 1.0 µg/min infusion; those assigned to high-dose lamifiban received a 750 µg bolus followed by a 5.0 µg/min infusion.

Lamifiban infusion was initiated and maintained according to initial treatment assignment; heparin was weight-adjusted and activated partial thromboplastin time (aPTT)-titrated. Systematic blinding of heparin administration and careful control of anticoagulation for all patients was achieved by use of a bedside aPTT device that produced encrypted results. A Hemochron® Jr. microcoagulation instrument automatically assayed whole blood collected and generated a multidigit code corresponding to the aPTT in seconds. Using the patient's study number and the coded aPTT result, the health care provider telephoned a central computer system, which deciphered the patient's aPTT and treatment assignment and then directed heparin or heparin-placebo infusion adjustments. The computer program titrated the heparin infusion according to a standardized nomogram to keep the aPTT to a laboratory equivalent of 60–85 s.

The primary endpoint was a composite of all-cause mortality and nonfatal MI (or reinfarction) in the first 30 d of follow-up. Secondary endpoints included death, myocardial (re)infarction, disabling stroke, and major and intermediate bleeding at 30 d; death and myocardial infarction at 6 mo; and death at 1-yr follow-up. Study group sizes, drug administration, and in-hospital cardiac procedures are detailed in Table 2. Demographic data and comparisons with the other 5-P trials are listed in Table 3. Principal safety and outcome data at 30 d and 6 mo are provided in Table 4. No difference in the composite of death or nonfatal MI was noted between the control group and any lamifiban group or the combination of all lamifiban-treated groups at 30 d. At 6-mo follow-up, a difference in the composite was present. Compared with the control group, three of the four lamifiban-treated groups had a lower event rate. Specifically, death or nonfatal MI at 6 mo was lowered 24% by low-dose lamifiban with or without heparin [odds ratio, 0.72; 95% confidence interval (CI), 0.54–0.96; $p = 0.027$] and 9% by high-dose lamifiban with or without heparin (odds ratio, 0.89; 95% CI, 0.68–1.16; $p = 0.450$) compared with control.

For uncertain reasons, the event rates diverged after 30 d. Between 30 and 180 d, the relative increase in myocardial (re)infarction was 36% for the control group, 19% for the high-dose lamifiban groups, and 15% for the low-dose lamifiban groups. Likewise, the relative increase in deaths during this time was 131% for the control group, 89% for the high-dose lamifiban groups, and 77% for the low-dose lamifiban groups. At 1 yr, all-cause mortality was 8.2, 8.4, and 6.9%, respectively ($p = 0.340$; Fig. 5). The overall incidences of bleeding complications and stroke are presented in Table 4. There were more bleeding-related events among those receiving high-dose lamifiban. The rates of major bleeding were 1.8, 0.6, and 0.8% for high-dose lamifiban groups, low-dose lamifiban groups, and control, respectively ($p = 0.058$).

An intriguing analysis from the PARAGON A trial was performed to understand better a potential dose-response relationship. The lamifiban plasma concentration was measured in 810 lamifiban-treated patients (34), and this was correlated *post hoc* with clinical outcome. The lamifiban level at steady state was directly related to the patient's renal function, and a middle concentration range (18–42 ng/mL: corresponding to 80–90% GPIIb/IIIa receptor occupancy) was associated with a 38% reduction in death and MI at 6 mo. Based on this information, the PARAGON B study was designed (35). In 29 countries, 5225 patients were randomized equally to placebo or to lamifiban. All lamifiban-treated patients received a 500 µg intravenous bolus. According to the creatinine clearance, estimated by the Cockcroft-Gault formula, patients were separated according to a creatinine clearance of 30–40, 40–70, or >70 mL/min and received a 1.0, 1.5, or 2.0 µg/min infusion of lamifiban, respectively (Table 2). All patients received aspirin and heparin. The primary endpoint of 30-d death, MI, or severe recurrent ischemia occurred in 11.8% of lamifiban-treated patients and 12.8% of placebo-treated patients ($p = 0.329$). Thus, despite the achievement of targeted plasma levels of lamifiban in the treated group, no over-all benefit was observed.

Tirofiban

Tirofiban (Aggrastat[TM], Merck, White House Station, NJ), a small-molecule, nonpeptide GPIIb/IIIa receptor antagonist, was initially studied in unstable angina in a Phase II, heparin-controlled study of 71 patients (36). Given for up to 48 h, tirofiban (MK-383) was well tolerated without significant bleeding. An encouraging reduction in the incidence of refractory angina was observed with tirofiban studied over a dose range of 0.075–0.15 µg/kg/min. These findings led to the designs of PRISM and PRISM-PLUS, two Phase III tirofiban

Table 2

Study Designs and Enrollment Details

Design/detail	PARAGON A	PRISM	PRISM-PLUS	PURSUIT	PARAGON B	GUSTO-IV
Enrollment dates	8/95–5/96	3/94–10/96	11/94–9/96	11/95–1/97	2/98–6/99	7/98–4/00
Drug	Lamifiban	Tirofiban	Tirofiban	Eptifibatide	Lamifiban	Abciximab
Patients enrolled Total	2282	3232	1915	10,948	5225	7800
Treatment groups (bolus + infusion)	755 @ 300 µg + 1 µg/min; 769 @ 750 µg + 5 µg/min; 758 @ placebo	1616 @ 0.6 µg/kg/min × 30 min + 0.15 µg/kg/min; 1616 @ placebo	773 @ 0.4 µg/kg/min × 30 min + 0.1 µg/kg/min; 345 @ 0.6 µg/kg/min × 30 min + 0.15 µg/kg/min; 797 @ placebo	1487 @ 180 µg/kg + 1.3 µg/kg/min; 4722 @ 180 µg/kg + 2.0 µg/kg/min; 4739 @ placebo	2628 @ 500 mg + 1.0–2.0 mg/min; 2597 @ placebo	2590 @ 0.25 mg/kg + 0.125 µg/kg/min × 24 h; 2612 @ 0.25 mg/kg + 0.125 µg/kg/min × 48 h; 2598 @ placebo
Infusion duration (h)	72	46	71	72	72	24 or 48
Heparin	Randomized, blinded aPTT 60–85 s	Randomized, blinded aPTT 1.5–2 × control	All patients aPTT 2 × control	Recommended (open-label) aPTT 50–70 s	All patients aPTT 50–70 s	All patients UFH @ aPTT 50–70 s or LMWH
Early drug discontinuation (%)	19	NA	14	36		
PTCA during study (%)	13	21	31	24	28	19
CABG during study (%)	11	17	23	14	15	11
1° Endpoint	Death or MI	Death, MI, or refractory ischemia composite	Death, MI, or refractory ischemia composite	Death or MI	Death, MI, or severe recurrent ischemia	Death or MI
Endpoint analysis (d)	30	2	7	30	30	30

Abbreviations: aPTT, activated partial thromboplastin time; CABG, coronary artery bypass graft; LMWH, low-molecular-weight heparin; MI, myocardial infarction; PTCA, percutaneous transluminal coronary angioplasty; UFH, unfractionated heparin.

Table 3
Characteristics of Study Groups at Enrollment (%)

Characteristic	PARAGON A	PRISM	PRISM-PLUS	PURSUIT	PARAGON B	GUSTO-IV
Age (yr)	66	62	63	64	64	65
Female	35	32	33	35	34	37
Diabetes	18	21	23	22	22	22
Hypertension	49	54	54	55	56	52
High cholesterol	42	47	49	42	50	30
Current smoker	23	26	NA	28	29	NA
Prior MI	35	47	43	32	30	31
Prior PTCA	11	15	10	13	14	10
Prior CABG	9	17	15	12	13	9
Presenting ECG						
ST depression	52	32	58	50	45	80
ST elevation	6	7	14	14	16	NA
T-wave inversion	54	51	53	52	46	NA
MI at enrollment	36	25	45	45	57[a]	59[a]

Abbreviations: MI, myocardial infarction; PTCA, percutaneous transluminal coronary angioplasty; CABG, coronary artery bypass graft surgery; ECG, electrocardiogram; NA, not available.

[a]Local laboratory positive troponin.

studies in unstable angina and non-Q-wave MI *(20,21)*. PRISM began enrollment in March 1994, and patients with accelerating or rest angina within 24 h and any clinical suspicion for ischemic heart disease were eligible (Table 2). Suspicion for ischemia included ST-segment or T-wave abnormalities consistent with ischemia; elevated cardiac enzymes; history of prior percutaneous transluminal coronary angioplasty (PTCA), coronary artery bypass graft (CABG), or positive stress test; or a known coronary arterial narrowing ≥50%. In PRISM, 3232 patients were randomized to tirofiban (0.6 µg/kg/min bolus followed by a 0.15 µg/kg/min infusion) or heparin. The tirofiban loading dose was actually given as a 30-min infusion, and the subsequent dose infusion was given for up to 47.5 h. The mean duration of infusion was 46 h, with 12% of infusions stopped early. All patients were to receive aspirin, and the target prolongation of aPTT among patients receiving heparin was twice the laboratory control value (Table 2). Patient management was prespecified in that angiography and coronary intervention during the first 48 h were discouraged.

Unlike other GPIIb/IIIa trials in unstable angina, the PRISM primary composite endpoint was at 48 h. The composite included death, MI, and refractory ischemia. The same endpoints plus rehospitalization for unstable angina were collected at 7 and 30 d. Refractory ischemia was defined as recurrent angina with (1) ST-T changes lasting for ≥20 min within a 1-h period despite full medical therapy, or (2) hemodynamic instability. The composite endpoint at 48 h was reduced 36% by tirofiban, with the greatest effect seen in the reduction of refractory ischemia events. At the time of endpoint ischemia, most patients were receiving both nitrates and β-blockers. At 7 d, the reduction in the composite endpoint by tirofiban was attenuated to a nonsignificant 8% lowering. Likewise, at 30-d follow-up, tirofiban still reduced the composite outcome, but only by 7% ($p = 0.34$). A similar decay of benefit or reversal of effect was seen in GUSTO-IV (Fig. 3).

Table 4
Clinical Outcome (%)

Characteristic	PARAGON A Placebo	PARAGON A Lamifiban 1 μg/min ± heparin	PARAGON A Lamifiban 5 μg/min ± heparin	PRISM Heparin	PRISM Tirofiban 0.15 μg/kg/min	PRISM-PLUS Heparin	PRISM-PLUS Heparin + tirofiban 0.10 μg/kg/min	PRISM-PLUS Tirofiban 0.15 μg/kg/min	PURSUIT Placebo	PURSUIT Eptifibatide 1.3 μg/kg/min	PURSUIT Eptifibatide 2.0 μg/kg/min	PARAGON B Placebo	PARAGON B Lamifiban 1–2 μg/kg/min	GUSTO-IV Placebo	GUSTO-IV Abciximab 24 h	GUSTO-IV Abciximab 48 h
No. of patients	758	755	769	1616	1616	797	773	345	4739	1487	4722	2597	2628	2598	2590	2612
30-d outcome																
Death	2.9	3.0	3.6	3.6	2.3	4.5	3.6	(6.1)	3.7	(3.4)	3.5	3.3	2.9	3.9	3.4	4.3
Nonfatal MI	10.6	9.4	10.9	4.3	4.1	9.2	6.6	(9.0)	13.5	(12.0)	12.6	9.8	8.8	5.1	5.6	5.9
Death or MI																
Overall	11.7	10.6	12.0	7.1	5.8	11.9	8.7	(13.6)	15.7	(13.4)	14.2	11.5	10.6	8.0	8.2	9.1
Relative reduction		9	−6		18		27				10		8		−3	−14
PTCA patients				9.1	7.2	10.2	5.9		16.8		11.8					
Non-PTCA patients				6.2	3.6	7.8	3.6		15.7		14.6	11.0	10.3			
6-mo outcome																
Death	6.6	5.2	6.8			7.0	6.9	(7.2)	6.2		6.4					
Nonfatal MI	14.3	10.8	12.9			10.5	8.3	(10.1)	15.7		14.7					
Death or MI	17.9	13.7	16.4			15.3	12.3	(15.9)	19.0		17.8					
Relative reduction		23	8				20				8					
Major bleeding[b]	3.0	3.0	6.0	0.4	0.4	0.8	1.4		1.3		3.0	0.9	1.3	0.3	0.6	1.0
Intracranial hemorrhage	0	0	0.1	0.1	0.1	0	0		0.1		0.1	0.1	0.1	0.04	0.2	0.1
RBC transfusion[c]	4.4	4.4	8.7	1.4	2.4	2.8	4.0		1.8		4.4	8.9	10.3	1.5	2.2	2.9
Thrombocytopenia[a]	1.1	1.5	1.3	0.1	0.4	0.3	0.5		0.4		0.6	0.5	0.7	1.0	4.7	7.0

Abbreviations: MI, myocardial infarction; PTCA, percutaneous transluminal coronary angioplasty; RBC, red blood cells.

[a] Thrombocytopenia defined as platelet count = 50,000/mm³. Numbers in parentheses are from discontinued treatment arms and are not contemporaneous; these are listed only for completeness, not direct comparisons.

[b] Major bleeding as defined by intracranial hemorrhage or decrease in hemoglobin of 5 g/dL not associated with coronary artery bypass grafting (CABG), except for PARAGON A.

[c] Transfusions reported are those not associated with CABG, except for PARAGON A.

% of Pts, Death

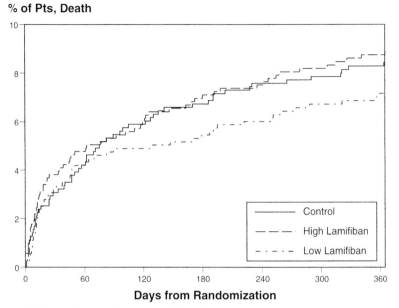

Days from Randomization

Fig. 5. Kaplan-Meier estimates of the probability of death during 1-yr follow-up in PARAGON with control compared with lamifiban patients grouped by low and high doses. All-cause mortality was 8.7, 7.3, and 8.9%, respectively ($p = 0.320$). (From ref. *19*, with permission.)

The PRISM-PLUS trial started enrollment in November, 1994 and randomized a total of 1915 patients. Compared with PRISM, patients in PRISM-PLUS were somewhat more unstable; they were required to have rest angina within 12 h plus electrocardiographic evidence of ischemia or serologic evidence of infarction. With these criteria, 45% of PRISM-PLUS patients had an infarction at enrollment compared with 25% in PRISM. Patients in PRISM-PLUS were randomized to tirofiban alone (0.6 µg/kg/min loading followed by 0.15 µg/kg/min), heparin, or tirofiban (0.4 mg/kg/min followed by 0.1 mg/kg/min) plus heparin. All patients were to receive aspirin, and the target prolongation of aPTT among patients receiving heparin was twice the laboratory control value. Patient management was prespecified in that angiography and coronary intervention before 48 h were discouraged, whereas they were encouraged to be performed between 48 and 96 h while continuing study drug infusion. Endpoint definitions were similar to those in PRISM, and the primary endpoint was a composite of death, MI, or refractory ischemia at 7 d.

An interim analysis revealed an increase in 7-d mortality among those randomized to high-dose tirofiban alone. Thus, after 1031 patients had been enrolled in the overall study, this treatment arm was discontinued. The 7-d mortality rates for the high-dose tirofiban, heparin, and moderate-dose tirofiban plus heparin groups were 4.6, 1.1, and 1.5%, respectively. The odds ratio for mortality at 7 d with high-dose tirofiban compared with heparin alone was 4.1 (95% CI, 1.4–12.3; $p = 0.012$). Although the 7-d, 30-d, and 6-mo rates of death as well as the death or MI composite were numerically highest for the high-dose tirofiban group, this difference was only statistically significant for 7-d mortality. Outcome information on this group is presented in Table 4 only for listing purposes and cannot be compared with the final data from the other two arms since it is not contemporaneous.

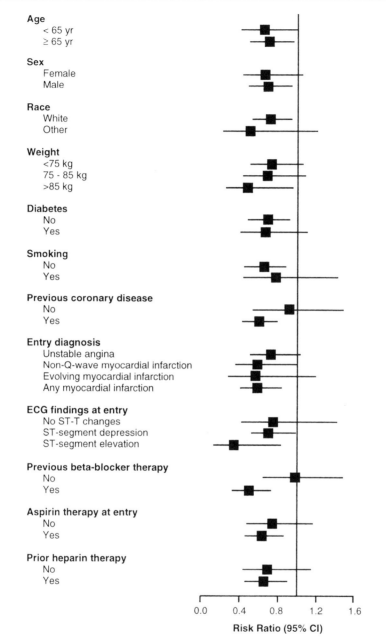

Fig. 6. Effect of treatment with heparin or tirofiban plus heparin on the composite primary endpoint at 7 d among various subgroups. Risk ratios <1 favor the subgroup receiving tirofiban plus heparin [horizontal lines represent the 95% confidence intervals (CI)]. There were no statistically significant interactions between the assigned treatment and any of the other factors shown except that effects of tirofiban were particular marked among those already taking β-blockers at enrollment. (From ref. *21*, with permission.)

The primary endpoint (7-d death, MI, refractory ischemia) was reduced 28% by tirofiban plus heparin compared with heparin alone (12.9 vs 17.9%, respectively). Impressively, this reduction in ischemic events was extended similarly to nearly all subgroups (Fig. 6).

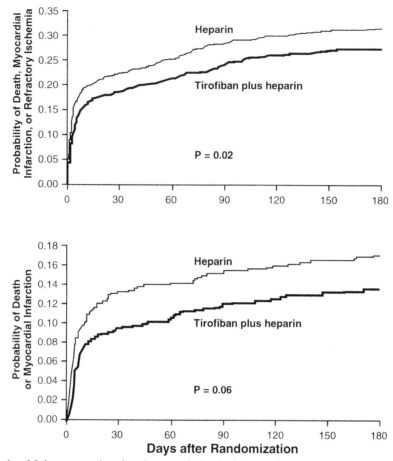

Fig. 7. Kaplan-Meier curves showing the cumulative incidence of events among patients randomly assigned to receive tirofiban plus heparin or tirofiban alone. The top panel is the composite of death, myocardial infarction, refractory ischemia, or rehospitalization for unstable angina. The bottom panel is the composite of death or myocardial infarction. *p* values were computed by Cox regression analysis. (From ref. *21*, with permission.)

Benefit from tirofiban was durable at 30 d, as the composite endpoint including rehospitalization for unstable angina was reduced 17% (18.5% vs 22.3%, *p* = 0.03) (Fig. 7). Considering the trend in event rate reduction provided by tirofiban, most of the benefit was present for preventing refractory ischemia and nonfatal MI. Even at 6-mo follow-up, both of these ischemic endpoints were reduced 21% in comparison with placebo.

Eptifibatide

Eptifibatide, (Integrilin™, COR Therapeutics, South San Francisco, CA) a cyclic heptapeptide, and competitive inhibitor of the GPIIb/IIIa receptor, was studied in a Phase II unstable angina trial published by Schulman et al. in 1996 *(37)*. This dose-finding trial randomized 227 patients to a low dose of eptifibatide (45 μg/kg bolus, 0.5 μg/kg/min infusion), "high-dose" eptifiabtide (90 μg/kg bolus, 1.0 μg/kg/min infusion), or placebo. The study drug was continued for 24–72 h, and all patients received heparin. The efficacy parameter was the frequency and duration of ischemic episodes as assessed by continuous electrocardiographic monitoring. A dose-dependent decrease in ischemic episodes was observed, although this only reached statistical significance in the high-dose group. During study drug infusion, no increase in bleeding events was noted with eptifibatide, and following drug cessation, no rebound phenomena occurred. Subsequent studies performed with eptifibatide during percutaneous coronary intervention used relatively higher doses of bolus plus infusion (135 µg/kg bolus and 0.5–0.75 µg/kg/min infusion). Even these doses, however, subsequently only inhibited platelet aggregation by 40–60% *(38)*.

The largest unstable angina study involving a GPIIb/IIIa inhibitor was the Platelet IIb/IIIa in Unstable Angina: Receptor Suppression Using Integrilin Therapy (PURSUIT) trial *(22)*. Between November 1995 and January 1997, 10,948 patients in 28 countries were randomized to one of two doses of eptifibatide or placebo (Table 2). All patients randomized to eptifibatide received a 180 µg/kg bolus and either a 1.3 µg/kg/min or 2.0 µg/kg/min infusion for 72 h. After 1487 patients received the moderate-dose infusion (1.3 µg/kg/min) of eptifibatide, this arm was discontinued since the higher dose arm had a similarly acceptable safety profile. Unlike PRISM-PLUS, the discontinued arm in PURSUIT was part of a prespecified plan, involved dropping the lower dose group, and was done because of acceptable safety. Except where noted, the following reported data are from the remaining 9461 patients equally randomized to placebo or high-dose eptifibatide. The study was designed to emulate although not interfere with the usual clinical treatment for patients with unstable angina. Hence, it was recommended, although not required, that all study patients receive oral aspirin and weight-adjusted intravenous heparin. Likewise, patients could have angiography and revascularization at any time during the study to conform with the attending physician's preference.

The primary endpoint was a composite of all-cause mortality and nonfatal MI (or reinfarction) at 30 d. Secondary endpoints included death and myocardial (re)infarction at 30 d, the composite at 96 h and 7 d, and safety and efficacy outcome in patients undergoing percutaneous coronary interventions. Demographic data, study drug administration, and in-hospital cardiac procedures are detailed in Tables 2 and 3. Principal safety and outcome data at 30 d and 6 mo are provided in Table 4. The outcome information for the discontinued treatment group is presented in Table 4 only for listing purposes and cannot be compared with the final data from the other two arms since it is not contemporaneous. At the time of enrollment, 45% of patients had a non-Q-wave myocardial infarction. Importantly, aspirin was used in 93% of patients, and heparin was used in 90%. Coronary angiography was performed in 60% of patients, and percutaneous coronary revascularization was performed in 24%.

Based on the site investigators' reports, the primary 30-d endpoint was reached in 10.0% of control patients and 8.0% of those receiving eptifibatide. Following adjudication by the Clinical Events Committee, the 12–28% relative reduction in events reported by sites among the four geographic regions was reduced to −7 to 22% (Fig. 8). Not surprisingly, the death rate did not change with adjudication, but rather, the number of patients considered to have non-Q-wave MI during follow-up was substantially increased. The study's overall adverse event rate climbed from 9 to 15% with adjudication of non-Q-wave MIs by elevated creatine kinase (CK)-MB. The overall study remained positive at 30 d, with a 10% reduction in death and nonfatal MI (Fig. 9) and a 22% reduction seen in North America. These data were durable at 6 mo (Table 4).

Irrespective of site report or Clinical Events Committee, geographic region, or early vs late follow-up, there was an approx 1.5% absolute reduction in death or nonfatal MI.

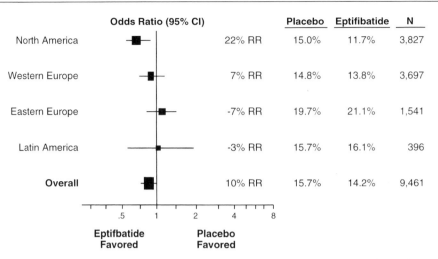

Fig. 8. Odds ratio for death or myocardial infarction according to the endpoints adjudicated by the Clinical Events Committee and separated according to geographic region in the PURSUIT trial. (Data from ref. *22*.)

This benefit was consistent among the subgroups except for women. As seen in Fig. 10, some of this discrepancy in gender-related outcome may have been geographically influenced by specific practice patterns. For example, early diagnostic catheterization (≤72 h) was performed in between 5 and 66% of patients according to location (Eastern Europe vs North America). Not surprisingly, the range of heparin usage (76–97%), early angioplasty (4–25%), and early bypass surgery (1–8%) was also associated with these regional differences.

CLINICAL OUTCOME: PARAGON A AND B, PRISM, PRISM-PLUS, PURSUIT (5 Ps), AND GUSTO-IV

The study designs of the 5 Ps and GUSTO-IV have many similarities, but also several important distinctions (Table 2) with regard to endpoint definitions, percentage of patients with infarction at enrollment, duration of therapy, concomitant use of heparin, use of percutaneous revascularization, and, importantly, timing of the primary endpoint analysis. Given these similarities and distinctions, several meta-analysis have already been considered *(39–42)*.

30-Day Mortality

Considering all patients enrolled into the first four ACS trials testing GPIIb/IIIa receptor blockade (Table 2), Kong et al. *(41)* performed a formal meta-analysis of approx 10,000 patients who were randomized to active therapy. They found that the odds ratio of death at 30 d was 0.90 (95% CI, 0.76–1.06) with GPIIb/IIIa treatment compared with placebo. Overall 30-d mortality for these patients was 3.4% compared with 3.7% for the 7910 patients assigned to receive placebo ($p = 0.27$). The lowest mortality was 2.3% for those receiving 0.15 µg/kg/min tirofiban in PRISM (36% relative reduction compared with placebo, $p = 0.02$) (Fig. 11). Ironically, the highest 30-d mortality among all treatment groups in all studies was also for 0.15 µg/kg/min tirofiban, in PRISM-PLUS (6.1% among

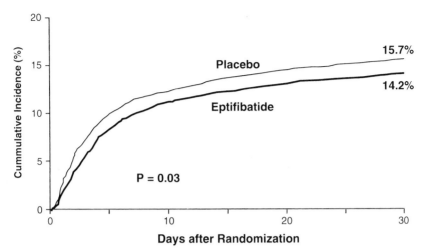

Fig. 9. Kaplan-Meier curves showing the incidence of death or nonfatal myocardial infarction at 30 d. Events were based on endpoints adjudicated by the Clinical Events Committee, and the *p* value is based on the log-rank test. (From ref. *22*, with permission.)

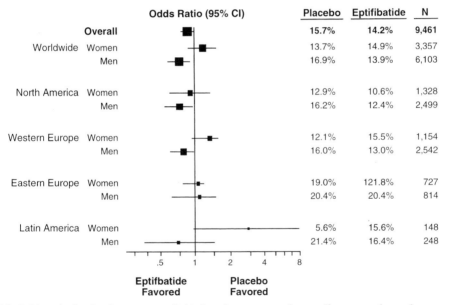

Fig. 10. Odds ratio for death or myocardial infarction separated according to gender and geographic region. Women overall showed no benefit from eptifibatide treatment, although this subgroup finding was primarily limited to outside North America. (Data from ref. *22*.)

345 patients). Thus, 30-d mortality was reduced with tirofiban in PRISM; however, this was not evident in any individual study, suggesting that any true reduction in overall mortality was minor.

Roffi and colleagues *(43)* also performed a meta-analysis considering mortality among all six large-scale GPIIb/IIIa inhibitor ACS trials. Their specific interest was in evaluating outcome among patients with and without diabetes mellitus. Interestingly, they observed

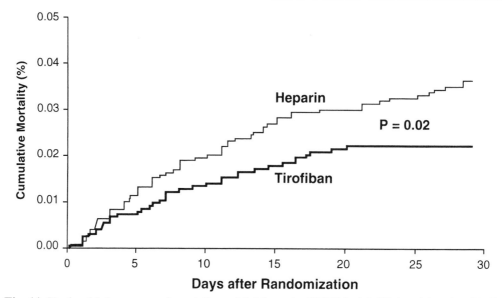

Fig. 11. Kaplan-Meier curves of mortality to 30 d from the PRISM trial. With a risk ratio of 0.62 favoring tirofiban, although wide confidence intervals, PRISM was the only study to show a survival benefit with GPIIb/IIIa therapy. (From ref. *20*, with permission.)

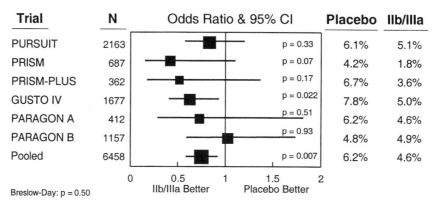

Fig. 12. Odds ratio and 95% confidence intervals for 30-d mortality among diabetic patients in GPIIb/IIIa ACS trials. Values <1.0 indicate a survival benefit from GPIIb/IIIa therapy. (From ref. *43*, with permission.)

mortality to be substantially reduced at 30 d among 6458 diabetic patients receiving active therapy vs placebo (6.2% vs 4.6%; odds ratio, 0.74; 95% CI, 0.59–0.92; $p = 0.007$; Fig. 12). Among the remaining patients (>23,000 without diabetes), no survival benefit was noted with platelet GPIIb/IIIa inhibition versus placebo (3.0% for both groups; Fig. 13). The largest and most systematic meta-analysis of these trials confirmed the finding of Roffi et al. *(43)* among diabetic patients. Boersma and colleagues *(42)* also evaluated the 31,402 patients from the six GPIIb/IIIa ACS trials listed in Table 2. This meta-analysis showed that 30-d mortality was 3.4% among the 18,297 patients receiving active therapy and 3.7% among the 13,105 patients receiving placebo. The odds ratio (0.91; 95% CI, 0.81–1.03)

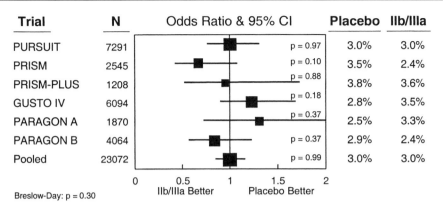

Trial	N	Odds Ratio & 95% CI	Placebo	IIb/IIIa
PURSUIT	7291	p = 0.97	3.0%	3.0%
PRISM	2545	p = 0.10	3.5%	2.4%
PRISM-PLUS	1208	p = 0.88	3.8%	3.6%
GUSTO IV	6094	p = 0.18	2.8%	3.5%
PARAGON A	1870	p = 0.37	2.5%	3.3%
PARAGON B	4064	p = 0.37	2.9%	2.4%
Pooled	23072	p = 0.99	3.0%	3.0%

Breslow-Day: p = 0.30   IIb/IIIa Better   Placebo Better

Fig. 13. Odds ratio and 95% confidence intervals for 30-d mortality among nondiabetic patients in GPIIb/IIIa ACS trials. Values <1.0 indicate a survival benefit from GPIIb/IIIa therapy. (From ref. *43*, with permission.)

again suggests a minor overall mortality benefit ($p = 0.14$) with GPIIb/IIIa therapy. In the smaller meta-analysis by Kong et al. *(41)*, the odds ratio for mortality at an early (48–96 h) timepoint was found to be 0.71 (95% CI, 0.50–1.01), favoring GPIIb/IIIa therapy. The odds ratio for mortality, shifting from 0.71 to 0.90 between two and 30 d in this meta-analysis, further strengthens the argument for considering one endpoint at a specific follow-up interval when comparing multiple trials. For example, had the primary endpoint of GUSTO-IV been at 7 d, abciximab would have been found to reduce the ischemic events by 10%, as opposed to increasing them by nearly 14% at 30 d (Fig. 3). Since most ACS trials have previously reported the treatment effect on death and nonfatal MI at 30 d as the primary endpoint, this may be the most appropriate point of comparison.

30-Day Myocardial Infarction

Enzymatic (serologic) evidence of myocardial infarction is not uncommonly present following percutaneous coronary intervention, especially among patients with an ACS. This must be kept in mind when interpreting unstable angina trials among patients also undergoing coronary interventions, since it can be unclear whether the increase in CK-MB or troponin occurred as a result of the primary disease process, the coronary intervention, or both. Among all patients randomized to GPIIb/IIIa therapy in the 5-P and GUSTO-IV trials, 7.4% had a nonfatal MI compared with 8.1% of the placebo cohort *(42)*.

30-Day Death or Myocardial Infarction

The composite rate of death or nonfatal MI among overall trial cohorts (i.e., treated and placebo groups) may be an indicator of the illness severity of the patients enrolled, the background medical treatment given, or the level of endpoint adjudication. The highest overall rate of 30-d death or MI was in PURSUIT (15.7%), and the lowest was in PRISM (5.8%). Among all patients receiving GPIIb/IIIa therapy in the Boersma et al. meta-analysis *(42)*, the 30-d death or MI composite was 10.8% compared with 11.8% for those receiving placebo ($p = 0.015$; Fig. 14). The 30-d odds ratio was 0.91 (95% CI, 0.85–0.98), or 10 fewer events per 1000 treated patients. Among the final or best GPIIb/IIIa treatment groups (PURSUIT and PRISM-PLUS had a treatment arm discontinued), the greatest

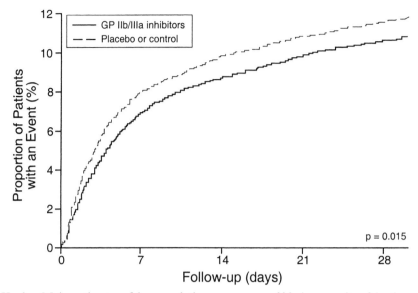

Fig. 14. Kaplan-Meier estimates of the cumulative occurrence of 30-d composite of death or myocardial infarction in a pooled analysis of 31,402 patients. (From ref. *42*, with permission.)

relative reduction (27% fewer events) was seen in PRISM-PLUS among patients receiving 0.10 µg/kg/min of tirofiban combined with heparin, but confidence intervals around this odds ratio are wide (OR = 0.70; 95% CI, 0.50–0.98), and the magnitude of risk reduction is not statistically different from that seen in other trials.

Considering multiple subgroups, Boersma and colleagues *(42)* showed that the benefit of GPIIb/IIIa inhibitors in reducing death or MI at 30 d was consistent across many demographic and baseline characteristics (Fig. 15). Patients receiving the absolute greatest treatment benefit were those with high-risk characteristics. An unexpected although statistically significant interaction was seen according to gender: men received a marked benefit, and women had a significantly worse outcome if receiving GPIIb/IIIa therapy. After stratifying patients according to evidence of myonecrosis (troponin elevation), no evidence remained for a gender effect in treatment response. The greatest relative risk reductions for 30-d death or MI with GPIIb/IIIa treatment has been repeatedly seen among patients who were troponin-positive on admission. For example, Newby and colleagues *(44)* prospectively studied 1160 patients in PARAGON B. Using a blinded core laboratory, they measured troponin levels before and during study treatment. Compared with placebo, lamifiban-treated patients who were troponin-positive had a significant reduction in 30-d death or MI (19.0% vs 11.0%). No treatment benefit was seen among troponin-negative patients (10.3% vs 9.6%, respectively). A similarly striking effect was seen with tirofiban in PRISM, as reported by Heeschen et al. *(45)*. Using CK-MB measurements in PURSUIT and troponin in GUSTO-IV, neither study showed a particular benefit for patients with an MI at enrollment.

Bleeding Events

An important side effect of GPIIb/IIIa inhibitors is bleeding (Table 4), and hence an overall estimate of bleeding parameters from the unstable angina trials is helpful. There

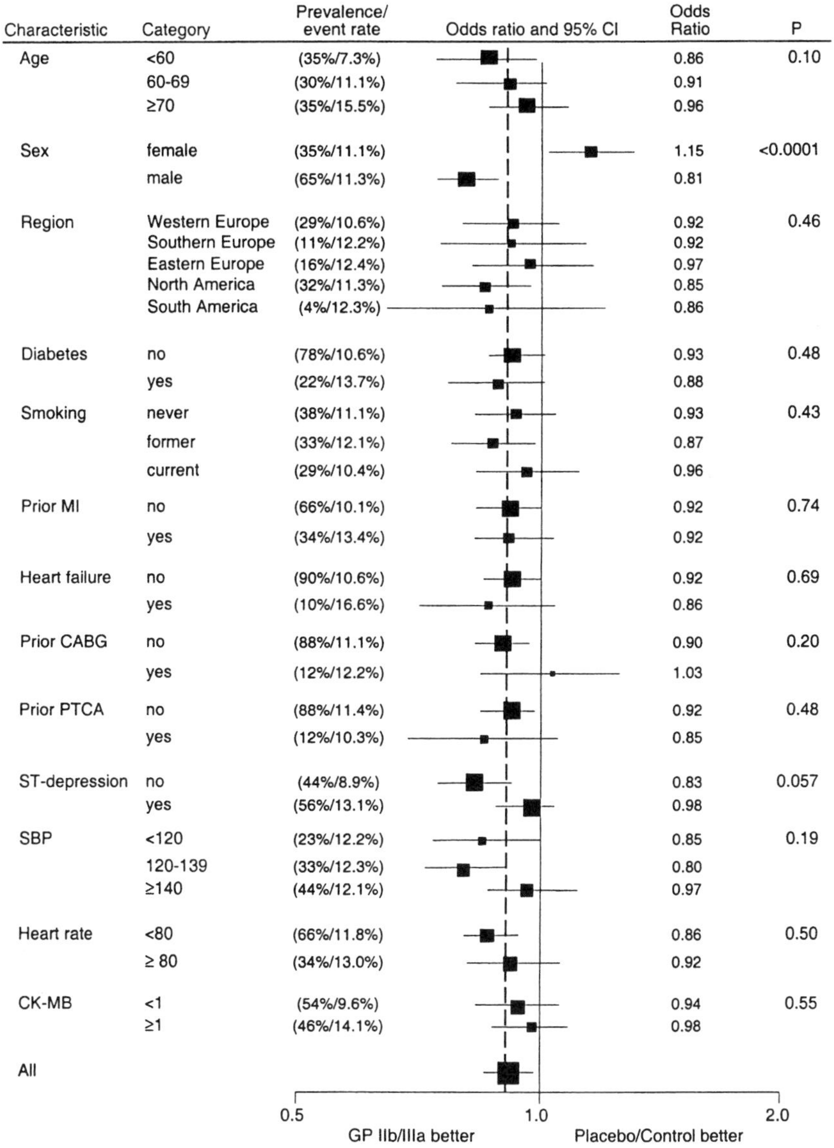

Characteristic	Category	Prevalence/ event rate	Odds ratio and 95% CI	Odds Ratio	P
Age	<60	(35%/7.3%)		0.86	0.10
	60-69	(30%/11.1%)		0.91	
	≥70	(35%/15.5%)		0.96	
Sex	female	(35%/11.1%)		1.15	<0.0001
	male	(65%/11.3%)		0.81	
Region	Western Europe	(29%/10.6%)		0.92	0.46
	Southern Europe	(11%/12.2%)		0.92	
	Eastern Europe	(16%/12.4%)		0.97	
	North America	(32%/11.3%)		0.85	
	South America	(4%/12.3%)		0.86	
Diabetes	no	(78%/10.6%)		0.93	0.48
	yes	(22%/13.7%)		0.88	
Smoking	never	(38%/11.1%)		0.93	0.43
	former	(33%/12.1%)		0.87	
	current	(29%/10.4%)		0.96	
Prior MI	no	(66%/10.1%)		0.92	0.74
	yes	(34%/13.4%)		0.92	
Heart failure	no	(90%/10.6%)		0.92	0.69
	yes	(10%/16.6%)		0.86	
Prior CABG	no	(88%/11.1%)		0.90	0.20
	yes	(12%/12.2%)		1.03	
Prior PTCA	no	(88%/11.4%)		0.92	0.48
	yes	(12%/10.3%)		0.85	
ST-depression	no	(44%/8.9%)		0.83	0.057
	yes	(56%/13.1%)		0.98	
SBP	<120	(23%/12.2%)		0.85	0.19
	120-139	(33%/12.3%)		0.80	
	≥140	(44%/12.1%)		0.97	
Heart rate	<80	(66%/11.8%)		0.86	0.50
	≥ 80	(34%/13.0%)		0.92	
CK-MB	<1	(54%/9.6%)		0.94	0.55
	≥1	(46%/14.1%)		0.98	
All					

0.5   1.0   2.0
GP IIb/IIIa better   Placebo/Control better

Fig. 15. Odds ratio and 95% confidence intervals for the occurrence of a 30-d composite of death or myocardial infarction among subgroups from a meta-analysis of the six large-scale GPIIb/IIIa-ACS trials. CABG, coronary artery bypass graft; SBP, systolic blood pressure; CK-MB, creative kinase MB; MI, myocardial infarction; PTCA, percutaneous transluminal coronary angioplasty. (From ref. *42*, with permission.)

are two different bleeding classifications (i.e., the one developed by the TIMI study group and the one developed by the GUSTO study group) and two different patient groups (those undergoing vascular surgery, such as CABG, and those not undergoing surgery). Major bleeding events by the TIMI criteria include a >5 g hemoglobin loss. This occurred in as few as 0.4% of GPIIb/IIIa-treated patients in PRISM and as many as 10% of GPIIb/IIIa-treated patients in PURSUIT when considering bleeding related to bypass surgery and

angioplasty. The highest bleeding among patients not undergoing CABG was understand-
ably among those receiving the highest doses of GPIIb/IIIa inhibitor, especially when combined with heparin. Severe bleeding according to the GUSTO classification (bleeding that
is life-threatening, leading to hemodynamic compromise, or an intracranial hemorrhage)
occurred in ≤1% of most trials study groups and was highest in the 2.0 µg/kg/min cohort
of PURSUIT (1.5%). Pooling all large-scale GPIIb/IIIa-ACS trial data, major bleeding
increased from 1.4% with heparin and aspirin (control), to 2.4% when adding a GPIIb/IIIa
antagonist *(42)*.

Blood product transfusion (usually RBC's and classified as moderate bleeding) occurred
in 8.3% of patients randomized to GPIIb/IIIa therapy and 6.5% of those receiving placebo.
Most transfusions were related to surgery or angioplasty procedures. Thrombocytopenia
(platelet count ≤ 100,000/mm^3) was infrequent, although it was more common with abciximab (Table 4). Major thrombocytopenia (platelet count ≤ 50,000/µL) was infrequent (≤1%)
in most study groups, as were platelet transfusions. Fortunately, intracranial hemorrhage
remains very rare with this class of drug, with no events occurring in many study groups.
The overall rate of intracranial hemorrhage was <0.1% for both the placebo and treatment
groups.

6-Month Death or Myocardial Infarction

Although information on events between 30-d and 6-mo follow-up are limited (i.e.,
there are no data on the number of patients who had revascularization procedures or were
maintained on β-blockers, angiotensin-converting enzyme inhibitors, or statins), most
trials collect a composite rate of death and nonfatal MI by survey. Quite encouragingly,
treatment benefit has been maintained at late follow-up. Even though there is an initial
decay in benefit (between the first week and first month of follow-up), the benefit at 30 d
is preserved at 6 mo. The relative reduction in death or MI present was 10% in the 30-d composite in PURSUIT and 8% at 6 mo. Likewise, the tirofiban plus heparin arm of PRISM-
PLUS reported a 20% relative reduction in the composite at late follow-up (Fig. 7). Somewhat
surprisingly, the 9% composite reduction at 30-d follow-up in PARAGON for low-dose
lamifiban was improved to a 23% reduction in death or MI over control. These data collectively suggest that although there is an initial decay of acute benefit, passivation probably
also occurs, which protects against intermediate-term events. The 6-mo odds ratio for death
or MI with GPIIb/IIIa treatment compared with placebo was 0.88 (95% CI, 0.79–0.97)
which translates into 16 fewer events per 1000 treated patients (−0.016; 95% CI, −0.027
to −0.004) *(41)*.

CURRENT ISSUES

A number of important issues remain to be discussed and understood regarding the
5-P and GUSTO-IV Trials, and their application to contemporary medical practice. It is
unarguable that GPIIb/IIIa receptor blockage provides an improved outcome during percutaneous coronary interventions. On the other hand, the small molecules that are highly
specific for the GPIIb/IIIa receptor, are distinct from the monoclonal antibody and have
differences among themselves. Questions therefore remain regarding the extent and timing of inhibition needed with these compounds, the importance of concomitant heparin,
the duration of receptor blockage required, and the importance of underlying renal function. Since the small-molecule GPIIb/IIIa receptor antagonists have an important plasma

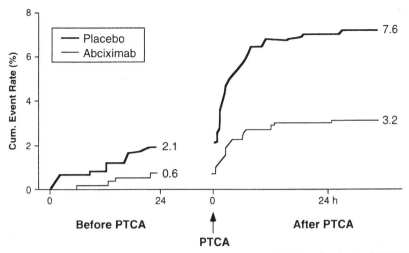

Fig. 16. Occurrence of preprocedural and periprocedural myocardial infarction in the CAPTURE study. Abciximab provided both a primary (preprocedural) and angioplasty-related reduction in the incidence of infarction. (From ref. *29*, with permission.)

phase (i.e., short half-life, need for continuous infusion, moderate dissociation constants), they are quite sensitive to renal function and excretion. Finally, as many patients with ACS undergo percutaneous revascularization, it is important to separate primary (medical) treatment effects from those associated with percutaneous coronary intervention.

Primary Therapy vs PCI Effect

In the CAPTURE trial, abciximab was given the day prior to angioplasty among patients with unstable angina. In this 24-h interim before PTCA, 2.1% of placebo patients had an MI compared with 0.6% of the abciximab group (71% relative reduction). A larger number of MI events occurred during and immediately after the procedure, and these were reduced 58% by abciximab (Fig. 16). This early observation suggested that GPIIb/IIIa inhibitors have both a primary and PTCA-related treatment effect. Therefore, in considering the results of PARAGON A and B, PURSUIT, PRISM, PRISM-PLUS, and GUSTO-IV, one must also consider the primary and PTCA-related effects separately.

By protocol design, PARAGON A and GUSTO-IV did not allow PTCA during the first 48 h and 60 h, respectively, unless the patient had medically refractory angina. PRISM and PRISM-PLUS discouraged procedures before 48 h, and the PURSUIT design allowed usual clinical practice. Between 48 and 96 h, angiography and (if appropriate) angioplasty were encouraged in the PRISM-PLUS protocol. With these protocol differences, the rate of PTCA among the studies varied from 13 to 31% (Table 2). Because only 13 and 19% of patients in PARAGON A and GUSTO-IV, respectively, underwent angioplasty, and few of these patients were still receiving study drug, the strength of subgroup analyses is limited. Meaningful information is available from the other trials.

In PURSUIT, 24% of patients underwent percutaneous coronary revascularization. Roughly half of these patients (12.7% of total cohort) underwent intervention within 72 h of randomization and were therefore still receiving study drug. Among these 1228 patients,

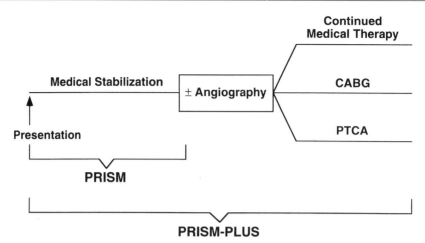

Fig. 17. Schematic of the study design timeline for the PRISM and PRISM-PLUS studies. In PRISM, percutaneous coronary revascularization (PTCA) was not recommended during the first 48 h, but was allowed thereafter, although administration of study drug was completed. PRISM-PLUS also did not recommend angiography in the first 48 h, although it was strongly recommended that angiography be performed along with angioplasty if possible during study drug infusion. (Data from refs. *20* and *21*.).

609 were in the eptifibatide group, and the composite of death and MI at 30-d follow-up was reduced by 30% compared with placebo (11.8% vs 16.8%, $p = 0.013$). As in the CAPTURE trial, the rate of preprocedural MIs was reduced by GPIIb/IIIa treatment (1.7% vs 5.5%). Considering then the remaining 8149 patients not undergoing early percutaneous revascularization in PURSUIT, the 30-d composite was relatively reduced 7% with eptifibatide (14.6% vs 15.7%, $p = 0.185$). Finally, patients who underwent late intervention (i.e., after discontinuation of eptifibatide) had no reduction in 30-d adverse events.

Since angiography and revascularization were discouraged in the first 48 h of PRISM, few of the 21% of the study cohort who had percutaneous revascularization were receiving study drug (Fig. 17). The 30-d composite of death and MI was reduced by 21% (7.2% vs 9.1%, p = NS) among those receiving prior or ongoing tirofiban. On the other hand, in those treated without percutaneous or surgical revascularization (i.e., medical management only), the composite was reduced 42% by tirofiban (3.6% vs 6.2%, $p < 0.05$). Finally, in PRISM-PLUS, in which percutaneous revascularization was encouraged during study drug infusion, 31% of the patients had angioplasty, and tirofiban reduced the 30-d death or MI composite by an impressive although nonsignificant 42% (5.9% vs 10.2%, p = NS) (Fig. 18). Among the 719 patients treated medically in PRISM-PLUS, tirofiban reduced the 30-d composite by 23% (7.8% vs 10.1%, p = NS). Overall, these data include 2357 patients undergoing PTCA, and prior or ongoing GPIIb/IIIa therapy reduced the 30-d composite of death or nonfatal MI by 30% (9.3% vs 13.3%). A smaller benefit was seen among the 10,867 patients treated without revascularization, as GPIIb/IIIa therapy relatively reduced the 30-d composite by 11% (12.1% vs 13.6%).

In the meta-analysis by Boersma and colleagues *(42)*, the six GPIIb/IIIa-unstable angina trials were analyzed for patients undergoing percutaneous coronary intervention within 5 d of enrollment versus those not undergoing percutaneous coronary intervention during

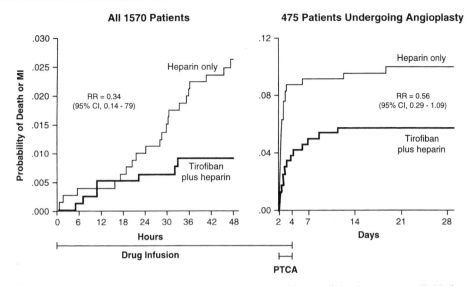

Fig. 18. Kaplan-Meier curves showing the cumulative incidence of death or myocardial infarction (MI) among patients randomly assigned to heparin or heparin plus tirofiban in PRISM-PLUS. The left panel shows events during the initial 48 h of medical stabilization and prior to recommended angiography and intervention. The right panel shows the incidence of death or myocardial infarction from the time of the procedure to 30 d. (From ref. *21*, with permission.)

this time. This analysis, therefore, reflects patients receiving a GPIIb/IIIa inhibitor at the time of percutaneous coronary intervention as well as those who had drug discontinued in the days prior. Regardless, patients who were randomized to GPIIb/IIIa therapy had a significantly lower likelihood of having an MI before revascularization. Of the 2421 patients undergoing percutaneous coronary intervention and receiving active therapy, 5.8% had a preprocedural MI vs 8.0% among the 1957 who underwent percutaneous coronary intervention and received placebo (odds ratio, 0.70; 95% CI, 0.55–0.89). These same subgroups had rates of 30-d death or MI of 11.8 and 14.5%, respectively (odds ratio, 0.77; 95% CI, 0.64–0.92). Thus, considering a somewhat selected cohort (i.e., those needing to undergo percutaneous coronary intervention during index hospitalization), there was an approx 28% reduction in preprocedural MI. A similar relative reduction was seen in 30-d death or MI. In assessing patients not undergoing percutaneous coronary intervention within 5 d, the meta-analysis included 15,876 patients receiving GPIIb/IIIa therapy and 11,148 patients receiving placebo. The 30-d death or MI composite for these two subgroups was 10.7 and 11.4%, respectively (odds ratio, 0.95; 95% CI, 0.87–1.02). This approx 6% relative risk reduction was not statistically significant.

The overall 9% relative reduction in death or MI at 30 d among these nearly 32,000 patients studied is similar to that reported for direct thrombin inhibitors or low-molecular-weight heparins tested against unfractionated heparin in ACSs. Likewise, the nearly 30% reduction seen in death or MI among those undergoing percutaneous revascularization is similar to that reported from other (interventional) studies testing GPIIb/IIIa inhibitors. Taken together, these observations confirm a primary treatment effect of GPIIb/IIIa on the ruptured plaque of unstable angina and an amplified benefit during further plaque disruption (i.e., angioplasty).

"Toxic Doses" vs Dose-Dependent Responses

Since most GPIIb/IIIa inhibitors are fully platelet-specific, "toxicity" has been manifest as excess bleeding. Fortunately, the overwhelming majority of bleeding is at the site of vascular puncture. Less commonly, gastrointestinal and genitourinary bleeding occur. On the other hand, the question has arisen of whether GPIIb/IIIa receptor antagonists can otherwise become "toxic." Several antithrombotics, such as heparin, hirudin, and fibrinolytics, have been associated with a narrow therapeutic window, and higher doses have been associated with both heightened bleeding and mortality. Among some GPIIb/IIIa trials, "high-dose" antagonism has been associated with an increase in bleeding and a neutral or negative effect on ischemic outcome. In IMPACT-II (*see* Chapter 6), angioplasty patients receiving the "higher dose" (0.75 µg/kg) eptifibatide infusion were found to have a similar or worse outcome compared with those receiving "lower dose" (0.5 µg/kg) eptifibatide or placebo. However, subsequent to this trial's completion, both eptifibatide doses were found to inhibit platelet function only modestly. Thus, rather than a toxic effect, the lack of demonstrated benefit from the higher dose regimen could be speculated to be from sampling error or toxic, procoagulant, or counterbalancing effects that remain to be illuminated.

The high-dose GPIIb/IIIa treatment arms of PARAGON A and PRISM-PLUS should have provided extensive platelet inhibition (>90% inhibition of ADP-induced aggregation). These also did not show benefit over low-dose treatment or placebo. Lamifiban at 5 µg/kg in the Canadian Lamifiban Study lowered 30-d death or nonfatal MI 70% compared with placebo. In this dose-exploring study, only 41 patients received the 5-µg/kg dose. In PARAGON, 769 patients received this dose, and the 30-d death or MI rate was 3% higher than placebo. A similar seeming discrepancy between trials with high-dose antagonists is seen with 0.6 µg/kg/min of tirofiban in PRISM and PRISM-PLUS. In PRISM, this high dose of antagonist without heparin reduced adverse events (death, MI, and refractory ischemia) by 32% at 48 h and by 7% at 30 d. These findings were considered favorable. On the other hand, this same dose of tirofiban in PRISM-PLUS was prematurely discontinued because of an increase in mortality at 7 d compared with placebo (4.6% vs 1.1%, respectively). At 30-d follow-up, the effect was statistically neutral (6.1% vs 4.0%, respectively) for this cohort. Thus, the question remains: why did high-dose tirofiban and lamifiban perform worse than their respective moderate doses and no better than placebo? These observations are in contrast to previous large studies of this class of antithrombotic therapy and suggests an upper limit of benefit or potential toxicity. Theoretical explanations for the apparent "toxicity" of high doses of tirofiban and lamifiban include intraplaque hemorrhage, paradoxic platelet activation, an interplay between excessive bleeding and clinical outcomes, or a question of chance.

The GUSTO-IV study importantly raised questions regarding toxicity of GPIIb/IIIa inhibitors. Similar to the administration of long-term oral GPIIb/IIIa inhibitors *(46)*, the 48-h administration of abciximab to medically treated patients with unstable angina led to a slightly worse outcome than those receiving placebo (Fig. 3). Of the 2612 patients receiving abciximab bolus and 48-h infusion, 9.1% died or had MI by 30 d. This was in contrast to the 8% rate among 2598 patients receiving placebo (odds ratio, 1.1; 95% CI, 0.94–1.39). Even patients who were troponin-positive at study enrollment received no benefit from the 48-h infusion of abciximab. Other than a reduction in mortality among diabetic patients, no other subgroup benefited (Fig. 12). These findings were quite disappointing and suggest again a partial agonist activity to these agents. Peter et al. *(47)* demonstrated antagonist-induced activation of the GPIIb/IIIa receptor with abciximab and small molecule agents. This occurs during trough periods or at low drug concentrations. Although this mechanism probably had an important consequence with oral therapy since recurrent trough levels occur between doses *(48)*, a similar phenomenon may have occurred with long-term abciximab administration. Steinhubl and colleagues *(48)* noted that a sizable proportion of patients fell to a relatively low level of aggregation inhibition at ≥8 h of abciximab infusion. These and other observations *(49)* suggest that there are counterbalancing forces associated with GPIIb/IIIa receptor antagonism, especially with longer term administration of these agents.

IIa/IIIa and Concomitant Heparin Thearpy

PARAGON was the only trial that factorially tested the benefit of antithrombin (heparin) therapy administered concomitantly with GPIIb/IIIa therapy. Overall, heparin provided no consistent benefit when combined with lamifiban. This may reflect the fact that bleeding events were increased among those receiving heparin with high-dose lamifiban but not with low-dose lamifiban. Likewise, at 30 d and 6 mo, the composite ischemic event rate was numerically highest among those receiving heparin with high-dose lamifiban and lowest for those receiving heparin with low-dose lamifiban. The group assigned to high-dose lamifiban with heparin had no improved parameter and had the highest percentage of patients discontinuing drug prematurely, usually because of bleeding or an ischemic event. In the 5-P trials, as well as in previous GPIIb/IIIa angioplasty studies, bleeding and adverse events were linked to the combination of potent platelet inhibition and full-dose heparin.

Although PARAGON A alone was not adequately powered to assess the extent of clinical benefit provided by concomitant heparin, collectively assessing these data in combination with other observations is helpful. These include the following findings: (1) the meta-analysis by Oler et al. *(50)*; (2) the largest relative benefit in the ACS trials was with moderate-dose tirofiban with heparin; (3) the intermediate-term benefit present in PRISM-PLUS with heparin added to tirofiban was not seen in PRISM's tirofiban without heparin group; and (4) PARAGON's low-dose lamifiban with heparin group had the best early, intermediate, and long-term outcomes. These findings suggest that heparin adds a modest benefit to antiplatelet therapy in ACS. Whether low-molecular-weight heparins added to GPIIb/IIIa antagonists will provide a more favorable risk/benefit ratio than unfractionated heparin, is the subject of ongoing clinical trials.

SUMMARY AND FUTURE DIRECTIONS

Despite contemporary medical therapies, patients presenting with unstable angina and electrocardiographic evidence of ischemia or serologic evidence of myocardial necrosis have a substantial 30-d rate of death or important nonfatal MI. Although antiplatelet agents such as aspirin, ticlopidine, and clopidogrel have substantially improved this outcome compared with placebo, intermediate and long-term follow-up shows that plaque passivation is not complete. The GPIIb/IIIa receptor antagonists are severalfold more potent than previous antiplatelet therapies, and they have been shown to be markedly beneficial in making the plaque disruption of percutaneous coronary revascularization quiescent. The PARAGON A and B, PRISM, PRISM-PLUS, and PURSUIT trials have alone and collectively demonstrated a reduction in ischemic events beyond that of aspirin and heparin therapy with intravenous GPIIb/IIIa antagonists. These agents reduce the 30-d occurrence of death or MI by approx 10% and this benefit is durable at late (6-mo to 1-yr) follow-up.

These concepts are embodied within the most recent ACC/AHA treatment guidelines for patients with an ACS *(51)*. Intravenous GPIIb/IIIa antagonists have a class I recommendation (majority of evidence and agreement supporting use) for patients in whom catheterization and percutaneous coronary intervention are planned. A class IIa recommendation (conflicting evidence or opinion although weight of evidence/opinion favors usefulness) is given for eptifibatide and tirofiban for high-risk patients (i.e., continuing ischemia or troponin-positive) in whom an invasive strategy is not planned or percutaneous coronary intervention patients who are already receiving aspirin and clopidogrel. Abciximab receives similar recommendation for percutaneous coronary intervention patients but receives a class III recommendation (evidence that it is not useful) for patients in whom percutaneous coronary intervention is not planned. In short, the benefit of GPIIb/IIIa agents appears to be highest among patients who have active atherothrombotic plaques, evidence of myonecrosis, or diabetes or who are treated aggressively with early percutaneous revascularization.

REFERENCES

1. Fuster V, Chesebro JH. Mechanisms of unstable angina. N Engl J Med 1986;315:1023–1025.
2. Moliterno DJ, Aguirre FV, Cannon CP, et al., for the GUARANTEE Investigators. The Global Unstable Angina Registry and Treatment Evaluation. Circulation 1996;94:I.
3. Willerson JT, Golino P, Eidt J, Campbell WB, Buja LM. Specific platelet mediators and unstable coronary artery lesions: experimental evidence and potential clinical implications. Circulation 1989;80: 198–205.
4. Coller BS. The role of platelets in arterial thrombosis and the rationale for blockade of platelet GP IIb/ IIIa receptors as antithrombotic therapy. Eur Heart J 1995;16(Suppl L):11–15.
5. Théroux P, Ouimet H, McCans J, et al. Aspirin, heparin, or both to treat acute unstable angina. N Engl J Med 1988;319:1105–1111.
6. The RISC Group. Risk of myocardial infarction and death during treatment with low dose aspirin and intravenous heparin in men with unstable coronary artery disease. Lancet 1990;336:827–830.
7. Wallentin LC, and the Research Group on Instability in Coronary Artery Disease in Southeast Sweden. Aspirin (75 mg/day) after an episode of unstable coronary artery disease: long-term effects on the risk for myocardial infarction, occurrence of severe angina and the need for revascularization. J Am Coll Cardiol 1991;18:1587–1593.
8. Cairns JA, Gent M, Singer J, et al. Aspirin, sulfinpyrazone, or both in unstable angina. N Engl J Med 1985; 313:1369–1375.
9. Lewis HDJ, Davis JW, Archibald DG, et al. Protective effects of aspirin against acute myocardial infarction and death in men with unstable angina. N Engl J Med 1983;309:396–403.
10. Antiplatelet Trialists' Collaboration. Collaborative overview of randomised trials of antiplatelet therapy —I. Prevention of death, myocardial infarction, and stroke by prolonged antiplatelet therapy in various categories of patients. BMJ 1994;308:81–106.
11. Antithrombotic Trialists' Collaboration. Collaborative meta-analysis of randomised trials of antiplatelet therapy for prevention of death, myocardial infarction, and stroke in high risk patients. BMJ 2002;324: 71–86.
12. Maffrand JP, Bernat A, Delebasse D, Defreyen G, Cazenave JP, Gordon JL. ADP plays a key role in thrombogenesis in rats. Thromb Haemost 1988;59:225–230.
13. De Minno G, Cerbone AM, Mattioli PL, Turco S, Iovine C, Mancini M. Functionally thrombosthenic state in normal platelets following the administration of ticlopidine. J Clin Invest 1985;75:328–338.
14. Panak E, Maffrand JP, Picard-Fraire C, Vallee E, Blanchard J, Roncucci R. Ticlopidine: a promise for the prevention and treatment of thrombosis and its complications. Haemostasis 1983;13(Suppl 1):1–54.
15. Balsano F, Rizzon P, Violi F, et al., and the Studio della Ticlopidina nell'Angina Instabile Group. Antiplatelet treatment with ticlopidine in unstable angina. A controlled multicenter clinical trial. Circulation 1990;82:17–26.

16. CAPRIE Steering Commitee. A randomised, blinded, trial of clopidogrel versus aspirin in patients at risk of ischaemic events (CAPRIE). Lancet 1996;348:1329–1339.

17. The Clopidogrel in Unstable Angina to Prevent Recurrent Events Trial Investigators. Effects of clopidogrel in addition to aspirin in patients with acute coronary syndromes without ST-segment elevation. N Engl J Med 2001;345:494–502.

18. The Platelet IIb/IIIa Antagonist for the Reduction of Acute Coronary Syndrome Events in a Global Organization Network (PARAGON)-B Investigators. Randomized, placebo-controlled trial of titrated intravenous lamifiban for acute coronary syndromes. Circulation 2002;105:316–321.

19. The PARAGON Investigators. An international, randomized, controlled trial of lamifiban, a platelet glycoprotein IIb/IIIa inhibitor, heparin, or both in unstable angina. Circulation 1998;97:2386–2395.

20. The Platelet Receptor Inhibition in Ischemic Syndrome Management (PRISM) Study Investigators. A comparison of aspirin plus tirofiban with aspirin plus heparin for unstable angina. N Engl J Med 1998; 338:1498–1505.

21. The Platelet Receptor Inhibition in Ischemic Syndrome Management in Patients Limited by Unstable Signs and Symptoms (PRISM-PLUS) Study Investigators. Inhibition of the platelet glycoprotein IIb/IIIa receptor with tirofiban in unstable angina and non-Q-wave myocardial infarction. N Engl J Med 1998; 338:1488–1497.

22. The PURSUIT Trial Investigators. Inhibition of platelet glycoprotein IIb/IIIa with eptifibatide in patients with acute coronary syndromes. N Engl J Med 1998;339:436–463.

23. The GUSTO IV-ACS Investigators. Effect of glycoprotein IIb/IIIa receptor blocker abciximab on outcome in patients with acute coronary syndromes without early coronary revascularisation: the GUSTO IV-ACS randomised trial. Lancet 2001;357:1915–1924.

24. The EPIC Investigators. Use of a monoclonal antibody directed against the platelet glycoprotein IIb/IIIa receptor in high-risk coronary angioplasty. N Engl J Med 1994;330:956–961.

25. The EPILOG Investigators. Platelet glycoprotein IIb/IIIa receptor blockade and low-dose heparin during percutaneous coronary revascularization. N Engl J Med 1997;336:1689–1696.

26. Lincoff AM, Califf RM, Anderson KM, et al. Evidence for prevention of death and myocardial infarction with platelet membrane glycoprotein IIb/IIIa receptor blockade by abciximab (c7E3 Fab) among patients with unstable angina undergoing percutaneous coronary revascularization. J Am Coll Cardiol 1997;30:149–156.

27. Topol EJ, Ferguson JJ, Weisman HF, et al., on behalf of the EPIC Investigators. Long term protection from myocardial ischemic events in a randomized trial of brief integrin β3 blockade wwith percutaneous intervention. JAMA 1997;278:479–484.

28. The EPISTENT Investigators. Randomised placebo-controlled and balloon-angioplasty-controlled trial to assess safety of coronary stenting with use of platelet glycoprotein-IIb/IIIa blockade. The EPISTENT Investigators. Evaluation of platelet IIb/IIIa inhibitor for stenting. Lancet 1998;352:87–92.

29. The CAPTURE Investigators. Randomised placebo-controlled trial of abciximab before and during coronary interventions in refractory unstable angina: the CAPTURE study. Lancet 1997;349:1429–1435.

30. Topol EJ, Moliterno DJ, Herrmann HC, et al. Comparison of two platelet glycoprotein IIb/IIIa inhibitors, tirofiban and abciximab, for the prevention of ischemic events with percutaneous coronary revascularization. N Engl J Med 2001;344:1888–1894.

31. Stone G, Moliterno D, Bertrand M, et al. Impact of clinical syndrome acuity on the differential response to 2 glycoprotein IIb/IIIa Inhibitors in patients undergoing coronary stenting. The TARGET Trial. Circulation 2002;105:2347–2354.

32. Théroux P, Kouz S, Roy L, et al., on behalf of the Investigators. Platelet membrane receptor glycoprotein IIb/IIIa antagonism in unstable angina. The Candian Lamifiban Study. Circulation 1996;94:899–905.

33. Topol EJ, Califf RM, Van de Werf F, et al. Perspectives on large-scale cardiovascular clinical trials for the new millennium. Circulation 1997;95:1072–1082.

34. Steiner B, Hofer U, Wittke B, et al. Plasma concentrations of lamifiban and glycoprotein IIb-IIIa receptor occupancy best predict clinical outcome in patients with unstable angina: results from PARAGON A. Eur Heart J 1998;19(abstract):598.

35. Moliterno DJ. Patient-specific dosing of IIb/IIIa antagonists during acute coronary syndromes: rationale and design of the PARAGON B study. The PARAGON B International Steering Committee. Am Heart J 2000;139:563–566.

36. Théroux P, Kouz S, Roy L., et al. Platelet membrane receptor glycoprotein IIb/IIIa antagonism in unstable angina. The Canadian Lamifiban Study. Circulation 1996;94:899–905.

37. Schulman SP, Goldschmidt-Clermont PJ, Topol EJ, et al. Effects of Integrelin, a platelet glycoprotein IIb/IIIa receptor antagonist, in unstable angina: a randomized multicenter trial. Circulation 1996;94:2083–2089.

38. Phillips DR, Teng W, Arfsten A, et al. Effect of Ca^{2+} on GP IIb-IIIa binding and inhibition of platelet aggregation by reductions in the concentration of ionized calcium in plasma anticoagulated with citrate. Circulation 1997;96:1488–1494.

39. Moliterno DJ, Topol EJ. Meta-analysis of platelet GP IIb/IIIa antagonist randomized clinical trials: consistent, durable, salutary effects. Circulation 1997;96:I–475.

40. Topol EJ. Toward a new frontier in myocardial reperfusion therapy: emerging platelet preeminence. Circulation 1997;97:211–218.

41. Kong DF, Califf RM, Miller DP, et al. Clinical outcomes of therapeutic agents that block the platelet glycoprotein inhibitor integrin in ischemic heart disease. Circulation 1998;98:2829–2935.

42. Boersma E, Harrington R, Moliterno D, et al. Platelet glycoprotein IIb/IIIa inhibitors in acute coronary syndromes: a meta-analysis of all major randomised clinical trials. Lancet 2002;359:189–198.

43. Roffi M, Chew D, Mukherjee D, et al. Platelet glycoprotein IIb/IIIa inhibitors reduce mortality in diabetic patients with non-ST-segment-elevation acute coronary syndromes. Circulation 2001;104:2767–2771.

44. Newby L, Ohman E, Christenson R, et al., for the PARAGON-B Investigators. Benefit of glycoprotein IIb/IIIa inhibition in patients with acute coronary syndromes and troponin T-positive status. The PARAGON-B Troponin T Substudy. Circulation 2001;103:2891–2896.

45. Heeschen C, Hamm CW, Goldmann B, Deu A, Langenbrink L, White HD. Troponin concentrations for stratification of patients with acute coronary syndromes in relation to therapeutic efficacy of tirofiban. PRISM Study Investigators. Platelet receptor inhibition in ischemic syndrome management. Lancet 1999; 354:1757–1762.

46. Chew DP, Bhatt DL, Sapp S, Topol EJ. Increased mortality with oral platelet glycoprotein IIb/IIIa antagonists: a meta-analysis of phase III multicenter randomized trials. Circulation 2001;103:201–206.

47. Peter K, Schwarz M, Ylanne J, et al. Induction of fibrinogen binding and platelet aggregation as a potential intrinsic property of various glycoprotein IIb/IIIa (alphaIIbbeta3) inhibitors. Blood 1998;92: 3240–3249.

48. Steinhubl SR, Kottke-Marchant K, Moliterno DJ, et al. Attainment and maintenance of platelet inhibition through standard dosing of abciximab in diabetic and nondiabetic patients undergoing percutaneous coronary intervention. Circulation 1999;100:1977–1982.

49. Chew DP, Moliterno DJ. A critical appraisal of platelet glycoprotein IIb/IIIa inhibition. J Am Coll Cardiol 2000;36:2028–2035.

50. Oler A, Whooley MA, Oler J, Grady D. Adding heparin to aspirin reduces the incidence of myocardial infarction and deat in patients with unstable angina: a meta-analysis. JAMA 1996;2276:811–815.

51. Braunwald E, Antman E, Beasley J, et al. ACC/AHA guideline update for the management of patients with unstable angina and non-ST-segment elevation myocardial infarction-2002: summary article: a report of the American College of Cardiology/American Heart Association Task Force on Practice Guidelines (Committee on the Management of Patients With Unstable Angina). Circulation 2002;106:1893–1900.

11

Platelet Glycoprotein IIb/IIIa Inhibitors and an Invasive Strategy

Christopher P. Cannon, MD

CONTENTS

INTRODUCTION
CLINICAL TRIALS
BENEFITS OF GPIIb/IIIa INHIBITION BY TREATMENT STRATEGY
TARGETING HIGH-RISK ACS PATIENTS
TACTICS-TIMI 18
ANGIOGRAPHIC OBSERVATIONS:
    ESTABLISHING THE MECHANISM OF BENEFIT
SAFETY ISSUES
COST EFFECTIVENESS
CONCLUSIONS
REFERENCES

INTRODUCTION

With the importance of plaque rupture and thrombosis in acute coronary syndromes (ACS) and the problem of distal embolization during percutaneous coronary intervention (PCI) *(1)*, inhibition of platelet aggregation by platelet glycoprotein (GP) IIb/IIIa receptor antagonists has taken on a central role. By preventing the final common pathway of platelet aggregation, i.e., fibrinogen-mediated crosslinkage of platelets via the GPIIb/IIIa receptor, these agents can potently inhibit platelet aggregation caused by all types of stimuli (e.g., thrombin, ADP, collagen, and others). Three agents, abciximab, tirofiban, and eptifibatide, are now approved for use in coronary angioplasty, and the latter two are also approved for treatment of unstable angina/non-ST elevation myocardial infarction (UA/NSTEMI) in patients not necessarily undergoing angioplasty. Abciximab is a monoclonal antibody Fab fragment directed at the GPIIb/IIIa receptor. Eptifibatide, a synthetic heptapeptide, and tirofiban, a nonpeptide molecule, are antagonists of the GPIIb/IIIa receptor whose structure mimics the arginine-glycine-aspartic acid (abbreviated RGD) amino acid sequence by which fibrinogen binds to the GPIIb/IIIa receptor.

From: *Contemporary Cardiology: Platelet Glycoprotein IIb/IIIa*
Inhibitors in Cardiovascular Disease, 2nd Edition
Edited by: A. M. Lincoff © Humana Press Inc., Totowa, NJ

CLINICAL TRIALS

Several trials have shown benefit of GPIIb/IIIa inhibition in UA/NSTEMI in patients managed predominantly with medical management *(2,3)*, early interventional management *(4)* or, both *(5–8)*. In the Platelet Receptor Inhibition for Ischemic Syndrome Management in Patients Limited by Unstable Signs and Symptoms (PRISM-PLUS) trial, tirofiban plus heparin and aspirin significantly reduced the odds of death, myocardial infarction (MI), or refractory ischemia at 7 d by 32% compared with heparin plus aspirin *(5)*. In the Platelet Glycoprotein IIb/IIIa in Unstable Angina: Receptor Suppression Using Integrilin Therapy (PURSUIT) trial, involving 10,948 patients, eptifibatide also significantly reduced the rate of death or MI at 30 d *(6)*. A meta-analysis of the first 10 trials, involving over 30,000 patients, found that treatment with a GPIIb/IIIa inhibitor led to a 21% reduction in death or MI at 30 d *(7,8)*.

More recently the Global Utilization of Strategies to Open Occluded Coronary Arteries (GUSTO) IV-ACS trial, no benefit was observed with abciximab treatment in patients managed conservatively *(9)*. One explanation put forth to explain these results is that the dose of the abciximab infusion may have been too low, which led to suboptimal levels of platelet inhibition. When this trial was added to the meta-analysis, along with the the Platelet IIb/IIIa Antagonist for the Reduction of Acute Coronary Syndrome Events in a Global Organization Network (PARAGON) B trial *(10)*, the overall benefit of the GPIIb/IIIa inhibitors in ACS became only 9% reduction in death or MI overall *(3)*. However, the GUSTO-IV-ACS trial and the recent meta-analysis have led some to question the overall efficacy of GPIIb/IIIa inhibition in patients treated medically.

BENEFITS OF GPIIb/IIIa
INHIBITION BY TREATMENT STRATEGY

In the overall trial results and the meta-analyses, it has been noted that in general, the relative treatment benefit of GPIIb/IIIa inhibition appears to be greater in those undergoing PCI vs those having medical therapy alone. For example, in the EPISTENT trial of abciximab, there was a relative 50% benefit regarding death or MI *(11)*, vs a 10% overall benefit in the PURSUIT trial *(6)*. Similarly, in the PURSUIT trial, in an unadjusted analysis, a greater benefit was observed in patients who underwent early PCI on eptifibatide (31% reduction in death or MI at 30 d, 16.7% vs 11.6%, $p = 0.01$), whereas the relative benefit was less (7% reduction, $p = 0.23$) in those treated medically, with late PCI or coronary artery bypass graft (CABG).

However, much of this apparent difference may have been caused by confounding, i.e., the patients selected for PCI may have been those with a greater thrombotic burden and thus more to gain from this antithrombotic therapy. Indeed, a more careful statistical analysis, counting all patients up to the time of a procedure, found no significant interaction of PCI vs no PCI in the relative benefit of the GPIIb/IIIa inhibitor *(12)*. In addition, a dramatic benefit has been seen in patients who eventually went on to bypass surgery *(13)*. In the PRISM-PLUS trial, the overall reduction in death or MI at 30 d was 30% ($p = 0.03$), with improvement being consistent across management strategies: medical therapy (25% reduction), PCI (35% reduction), and bypass surgery (30% reduction).

The relative benefits of GPIIb/IIIa inhibition in regard to medical vs interventional treatment have been examined in a pooling of data from PRISM-PLUS, PURSUIT, and CAP-

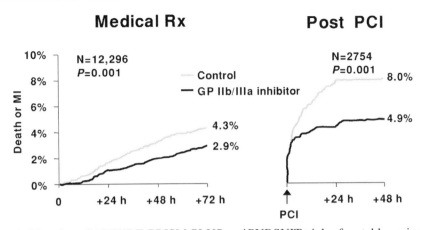

Fig. 1. Pooled data from CAPTURE, PRISM-PLUS, and PURSUIT trials of unstable angina, showing benefit of GPIIb/IIIa inhibition during medical therapy only (left) and during and immediately following PCI (right). (From ref. *14*, with permission.)

TURE involving 12,296 patients; there was a 34% relative reduction in death or MI during a period of 24 h of medical management only (3.8% vs 2.5%, *p* = 0.001) (Fig. 1) *(14)*. An additional benefit was seen when the agents were continued during angioplasty (8.0% vs 4.9%, *p* = 0.001). Looking more broadly at the trials, among patients who undergo PCI, in those with ACS the benefit of GPIIb/IIIa inhibition is quite dramatic, with reductions of death or MI ranging from 30 to 70% (Fig. 2). Thus, GPIIb/IIIa inhibition is beneficial for the medically treated patients and appears to have an additional benefit in patients in whom the drug is continued through PCI.

TARGETING HIGH-RISK ACS PATIENTS

The overall benefit of early GPIIb/IIIa inhibition in UA/NSTEMI can be increased when it is applied to appropriately risk-stratified patients. This has been seen most dramatically in patients with elevated troponin values. These patients are at a two- to threefold higher risk of subsequent cardiac complications, including mortality *(15–20)*. Elevated markers have been shown to correlate with a higher rate of thrombus at angiography *(21,22)*, and worse TIMI flow grade in the culprit artery, as well as worse myocardial perfusion *(22)*. It has further been observed that a greater antithrombotic effect is observed in these groups: for example, the degree of resolution of thrombus after 24 h of therapy with abciximab in the CAPTURE trial was greater in those who were troponin-T-positive vs negative *(19)*.

Clinical benefits have followed the same pattern. The reduction in death or MI at 6 mo in the CAPTURE trial was 70% in those who were troponin-T-positive vs no significant benefit for those who were troponin-T-negative (*p* < 0.001) *(19)* (Fig. 3A). These findings have been duplicated with tirofiban vs heparin in the PRISM trial (Fig. 3B) *(23,24)*. Idenical findings of a 50–70% reduction in death or MI was seen in the PARAGON B and PRISM-PLUS troponin substudies *(24,25)*. Thus, four independent trials confirmed the very large (approx 70%) benefit of GPIIb/IIIa inhibition in troponin-positive patients.

A similar pattern of benefit has been seen with other markers of increased risk, including the TIMI risk score, ST-segment changes, and diabetes in the PRISM-PLUS trial *(5,26,27)*.

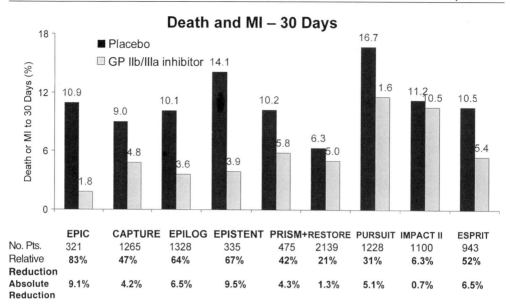

Fig. 2. Benefit of GPIIb/IIIa inhibition among patients with UA/NSTEMI treated with percutaneous coronary intervention across all large trials. As shown, both the relative benefit and the absolute benefit are quite substantial, ranging from 50 to 100 deaths or MIs prevented for every 1000 patients treated. (Adapted from ref. *50*, with data from ref. *51*.)

Another important point, however, is that the dramatic benefit of GPIIb/IIIa inhibition found in the high-risk patient groups is seen regardless of the treatment strategy. In the PRISM study, there was the same approx 70% reduction in death or MI at 30 d in patients who had baseline positive troponin values, regardless of whether or not they underwent revascularization *(23)*. Similarly, and more recently, the benefit of GPIIb/IIIa inhibition was seen in those with a TIMI risk score of 4 or higher, regardless of whether they had PCI or not *(26)*. Thus, in ACS, the benefit of GPIIb/IIIa inhibition appears to relate to the patient's risk and not necessarily to the treatment strategy used.

TACTICS-TIMI 18

Further validation of the benefit of GPIIb/IIIa inhibition in the overall management of UA/NSTEMI comes from the Treat Angina with Aggrastat® and Determine Cost of Therapy with an Invasive or Conservative Strategy (TACTICS)-TIMI 18 trial. In this trial, patients with a typical history of UA/NSTEMI, with either electrocardiographic changes, positive cardiac markers, or a history of coronary disease were all treated with aspirin, heparin, and the GPIIb/IIIa inhibitor tirofiban for 48 h, including ≥12 h following PCI. Patients were randomized to either an early invasive strategy with coronary angiography between 4 and 48 h after randomization and revascularization when feasible, or to a conservative strategy whereby angiography was reserved only for patients with rest ischemia or a positive stress test (which included nuclear perfusion imaging or echocardiography in approx 85% of patients).

Overall, there was a significant reduction with the invasive approach in the primary endpoint, death, MI, or rehospitalization for an ACS at 6 mo: 15.9% in early invasive strategy

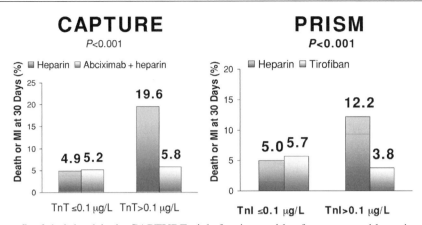

Fig. 3. Benefit of abciximab in the CAPTURE trial of patients with refractory unstable angina treated with angioplasty in those with positive vs negative troponin T (TnT) levels at study entry (left). Greater benefit of tirofiban vs heparin in patients with UA/NSTEMI was also seen those with positive troponin I values in the PRISM trial, with a nearly 70% reduction in death or MI at 30 d with the GPIIb/IIIa inhibitor (right). (Data from refs. *19* and *23*.)

vs 19.4% in the conservative group [odds ratio (OR) 0.78, $p = 0.025$] *(28)*. Death or MI at 30 d was also significantly reduced at 30 d, (4.7% vs 7.0%, respectively, $p = 0.02$), as well as at 6 mo ($p = 0.0498$).

When comparing these data with those of the four prior randomized trials of invasive vs conservative strategies *(29–34)*, an interesting difference emerges. In the trials without GPIIb/IIIa inhibition, the rate of MI tended to be higher in the invasive group over the first 2 wk, consistent with an "early hazard" associated with coronary interventions. In contrast, in TACTICS-TIMI 18, there was a significantly *lower* rate of MI over the first weeks, an effect that is probably owing to the well-documented protection afforded by GPIIb/IIIa inhibition during PCI *(8)*.

As seen for GPIIb/IIIa inhibition, a significantly greater benefit was found in patients with positive troponin values compared with those who had negative values *(28)*. In patients with a troponin T > 0.01 ng/mL (54% of the population) or in those with troponin T ≥ 0.1 ng/mL (60% of the population), there was a relative 39% risk reduction in the primary endpoint with the invasive vs conservative strategy (each $p < 0.001$), whereas patients with a negative troponin level had similar outcomes with either strategy *(35)*. Death or nonfatal MI also followed the same pattern, with a significant reduction with the invasive strategy in patients with positive troponin levels vs no benefit in those with negative troponin levels. The same pattern of benefit was seen in higher risk patients, defined by the presence of ST-segment changes or a TIMI risk score of 3 or higher.

This study demonstrates that among patients with UA/NSTEMI who were treated with the GPIIb/IIIa inhibitor tirofiban, an early invasive strategy was superior to a conservative strategy in reducing major cardiac events at 30 d and 6 mo. In addition, the absolute rate of death or MI at 30 d in the invasive group, 4.7%, is the lowest observed rate in any UA/NSTEMI trial to date *(5,6,8,36)*. Thus, this strategy of using "upstream" GPIIb/IIIa inhibition with tirofiban in combination with early invasive treatment leads to excellent outcomes and could be considered the treatment of choice for most UA/NSTEMI patients.

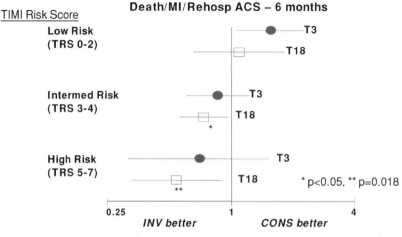

Fig. 4. Comparison of event rates in the TIMI 3 vs TACTICS-TIMI 18 trials stratified by the TIMI risk score (TRS). ACS, acute coronary syndrome; CONS, conservative; INV, invasive; MI, myocardial infarction. (Data from ref. *37*.)

An analysis of the contribution of GPIIb/IIIa inhibition toward improving outcomes in high-risk ACS patients was done by comparing results from TIMI III (the first trial of an invasive vs conservative strategy) with those from TACTICS-TIMI 18. In both TIMI III and TACTICS-TIMI 18, inclusion and exclusion criteria were similar, but in TIMI III, the medical treatment consisted of only aspirin, heparin, and antiischemic therapy. In TACTICS-TIMI 18, patients also received tirofiban. In addition, stents were used in 85% of the patients undergoing PCI in TACTICS-TIMI 18 vs none of the patients in TIMI III.

When patients were stratified by the TIMI risk score, an interesting pattern emerged: a consistently better outcome was seen in the TACTICS-TIMI 18 trial compared with the TIMI III trial in each of the risk strata (Fig. 4) *(37)*. In low-risk patients in TIMI III, the incidence of death, MI, or rehospitalization after 6 mo was significantly worse among patients randomized to the invasive strategy arm, whereas in TACTICS-TIMI 18, event rates among low-risk patients were approximately the same for both treatment strategies. For intermediate-risk patients, outcomes for the invasive vs the conservative group were roughly equal in TIMI III, whereas they were significantly better for the invasive vs conservative strategy in TACTICS-TIMI 18. Finally, although a trend was seen for improved outcomes among high-risk patients treated invasively in the TIMI III trial, in TACTICS-TIMI 18, there was a dramatic, 10% absolute reduction in events. These differences are consistent with the main hypothesis of the trial, that the new advances in cardiology of coronary stenting and GPIIb/IIIa inhibition would improve the safety of the early invasive strategy and lead to an overall benefit compared with a conservative approach.

ANGIOGRAPHIC OBSERVATIONS: ESTABLISHING THE MECHANISM OF BENEFIT

Angiographic data from three trials show that the GPIIb/IIIa inhibitors lead to greater resolution of thrombus and improved coronary flow compared with aspirin and heparin alone *(38–40)*. In the PRISM-PLUS trial, the percentage of patients who had definitive thrombus was reduced from 24 to 17%, and there was a 23% improvement in overall thrombus grade ($p = 0.022$) *(39)*. In addition, administration of tirofiban led to a 35% overall improvement in TIMI flow grade ($p = 0.002$), with TIMI grade 3 flow improving from 74.5 to 81.9% *(39)*. Similar data have recently been found in the TACTICS-TIMI 18 trial, in which longer duration of therapy produced greater resolution of thrombus *(40)*. Together, these data establish the pathophysiologic link among the potent platelet inhibition achieved by the GPIIb/IIIa inhibitors, reduction in thrombus, improvement in coronary blood flow, and consequent improvement in clinical outcome for patients.

GPIIb/IIIa inhibitors have also been shown to reduce the size of an evolving non-ST-elevation MI, with evidence from three trials. In the PRISM-PLUS troponin substudy, among patients with a positive troponin at study entry, those randomized to tirofiban plus heparin had a significantly lower peak troponin *(41)*. In the PURSUIT trial, when looking at either index or recurrent MI during the first 72 h, it was observed that the size of the MI, measured by peak creatine kinase (CK)-MB, was significantly smaller in patients treated with eptifibatide *(42)*. In the prospective EARLY trial, preliminary data show that among those treated within the first 8 h, the infarct size determined by CK-MB curve fitting was smaller in those treated with early eptifibatide *(43)*. Thus, aggressive GPIIb/IIIa inhibition appears to be able to reduce the size of the infarct among patients with evolving non-ST-elevation MI.

Interestingly, GPIIb/IIIa inhibition appears to have a greater benefit when treatment is initiated earlier relative to the onset of pain. In an analysis from PURSUIT, the absolute reduction in death or MI of eptifibatide was 2.8% for patients treated within 6 h from the onset of pain and was lower for those treated between 6 and 12 and 12 and 24 h after onset of pain *(44)*. No benefit was observed in patients treated 24 h after onset of pain.

SAFETY ISSUES

As for all antithrombotic agents, the risk of major hemorrhage is modestly increased for patients treated with GPIIb/IIIa inhibitors. In PRISM-PLUS, major bleeding occurred in 4.0% of patients treated with tirofiban plus heparin plus aspirin vs 3.0% for heparin plus aspirin, $p = $ NS *(5)*. For eptifibatide, the rates of severe or moderate bleeding for eptifibatide vs placebo were 12.8% vs 9.9% ($p < 0.001$) *(6)*.

Thrombocytopenia is another side effect with GPIIb/IIIa inhibitors. For tirofiban in PRISM-PLUS, the rate of severe thrombocytopenia (<50,000 cells/mm^3) was 0.5% vs 0.3% for heparin, $p = 0.44$). The latter event is associated with increased bleeding and (in a smaller proportion of patients) recurrent thrombotic events *(45,46)*. This syndrome bears a resemblance to heparin-induced thrombocytopenia and indicates a need to monitor platelet count daily during the GPIIb/IIIa infusion.

COST EFFECTIVENESS

Thus, evidence from the major trials has shown that GPIIb/IIIa inhibition in patients with UA/NSTEMI leads to significant reductions in major cardiac events, regardless of whether an invasive or conservative strategy is employed. In the trials to date, patients enrolled have been at medium to higher risk, on the basis of rest pain and either electrocardiographic changes or positive cardiac markers. Although these agents are more expensive than heparin therapy, the cost is balanced by a reduction in recurrent cardiac events. A cost-effectiveness analysis from PURSUIT found that the cost per year of life saved was approx $16,000, well within the generally acceptable range for medical interventions *(47)*. As noted above in the section on risk stratification, benefit appears to be greatest in patients at higher risk, as evidenced by those who have a positive troponin level at baseline *(19,23)*, those with diabetes *(27)*, or recurrent angina, or those with prior aspirin use *(48)*. In these high-risk subgroups of patients, the absolute benefit is greater and the therapy is even more cost-effective.

A recent analysis from TACTICS-TIMI 18 has shown that the overall strategy of early GPIIb/IIIa inhibition and an invasive strategy was very cost-effective relative to a conservative strategy *(49)*. Estimated cost per year of life gained for the invasive strategy, based on projected life expectancy, was approx $17,000. In high-risk patients with a positive troponin level or ST-segment changes, these figures were. Thus, in patients with UA/NSTEMI treated with the GPIIb/IIIa inhibitor tirofiban, the clinical benefit of an early invasive strategy is achieved with a small increase in cost, yielding very favorable projected estimates of cost per year of life gained. These results provide further support for the broader use of an early invasive strategy utilizing early GPIIb/IIIa inhibition with tirofiban.

CONCLUSIONS

GPIIb/IIIa inhibition has been shown to be beneficial in patients with UA/NSTEMI, regardless of the treatment strategy ultimately used. However, those who are managed invasively have a double benefit—that achieved during the medical treatment phase and that achieved during a PCI. Accordingly, the 2002 American College of Cardiology/American Heart Association Guidelines for UA/NSTEMI present a class I recommendation (and level of evidence A) that GPIIb/IIIa inhibition be used in patients managed with an invasive strategy. For high-risk patients, these guidelines recommend an invasive strategy, and thus GPIIb/IIIa inhibition should be used. However, if a high-risk patient is managed conservatively, the guidelines give a class IIa recommendation for the use of GPIIb/IIIa inhibition.

REFERENCES

1. Topol EJ, Yadav JS. Recognition of the importance of embolization in atherosclerotic vascular disease. Circulation 2000;101:570–580.
2. The Platelet Receptor Inhibition for Ischemic Syndrome Management (PRISM) Study Investigators. A comparison of aspirin plus tirofiban with aspirin plus heparin for unstable angina. N Engl J Med 1998; 338:1498–1505.
3. Boersma E, Harrington RA, Moliterno DJ, et al. Platelet glycoprotein IIb/IIIa inhibitors in acute coronary syndromes: a meta-analysis of all major randomised clinical trials. Lancet 2002;359:189–198.
4. The CAPTURE Investigators. Randomised placebo-controlled trial of abciximab before and during coronary intervention in refractory unstable angina: the CAPTURE study. Lancet 1997;349:1429–1435 [published erratum appears in Lancet 1997;350:744].
5. The Platelet Receptor Inhibition for Ischemic Syndrome Management in Patients Limited by Unstable Signs and Symptoms (PRISM-PLUS) Trial Investigators. Inhibition of the platelet glycoprotein IIb/IIIa receptor with tirofiban in unstable angina and non-Q-wave myocardial infarction. N Engl J Med 1998; 338:1488–1497.
6. The PURSUIT Trial Investigators. Inhibition of platelet glycoprotein IIb/IIIa with eptifibatide in patients with acute coronary syndromes. N Engl J Med 1998;339:436–443.
7. Topol EJ, Byzova TV, Plow ER. Platelet GPIIb-IIIa blockers. Lancet 1999;353:227–231.
8. Kong DF, Califf RM, Miller DP, et al. Clinical outcomes of therapeutic agents that block the platelet glycoprotein IIb/IIIa integrin in ischemic heart disease. Circulation 1998;98:2829–2835.

9. The GUSTO IV-ACS Investigators. Effect of glycoprotein IIb/IIIa receptor blocker abciximab on out-come in patients with acute coronary syndromes without early coronary revascularisation: the GUSTO IV-ACS randomised trial. Lancet 2001;357:1915–1924.

10. The Platelet IIb/IIIa Antagonist for the Reduction of Acute Coronary Syndrome Events in a Global Organization Network (PARAGON)-B Investigators. Randomized, placebo-controlled trial of titrated intra-venous lamifiban for acute coronary syndromes. Circulation 2002;105:316–321.

11. The EPISTENT Investigators. Randomised placebo-controlled and balloon-angioplasty-controlled trial to assess the safety of coronary stenting with use of platelet glycoprotein-IIb/IIIa blockade. Lancet 1998; 352:87–92.

12. Kleiman NS, Lincoff AM, Flaker GC, et al., for the PURSUIT Investigators. Early percutaneous coro-nary intervention, platelet inhibition with eptifibatide, and clinical outcomes in patients with acute coro-nary syndromes. Circulation 2000;101:751–757.

13. Marso SP, Bhatt DL, Roe MT, et al. Enhanced efficacy of eptifibatide administration in patients with acute coronary syndrome requiring in-hospital coronary artery bypass grafting. Circulation 2000;102: 2952–2958.

14. Boersma E, Akkerhuis KM, Theroux P, Califf RM, Topol EJ, Simoons ML. Platelet glycoprotein IIb/IIIa receptor inhibition in non-ST-elevation acute coronary syndromes: early benefit during medical treat-ment only, with additional protection during percutaneous coronary intervention. Circulation 1999;100: 2045–2048.

15. Hamm CW, Ravkilde J, Gerhardt W, et al. The prognostic value of troponin T in unstable angina. N Engl J Med 1992;327:146–150.

16. Ohman EM, Armstrong P, Christenson RH, et al., GUSTO-IIa Investigators. Cardiac troponin T levels for risk stratification in unstable myocardial ischemia. N Engl J Med 1996;335:1333–1341.

17. Hamm CW, Goldmann BU, Heeschen C, Kreymann G, Berger J, Meinertz T. Emergency room triage of patients with acute chest pain by means of rapid testing for cardiac troponin T or troponin I. N Engl J Med 1997;337:1648–1653.

18. Newby LK, Christenson RH, Ohman EM, et al. Value of serial troponin T measures for early and late risk stratification in patients with acute coronary syndromes. The GUSTO-IIa Investigators. Circulation 1998;98:1853–1859.

19. Hamm CW, Heeschen C, Goldmann B, et al., for the c7E3 Fab Antiplatelet Therapy in Unstable Refrac-tory Angina (CAPTURE) Study Investigators. Benefit of abciximab in patients with refractory unstable angina in relation to serum troponin T levels. N Engl J Med 1999;340:1623–1629.

20. Antman EM, Tanasijevic MJ, Thompson B, et al. Cardiac-specific troponin I levels to predict the risk of mortality in patients with acute coronary syndromes. N Engl J Med 1996;335:1342–1349.

21. Heeschen C, van Den Brand MJ, Hamm CW, Simoons ML. Angiographic findings in patients with refrac-tory unstable angina according to troponin T status. Circulation 1999;100:1509–1514.

22. Wong GC, Morrow DA, Murphy S, et al., for the TACTICS-TIMI 18 Study Group. Elevations in tropo-nin T and I are associated with abnormal tissue level perfusion: a TACTICS-TIMI 18 substudy. Circulation 2002;106:202–207.

23. Heeschen C, Hamm CW, Goldmann B, Deu A, Langenbrink L, White HD, for the PRISM Study Investi-gators. Troponin concentrations for stratification of patients with acute coronary syndromes in relation to therapeutic efficacy of tirofiban. Lancet 1999;354:1757–1762.

24. Januzzi JL, Chai CU, Sabatine MS, Jang IK. Elevation in serum troponin I predicts the benefit of tirofi-ban. J Thromb Thrombolysis 2001;11:211–215.

25. Newby LK, Ohman EM, Christenson RH, et al. Benefit of glycoprotein IIb/IIIa inhibition in patients with acute coronary syndromes and troponin T-positive status: the PARAGON-B troponin T substudy. Circulation 2001;103:2891–2896.

26. Morrow DA, Antman EM, Snapinn SM, McCabe CH, Theroux P, Braunwald E. An integrated clinical approach to predicting the benefit of tirofiban in non-ST elevation acute coronary syndromes: applica-tion of the TIMI risk score for UA/NSTEMI in PRISM-PLUS. Eur Heart J 2002;23:223–229.

27. Theroux P, Alexander J Jr, Pharand C, et al. Glycoprotein IIb/IIIa receptor blockade improves outcomes in diabetic patients presenting with unstable angina/non-ST-elevation myocardial infarction: results from the Platelet Receptor Inhibition in Ischemic Syndrome Management in Patients Limited by Unstable Signs and Symptoms (PRISM-PLUS) study. Circulation 2000;102:2466–2472.

28. Cannon CP, Weintraub WS, Demopoulos LA, et al. Comparison of early invasive and conservative strategies in patients with unstable coronary syndromes treated with the glycoprotein IIb/IIIa inhibitor tirofiban. N Engl J Med 2001;344:1879–1887.

29. The TIMI IIIB Investigators. Effects of tissue plasminogen activator and a comparison of early invasive and conservative strategies in unstable angina and non-Q-wave myocardial infarction: results of the TIMI IIIB trial. Circulation 1994;89:1545–1556.

30. Anderson HV, Cannon CP, Stone PH, et al., for the TIMI-IIIB Investigators. One-year results of the Thrombolysis in Myocardial Infarction (TIMI) IIIB clinical trial. A randomized comparison of tissue-type plasminogen activator versus placebo and early invasive versus early conservative strategies in unstable angina and non-Q-wave myocardial infarction. J Am Coll Cardiol 1995;26:1643–1650.

31. McCullough PA, O'Neill WW, Graham M, et al. A prospective randomized trial of triage angiography in acute coronary syndromes ineligible for thrombolytic therapy. Results of the medicine versus angiography in thrombolytic exclusion (MATE) trial. J Am Coll Cardiol 1998;32:596–605.

32. Boden WE, O'Rourke RA, Crawford MH, et al., for the Veterans Affairs Non-Q-Wave Infarction Strategies in Hospital (VANQWISH) Trial Investigators. Outcomes in patients with acute non-Q-wave myocardial infarction randomly assigned to an invasive as compared with a conservative strategy. N Engl J Med 1998;338:1785–1792.

33. FRagmin and Fast Revascularisation during Instability in Coronary Artery Disease Investigators. Invasive compared with non-invasive treatment in unstable coronary-artery disease: FRISC II prospective randomised multicentre study. Lancet 1999;354:708–715.

34. Wallentin L, Lagerqvist B, Husted S, Kontny F, Stahle E, Swahn E. Outcome at 1 year after an invasive compared with a non-invasive strategy in unstable coronary-artery disease: the FRISC II invasive randomised trial. FRISC II Investigators. Fast Revascularisation during Instability in Coronary Artery Disease. Lancet 2000;356:9–16.

35. Morrow DA, Cannon CP, Rifai N, et al., for the TACTICS-TIMI 18 Investigators. Ability of minor elevations of troponin I and T to predict benefit from an early invasive strategy in patients with unstable angina and non-ST elevation myocardial infarction: results from a randomized trial. JAMA 2001;286: 2405–2412.

36. Antman EM, McCabe CH, Gurfinkel EP, et al. Enoxaparin prevents death and cardiac ischemic events in unstable angina/non-Q-wave myocardial infarction: results of the Thrombolysis in Myocardial Infarction (TIMI) 11B trial. Circulation 1999;100:1593–1601.

37. Sabatine MS, Cannon CP, Murphy SA, DiBattiste PM, Demopoulos LA, Braunwald E. Implications of upstream GP IIb/IIIa inhibition and stenting in the invasive management of UA/NSTEMI: a comparison of TIMI IIIB and TACTICS-TIMI 18. Circulation 2001;104(Suppl II):II–549.

38. van den Brand M, Laarman GJ, Steg PG, et al. Assessment of coronary angiograms prior to and after treatment with abciximab, and the outcome of angioplasty in refractory unstable angina patients. Angiographic results from the CAPTURE trial. Eur Heart J 1999;20:1572–1578.

39. Zhao X-Q, Theroux P, Snapinn SM, Sax FL, for the PRISM-PLUS Investigators. Intracoronary thrombus and platelet glycoprotein IIb/IIIa receptor blockade with tirofiban in unstable angina or non-Q-wave myocardial infarction. Angiographic results from the PRISM-PLUS trial (Platelet Receptor Inhibition for Ischemic Syndrome Management in Patients Limited by Unstable Signs and Symptoms). Circulation 1999;100:1609–1615.

40. Gibson M, Murphy SA, Weisberg S, Pai R, et al. Early initiation of tirofiban therapy before percutaneous coronary intervention is associated with improved flow and tissue level perfusion: a TACTICS-TIMI 18 substudy. Circulation 2001;104(Suppl II):II-548–549.

41. Januzzi JL, Hahn SS, Chae CU, et al. Effects of tirofiban plus heparin versus heparin alone on troponin I levels in patients with acute coronary syndromes. Am J Cardiol 2000;86:713–717.

42. Alexander JH, Sparapani RA, Mahaffey KW, et al., for the PURSUIT Investigators. Eptifibatide reduces the size and incidence of myocardial infarction in patients with non-ST-elevation acute coronary syndromes. J Am Coll Cardiol 1999;33(Suppl A):331A.

43. Roe MT. The EARLY trial. Eur Heart J 2001;22(Abstr Suppl):592.

44. Bhatt DL, Marso SP, Houghtaling P, Labinaz M, Lauer MA. Does earlier administration of eptifibatide reduce death and MI in patients with acute coronary syndromes? Circulation 1998;98(Suppl I):I–561.

45. Mahaffey KW, Harrington RA, Simoons ML, et al., for the PURSUIT Investigators. Stroke in patients with acute coronary syndromes: incidence and outcomes in the Platelet Glycoprotein IIb/IIIa in Unstable Angina Receptor Suppression Using Integrilin Therapy (PURSUIT) trial. Circulation 1999;99:2371–2377.

46. Coulter SA, Cannon CP, Cooper RA, et al. Thrombocytopenia, bleeding, and thrombotic events with oral glycoprotein IIb/IIIa inhbition: results from OPUS-TIMI 16. J Am Coll Cardiol 2000;35(Suppl A):393A.

47. Mark DB, Harrington RA, Lincoff AM, et al. Cost-effectiveness of platelet glycoprotein IIb/IIIa inhibition with eptifibatide in patients with non-ST-elevation acute coronary syndromes. Circulation 2000;101: 366–371.

48. Alexander JH, Harrington RA, Tuttle RH, et al. Prior aspirin use predicts worse outcomes in patients with non-ST-elevation acute coronary syndromes. PURSUIT Investigators. Platelet IIb/IIIa in Unstable angina: Receptor Suppression Using Integrilin Therapy. Am J Cardiol 1999;83:1147–1151.

49. Mahoney EM, Jurkovitz CT, Chu H, et al., for the "Treat Angina with Aggrastat and Determine Cost of Therapy with an Invasive or Conservative Strategy (TACTICS)-TIMI 18" Investigators. Cost and cost-effectiveness of an early invasive versus conservative strategy for the treatment of unstable angina and non-ST elevation myocardial infarction. JAMA 2002;288:1851–1858.

50. Braunwald E, Antman EM, Beasley JW, et al. ACC/AHA guidelines for the management of patients with unstable angina and non-ST segment elevation myocardial infarction: a report of the American College of Cardiology/American Heart Association Task Force on Practice Guidelines (Committee on the Management of Unstable Angina and Non-ST Segment Elevation Myocardial Infarction). J Am Coll Cardiol 2000;36:970–1056.

51. The ESPRIT Investigators. Enhanced Suppression of the Platelet IIb/IIIa Receptor with Integrilin Therapy. Novel dosing regimen of eptifibatide in planned coronary stent implantation (ESPRIT): a randomised, placebo-controlled trial. Lancet 2000;356:2037–2044.

12

Glycoprotein IIb/IIIa Receptor Blockade in Myocardial Infarction

Adjunctive Therapy to Percutaneous Coronary Interventions

Franz-Josef Neumann, MD

CONTENTS

INTRODUCTION
THE ILLUSION OF TIMI GRADE 3 FLOW
ROLE OF PLATELETS IN LIMITING REPERFUSION
EFFECT OF GPIIb/IIIa BLOCKADE ON MICROVASCULAR REPERFUSION,
    RECOVER OF CONTRACTILE FUNCTION, AND MYOCARDIAL SALVAGE
EFFECT OF GPIIb/IIIa BLOCKADE ON CLINICAL OUTCOME
FUTURE PROSPECTS
SUMMARY
REFERENCES

INTRODUCTION

In acute myocardial infarction, early, complete, and sustained restoration of blood flow in the occluded coronary artery can salvage myocardium at risk and improve survival. Randomized trials *(1)* as well as large registries *(2,3)* have shown that direct percutaneous transluminal coronary angioplasty (PTCA) is more efficacious in achieving this goal than thrombolysis. Additional placement of a stent improves long-term clinical outcome by reducing the need for target lesion revascularization but has no beneficial effect on the quality of reperfusion or the risk of early complications, such as death and reinfarction *(4–6)*.

For percutaneous coronary interventions (PCIs) in the absence of acute myocardial infarction, glycoprotein (GP) IIb/IIIa receptor blockade has been shown to reduce the early hazard of ischemic complications by up to about one-half (*see* Chapters 5–8). This peri-interventional effect translates into a long-term clinical benefit that can be verified as late as 3 yr after the intervention *(7)*. If GPIIb/IIIa blockade is equally effective in acute myocardial infarction, the combination of stenting with GPIIb/IIIa blockade may afford a highly efficient and durable reperfusion strategy.

From: *Contemporary Cardiology: Platelet Glycoprotein IIb/IIIa
Inhibitors in Cardiovascular Disease, 2nd Edition*
Edited by: A. M. Lincoff © Humana Press Inc., Totowa, NJ

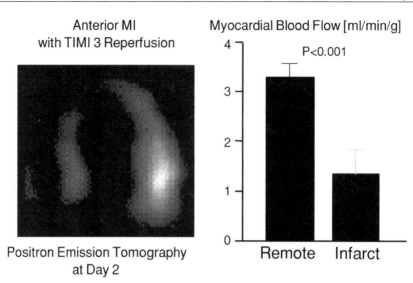

Fig. 1. Impairment of microvascular reperfusion in acute myocardial infarction (MI) despite TIMI grade 3 flow as assessed by positron emission tomography *(11)*. (Left) Example of patient with anterior myocardial infarction (courtesy of Professor M. Schwaiger, Nuclear Medicine, Technical University of Munich.) (Right) Mean adenosine-induced myocardial blood (SD) in the remote region and in the infarct region.

This chapter discusses the role of GPIIb/IIIa blockade as an adjunct to PCI in acute myocardial infarction. Among the three agents approved for clinical use with PCI, abciximab is the only agent for which randomized clinical studies in the setting of acute myocardial infarction have yet been published. Therefore, this review focuses on the role of abciximab for PCI in acute myocardial infarction.

THE ILLUSION OF TIMI GRADE 3 FLOW

In acute myocardial infarction, myocardial salvage after timely recanalization of the infarct-related artery is critically dependent on coronary blood flow to the area at risk. Only in patients in whom Thrombolysis in Myocardial Infarction (TIMI) grade 3 flow can be achieved can recanalization of the coronary artery occlusion improve regional ejection fraction in the infarct area and afford a clinical benefit *(8–10)*.

Normalization of large vessel flow by angiographic criteria, however, does not mean complete recovery of microvascular perfusion. Even in the presence of large-vessel TIMI grade 3 flow, positron emission tomography (Fig. 1) or myocardial contrast echocardiography frequently reveal substantial perfusion defects *(11–14)*. Likewise, Doppler flow velocity measurements show depressed coronary flow velocities and flow reserve during early reperfusion despite optimal vessel patency *(11)*. In general, the initial microvascular incompetence in the infarct region is partially reversible within the first 2 wk of reperfusion. However, the pattern of reperfusion varies considerably between patients, from complete normalization in some to even deterioration in others *(11)*. Variations of tissue reperfusion within the spectrum of TIMI grade 3 flow, as assessed by flow velocity measurements *(11, 15–18)*, TIMI frame counts *(19,20)*, or myocardial blush *(21,22)*, are important predictors of myocardial recovery and clinical outcome. Reversal of the early microvascular incom-

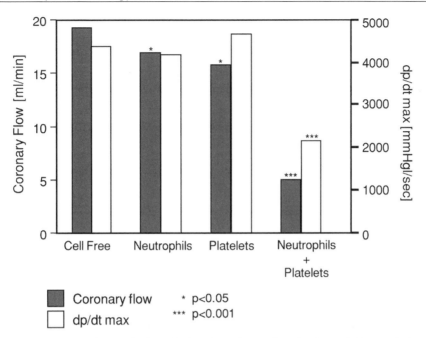

Fig. 2. Myocardial blood flow in isolated ischemic and reperfused guinea pig hearts during reperfusion with cell-free perfusate and suspensions of platelets, leukocytes, or both *(30)*.

petence is thus an important prerequisite for recovery of contractile function in the infarct region. These considerations underscore the need to address not only large-vessel patency but also microvascular perfusion when treating acute myocardial infarction.

ROLE OF PLATELETS IN LIMITING REPERFUSION

Previous investigations on experimental models of myocardial infarction documented the preeminent role of platelets in limiting blood flow during reperfusion in acute myocardial infarction *(23)*. By occlusive thrombus formation, distal embolization of small aggregates, and release of vasoconstrictive mediators, platelets interfere with both large-vessel patency and microvascular flow *(23)*.

Activated platelets can also adhere to the endothelial cells in the reperfused region *(24–27)*. During reperfusion in experimental myocardial infarction, platelets accumulate in the microvasculature of the infarct region *(28)*. In isolated guinea pig hearts, this platelet accumulation was associated with impaired recovery of external work after ischemia *(29)*. It was concluded that platelet adhesion to the coronary endothelium during reperfusion after myocardial ischemia impairs cardiac recovery. The potential of platelets to contribute to both impaired reperfusion and cardiac dysfunction after myocardial ischemia is also demonstrated by experiments in isolated perfused rat hearts *(30)*. In these experiments, reperfusion with either platelet or neutrophil suspensions reduced coronary flow and contractile function (dP/dt_{max}) during reperfusion after ischemia by <12% compared with cell-free perfusate. However, ischemic hearts reperfused with both neutrophils and platelets exhibited decreases of 50–60% in all measurements of coronary flow and cardiac function ($p < 0.001$) (Fig. 2). These results provided strong evidence that platelets and neutrophils act synergistically in provoking post-reperfusion cardiac microvascular and contractile dysfunction.

Tethering of platelets to activated endothelium is P-selectin-mediated, and subsequent firm adhesion is caused by interaction of GP IIb/IIIa-bound fibrinogen with endothelial vitronectin receptors and intercellular adhesion molecule-1 (ICAM-1) *(25–27)*. In activated endothelium, expression of vitronectin receptors is enhanced on the luminal aspect *(25)*. Through stimulation by CD40L and platelet-bound interleukin-1 activity, binding of activated platelets to endothelial cells stimulates the expression of monocyte chemo-attractant protein-1 and of ICAM-1 via an NF-κB-dependent mechanism *(25,31,32)*. Activated platelets thus modulate chemotactic and adhesive properties of endothelial cells and direct leukocyte attachment, as shown in cell culture studies *(33)*.

Platelets can also directly support leukocyte adhesion. Heterotypic interactions of endothelium-bound platelets appear to play an important role in the recruitment of leukocytes to the site of vascular injury *(34)*. In these interactions, primary attachment of platelets to myeloid leukocytes occurs by tethering of the platelet P-selectin to P-selectin glycoprotein ligand-1 (PSGL-1) on leukocytes *(35–40)*. Secondarily, the heterotypic adhesion is stabilized by binding of Mac-1 to an unknown counter-receptor on the platelet *(38–41)*. This is enabled by Mac-1 activation as a consequence of tyrosine phosphorylation and mitogen-activated protein (MAP) kinase activation owing to PSGL-1 ligation *(39,42)*. Leukocyte activation by binding of stimulated platelets is further enhanced by CD40L-dependent signal transduction pathways *(31)*. In vitro, binding of activated platelets to myeloid leukocytes induces expression of proinflammatory cytokines, oxidative burst, and increased surface expression of tissue factor and Mac-1 *(43–46)*. Mac-1 is known to play a key role in leukocyte-dependent reperfusion injury *(47–49)*.

In patients with acute myocardial infarction, there are abundant platelet-leukocyte aggregates in peripheral blood *(44)*. GPIIb/IIIa receptor blockade with abciximab in patients with acute myocardial infarction reduces platelet-monocyte interaction by decreasing the mass of platelets attached to monocytes *(50)*. Through this mechanism, abciximab decreases Mac-1 surface expression on circulating monocytes *(50)*. This effect is complemented by the direct Mac-1-blocking properties of abciximab *(51)*. In addition, cell culture experiments show that abciximab can prevent firm adhesion of platelets to activated endothelial cells by blockage of both GPIIb/IIIa and the vitronectin receptor *(25,52)*. The inhibitory effect of abciximab on heterotypic platelet interactions during ischemia and reperfusion could be confirmed by experiments in isolated guinea pig hearts *(53)*. In these experiments, inhibition of heterotypic platelet interactions by abciximab improved the recovery of contractile function *(53)*. These studies demonstrate the functional importance of heterotypic platelet interactions during ischemia and reperfusion.

EFFECT OF GPIIb/IIIa BLOCKADE
ON MICROVASCULAR REPERFUSION, RECOVERY
OF CONTRACTILE FUNCTION, AND MYOCARDIAL SALVAGE

The principle goal of reperfusion therapy is preservation of contractile function by myocardial salvage. Optimization of both large-vessel patency and microvascular perfusion is pivotal to this goal. Modern interventional techniques are highly successful in restoring large-vessel patency. To improve distal circulation, additional measures need to be taken. GPIIb/IIIa blockade is highly promising for this end. GPIIb/IIIa blockade appears to pre-

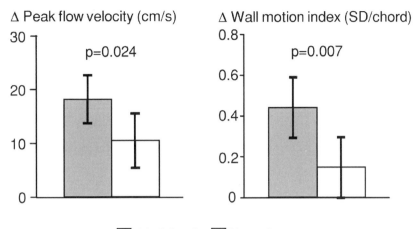

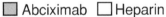

Fig. 3. Increase between 14-d follow-up and initial postinterventional study in papaverine-induced peak flow velocity in the recanalized and stented infarct-related artery (left) and in wall motion index within the infarct region (right). Columns represent the mean difference. Error bars indicate the 95% confidence interval. Error bars not including zero indicate that the change between initial study and follow-up is statistically significant at the 0.05 level. *p* values above the columns refer to the difference between the two treatment groups. (From ref. *18*, with permission.)

vent distal embolization of platelet aggregates from the treated plaque. Moreover, abciximab, because of its ability to block not only GP IIb/IIIa but also vitronectin receptors and Mac-1 *(51,52)*, can interfere with heterotypic platelet and leukocyte interactions that limit microvascular reflow.

The role of GPIIb/IIIa receptor blockade in optimizing microvascular reperfusion could be confirmed clinically in ISAR-2 (Intracoronary Stenting and Antithrombotic Regimen) *(18,54)*. In this prospective study, patients undergoing stenting in acute ST-elevation and non-ST-elevation myocardial infarction within 48 h after onset of symptoms were randomly assigned to receive either open-label standard-dose heparin or abciximab plus low-dose heparin. In the first 200 patients of ISAR-2, flow velocities in the recanalized vessel were assessed with the Doppler wire immediately after the procedure and at 14-d angiographic follow-up *(18)*. At the same time points, regional wall motion was analyzed in left ventricular angiograms by the centerline method. Abciximab significantly improved the recovery of peak flow velocity in the recanalized vessel compared with standard heparin treatment (Fig. 3) *(18)*. As quantitative coronary angiography did not reveal any difference in angiographic outcome between the two treatment groups, the beneficial effect of abciximab reflected improvement of microvascular function. Consistent with the close relation between microvascular and contractile recovery, the improvement of wall motion index in the infarct region was significantly greater in patients assigned to abciximab than in those on heparin alone (Fig. 3) *(18)*. At 14-d follow-up, the abciximab treatment group had a higher global left ventricular (LV) ejection fraction than the heparin treatment group [mean (95% confidence interval), 62 (59–65) % vs 56 (53–59) %, *p* = 0.003].

The study demonstrated that in acute myocardial infarction abciximab has important effects beyond the maintenance of large-vessel patency. It improves the recovery coronary perfusion at the level of the distal vascular bed and concomitantly enhances the restoration of left ventricular function in the infarct area. These findings are consistent with the results of the ADMIRAL (Abciximab before Direct Angioplasty and Stenting in Myocardial Infarction Regarding Acute and Long Term Follow-Up) trial (*see* the following section), which found better TIMI flow grades after PCI in the abciximab-treated group compared with the placebo group, as well as higher global LV function ejection fractions *(55)*. In CADILLAC (Controlled Abciximab and Device Investigation to Lower Late Angioplasty) *(6)*, another trial that assessed abciximab as an adjunct to PCI in acute myocardial infarction (*see* the following section), LV ejection fractions and regional wall motions at 7-mo follow-up showed no statistically significant difference, although the point estimates favored abciximab. Detection of such long-term benefit is probably hampered by considerable scatter caused by variations in restenosis, medication, and individual LV loading conditions.

The improved recovery of contractile function in ISAR-2 and ADMIRAL provided circumstantial evidence for improved myocardial salvage by stents plus abciximab compared with stents plus traditional antithrombotic treatment. The issue of myocardial salvage was directly addressed in the two STOP-AMI (Stent versus Thrombolysis for Occluded Coronary Arteries in Patients with Acute Myocardial Infarction) trials *(56–58)*. Prior to the STOP-AMI trials, it had never been shown that PCI confers larger myocardial salvage than fibrinolysis *(59)*. The prospective randomized STOP-AMI trials thus pursued the question, of whether PCI optimized with stenting plus abciximab can improve myocardial salvage over what can be achieved with thrombolysis. Both trials enrolled patients with acute myocardial infarction who presented within 12 h of onset of symptoms and were eligible for thrombolysis. The thrombolytic regimen was front-loaded alteplase in STOP-AMI *(56,57)* and half-dose alteplase plus full-dose abciximab in STOP-AMI-2 *(58)*. STOP-AMI comprised 140 patients and STOP-AMI-2 162 patients. Technetium-99m sestamibi scintigraphy was performed on admission to delineate the area at risk (initial perfusion defect) and after a median of 10 (STOP-AMI) or 11 (STOP-AMI-2) d to assess the final infarct size (late perfusion defect). In both studies, the primary endpoint was the salvage index, reflecting the proportion of the area at risk that could be salvaged [(initial perfusion defect–late perfusion defect)/initial perfusion defect].

In both STOP-AMI trials, the mechanical intervention optimized by abciximab yielded a larger salvage index than the purely pharmacologic reperfusion strategies (Fig. 4). Corroborating the primary endpoint, in both trials absolute infarct sizes were smaller after PCI than after thrombolysis, and absolute myocardial salvages were larger. Although none of the STOP-AMI trials was powered to look at clinical outcome, both suggest that better salvage confers better clinical outcome. In STOP-AMI, 1-yr mortality in the PCI arm was significantly lower than in the fibrinolysis arm (15.9% vs 4.2%, $p = 0.02$) *(57)*, and in STOP-AMI-2 the combined 6-mo rate of death, reinfarction, and stroke was 8.6% in the PCI arm compared with 18.5% in the thrombolysis arm ($p = 0.06$) *(58)*.

When comparing the two STOP-AMI trials, it is conspicuous that the benefit of optimized PCI over fibrinolysis in STOP-AMI is diluted by addition of abciximab to fibinolysis in STOP-AMI-2 (Fig. 4). Hence, abciximab appears to exert a specific contribution to the maximization of myocardial salvage by the optimized PCI. This interpretation is supported by findings from the TIMI 14 study comparing thrombolytic regimens with and without abciximab *(60)*. In TIMI 14, ST-segment resolution as a surrogate for tissue perfusion in patients with TIMI grade 3 reperfusion was better in the abciximab regimens than in the fibrinolytic regimen without abciximab *(60)*.

Salvage Index (%)

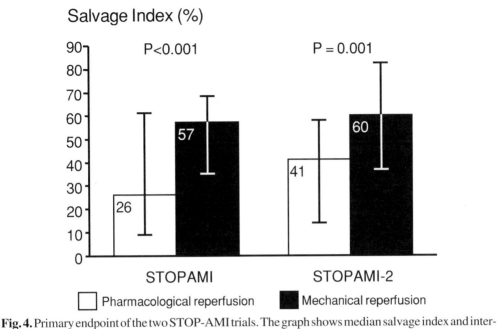

Fig. 4. Primary endpoint of the two STOP-AMI trials. The graph shows median salvage index and interquartile range *(56,58)*.

EFFECT OF GPIIb/IIIa BLOCKADE ON CLINICAL OUTCOME

Subgroup analysis of the 55 patients with acute myocardial infarction in EPIC (Evaluation of c7E3 for the Prevention of Ischemic Complications) suggested a major benefit from abciximab with PCI for acute myocardial infarction *(61)*. Subsequently, four major studies investigated the effect of GPIIb/IIIa blockade on clinical outcome in this setting: RAPPORT *(62)* (ReoPro and Primary PTCA Organization and Randomized Trial), ISAR-2 *(54)*, ADMIRAL *(55)*, and CADILLAC *(6)* (Fig. 5).

The first of these studies, RAPPORT *(62)*, randomized 483 patients with acute ST-elevation myocardial infarction of <12-h duration on a double-blind basis, to placebo or abciximab if they were deemed candidates for primary PTCA. Abciximab compared with placebo significantly reduced the 30-d incidence of death, reinfarction, or urgent target vessel revascularization (TVR) by 51% (Fig. 5). This benefit was maintained during 6-mo follow-up. The rate of nonurgent TVR, however, was not significantly affected by abciximab (17.4% at 6 mo with abciximab vs 13.6% with placebo). Thus, the primary efficacy endpoint of the study, the composite of death, reinfarction, or TVR at 6 mo showed no difference (28.2% vs 28.1%, $p = 0.97$). Because the heparin dosing was not reduced in the abciximab arm, major bleeding occurred significantly more frequently in the abciximab group, mostly at the arterial access site. It was concluded that abciximab during primary PTCA for acute myocardial infarction yielded a substantial reduction in the acute cardiac complications.

ISAR-2 *(54)* and ADMIRAL *(55)* specifically addressed the effect of abciximab on clinical outcome with stenting in acute myocardial infarction. ISAR-2 included 401 patients undergoing stenting within 48 h after onset of ST-elevation and non-ST-elevation acute

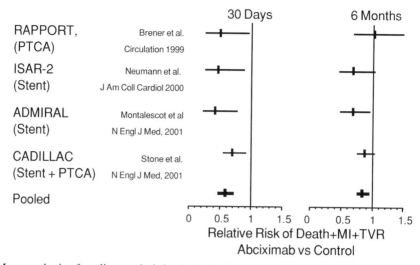

Fig. 5. Meta-analysis of studies on abciximab during percutaneous coronary intervention for acute myocardial infarction (MI). PTCA, percutaneous transluminal coronary angioplasty; TVR, target vessel revascularization. (From ref. *70*, with permission.)

myocardial infarction *(54)*. In an open-label design, patients were randomized to abciximab plus reduced-dose heparin or to high-dose heparin. By 30 d, the composite clinical endpoint of death, reinfarction, and target lesion revascularization was reached in 5.0% of the abciximab group and in 10.5% of the control group (Fig. 5) *(54)*. Abciximab thus achieved a relative reduction of the early risk by 53% (Fig. 5) *(54)*. At 1 yr, absolute reduction in the composite clinical endpoint by abciximab was still 5.7% but had lost its statistical significance. This was caused by a rate of TVR that was unaffected by abciximab *(54)*. As in ERASER *(63)* and EPISTENT *(64)*, binary in-stent restenosis rates at angiographic follow-up were not significantly different between abciximab and control in ISAR-2 (31.1 and 30.6%, $p = 0.92$) *(54)*.

ADMIRAL tested abciximab in a double-blind, placebo-controlled design that included 300 patients with ST-elevation myocardial infarction within 24 h after onset of pain *(55)*. In this trial, the 30-d rates of death, reinfarction, and TVR were 6.0% in the abciximab group but 14.6% in the placebo group ($p=0.01$) (Fig. 5) *(55)*. At 6 mo, the risk reduction by abciximab compared with placebo was still statistically significant with respect to the composite endpoint [relative risk (95% confidence interval) 0.68 (0.48–0.95); $p = 0.035$] (Fig. 5) *(55)*. An important new aspect of ADMIRAL, compared with other trials using abciximab for PCI in acute myocardial infarction, is the upstream use of GPIIb/IIIa blockade. In ADMIRAL, randomization and study drug administration were performed immediately after the decision for catheter intervention in acute myocardial infarction. Thus, 26% of the patients received their study medication upstream, that is, in the mobile intensive care unit or the emergency room. These patients had substantially better 30-d and 6-mo outcomes than those who received their study drug in the intensive cardiac care unit or the catheterization laboratory (Fig. 6). ADMIRAL adds weight to the concept that abciximab, in particular when administered upstream, improves the outcome of patients being stented for acute myocardial infarction.

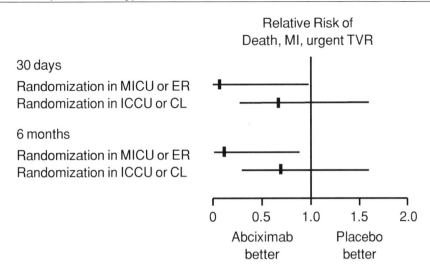

Fig. 6. Relative risk of death, reinfarction, or urgent target vessel revascularization (TVR) according to the timing of study drug administration *(55)*. MI, recurrent myocardial infarction; MICU; mobile intensive care unit; ER, emergency room; ICCU, intensive cardiac care unit; CL, catheterization laboratory.

CADILLAC investigated stent versus PTCA and abciximab vs heparin alone in a 2-by-2 factorial design *(6)*. CADILLAC, thus far, is the largest trial using abciximab for PCI in AMI. It comprised 2082 patients with ST-elevation myocardial infarction within the first 12 h after onset of pain *(6)*. Abciximab compared with control reduced the composite of death, myocardial infarction, and TVR by 30% (5.0% vs 7.1%, $p = 0.04$) at 30 d and by 14% (13.0% vs 15.1%, $p = 0.17$) at 6 mo (Fig. 5) *(6)*. Thus, the effect of abciximab in CADILLAC was consistent with the other trials, although the risk reduction was somewhat lower than expected based on the earlier studies. This may be because CADILLAC recruited a low-risk cohort with an unprecedented low overall mortality of 3.3% *(6)*. Of the 2681 patients who were screened for inclusion in CADILLAC, 599 (22.3%) were excluded based on high-risk angiographic features or because noninterventional management was the proper approach. Exclusion of these patients will have reduced the overall risk in CADILLAC.

If CADILLAC is broken down into subgroups with and without stent, the benefit of abciximab with respect to the composite endpoint at 6 mo was nearly significant in the PTCA group (15.2% vs 19.3%, $p = 0.07$), whereas in the stent groups event rates were almost identical (10.9% vs 10.8%). However, since an interaction of the effect of abciximab with the type of percutaneous coronary intervention has not been shown in any previous trial (*see* previous chapters), it is questionable whether the groups with and without stents deserve separate analysis. Metaanalysis of all studies owing abciximab for PCI in acute myocardial infarction reveals a significant reduction in 30-d and 6-mo event rates (Fig. 5).

FUTURE PROSPECTS

Confirming earlier smaller studies *(65,66)*, the large randomized DANAMI-2 trial has recently shown that transport to PCI in acute myocardial infarction gives a better outcome than local thrombolysis, if the patient can be brought to the catheterization laboratory within 3 h *(67)*. In 1129 patients with acute myocardial infarction admitted to hospitals without catheterization facilities and randomized to transport to PCI in a center, the 30-d rate of death, reinfarction, and stroke was 8.5%, whereas it was 14.2% ($p = 0.002$) for those randomized to local thrombolysis. DANAMI-2 suggests that, from a population perspective, the prospects for patients with acute myocardial infarction can be substantially improved by the implementation of networks that allow rapid allocation and transport of patients to infarct centers that provide PCI.

With a treatment strategy of systematic transport to PCI in acute myocardial infarction, the concept of upstream treatment will gain importance. Thus far, evidence from ADMIRAL suggests that administration of abciximab well before the start of PCI improves acute and long-term outcome. Subgroup analyses from both SPEED *(68)* and PACT *(69)* indicate that the outcome in acute myocardial infarction can be improved, if prior to PCI at least partial reperfusion is achieved by thrombolysis. In this respect, combination of full-dose abciximab with half-dose fibrinolytic agents (*see* Chapter 13) appears particularly attractive. The concept of "facilitated PCI" by upstream use of GPIIb/IIIa blockade, either alone or in combination with a half-dose fibrinolytic agent, needs to be tested in future randomized trials, such as FINESSE (Facilitated Intervention with Enhanced Reperfusion Speed to Stop Events).

SUMMARY

GPIIb/IIIa receptor blockade with abciximab interferes with several mechanism that limit reperfusion in acute myocardial infarction. Clinical studies have shown that abciximab improves recovery of microvascular and contractile function. Stenting in combination with abciximab confers a substantially larger myocardial salvage than thrombolysis. Circumstantial evidence suggests that abciximab makes an important contribution to this beneficial effect. Metaanalysis of the four randomized clinical trials using abciximab as an adjunct to PCI in acute myocardial infarction, RAPPORT, ISAR-2, ADMIRAL, and CADILLAC, reveals a reduction in the composite of death, reinfarction, and reintervention during 30-d and 6-mo follow-up. This benefit is particularly large if abciximab is administered upstream, as suggested by ADMIRAL, and may be negligible in low-risk settings, as suggested by analysis of the stent group in CADILLAC. The concept of facilitated PCI either by upstream GPIIb/IIIa blockade alone or in combination with a half-dose fibrinolytic agent awaits confirmation by future studies. Further studies are also needed to address the efficacy of GPIIb/IIIa blockers other than abciximab in the setting of PCI in acute myocardial infarction.

REFERENCES

1. Weaver WD, Simes RJ, Betriu A, et al. Comparison of primary coronary angioplasty and intravenous thrombolytic therapy for acute myocardial infarction: a quantitative review [published erratum appears in JAMA 1998;279:1876]. JAMA 1997;278:2093–2098.
2. Magid DJ, Calonge BN, Rumsfeld JS, et al. Relation between hospital primary angioplasty volume and mortality for patients with acute MI treated with primary angioplasty vs thrombolytic therapy. JAMA 2000;284:3131–3138.
3. Zahn R, Schiele R, Schneider S, et al. Primary angioplasty versus intravenous thrombolysis in acute myocardial infarction: can we define subgroups of patients benefiting most from primary angioplasty? Results from the pooled data of the Maximal Individual Therapy in Acute Myocardial Infarction Registry and the Myocardial Infarction Registry. J Am Coll Cardiol 2001;37:1827–1835.
4. Suryapranata H, van't Hof AW, Hoorntje JC, de Boer MJ, Zijlstra F. Randomized comparison of coronary stenting with balloon angioplasty in selected patients with acute myocardial infarction. Circulation 1998;97:2502–2505.

5. Grines CL, Cox DA, Stone GW, et al. Coronary angioplasty with or without stent implantation for acute myocardial infarction. N Engl J Med 1999;341:1949–1956.
6. Stone GW, Grines CL, Cox DA, et al. Comparison of angioplasty with stenting, with or without abciximab, in acute myocardial infarction. N Engl J Med 2002;346:957–966.
7. Topol EJ, Ferguson JJ, Weisman HF, et al. Long-term protection from myocardial ischemic events in a randomized trial of brief integrin beta3 blockade with percutaneous coronary intervention. JAMA 1997; 278:479–484.
8. Vogt A, von Essen R, Tebbe U, Feuerer W, Appel KF, Neuhaus KL. Impact of early perfusion status of the infarct-related artery on short-term mortality after thrombolysis for acute myocardial infarction: retrospective analysis of four German multicenter studies. J Am Coll Cardiol 1993;21:1391–1395.
9. Simes RJ, Topol EJ, Holmes DR Jr, et al. Link between the angiographic substudy and mortality outcomes in a large randomized trial of myocardial reperfusion. Importance of early and complete infarct artery reperfusion. GUSTO-I Investigators. Circulation 1995;91:1923–1928.
10. Anderson JL, Karagounis LA, Becker LC, Sorensen SG, Menlove RL. TIMI perfusion grade 3 but not grade 2 results in improved outcome after thrombolysis for myocardial infarction. Ventriculographic, enzymatic, and electrocardiographic evidence from the TEAM-3 study. Circulation 1993;87:1829–1839.
11. Neumann FJ, Kosa I, Dickfeld T, et al. Recovery of myocardial perfusion in acute myocardial infarction after successful balloon angioplasty and stent placement in the infarct-related coronary artery. J Am Coll Cardiol 1997;30:1270–1276.
12. Ito H, Iwakura K, Oh H, et al. Temporal changes in myocardial perfusion patterns in patients with reperfused anterior wall myocardial infarction. Their relation to myocardial viability. Circulation 1995;91:656-662.
13. Ito H, Maruyama A, Iwakura K, et al. Clinical implications of the 'no reflow' phenomenon. A predictor of complications and left ventricular remodeling in reperfused anterior wall myocardial infarction. Circulation 1996;93:223–228.
14. Ito H, Tomooka T, Sakai N, et al. Lack of myocardial perfusion immediately after successful thrombolysis. A predictor of poor recovery of left ventricular function in anterior myocardial infarction. Circulation 1992;85:1699–1705.
15. Wakatsuki T, Nakamura M, Tsunoda T, et al. Coronary flow velocity immediately after primary coronary stenting as a predictor of ventricular wall motion recovery in acute myocardial infarction. J Am Coll Cardiol 2000;35:1835–1841.
16. Tsunoda T, Nakamura M, Wakatsuki T, et al. The pattern of alteration in flow velocity in the recanalized artery is related to left ventricular recovery in patients with acute infarction and successful direct balloon angioplasty. J Am Coll Cardiol 1998;32:338–344.
17. Mazur W, Bitar JN, Lechin M, et al. Coronary flow reserve may predict myocardial recovery after myocardial infarction in patients with TIMI grade 3 flow. Am Heart J 1998;136:335–344.
18. Neumann FJ, Blasini R, Schmitt C, et al. Effect of glycoprotein IIb/IIIa receptor blockade on recovery of coronary flow and left ventricular function after the placement of coronary-artery stents in acute myocardial infarction. Circulation 1998;98:2695–2701.
19. French JK, Hyde TA, Straznicky IT, et al. Relationship between corrected TIMI frame counts at three weeks and late survival after myocardial infarction. J Am Coll Cardiol 2000;35:1516–1524.
20. Gibson CM, Murphy SA, Rizzo MJ, et al. Relationship between TIMI frame count and clinical outcomes after thrombolytic administration. Thrombolysis in Myocardial Infarction (TIMI) Study Group. Circulation 1999;99:1945–1950.
21. Gibson CM, Cannon CP, Murphy SA, et al. Relationship of TIMI myocardial perfusion grade to mortality after administration of thrombolytic drugs. Circulation 2000;101:125–130.
22. van't Hof AW, Liem A, Suryapranata H, Hoorntje JC, de Boer MJ, Zijlstra F. Angiographic assessment of myocardial reperfusion in patients treated with primary angioplasty for acute myocardial infarction: myocardial blush grade. Zwolle Myocardial Infarction Study Group. Circulation 1998;97:2302–2306.
23. Topol EJ. Toward a new frontier in myocardial reperfusion therapy. Emerging platelet preeminence. Circulation 1998;1997:211–218.
24. Gawaz M, Neumann FJ, Ott I, Schiessler A, Schömig A. Platelet function in acute myocardial infarction treated with direct angioplasty. Circulation 1996;93:229–237.
25. Gawaz M, Neumann FJ, Dickfeld T, et al. Vitronectin receptor (αvβ3) mediates platelet adhesion to the luminal aspect of endothelial cells. Implications for reperfusion in acute myocardial infarction. Circulation 1997;96:1809–1818.
26. Massberg S, Enders G, Matos FC, et al. Fibrinogen deposition at the postischemic vessel wall promotes platelet adhesion during ischemia-reperfusion in vivo. Blood 1999;94:3829–3838.

27. Massberg S, Enders G, Leiderer R, et al. Platelet-endothelial cell interactions during ischemia/reperfusion: the role of P-selectin. Blood 1998;92:507–515.
28. Laws KH, Clanton JA, Starnes VA, et al. Kinetics and imaging of indium-11-labeled autologous platelets in experimental myocardial infarction. Circulation 1983;67:110–116.
29. Heindl B, Zahler S, Welsch U, Becker BF. Disparate effects of adhesion and degranulation of platelets on myocardial and coronary function in postischaemic hearts. Cardiovasc Res 1998;38:383–394.
30. Lefer AM, Campbell B, Scalia R, Lefer DJ. Synergism between platelets and neutrophils in provoking cardiac dysfunction after ischemia and reperfusion. Circulation 1998;98:1322–1328.
31. Henn V, Slupsky JR, Grafe M, et al. CD40 ligand on activated platelets triggers an inflammatory reaction of endothelial cells. Nature 1998;391:591–594.
32. Gawaz M, Neumann FJ, Dickfeld T, et al. Activated platelets induce monocyte chemotactic protein-1 secretion and surface expression of intercellular adhesion molecule-1 on endothelial cells. Circulation 1998;98:1164–1171.
33. Kuijper PH, Gallardo Torres HI, van der Linden JA, et al. Platelet-dependent primary hemostasis promotes selectin- and integrin-mediated neutrophil adhesion to damaged endothelium under flow conditions. Blood 1996;87:3271–3281.
34. Kirchhofer D, Riederer MA, Baumgartner HR. Specific accumulation of circulating monocytes and polymorphonuclear leukocytes on platelet thrombi in a vascular injury model. Blood 1997;89:1270–1278.
35. Hamburger S, McEver RP. GMP-140 mediates adhesion of stimulated platelets to neutrophils. Blood 1990;75:550–554.
36. Rinder HM, Bonan JL, Rinder CS, Ault KA, Smith BR. Dynamics of leukocyte-platelet adhesion in whole blood. Blood 1991;78:1730–1737.
37. Rinder HM, Bonan JL, Rinder CS, Ault KA, Smith BR. Activated and unactivated platelet adhesion to monocytes and neutrophils. Blood 1991;78:1760–1769.
38. Diacovo TG, Roth SJ, Buccola JM, Bainton DF, Springer TA. Neutrophil rolling, arrest, and transmigration across activated, surface-adherent platelets via seqential action of P-selectin and the β2-integrin CD11b/CD18. Blood 1996;88:146–157.
39. Evangelista VE, Manarini S, Rotondo S, et al. Platelet/polymorphonuclear leukocyte interaction in dynamic conditions: evidence of adhesion cascade and cross talk between P-selectin and the β2 integrin CD11b/CD18. Blood 1996;88:4183–4194.
40. Konstantopoulos K, Neelamegham S, Burns AR, et al. Venous levels of shear support neutrophil-platelet adhesion and neutrophil aggregation in blood via P-selectin and β2-integrin. Circulation 1998;98:873–882.
41. Sheikh S, Nash GB. Continuous activation and deactivation of integrin CD11b/CD18 during de novo expression enables rolling neutrophils to immobilize on platelets. Blood 1996;87:5040–5050.
42. Hidari KI, Weyrich AS, Zimmerman GA, McEver RP. Engagement of P-selectin glycoprotein ligand-1 enhances tyrosine phosphorylation and activates mitogen-activated protein kinases in human neutrophils. J Biol Chem 1997;272:28,750–28,756.
43. Neumann FJ, Marx N, Gawaz M, et al. Induction of cytokine expression in leukocytes by binding of thrombin-stimulated platelets. Circulation 1997;95:2387–2394.
44. Ott I, Neumann FJ, Gawaz M, May A, Schmitt M, Schömig A. Increased neutrophil-platelet interaction in patients with unstable angina. Circulation 1996;94:1239–1246.
45. Barry OP, Pratico D, Savani RC, Fitzgerald GA. Modulation of monocyte-endothelial cell interactions by platelet microparticles. J Clin Invest. 1998;102:136–144.
46. Nagata K, Tsuji T, Todoroki N, et al. Activated platelets induce superoxide anion release by monocytes and neutrophils through P-selectin (CD62). J Immunol 1993;151:3267–3273.
47. Nolte D, Hecht R, Schmid P, et al. Role of Mac-1 and ICAM-1 in ischemia-reperfusion injury in a microcirculation model of BALB/C mice. Am J Physiol 1994;267:H1320–H1328.
48. Ma XL, Tsao PS, Lefer AM. Antibody to CD-18 exerts endothelial and cardiac protective effects in myocardial ischemia and reperfusion. J Clin Invest 1991;88:1237–1243.
49. Neumann FJ, Ott I, Gawaz M, et al. Cardiac release of cytokines and inflammatory responses in acute myocardial infarction. Circulation 1995;92:748–755.
50. Neumann FJ, Zohlnhöfer D, Fakhoury L, Ott I, Gawaz M, Schömig A. Effect of glycoprotein IIb/IIIa receptor blockade on platelet-leukocyte interaction and surface expression of the leukocyte integrin Mac-1 in acute myocardial infarction. J Am Coll Cardiol 1999;34:1420–1426.
51. Simon DI, Xu H, Ortlepp S, Rogers C, Rao NK. 7E3 monoclonal antibody directed against the platelet glycoprotein IIb/IIIa cross-reacts with the leukocyte integrin Mac-1 and blocks adhesion to fibrinogen and ICAM-1. Arterioscler Thromb Vasc Biol 1997;17:528–535.

52. Tam SH, Sassoli PM, Jordan RE, Nakada MT. Abciximab (ReoPro, chimeric 7E3 Fab) demonstrates equivalent affinity and functional blockade of glycoprotein IIb/IIIa and alpha(v)beta3 integrins. Circulation 1998;98:1085–1091.

53. Kupatt C, Habazettl H, Hanusch P, et al. c7E3Fab reduces postischemic leukocyte-thrombocyte interaction mediated by fibrinogen. Implications for myocardial reperfusion injury. Arterioscler Thromb Vasc Biol 2000;20:2226–2232.

54. Neumann FJ, Kastrati A, Schmitt C, et al. Effect of glycoprotein IIb/IIIa receptor blockade with abciximab on clinical and angiographic restenosis rate after the placement of coronary stents following acute myocardial infarction. J Am Coll Cardiol 2000;35:915–921.

55. Montalescot G, Barragan P, Wittenberg O, et al. Platelet glycoprotein IIb/IIIa inhibition with coronary stenting for acute myocardial infarction. N Engl J Med 2001;344:1895–1903.

56. Schömig A, Kastrati A, Dirschinger J, et al. Coronary stenting plus platelet glycoprotein IIb/IIIa blockade compared with tissue plasminogen activator in acute myocardial infarction. N Engl J Med 2000;343: 385–391.

57. Schömig A, Kastrati A, Schricke U, et al. Stents versus thrombolysis for occluded coronary arteries in patients with AMI—1-year update of the STOPAMI trial results (abstract). Circulation 2000;102(Suppl I).

58. Kastrati A, Mehilli J, Dirschinger J, et al. Myocardial salvage after coronary stenting plus abciximab versus fibrinolysis plus abciximab in patients with acute myocardial infarction: a randomised trial. Lancet 2002;359:920–925.

59. Gibbons RJ, Holmes DR, Reeder GS, Bailey KR, Hopfenspirger MR, Gersh BJ. Immediate angioplasty compared with the administration of a thrombolytic agent followed by conservative treatment for myocardial infarction. N Engl J Med 1993;328:685–691.

60. de Lemos JA, Antman EM, Gibson CM, et al. Abciximab improves both epicardial flow and myocardial reperfusion in ST-elevation myocardial infarction. Observations from the TIMI 14 trial. Circulation 2000; 101:239–243.

61. Lefkovits J, Ivanhoe RJ, Califf RM, et al. Effects of platelet glycoprotein IIb/IIIa receptor blockade by a chimeric monoclonal antibody (abciximab) on acute and six-month outcomes after percutaneous transluminal coronary angioplasty for acute myocardial infarction. EPIC investigators. Am J Cardiol 1996;77: 1045–1051.

62. Brener SJ, Barr LA, Burchenal JE, et al. Randomized, placebo-controlled trial of platelet glycoprotein IIb/IIIa blockade with primary angioplasty for acute myocardial infarction. Circulation 1998;98:734–741.

63. Ellis GS, Serruys PW, Popma JJ, et al. Can abciximab prevent neointimal proliferation in Palmaz-Schatz stents? The final ERASER results (abstract). Circulation 1997;96(Suppl I):I–87.

64. Lincoff AM, Califf RM, Moliterno DJ, et al. Complementary clinical benefits of coronary-artery stenting and blockade of platelet glycoprotein IIb/IIIa receptors. N Engl J Med 1999;341:319–327.

65. Widimsky P, Groch L, Zelizko M, Aschermann M, Bednar F, Suryapranata H. Multicentre randomized trial comparing transport to primary angioplasty vs immediate thrombolysis vs combined strategy for patients with acute myocardial infarction presenting to a community hospital without a catheterization laboratory. The PRAGUE study. Eur Heart J 2000;21:823–831.

66. Vermeer F, Oude Ophuis AJ, vd Berg EJ, et al. Prospective randomised comparison between thrombolysis, rescue PTCA, and primary PTCA in patients with extensive myocardial infarction admitted to a hospital without PTCA facilities: a safety and feasibility study. Heart 1999;82:426–431.

67. Anderson R. Late breaking trials: DANAMI-2. In: 51st Annual Scientific Session of the American College of Cardiology, Atlanta, GA, March 17–20, 2002.

68. Herrmann HC, Moliterno DJ, Ohman EM, et al. Facilitation of early percutaneous coronary intervention after reteplase with or without abciximab in acute myocardial infarction: results from the SPEED (GUSTO-4 pilot) trial. J Am Coll Cardiol 2000;36:1489–1496.

69. Ross AM, Coyne KS, Reiner JS, et al. A randomized trial comparing primary angioplasty with a strategy of short-acting thrombolysis and immediate planned rescue angioplasty in acute myocardial infarction: the PACT trial. PACT investigators. Plasminogen-Activator Angioplasty Compatibility Trial. J Am Coll Cardiol 1999;34:1954–1962.

70. Neumann FJ, Schömig A. Stent anticoagulation and technique. In: Topol EJ, ed. Textbook of Interventional Cardiology, 4th edition. WB Saunders, Philadelphia, PA, 2002, p. 752.

13

Glycoprotein IIb/IIIa Receptor Blockade in Acute Myocardial Infarction

Adjunctive Therapy to Fibrinolysis

Sorin J. Brener, MD

CONTENTS

INTRODUCTION
EARLY EXPERIENCE WITH ADJUCTIVE PLATELET INHIBITION
REDUCED-DOSE FIBRINOLYSIS WITH GPIIb/IIIa ANTAGONISM:
    PHASE II ANGIOGRAPHIC STUDIES
REDUCED-DOSE FIBRINOLYSIS WITH GPIIb/IIIa ANTAGONISM:
    PHASE III STUDIES
SUMMARY AND RECOMMENDATIONS
REFERENCES

INTRODUCTION

Pharmacologic reperfusion with fibrinolytic therapy remains the principal method of infarct-artery recanalization for patients with acute myocardial infarction (AMI). Its universal availability, ease of administration, and effectiveness have been demonstrated in an impressive array of clinical trials in the last two decades *(1–3)*. Nevertheless, significant limitations and unfulfilled expectations continue to render this therapy less than perfect. Three generations of fibrinolytic agents have not been able to solve three vexing problems: restoration of normal flow [Thrombolysis in Myocardial Infarction (TIMI) grade 3] in the infarct artery is achieved in fewer than half the patients at 60 min from drug administration: one-fourth of those with epicardial reperfusion have impaired microvascular perfusion *(4,5)*; and finally, major bleeding [particularly intracranial hemorrhage (ICH)] remains high and has a major impact on outcome. Three recent megatrials *(6–8)* comparing the parent tissue plasminogen activator (t-PA) molecule with novel compounds, specifically designed to address some of t-PA's deficiencies, have failed to demonstrate, in general, superior efficacy (mortality reduction) or safety (ICH reduction). Some progress has been made with respect to major, nonintracranial, hemorrhage *(9)* and treatment of patients presenting beyond 4 h from symptom onset *(8)*.

From: *Contemporary Cardiology: Platelet Glycoprotein IIb/IIIa*
Inhibitors in Cardiovascular Disease, 2nd Edition
Edited by: A. M. Lincoff © Humana Press Inc., Totowa, NJ

Intensive examination of the failure of fibrinolytic agents to produce a higher rate of infarct-artery reperfusion has focused on the prothrombotic milieu engendered by these agents upon lysis of fibrin and liberation of clot-bound thrombin. Furthermore, as platelets are the initial element to accumulate at the site of plaque rupture and support rethrombosis, potent inhibitors of this mechanism became a logical target of investigation *(10,11)*. The most profound blockade of platelet activation and subsequent aggregation can be achieved by inhibitors of the final common pathway of platelet stimulation, glycoprotein (GP) IIb/ IIIa receptor *(12)*. Their pharmacology and properties are discussed elsewhere in this textbook. Experimental evidence in animals and humans pointed to the ability of these platelet antagonists to cause "dethrombosis," or reverse the process of fibrin deposition on a biologic template provided by the cellular membrane of aggregating platelets *(13)*.

Thus, application of these principles to reperfusion therapy using combination fibrin and platelet lysis was expected to yield the following advantages:

1. Arrest and modify the process of coronary thrombosis, thus promoting faster and more complete restoration of flow in a larger proportion of patients.
2. Improve tissue perfusion by minimizing the deleterious effects of thrombus embolization, which are often related to platelet degranulation and activation.
3. Obviate the need for, or facilitate the performance of, immediate percutaneous revascularization in patients who fail to reperfuse or are selected for immediate mechanical revascularization on clinical grounds.
4. By employing a lower dose of fibrinolytics, reduce the most severe complications of full-dose lytics, particularly intracranial hemorrhage.

This chapter will examine these expectations in light of the accumulated data and will map the road for future research.

EARLY EXPERIENCE WITH ADJUCTIVE PLATELET INHIBITION

The initial efforts to combine fibrin and platelet lytics were directed mostly at preventing reocclusion following initial patency and revolved around a full dose of a plasminogen activator-based regimen, to which GPIIb/IIIa inhibition was added in increasing doses. This approach was based on the assumption that a large amount of plasminogen activator is needed for clot lysis, while assigning lesser importance to the prothrombotic effect of these agents.

The Thrombolysis and Angioplasty in Myocardial Infarction (TAMI) 8 Trial

Kleiman et al. *(14)* conducted a pilot study in 60 patients treated with t-PA, aspirin, and heparin (control group) and ascending doses of the monoclonal antibody 7E3 (abciximab precursor) initiated at 3–15 h after fibrinolysis. Arterial patency (TIMI grade 2 or 3 flow) was detected in 56% of the control group and 92% of the 7E3 patients without a significant increase in major bleeding complications. Optimal platelet inhibition was obtained at a bolus dose of 0.25 mg/kg, consistent with the current dosing of abciximab.

The Integrilin to Minimize Platelet Aggregation and Coronary Thrombosis in Acute Myocardial Infarction (IMPACT-AMI) Trial

The IMPACT-AMI investigators *(15)* extended this concept to a dose-ranging trial in which 180 patients with AMI were treated with accelerated full-dose t-PA and a peptide inhibitor of the GPIIb/IIIa receptor, eptifibatide, given in escalating doses. The primary endpoint was the rate of TIMI grade 3 flow at 90 min. The highest dose of eptifibatide used (180 µg/kg bolus and 0.75 µg/kg/min infusion for 24 h) achieved TIMI 3 grade flow in 66%, compared with 39% in t-PA-alone patients ($p = 0.006$). There was a significant reduction in the time to complete ST-segment deviation resolution in the optimal eptifibatide group, from a median of 116 min for t-PA to 65 min ($p = 0.05$), indicating superior myocardial reperfusion. Severe bleeding complications occurred in 4% of the high-dose eptifibatide (one patient had intracranial hemorrhage) and 5% of t-PA control patients, whereas severe thrombocytopenia was found in 4 and 6%, respectively.

Eptifibatide and Streptokinase in Acute Myocardial Infarction

Streptokinase and eptifibatide were combined in a similar study *(16)*. One hundred eighty-one patients with AMI received aspirin, heparin, and full-dose streptokinase (1.5 million U) and were randomized to additional eptifibatide or placebo. The doses of eptifibatide tested were 180 µg/kg bolus followed by an infusion of 0.75 (IMPACT-AMI dose), 1.33, or 2.0 (PURSUIT dose) *(17)* µg/kg/min. The primary endpoint (TIMI grade 3 flow at 90 min) was achieved in 38% of the streptokinase alone group and 53, 44, and 52% of the eptifibatide groups, respectively. The two higher doses of the platelet inhibitor were associated with an incidence of moderate or severe bleeding of 40%, compared with 16% and 3% for the low-dose eptifibatide- and streptokinase-alone groups, respectively. The lack of a significant dose-effect response in arterial patency and the high rate of bleeding led to discontinuation of enrollment in the high-dose group.

The Platelet Aggregation Receptor Antagonist Dose Investigation and Reperfusion Gain in Myocardial Infarction (PARADIGM) Trial

The PARADIGM investigators enrolled 353 patients with AMI of <12 h in three phases of a dose-finding study *(18)*. All patients received aspirin and heparin. t-PA (75% of patients) or streptokinase (25%) were administered in the usual fashion. Placebo or lamifiban (a highly selective nonpeptide inhibitor of the GPIIb/IIIa receptor) in escalating doses of 300–400 µg/kg bolus and infusions of 1.0, 1.5, or 2.0 µg/kg/min for 24 h were added. The primary efficacy endpoint was achievement of >85% platelet inhibition in response to ADP and thrombin receptor agonist peptide (TRAP). Lamifiban at the highest dose induced marked platelet inhibition both after the bolus and at steady state. The effects of lamifiban were more pronounced in the streptokinase-treated patients. As in IMPACT-AMI, time to steady-state recovery of the ST-segment deviation was shortened by lamifiban from 122 to 88 min ($p = 0.003$). There was no systematic angiography in this trial. Adverse clinical events occurred insignificantly less often in the patients treated with lamifiban than with placebo, and major bleeding was noted in 3.0 and 1.7%, respectively.

REDUCED-DOSE FIBRINOLYIS WITH GPIIb/IIIa ANTAGONISM: PHASE II ANGIOGRAPHIC STUDIES

Six phase two clinical trials have completed enrolling approx 3500 AMI patients in angiographically controlled evaluations of the optimal combination of fibrinolytic agents [tissue plasminogen activator (t-PA), streptokinase, reteplase (r-PA), and tenecteplase (TNK)-t-PA] and a GPIIb/IIIa antagonist (abciximab, eptifibatide or tirofiban) *(19–23)*. Earlier studies consisted of dose-finding and dose-confirmation phases. All were similar with

Table 1
Trials of Reduced-Dose Fibrinolysis
and Platelet Glycoprotein (GP) Inhibition

Acronym (ref.)	No.	Lytic	GP inhibitor	1st angiogram (min)
TIMI 14 (19)	888	t-PA	Abciximab	90
SPEED (20)	528	r-PA	Abciximab	60–90
INTRO-AMI (21)	649	t-PA	Eptifibatide	60
INTEGRITI (22)	438	TNK	Eptifibatide	60
ENTIRE (23)	483	TNK	Abciximab	60
FASTER	408	TNK	Tirofiban	60

Abbreviations: r-PA, reteplase; TNK, tenecteplase; t-PA, tissue plasminogen activator.

respect to inclusion (6–12 h from symptom onset, eligibility for fibrinolysis) and exclusion criteria (cardiogenic shock) and angiographic endpoint, as shown in Table 1. One study (23) also evaluated the contribution to reperfusion of low-molecular-weight heparin (enoxaparin) compared with unfractionated heparin. The principal assumptions tested were that:

1. Reduced-dose fibrinolysis (50–75%) will not compromise efficacy and will enhance safety, in particular reducing the incidence of ICH.
2. The addition of GPIIb/IIIa antagonism will enhance efficacy compared with full-dose fibrinolysis alone without a significant increase in major bleeding complications.
3. The combination of the two agents will improve, beyond epicardial flow restoration, other parameters of reperfusion, such as resolution of ST-segment elevation and myocardial blush score.
4. The combination regimen will facilitate percutaneous revascularization, usually performed at the time of the protocol-mandated angiography.

None of the studies were powered to detect differences in 30-d ischemic endpoints and thus served as hypothesis-generating efforts, rather than as a definitive shift in the paradigm of reperfusion therapy.

The principal angiographic results of the six trials are shown in Figs. 1 and 2, including only direct comparisons between a full-dose fibrinolytic agent and a combination regimen. The brief attempt to administer streptokinase and abciximab resulted in a high incidence of bleeding, similar to the combination with eptifibatide, and is not included in this compilation (19). The impact on ST-segment elevation resolution is shown in Fig. 3 for trials that reported this outcome. In small subsets of patients treated with combination therapy, there was also improvement in the TIMI myocardial perfusion grade (blush score) (24). There were no significant differences in the incidence of death or reinfarction at 30 d in any of the trials between combination and monotherapy. Death occurred in approx 4% of patients and reinfarction in approx 3%. Major bleeding, including ICH, was reported using the TIMI definition (25) for all trials except SPEED, for which the GUSTO formula was utilized (20). The incidence of important bleeding was in general higher in the combination than the monotherapy regimen, although this difference did not reach statistical significance. The incidence of ICH varied between 0 and 3%, representing very few patients in many small groups allocated to various regimens.

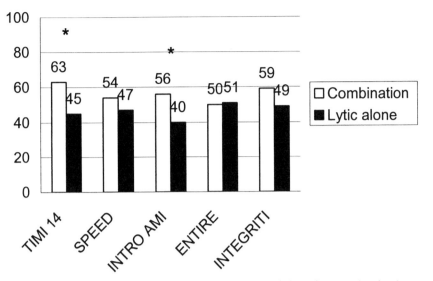

Fig. 1. Incidence of TIMI grade 3 flow at 60 min from drug administration (randomized comparison of combination therapy vs monotherapy). *, $p < 0.05$.

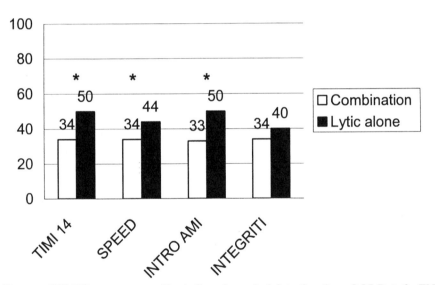

Fig. 2. Corrected TIMI frame counts at 60 min from drug administration. *, $p < 0.05$. Data for ENTIRE are not yet available.

The recommendations for immediate percutaneous revascularization following control angiography were not standardized in the various trials. In some, it was recommended for less than optimal pharmacologic reperfusion (rescue angioplasty), whereas in others it was encouraged (when feasible) even for patients with TIMI grade 3 flow (facilitated angioplasty). The most comprehensive analysis on this subject was performed in SPEED *(26)*. Patients treated with immediate angioplasty ($n = 322$, 71% of enrolled patients) had a significantly higher incidence of freedom from ischemic events at 30 d than those not

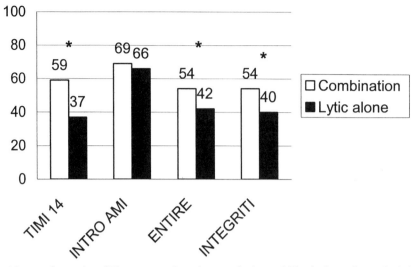

Fig. 3. Incidence of complete ST-segment elevation resolution at 180 min from drug administration. *$p < 0.05$.

undergoing revascularization. (Fig. 4) Similar results were reported from a subgroup of patients in TIMI 14 undergoing immediate angioplasty *(27)*. Among 113 patients undergoing immediate PCI after reperfusion therapy in TIMI 14, mean ST-segment deviation resolution was 8% in recipients of lytic monotherapy and 49% in those treated with combination abciximab and t-PA ($p = 0.002$).

To interpret results properly across different therapeutic regimens, some methodologic aspects of the trials merit attention. Early (60 min) angiographic evaluation, although clinically important, penalizes lytic regimens based on t-PA, whose completion requires the whole interval up to angiography. In contrast, single- (TNK) or double-bolus (r-PA) regimens are completed well in advance of the angiographic evaluation. In some instances *(21)*, angioplasty following the 60-min evaluation, although not recommended, was performed, complicating the assessment of TIMI grade 3 flow at 90 min and comparison with other regimens. This is also relevant to ST-segment elevation resolution at 180 min, which, in many cases, was measured after percutaneous revascularization. Finally, the concept of facilitated angioplasty after pharmacologic reperfusion cannot be clearly assessed in these trials, as the performance, timing, and indications for percutaneous revascularization were not standardized and tended to reflect the investigators' preference.

Despite these limitations, several broad conclusions can be drawn:

1. Combination fibrin and platelet-lysis tends to increase the incidence of TIMI grade 3 flow at 60 and 90 min, compared with fibrinolytic monotherapy. The absolute difference varies across regimens and studies between 10 and 20%. Based on the findings from the Global Utilization of Strategies to Open Occluded Arteries (GUSTO) I trial *(3)*, such an advantage is unlikely to translate into a significant reduction in mortality in small trials, particularly in a low-risk population with mortality rates of <5%.

2. The combination regimens tend to improve myocardial reperfusion, as measured by ST-segment elevation resolution and myocardial blush score.

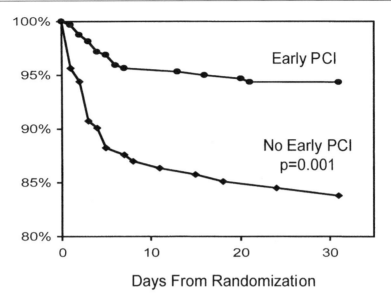

Days From Randomization

Fig. 4. Facilitated or rescue angioplasty in SPEED. PCI, percutaneous coronary intervention. (From ref. *26*.)

3. Bleeding complications, including ICH, have not been reduced by combination therapy. In fact, there were nominally more episodes of major bleeding in the combination regimens.
4. Rescue (for failed reperfusion) or facilitated (for residual stenosis with TIMI grade 3 flow) angioplasty was in general associated with acceptable results, particularly when compared with historical controls *(28–30)*. The excess ischemic complications observed earlier, particularly the high incidence of death in patients with failed PCI, did not occur in the context of frequent stenting and use of potent platelet antagonists.

REDUCED-DOSE FIBRINOLYIS
WITH GPIIb/IIIa ANTAGONISM: PHASE III STUDIES

Two large clinical trials, powered to detect differences in mortality and other important ischemic and bleeding complications at 30 d between regimens, have examined the role of combination anti-fibrin and platelet therapy in AMI.

Global Utilization of Strategies
to Open Occluded Coronary Arteries (GUSTO) V

Eight-hundred twenty hospitals randomized in an open-label design 16,588 patients with AMI within 6 h of symptom onset to full-dose r-PA or half-dose r-PA (5 MU twice, 30 min apart) and full-dose abciximab (0.25 µg/kg bolus and 0.125 µg/kg/minute infusion for 12 h) *(31)*. Patients selected for primary angioplasty were excluded. The important baseline characteristics are shown in Table 2. The primary endpoint was all-cause mortality at 30 d. Data were collected by investigators with respect to reinfarction and 15 other complications of AMI up to 7 d or hospital discharge. Bleeding and neurologic complications were assessed independently.

At 30 d (Fig. 5), the incidence of death in the mono- and dual-therapy groups was 5.9 and 5.6%, respectively ($p = 0.43$ for superiority and $p = 0.95$ for noninferiority), relative risk 0.95 (0.84–1.08). Mortality rates in prespecified subgroups are shown in Fig. 6. With

Table 2
Baseline Characteristics (%) of Patients in GUSTO V

	r-PA (n = 8260)	r-PA+ abciximab (n = 8328)
Age (yr)	61 ± 12	62 ± 12
Women	24	25
Diabetes	16	16
Previous MI	15	16
Hypertension	33	35
Prior PCI/CABG	10	10
Anterior MI	37	38
Time to therapy (h)	2.9 ± 1.6	3.1 ± 2.2

Abbreviations: CABG, coronary artery bypass graft; MI, myocardial infarction; PCI, percutaneous coronary intervention; r-PA, reteplase.

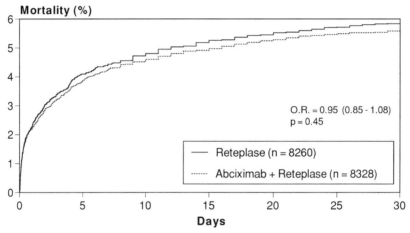

Fig. 5. Thirty-day mortality in GUSTO V.

the exception of pulmonary embolism and pericardial effusion, all other 14 prespecified post-MI complications were less common in the combination therapy arm. Reinfarction by d 7, manifested by enzyme reelevation and new electrocardiographic changes, was significantly less common in the combination arm than in the monotherapy group (2.3% vs 3.5%, $p < 0.0001$. Urgent (<6 h) percutaneous revascularization was significantly less often needed in the combination arm than in the monotherapy group (5.6% vs 8.6%, $p = 0.001$).

In contrast, bleeding complications were more common in the dual-therapy group; severe bleeding (1.1% vs 0.5%), any bleeding (24.6% vs 13.7%), and requirement for transfusion (5.7% vs 4.0%) were significantly increased in the combination arm ($p < 0.0001$ for all). This excess was related to spontaneous bleeding and not to surgical or percutaneous revascularization procedures.

The overall rate of any stroke (0.9% vs 1.0%) and ICH (0.6% vs 0.6%) was similar between the two groups. Nevertheless, there was a statistically significant interaction between treat-

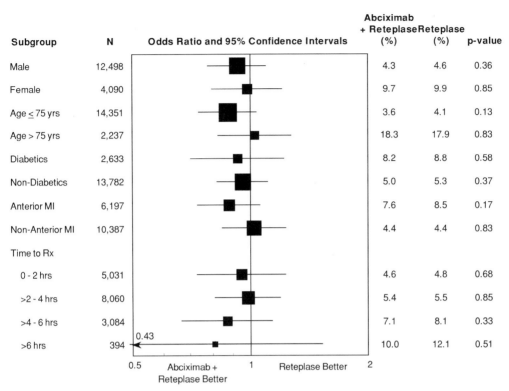

Subgroup	N	Odds Ratio and 95% Confidence Intervals	Abciximab + Reteplase (%)	Reteplase (%)	p-value
Male	12,498		4.3	4.6	0.36
Female	4,090		9.7	9.9	0.85
Age ≤ 75 yrs	14,351		3.6	4.1	0.13
Age > 75 yrs	2,237		18.3	17.9	0.83
Diabetics	2,633		8.2	8.8	0.58
Non-Diabetics	13,782		5.0	5.3	0.37
Anterior MI	6,197		7.6	8.5	0.17
Non-Anterior MI	10,387		4.4	4.4	0.83
Time to Rx					
0 - 2 hrs	5,031		4.6	4.8	0.68
>2 - 4 hrs	8,060		5.4	5.5	0.85
>4 - 6 hrs	3,084		7.1	8.1	0.33
>6 hrs	394		10.0	12.1	0.51

0.43 · 0.5 Abciximab + Reteplase Better · 1 · Reteplase Better · 2

Fig. 6. Thirty-day mortality in GUSTO V in prespecified subgroups. MI, myocardial infarction.

ment assignment and age with respect to ICH. Patients older than 75 yr had a significantly higher incidence of ICH with combination therapy than with monotherapy (2.1% vs 1.1%), compared with 0.4% vs 0.5%, respectively, for younger patients ($p = 0.033$ for interaction). This excess in ICH is probably responsible for the lack of any benefit of the combination regimen in elderly patients.

Although this trial did not show improved survival at 30 d for patients treated with combination fibrin and platelet antagonists, it is noteworthy that the overall mortality was much lower than expected (5.9% vs 7.5% for the r-PA groups in GUSTO V and GUSTO III, respectively). This may represent a secular trend of improvement in AMI outcome or selection of patients at lower risk than in previous fibrinolytic trials. The latter appears plausible, as the incidence of ICH in the r-PA monotherapy arms in GUSTO V was 0.6%, compared with 0.9% in GUSTO III. Within this context, the power of the study to detect noninferiority is <80%, and it is possible that the combination regimen could be associated with a 7% increase or a 15% decrease in mortality, compared with r-PA monotherapy. It is also important to note that many other complications of AMI, particularly reinfarction, were reduced by the dual-therapy regimen, an advantage that may translate into survival advantage at 1 yr. In previous fibrinolytic trials, reinfarction was associated with at least doubling of mortality, compared with patients without reinfarction *(32)*. Nevertheless, 1-yr mortality was identical (8.38%) in both groups *(32a)*. Preliminary analyses did not suggest that rescue PCI was favorably impacted by combination therapy, although it is difficult to eliminate the selection bias and the knowledge of the treatment assigned (A. M. Lincoff, personal communication).

Table 3
Baseline Characteristics (%) of Patients in ASSENT-3

	TNK+Enox (n = 2040)	TNK+Abcix (n = 2017)	TNK+UFH (n = 2038)
Age (yr)	61 ± 12	61 ± 12	61 ± 13
Women	23	24	23
Diabetes	19	18	18
Previous MI	14	13	14
Hypertension	41	41	41
Prior PCI/CABG	10	9	9
Anterior MI	39	39	38
Time to therapy (h)	3.0 ± 1.7	3.1 ± 1.4	3.1 ± 1.6

Abbreviations: Enox, enoxaparin; Abcix, abciximab; TNK, tenecteplase; UFH, unfractionated heparin. For other abbreviations, *see* Table 2 footnote.

The Assessment of Safety and Efficacy of a New Thrombolytic Regimen (ASSENT)-3 Trial

Following the demonstration that TNK-t-PA and t-PA are equivalent as monotherapy for AMI, this trial tested in an open-label design two new combination regimens against TNK monotherapy *(33)*. At 575 hospitals, 6095 patients within 6 h of onset of AMI were randomized to full-dose TNK with enoxaparin (continued for up to 7 d), half-dose TNK with abciximab and low-dose unfractionated heparin (UFH; for 48 h), or full-dose TNK with weight-adjusted UFH (for 48 h). The activated partial thromboplastin time (aPTT) for patients receiving UFH was maintained at 50–70 s and was first adjusted 3 h after TNK administration. The primary efficacy endpoint was the 30-d composite of death, in-hospital reinfarction, or in-hospital refractory ischemia. The same endpoints plus in-hospital major bleeding or ICH constituted the primary efficacy and safety endpoint.

The baseline characteristics of the patients enrolled in ASSENT-3 are shown in Table 3. At 30 d, the incidence of the primary efficacy (Fig. 7) and efficacy and safety endpoints (Fig. 8) were significantly reduced in comparison with the standard TNK therapy in both experimental arms. This difference in efficacy was already evident by 48 h, the time of discontinuation of UFH (6.1, 5.2, and 8.8%, respectively, $p < 0.0001$). Death (5.4, 6.6, and 6.0%, respectively, $p = 0.25$) and ICH (0.88, 0.94, and 0.93%, $p = 0.98$) were similar among the three groups. In contrast, in-hospital reinfarction (2.7, 2.2, and 4.2%, $p = 0.0009$) and refractory ischemia (4.7, 3.2, and 6.5%, respectively, $p < 0.0001$) occurred significantly less frequently in the experimental arms, particularly in the abciximab-treated cohort. Non-ICH major bleeding was more common in the abciximab group (3.0, 4.3, and 2.2%, respectively, $p = 0.0005$).

Prespecified subgroup analysis based on gender, age, diabetes, infarct location, and time-to-treatment identified two interesting findings: there was a significant interaction ($p = 0.0004$) between diabetes and treatment allocation for efficacy (Fig. 9) and between diabetes ($p = 0.0007$) and age ($p = 0.001$) and treatment allocation for efficacy and safety (Fig. 10). Whereas the age-treatment interaction was similar to that observed in GUSTO V, the findings in the diabetic patients are puzzling and unexpected. The need for urgent PCI was reduced in the experimental arms, particularly in the abciximab group (11.9, 9.1, and 14.4%, respectively, $p < 0.001$).

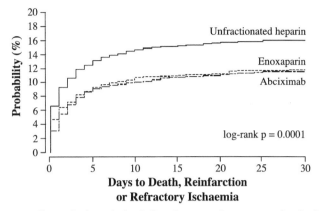

Fig. 7. Thirty-day mortality or in-hospital reinfarction or refractory angina in ASSENT-3. (From ref. *33*, with permission.)

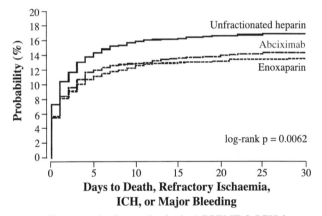

Fig. 8. Thirty-day primary efficacy and safety endpoint in ASSENT-3. ICH, intracranial hemorrhage. (From ref. *33*, with permission.)

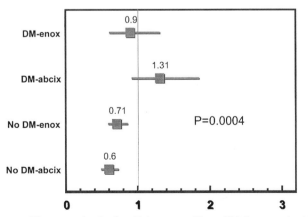

Fig. 9. Primary efficacy endpoint by diabetes mellitus (DM) status in ASSENT-3.

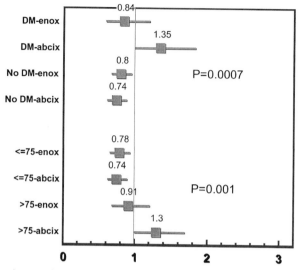

Fig. 10. Thirty-day primary efficacy and safety endpoint by diabetes mellitus (DM) status and age in ASSENT-3.

The standard TNK arm in ASSENT-2 and ASSENT-3 had a very similar outcome, suggesting that the population enrolled in the two trials was comparable. The incidence of non-ICH major bleeding was markedly lower in ASSENT-3 (2.2% vs 4.7%, $p < 0.01$), probably reflecting the earlier adjustment of aPTT after fibrinolysis in the latter trial.

SUMMARY AND RECOMMENDATIONS

Reperfusion therapy for AMI has changed significantly in the last half decade. The new paradigm has shifted the emphasis from epicardial reperfusion (which remains necessary) to myocardial reperfusion, which has become the ultimate goal. To this end, pharmacologic reperfusion regimens based on dual fibrin and platelet antagonists seemed to promise both enhanced epicardial reperfusion and substantial improvement in myocardial perfusion. Six small trials with angiographic endpoints have confirmed that, in general, the combination of half the dose of a fibrinolytic agent and a GPIIb/IIIa platelet antagonist improves epicardial and myocardial reperfusion, compared with standard-dose fibrinolysis, on the background of aspirin and UFH.

Larger trials designed to detect differences in critical ischemic complications have failed to confirm the advantage of these regimens over fibrinolysis monotherapy with respect to short-term mortality. Nevertheless, important secondary endpoints, such as reinfarction, refractory ischemia, and complications of the original infarction have been favorably affected by these new regimens. A number of questions remain unanswered:

1. Will improved background antithrombin therapy, such as low-molecular-weight heparin or direct thrombin inhibitors, interact positively with combination fibrin and platelet lysis to reduce ischemic complications of AMI further?
2. Are certain combination and dosing regimens better than others, and is there a correlation between the level of platelet inhibition and outcome? Particularly germane is the possibility that certain lytic agents, such as TNK, are better suited for lightweight patients and for those presenting at considerable delay from symptom onset.

3. Will a reduction in ischemic complications and an improvement in functional status or myocardial salvage justify the incremental cost of combination therapy?
4. Will combination therapy reduce the need for rescue PCI and facilitate definitive mechanical revascularization, or will primary PCI remain the optimal, yet logistically difficult, therapy for AMI? This important issue is addressed by two randomized clinical trials comparing primary PCI with GPIIb/IIIa inhibition vs combination fibrin and platelet lysis followed by PCI for high-risk AMI patients.

Until more data become available, it appears that combination therapy with a potent antiplatelet agent and reduced-dose fibrinolysis is a viable alternative to fibrinolysis monotherapy in patients younger than 75 yr. Longer term follow-up will clarify whether reductions in immediate ischemic complications eventually improve survival.

REFERENCES

1. GISSI Investigators. Effectiveness of intravenous thrombolytic treatment in acute myocardial infarction. Lancet 1986;1:397–401.
2. ISIS-3 (Third International Study of Infarct Survival) Collaborative Group. ISIS-3: a randomised comparison of streptokinase vs tissue plasminogen activator vs anistreplase and of aspirin plus heparin vs aspirin alone among 41,299 cases of suspected acute myocardial infarction. Lancet 1992;339:753–770.
3. GUSTO-I Investigators. An international randomized trial comparing four thrombolytic strategies for acute myocardial infarction. N Engl J Med 1993;329:673–682.
4. Lincoff AM, Topol EJ. Illusion of reperfusion. Does anyone achieve optimal reperfusion during acute myocardial infarction? [corrected and republished article originally printed in Circulation 1993;87: 1792–1805]. Circulation 1993;88:1361–1374.
5. Ito H, Okamura A, Iwakura K, et al. Myocardial perfusion patterns related to thrombolysis in myocardial infarction perfusion grades after coronary angioplasty in patients with acute anterior wall myocardial infarction. Circulation 1996;93:1993–1999.
6. The GUSTO III Investigators. A comparison of reteplase and alteplase for acute myocardial infarction. N Engl J Med 1997;337:1118–1123.
7. INTIME-II Investigators. Intravenous n-PA for the treatment of infarcting myocardium early. InTIME-II, a double-blind comparison of single-bolus lanoteplase vs accelerated alteplase for the treatment of patients with acute myocardial infarction. Eur Heart J 2000;21:2005–2013.
8. Assessment of the Safety and Efficacy of a New Thrombolytic (ASSENT-2) Investigators. Single-bolus tenecteplase compared with front-loaded alteplase in acute myocardial infarction: the ASSENT-2 double-blind randomised trial. Lancet 1999;354:716–722.
9. Lesaffre E, Bluhmki E, Wang-Clow F, et al. The general concepts of an equivalence trial, applied to ASSENT-2, a large-scale mortality study comparing two fibrinolytic agents in acute myocardial infarction. Eur Heart J 2001;22:898–902.
10. Weinberger I, Fuchs J, Davidson E, Rotenberg Z. Circulating aggregated platelets, number of platelets per aggregate, and platelet size during acute myocardial infarction. Am J Cardiol 1992;70:981–983.
11. Topol EJ. Toward a new frontier in myocardial reperfusion therapy: emerging platelet preeminence. Circulation 1998;97:211–218.
12. Coller B, Folts J, Smith S, Scudder L, Jordan R. Abolition of in vivo platelet thrombus formation in primates with monoclonal antibodies to the platelet GPIIb/IIIa receptor (correlation with bleeding time, platelet aggregation, and blockade of GPIIb/IIIa receptors). Circulation 1989;80:1766–1774.
13. Gold HK, Garabedian HD, Dinsmore RE, et al. Restoration of coronary flow in myocardial infarction by intravenous chimeric 7E3 antibody without exogenous plasminogen activators. Observations in animals and humans. Circulation 1997;95:1755–1759.
14. Kleiman NS, Ohman ME, Califf RM, et al. Profound inhibition of platelet aggregation with monoclonal antibody 7E3 fab after thrombolytic therapy. Results of the thrombolysis and angioplasty in myocardial infarction (TAMI) 8 pilot study. J Am Coll Cardiol 1993;22:381–389.
15. Ohman EM, Kleiman NS, Gacioch G, et al., for the IMPACT-AMI Investigators. Combined accelerated tissue-plasminogen activator and platelet glycoprotein IIb/IIIa integrin receptor blockade with Integrilin in acute myocardial infarction. Results of a randomized, placebo-controlled, dose-ranging trial. Circulation 1997;95:846–854.

16. Ronner E, van Kesteren HA, Zijnen P, et al. Safety and efficacy of eptifibatide vs placebo in patients receiving thrombolytic therapy with streptokinase for acute myocardial infarction. A phase II dose escalation, randomized, double-blind study. Eur Heart J 2000;21:1530–1536.

17. The PURSUIT Trial Investigators. Inhibition of platelet glycoprotein IIb/IIIa with eptifibatide in patients with acute coronary syndromes. Platelet Glycoprotein IIb/IIIa in Unstable Angina: Receptor Suppression Using Integrilin Therapy. N Engl J Med 1998;339:436–443.

18. PARADIGM Investigators. Combining thrombolysis with the platelet glycoprotein IIb/IIIa inhibitor lamifiban: results of the Platelet Aggregation Receptor Antagonist Dose Investigation and Reperfusion Gain in Myocardial Infarction (PARADIGM) trial. J Am Coll Cardiol 1998;32:2003–2010.

19. Antman EM, Giugliano RP, Gibson CM, et al. Abciximab facilitates the rate and extent of thrombolysis: results of the thrombolysis in myocardial infarction (TIMI) 14 trial. The TIMI 14 Investigators. Circulation 1999;99:2720–2732.

20. The SPEED Investigators. Trial of abciximab with and without low-dose reteplase for acute myocardial infarction. Strategies for Patency Enhancement in the Emergency Department (SPEED) Group. Circulation 2000;101:2788–2794.

21. Brener SJ, Zeymer U, Adgey AAJ, et al. Eptifibatide and low-dose tissue plasminogen activator in acute myocardial infarction: the INtegrilin and low-dose ThRombolysis in Acute Myocardial Infarction—INTRO AMI Trial. J Am Coll Cardiol 2002;39:377–386.

22. Giugliano RP, Roe MT, Zeymer U, et al. Restoration of epicardial and myocardial perfusion in acute ST-elevation myocardial infarction with combination eptifibatide+reduced-dose tenecteplase: dose-finding results from the INTEGRITI trial. Circulation 2001;104:II–538 (abstract).

23. Antman EM, Louwerenburg HW, Baars HF, et al., for the ENTIRE-TIMI 23 Investigators. Enoxaparin as adjunctive antithrombin therapy for ST-elevation myocardial infarction: results of the ENTIRE-Thrombolysis in Myocardial Infarction (TIMI) 23 Trial. Circulation 2002;105:1642–1649.

24. Gibson CM, Cannon CP, Murphy SA, et al. Relationship of TIMI myocardial perfusion grade to mortality after administration of thrombolytic drugs. Circulation 2000;101:125–130.

25. Chesebro J, Knatterud G, Roberts R, et al. Thrombolysis in Myocardial Infarction (TIMI) Trial, phase I: a comparison between intravenous tissue plasminogen activator and intravenous streptokinase. Clinical findings through hospital discharge. Circulation 1987;76:142–154.

26. Herrmann HC, Moliterno DJ, Ohman EM, et al. Facilitation of early percutaneous coronary intervention after reteplase with or without abciximab in acute myocardial infarction: results from the SPEED (GUSTO-4 pilot) trial. J Am Coll Cardiol 2000;36:1489–1496.

27. Schweiger MJ, Cannon CP, Murphy SA, et al. Early coronary intervention following pharmacologic therapy for acute myocardial infarction (the combined TIMI 10B-TIMI 14 experience). Am J Cardiol 2001;88:831–836.

28. Ellis S, Van de Werf F, Ribeiro-daSilva E, Topol E. Present status of rescue coronary angioplasty: current polarization of opinion and randomized trials. J Am Coll Cardiol 1992;19:681–686.

29. Abbottsmith CW, Topol EJ, George BS, et al. Fate of patients with acute myocardial infarction with patency of the infarct-related vessel achieved with successful thrombolysis versus rescue angioplasty. J Am Coll Cardiol 1990;16:770–778.

30. Ellis SG, Da Silva ER, Spaulding CM, Nobuyoshi M, Weiner B, Talley JD. Review of immediate angioplasty after fibrinolytic therapy for acute myocardial infarction: insights from the RESCUE I, RESCUE II, and other contemporary clinical experiences. Am Heart J 2000;139:1046–1053.

31. GUSTO V Investigators. Reperfusion therapy for acute myocardial infarction with fibrinolytic therapy or combination reduced fibrinolytic therapy and platelet glycoprotein IIb/IIIa inhibition: the GUSTO V randomised trial. Lancet 2001;357:1905–1914.

32. Barbash GI, Birnbaum Y, Bogaerts K, et al. Treatment of reinfarction after thrombolytic therapy for acute myocardial infarction: an analysis of outcome and treatment choices in the Global Utilization of Streptokinase and Tissue Plasminogen Activator for Occluded Coronary Arteries (GUSTO I) and Assessment of the Safety of a New Thrombolytic (ASSENT 2) Studies. Circulation 2001;103:954–960.

32a. Lincoff AM, Califf RM, Van De Werf F, et al. Mortality at 1 year with combination platelet glycoprotein IIb/IIIa inhibition and reduced-dose fibrinolytic therapy vs conventional fibrinolytic therapy for acute myocardial infarction: GUSTO V randomized trial. JAMA 2002;288:2130–2135.

33. ASSENT-3 Investigators. Efficacy and safety of tenecteplase in combination with enoxaparin, abciximab, or unfractionated heparin: the ASSENT-3 randomized trial in acute myocardial infarction. Lancet 2001;358:605–613.

IV PRACTICAL ISSUES AND FUTURE APPLICATIONS

14   Economics
of Glycoprotein IIb/IIIa Inhibition

Daniel B. Mark, MD, MPH

CONTENTS

INTRODUCTION
ECONOMIC ANALYSIS OF GLYCOPROTEIN IIb/IIIa RECEPTOR
    ANTAGONISTS
SUMMARY
REFERENCES

INTRODUCTION

Basic Concepts of Economic Analysis

Medical cost analysis is a hybrid field that incorporates concepts from both accounting and economics *(1)*. Economics provides much of the theoretical and conceptual framework for cost analysis while accounting provides us with practical measurement tools and concepts. One consequence of this admixture is that there are several distinct but overlapping sets of terminology used in cost analysis. We will start our review of this area by considering some of the basic concepts and terms that the clinician is likely to encounter in reading the medical cost literature.

When most people hear the term "cost," they think of money. An economist, on the other hand, thinks of cost in a much more theoretical way *(2,3)*. A major precept of economics is that any societal decision to employ the resources of society in the production of goods and services is necessarily accompanied by lost opportunities to do something else with those resources *(4,5)*. Health care services and programs engender a "cost" through their consumption of resources, which are then lost to other uses. The technical term for this concept is "opportunity cost" *(1,6)*. Economists are far more concerned with this notion of opportunity cost than they are with measuring dollars spent.

Another important related concept from economics holds that society's collective resources are finite. Consequently, there will not be sufficient resources to fulfill all of society's goals, forcing the need for choices to be made among competing priorities. Economics therefore strives to provide a set of tools to help policy and other decision makers decide how to allocate societal resources efficiently. In the most general terms,

From: *Contemporary Cardiology: Platelet Glycoprotein IIb/IIIa
Inhibitors in Cardiovascular Disease, 2nd Edition*
Edited by: A. M. Lincoff © Humana Press Inc., Totowa, NJ

resources are divided into large categories such as land, labor, and capital (e.g., stores of raw material, factories, machines). Technology allows society to convert these raw resources into desired goods and services, including medical care. In order to understand societal alternatives for the use of such resources, it is necessary to assess the opportunity cost of various types of health care as well as that of investments in defense, public education, transportation, and other societal priorities. To compare the resource requirements of these needs, a common metric must be found. Some societies still use barter to match goods and services, but most industrialized societies employ markets (collections of sellers and buyers), with money used as the standard exchange intermediary. The market price in these societies represents the monetary equivalent in value of the total resource inputs used in the production of the particular good or service. Money then is a convenient shorthand for valuing all these resources, but the underlying resources themselves are the primary concern for the economist.

Unfortunately, the economic concept of opportunity cost, while representing the purest definition of "true cost," is actually a theoretical construct that does not have a practical measurement analog *(1)*. Accountants, being more concerned with measurement than economists, have made some important simplifications to allow approximation of opportunity cost. In each costing exercise, because the cost information itself has a cost, the analyst must decide how much detail is necessary to satisfy the particular study requirement. In addition, cost needs to be assessed from an explicitly defined perspective. In health care, a variety of valid perspectives are possible. If a patient receives a $10,000 cardiac procedure but only pays her deductible and copayment amounting to $1000 (with the remainder paid by insurance), then for that patient the cost of the procedure is $1000. The cost to the insurance company may be only $6000 if they have negotiated discounted payments with the hospital. The cost to the hospital of delivering the care in question is different from both these figures. The societal perspective is the one most often used by cost analysts in medicine. This is the broadest possible perspective since it incorporates all costs and health benefits created by the contemplated change in medical care *(5)*.

Costs can be classified according to their behavior as production is increased or decreased (variable vs fixed costs) and in terms of their traceability to the production of health care services (direct vs indirect costs). *Variable costs* increase in direct proportion to production of extra health care. Disposable supplies in a catheterization laboratory are an example of variable costs. *Fixed costs*, as the name implies, do not change with the volume of care provided (e.g., the depreciation of the catheterization facility itself) *(1)*. *Direct costs* can be readily linked to the production of a particular health care product or service (e.g., disposable supplies, labor), whereas *indirect costs* (or overhead) cannot (e.g., heating, electricity, laundry, medical records, hospital administrators).

Two terms are used to describe the effect on costs resulting from shifts in the use of health services. *Marginal cost* refers to the extra cost involved in generating one extra unit of a good or service within the context of a given health care intervention [e.g., performing one extra coronary angioplasty (PTCA)] and is equivalent to variable cost. *Incremental cost* is the cost involved in shifting from one health care intervention to an alternative (e.g., from thrombolysis to direct angioplasty); this is a fundamental notion that underlies cost-effectiveness analysis.

Another important economic concept for the clinician is that of *induced cost or induced saving*. If one performs a cardiovascular procedure, it is clear that the cost of that procedure includes the cost of the equipment consumed in the procedure (such as coronary stents or balloon catheters). It may be less clear that the cost of the procedure also includes things that happen later in the patient's follow-up as a consequence of the decision to do that procedure. For example, the need to have a second procedure to treat restenosis is an induced cost of the initial procedure. The reduced need for a repeat procedure when a coronary stent is substituted for a standard balloon catheter procedure is an induced saving of the coronary stent procedure. The key concept is that it is not sufficient in most cases of medical care to look only at the immediate costs of care. Downstream costs and cost savings must also be assessed in order to provide an accurate picture of the total economic effects of a particular technology or strategy.

One other term that is often used in economic analysis is *indirect cost*. This term actually has two meanings, an accounting meaning in which it refers to overhead (as described above) and an economic meaning in which it refers to costs associated with lost productivity. Because of this confusion of terminology, many modern investigators substitute the term *productivity costs* when they are referring to the latter type of indirect costs *(5)*. In medical care, typical productivity costs include those associated with time lost from work. Difficulties encountered in assessing productivity costs relate in part to the proper methods of assessing such costs for individuals who are retired from the workforce or those who are working at home (not for pay). In practice, productivity costs are infrequently examined in medical economic studies.

In an ideal competitive economic market, prices for goods and services are established by the dynamic interplay between sellers and buyers. Such markets are characterized by competition on price among many sellers (none of whom is large enough to control prices), easy entry into the market by new sellers, and knowledgeable buyers who themselves pay for the goods and services they consume *(2)*. The "medical marketplace" has none of these features. Patients are usually insulated from most of the cost of the care they consume by insurance, and they do not have the technical knowledge to discriminate among the care options they face. In most local health care markets, there are only a few buyers (insurance companies) and sellers (medical care systems) of health care. Although managed care has introduced price competition to medicine, it is not the ideal competition of economic textbooks. During the peak of the managed care era, managed care companies often controlled large blocks of business, and providers were forced to accept a heavily discounted price in order to retain this portion of their patient population. Because of these and related issues and because of the fragmentation of the medical marketplace, providers may have one price for self-pay patients (full charges, usually their highest price), another price for discounted fee-for-service business, and yet another price for managed care. Typically, none of these reflect the opportunity cost of the care provided. Thus, there is no market price for medical care in the way that automobiles and refrigerators have a market price. Consequently, several different approaches have been developed to estimate medical costs (or prices). These are reviewed briefly in the next section.

Cost Measurement

Two general approaches are available to measure the costs of medical care services: bottom-up and top-down. The bottom-up methods are all based on counting individual resources consumed in a particular episode of care and assigning appropriate cost weights. The gold standard bottom-up method is known as microcosting and involves a very detailed enumeration of all resources consumed, estimation of cost weights for each individual resource, and calculation of total costs through multiplication of the individual resources by their cost weights. Although microcosting analysis is possible for simple types of medical care, such as administration of an intravenous antibiotic, it can be very laborious and expensive for complex forms of care. Even things such as an admission for coronary angioplasty or acute myocardial infarction are relatively complex when considering doing a microcosting analysis. Fortunately, increasing numbers of hospitals in the United States have installed detailed computer-based cost accounting systems that provide an approximate version of the gold standard bottom-up cost analysis. These systems have not been well studied from a research point of view, but they do appear to offer a better estimate of true underlying costs than is available through alternatives. Like any costing methodology, they should not be accepted without question, and component inputs should be carefully scrutinized for reasonableness whenever possible.

The simplest version of the bottom-up approach is the so-called *big ticket method*. This is based on an identification of a subset of resources consumed that are considered the most important and/or costly (the big tickets). This approach is the most inexpensive method of costing and allows the analyst to concentrate on generating cost estimates for a small subset of the entire portfolio of resources consumed. There are several potential disadvantages to this simple method, however. Most importantly, the analysis may oversimplify the true resource effects of the strategies under study and therefore may miss important cost differences. There are rarely sufficient prior data available to assure the analyst that he or she has captured all the important resources in the appropriate amount of detail. This approach also assumes that all big ticket resources of a particular type have the same cost, which of course is clearly not true. Cost weights for this type of analysis are often chosen more for convenience than established suitability for the task.

The other major approach to cost estimation is the top-down approach. Two different methods can be used here. The most common method used in medical cost research applications involving hospital-based care is the collection of hospital billing information and the conversion of the charges on the hospital bills into costs using correction factors that are published in each hospital's annual cost report. The vast majority of hospitals in the United States generate the type of bills (UB-92) and the Medicare Cost Reports that are necessary to accomplish this conversion. (Notable exceptions are Veterans Administration Hospitals and some fully capitated HMOs.) Physician costs can also be collected as billing information, although this is generally onerous because physician billing for a particular medical center is often done from individual offices rather than from a centralized billing office. In addition, there are no standardized conversion factors to correct physician charges back to costs. For that reason, many current analysts use the Medicare Fee Schedule as a national standard for physician costs.

The Medicare Fee Schedule also provides the best current source for costs of outpatient visits and testing. A much simpler top-down approach that is used primarily when there are limited details available in the database about resources consumed is to assign each inpatient episode of patient care to a diagnosis-related group (DRG) category and assign price weights to the entire episode of care based on this type of aggregating classification. This approach has many of the same limitations described earlier for the big ticket bottom-up approach. Clearly not all episodes of hospitalization for coronary angioplasty involve the same amount of resources or should be given the same cost weight, just as different hospitalizations for myocardial infarction or coronary bypass surgery should not be viewed as economically uniform.

Cost Measurement in Clinical Trials

Over the last decade, several groups have pioneered the use of empirical cost data collection in large-scale randomized trials and in large, single-site observational studies as the principal method for estimating medical costs *(7–11)*. By generating an empirical database of costs similar to the empirical clinical database that is typically generated in clinical trials and outcome studies, we have a much richer source of investigation and can perform analyses that do not appear as arbitrary and subject to analyst biases as earlier literature and expert-based opinion analyses often did. We have shown that it is feasible to collect hospital billing information on large numbers of patients enrolled in the United States and that these data can reliably provide an estimate of medical costs. Ideally, we would prefer to have access to a detailed hospital accounting system in every hospital in which we enroll patients in a particular study, but this is rarely feasible. Consequently, we anticipate that for at least the next 5 years we will continue to be measuring hospital costs through the use of medical bills and correction factors as described above.

Cost-Effectiveness Analysis

Many clinicians tend to confuse cost-effectiveness analysis with economic analysis in general, but these two concepts are not equivalent. Cost-effectiveness analysis is a specific type of economic analysis that attempts to assess the value of medical care by relating in a structured fashion the added costs of a particular strategy to its added medical benefits. Typically, cost-effectiveness analyses express their results in terms such as the extra dollars required to add an additional life year with the new strategy relative to standard care. The goal of cost-effectiveness analysis is not to assist the clinician at the bedside, but rather to give policy analysts a tool to use in allocating societal resources. Although theoretically attractive, this use of cost effectiveness is rarely attempted in actual practice and the challenge for modern analysts is to find ways of doing cost-effectiveness analysis that are more relevant to the challenges and concerns of practitioners, administrators, health plans, and patients in the modern era. Additional details on cost-effectiveness methodologies are provided elsewhere *(1,5)*.

ECONOMIC ANALYSIS OF GLYCOPROTEIN IIb/IIIa RECEPTOR ANTAGONISTS

Studies of Percutaneous Coronary Revascularization

The three currently available intravenous glycoprotein (GP) IIb/IIIa platelet receptor blockers have all been studied in large-scale clinical trials involving percutaneous revascularization patients, as described in earlier chapters in this book. Six trials with prospective economic analysis of GPIIb/IIIa inhibitors in percutaneous intervention populations have been completed: EPIC, EPILOG, and EPISTENT (involving abciximab); IMPACT II and ESPRIT (eptifibatide); and RESTORE (tirofiban).

ABCIXIMAB

The Evaluation of Monoclonal Antibody to Prevent Ischemic Complications (EPIC) trial randomized 2099 high-risk PTCA patients to one of three arms: placebo, bolus abciximab, and bolus plus infusion abciximab. All patients received aspirin and a fixed dose regimen of intravenous heparin. At 30 d, bolus plus 12-h infusion abciximab reduced ischemic

Table 1
Major Baseline Hospital Resource Consumption and Hospital Costs in the EPIC Study

	Placebo (n = 696)	*Bolus only* (n = 695)	*Bolus plus infusion* (n = 708)
Resource consumption (%)			
Urgent re-PTCA	3.6	2.6	0.7
Nonurgent re-PTCA	3.3	2.3	3.7
Coronary stent	0.6	1.7	0.6
Urgent CABG	3.6	2.0	2.4
Nonurgent CABG	1.1	1.4	2.3
Intraaortic balloon pump	3.3	2.4	2.9
RBC transfusion	7	13	15
Medical costs and length of stay (means $)			
Hospital costs	11,430	11,141	11,562
Physician fees	2004	1993	2015
Total medical costs	13,434	13,135	13,577
Total length of stay (d)	5.9	6.1	6.4

Abbreviations: PTCA, coronary angioplasty; CABG, coronary bypass surgery; RBC, red blood cell. From ref. 7.

endpoints by 35% relative to placebo but doubled major in-hospital bleeding episodes (from 7 to 14%) *(12)*. Six-month ischemic episodes were further reduced by 23% *(13)*. The economic substudy of EPIC was conducted prospectively as part of the overall EPIC research effort *(7)*. Hospital costs were estimated using hospital bills and Medicare conversion factors, as described above. Physician fees were estimated from the Medicare Fee Schedule and the record of physician services contained in the case report form. The cost of abciximab was estimated from the per vial cost of the drug and the weight of the patients in the EPIC trial, assuming that unused portions of vials would be wasted.

During the index hospitalization, the baseline costs in EPIC (excluding the cost of abciximab) were not significantly different (Table 1). Including the cost of abciximab ($1407), the baseline hospital plus physician costs were $14,984 for the bolus plus infusion abciximab arm and $13,434 for the placebo arm. To understand the dissociation evident between the beneficial effect of abciximab on the primary study endpoint (which reflected a composite of adverse ischemic events) and the absence of a related economic benefit, we developed an "explanatory" regression model. This model demonstrated that during the initial hospitalization, the decrease in ischemic events owing to abciximab generated a potential cost saving that was estimated at $622 per patient (Table 2). However, the excess major bleeding in the bolus plus infusion abciximab arm generated a $521 excess in costs for this arm.

During the 6-mo follow-up, the abciximab arm experienced a 23% decrease in rehospitalization and a 22% decrease in repeat revascularization procedures *(7)*. The associated cost savings from these resource reductions averaged $1270 per patient ($p = 0.02$). Combining the baseline and follow-up costs for each treatment arm yielded a net 6-mo cost for the abciximab bolus and infusion arm of $293 per patient. Based on these data, we projected that if EPIC results could be replicated in terms of efficacy of therapy, with a simultaneous reduction in the rate of major bleeding, then abciximab had the potential to pay for itself over the 6-mo observation period.

Table 2
Multivariable Linear Regression Model from the EPIC Economic Substudy[a]

Event	Estimated cost[b] ($)	Placebo incidence (%)		Bolus plus infusion incidence (%)		Savings (costs) associated with bolus plus infusion treatment ($)	
		Intent to treat	Rx received	Intent to treat	Rx received	Intent to treat	Rx received
Efficacy							
Non-urgent PTCA	4973	3.3	3.4	3.7	3.4	(25)	(1)
Urgent PTCA	8852	3.6	3.8	0.7	0.7	268	273
Non-urgent CABG	14,750	1.1	0.9	2.3	1.8	(164)	(130)
Urgent CABG	27,349	3.6	3.8	2.4	2.1	365	479
Total	—	—	—	—	—	444	622
Bleeding[c]							
Major bleeding	5896	3.3	3.4	10.6	10.5	(430)	(418)
Minor bleeding	1327	9.2	9.4	16.8	17.1	(101)	(102)
Total						(531)	(521)

Abbreviations: PTCA, coronary angioplasty; CABG, coronary bypass surgery; Rx, treatment.
[a]All variables coded 0 (condition absent)/1 (condition present).
[b]Predicted costs from regression model.
[c]Bleeding not associated with CABG.
Note that the incidence of urgent PTCA, urgent CABG, and major and minor bleeding reflects outcomes as of hospital discharge, whereas the clinical reports from this study provide 30-d outcomes.

EPIC was the first large-scale trial of a GPIIb/IIIa platelet inhibitor and demonstrated that this class of drugs provided a major therapeutic advance as adjunctive therapy for PTCA. However, the doubled risk of major bleeding provided a significant damper on the clinical and economic attractiveness of this therapy. The EPILOG trial was conducted to validate and extend the findings of EPIC to a broader percutaneous intervention population *(14)*. Importantly, it used a weight-adjusted lower dose heparin regimen to evaluate whether bleeding could be controlled with preserved efficacy. A total of 2792 urgent or elective percutaneous coronary intervention patients were enrolled in EPILOG before the study was stopped early by the Data and Safety Monitoring Board. Clinically, the trial demonstrated a 57% reduction in major ischemic complications consisting of death, myocardial infarction (MI), or urgent revascularization in the abciximab/low-dose heparin arm by 30 d. The modified heparin regimen was successful in reducing the rate of major bleeding to that of the placebo arm (2% for abciximab vs 3.1% for placebo plus standard-dose heparin).

A prospective cost analysis was performed in EPILOG using the same methods previously described for EPIC *(15)*. The analysis showed that total baseline medical costs for the abciximab arm (including $1457 for the abciximab regimen itself) was $10,215 vs $9632 for placebo, a $583 net excess cost for the abciximab strategy (Table 3). Thus, EPILOG confirmed the prediction made in the EPIC economic analysis, videlicet, that a reduction in ischemic complications with control of the excess bleeding risk would result in a cost offset of about $600 during the initial hospitalization.

Table 3
Baseline Medical Resources and Costs in the EPILOG Trial

	Heparin *(n = 939)*	*Abciximab plus* *low-dose heparin* *(n = 935)*
Resources		
Repeat PTCA (%)	4.0	2.0
Stent placed (%)	26	16.7
CABG (%)	2.9	1.2
ICU LOS (d)	1.4 d	1.3 d
Total LOS (d)	3.5 d	3.4 d
Costs ($)		
Hospital Costs	8291	7485
MD fees	1341	1273
Total	9632	8758
Total plus abciximab	9632	10,215

Abbreviations: CABG, coronary artery bypass graft; ICU, intensive care unit; LOS, length of stay; PTCA, coronary angioplasty.
From ref. *15.*

The follow-up picture from EPILOG was significantly different from that seen in EPIC *(15).* Unlike the earlier trial, EPILOG did not show any reduction in subsequent hospitalizations or cardiac procedures. In fact, there was a nonsignificant increase in hospitalizations and medical costs for the abciximab/low-dose heparin arm relative to placebo. Thus, the net cost of abciximab in the more modern EPILOG study (approx $600) is approximately twice that initially predicted by EPIC (approx $300) *(15).*

The CAPTURE trial compared abciximab bolus plus infusion for 24 h versus placebo in 1265 unstable angina patients scheduled for PTCA *(16).* Unlike EPIC and EPILOG, in which the abciximab bolus was given just prior to the procedure, CAPTURE patients received almost all their abciximab prior to the procedure, with drug continued for only 1 h after the procedure. At 30 d, the abciximab arm showed a 29% reduction in the primary endpoint of death, MI, or urgent revascularization ($p = 0.012$). Unfortunately, no economic data were collected in this European trial. On the basis of the resource use data published, it seems likely that the economics of abciximab use during the index hospitalization would be consistent with the results of EPIC and EPILOG, namely, a partial offset of the cost of abciximab owing to reduced ischemic events.

The Evaluation of Platelet IIb/IIIa Inhibitor for Stenting (EPISTENT) trial randomized 2399 patients scheduled for elective or urgent percutaneous revascularization to stenting plus placebo ($n = 809$), stenting plus abciximab ($n = 794$), or balloon angioplasty plus abciximab ($n = 796$) *(17).* At 30 d, mortality was 0.6% in the stent-alone arm, 0.3% in the stent-abciximab arm, and 0.8% in the balloon-abciximab arm. The corresponding MI rates were 9.6, 4.5, and 5.3%, respectively. Major bleeding occurred in 2.2% of stent-alone patients, 1.5% of stent-abciximab patients, and 1.4% of balloon-abciximab patients. After 1 yr of follow-up, 2.4% of the stent-alone patients had died compared with 1% of the stent-abciximab patients and 2.1% of the balloon-abciximab patients *(18).* Corresponding 1-yr MI rates were 11.3, 5.9, and 7.7%, respectively.

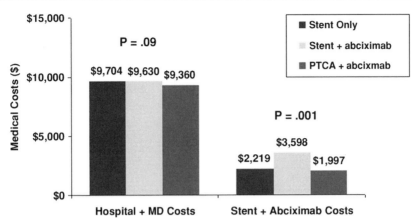

Fig. 1. Baseline hospital costs in the EPISTENT economic substudy.

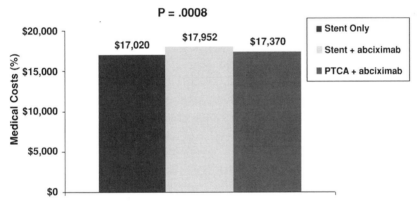

Fig. 2. Cumulative 1-yr medical costs in the EPISTENT economic substudy.

Economic analysis of EPISTENT was performed using the US cohort from the trial (*n* = 1438) *(18)*. As shown in Fig. 1, the baseline hospital costs for the three treatment groups differed only in the cost of the experimental interventions, with the combination stent-abciximab arm being $1400–$1600 more expensive than the other two groups. Follow-up rehospitalization was higher in the balloon-abciximab arm than the other two arms owing to a greater need for repeat revascularizations. Thus, follow-up medical costs were $5096 in the stent-only arm, $4723 in the stent-abciximab arm, and $6013 in the balloon-abciximab arm. Cumulative 1-yr medical costs remained higher in the stent-abciximab arm (Fig. 2), but the increment was considerably smaller ($600–900) than after the index hospitalization. Table 4 shows the cost-effectiveness ratios for stent-abciximab compared with stent alone ($6213 per life-year added) and with balloon-abciximab ($5291 per life-year added). Thus, although stenting with abciximab has considerably higher up-front procedural costs, a significant portion of the incremental costs is recouped in the first year following the procedure. Furthermore, this combination therapy is a very economically attractive way of increasing health benefits for coronary artery disease (CAD) patients.

Table 4
EPISTENT Cost-Effectiveness Analysis

| | Stent plus abciximab compared with | |
	Stent alone	PTCA plus abciximab
Incremental costs	$932	$582
Incremental LE (3% discount)	0.15 life-yr	0.11 life-yr
Incremental CE	$6213 per added life-yr	$5291 per added life-yr

Abbreviations: CE, cost effectiveness; LE, life expectancy.

EPTIFIBATIDE

The Integrilin to Minimize Platelet Aggregation and Coronary Thrombosis (IMPACT II) trial tested two doses of eptifibatide (Integrilin) against placebo in a cohort of 4010 PTCA patients *(19)*. At 30 d, the lower dose eptifibatide bolus plus infusion regimen demonstrated a reduction in 30-d ischemic events (death, MI, urgent revascularization) ($p=0.06$), whereas a somewhat smaller effect was seen in the high-dose regimen ($p=0.22$). When it was reanalyzed by treatment received (instead of intention-to-treat), the 30-d event rate for the lower dose regimen was significantly lower than for the placebo group ($p=0.035$). At 30 d, the low-dose eptifibatide group had a very modest reduction in urgent/emergent percutaneous revascularization (2.6% vs 2.8% for placebo), bailout stent use (0.5% vs 1.4% for placebo), and urgent/emergency coronary artery bypass surgery (1.6% vs 2.8% for placebo) *(19)*. The associated cost offset was small and not statistically significant. Importantly, there was no increase in major bleeding seen. In follow-up, there was no evidence of a differential effect of eptifibatide on rehospitalization or repeat procedures. As discussed elsewhere in this volume, analysis of the platelet effects achieved by the two eptifibatide doses used in IMPACT II revealed an inhibition level of 40–60%, substantially lower than the target of ≥80% inhibition. These findings led to the change in dosing of eptifibatide used in PURSUIT (discussed below).

The Enhanced Suppression of the Platelet IIb/IIIa Receptor with Integrilin Therapy (ESPRIT) trial randomized 2064 patients undergoing PCI with stenting to either eptifibatide or placebo *(20)*. The eptifibatide arm received two 180 µg/kg boluses 10 min apart. After the first bolus, a 2.0 µg/kg/min intravenous drip was started and maintained for up to 18–24 h. This dosing regimen provides a higher level of platelet inhibition than was seen in IMPACT II. ESPRIT was terminated early by the Data and Safety Monitoring Board for efficacy. At 30 d, the eptifibatide regimen reduced the death/MI rate from 9.2% in the placebo arm to 5.5% ($p=0.001$). MI was reduced from 9 to 5.4% ($p=0.002$). Death was 0.2% in the placebo group and 0.1% in the eptifibatide group ($p=0.55$). Major bleeding was seen in 0.4% of placebo patients and 1% of eptifibatide patients. During the index hospitalization, there was no significant difference in major resource use including hospital days and repeat revascularization *(20)*.

The cost of the eptifibatide regimen in the ESPRIT population was $495. Total hospital costs, including eptifibatide, were $10,721 in the eptifibatide arm and $10,430 in the placebo arm, leaving a net cost for the eptifibatide strategy of $291 per patient. Follow-up costs out to 1 yr were $2121 vs $2254, leaving a net 1-yr cost for the eptifibatide strategy of $146. At 1 yr, the death rate was 1.4% for eptifibatide vs 2% for placebo ($p = 0.28$), and the MI rate was 7.2% for eptifibatide versus 10.7% ($p = 0.004$) for placebo. Using long-term Duke data to project out life expectancy for the two strategies, eptifibatide as used in the ESPRIT trial added 0.10 life-years (discounted at 3%) per patient. The corresponding cost-effectiveness ratio was $1407 per year of life saved, which is very economically attractive by conventional criteria.

TIROFIBAN

The Randomized Efficacy Study of Tirofiban for Outcomes and Restenosis (RESTORE) trial randomized 2139 patients with an acute coronary syndrome (acute MI, unstable angina) who were referred within 72 h of presentation for percutaneous coronary intervention to either tirofiban or placebo *(21)*. The drug was given as a bolus plus 36-h infusion. There was a significant 38% reduction in the combined ischemic endpoint at 48 h, but at 30 d the results had converged somewhat, leading to a net 16% reduction by tirofiban ($p = 0.16$). When the primary endpoint was redefined as death, MI, or urgent revascularization, the tirofiban arm demonstrated a 24% reduction at 30 d ($p = 0.052$). There was no excess of major bleeding seen with tirofiban *(21)*. Thus, the results of RESTORE and IMPACT II are similar. The 6-mo follow-up data from RESTORE showed no evidence of a post-30-d effect of the drug on outcomes *(22)*. Economic analysis of this trial was performed using hospital billing data for a subset of patients in the United States with imputation of cost for the remaining US patients *(23)*. The cost of the tirofiban regimen was estimated at $700. In-hospital costs (including tirofiban costs) were $12,230 for the tirofiban arm and $12,145 for placebo. The offset of the costs of the tirofiban regimen was created by reduced repeat revascularization procedures.

Studies of Patients with Acute Coronary Syndromes

Of the major studies that have been completed using intravenous GPIIb/IIIa receptor blockers in acute coronary syndrome patients, only PURSUIT has included an economic analysis. PURSUIT randomized 10,948 patients with an acute coronary syndrome (unstable angina, non-ST-segment elevation MI) between November 1995 and January 1997 *(24)*. As described elsewhere in this text, PURSUIT had three treatment arms, two with bolus plus 72-h infusion of eptifibatide regimen and one with bolus placebo plus infusion placebo. As mandated by protocol, the Data and Safety Monitoring Board determined that the higher dose eptifibatide regimen had an acceptable safety profile, and the lower dose regimen was dropped after 3126 patients had been randomized *(24)*. Adjunctive therapy and use of invasive procedures were left to the discretion of the individual investigators, but all were encouraged to use daily aspirin (80–325 mg) and some form of heparin therapy.

At 30 d, the bolus plus 72-h infusion eptifibatide regimen produced a 1.5% absolute reduction in the composite primary endpoint (death or MI; 15.7% in the placebo arm vs 14.2% in the eptifibatide arm, $p = 0.042$) *(24)*. The therapeutic benefit of eptifibatide was fully established by 96 h and was preserved out to 30 d. Using investigator-defined rather than Clinical Events Committee-defined MIs in the primary endpoint yielded a slightly larger treatment effect (placebo event rate 10% vs 8.1% for eptifibatide, $p = 0.001$). Major bleeding was increased in the eptifibatide arm (10.6% vs 9.1% for placebo, $p = 0.016$), but strokes were not increased.

Table 5
Index Hospitalization Resource
Consumption and Costs from the PURSUIT Trial

	Eptifibatide (n = 1754)	Placebo (n = 1765)
Medical resource consumption (%)		
Dx cardiac catheterization	85	85
Percutaneous intervention	35	36
Coronary bypass surgery	20	20
ICU LOS (mean d)	3.7	3.7
Total LOS (mean d)	6.5	6.5
Medical costs ($)		
Hospital costs	12,420	12,617
MD costs	2309	2340
Total costs	14,729	14,957

Abbreviations: ICU, intensive care unit; LOS, length of stay.
From ref. *25.*

As a prospective part of the PURSUIT research effort, we collected medical cost data in 2464 of the 3519 patients enrolled in the United States using the methods described earlier in this chapter *(25)*. The cost of eptifibatide was estimated from the drug's average wholesale price (AWP) and the amount of drug actually administered to each US patient. For the 1055 US patients without hospital billing data, we used a resource-based regression model to impute their costs. Thus, the primary cost comparisons in PURSUIT were based on the entire US cohort (measured plus imputed).

During the index hospitalization, we found no evidence of an effect of eptifibatide on major resource consumption (Table 5). Diagnostic catheterization was performed in 85% of both groups, percutaneous revascularization in one-third, and coronary bypass surgery in 20%. Thus, the baseline medical costs in the two arms (excluding the costs for the eptifibatide regimen) were equivalent, at approximately $14,800 ($p = 0.78$).

Resource consumption after discharge and out to the 6-mo anniversary of enrollment (when follow-up was terminated) also did not show any treatment-related differences. Diagnostic cardiac catheterization was used in 14% of both groups, percutaneous intervention in 7%, and bypass surgery in 4%. The corresponding medical costs averaged about $3800 ($p = 0.60$), whereas the cumulative 6-mo costs were approx $18,600 ($p = 0.78$).

In the second phase of the economic analysis of PURSUIT, we created a cost-effectiveness model to relate the incremental clinical benefits demonstrated for eptifibatide by PURSUIT to its incremental costs. The cost-effectiveness (CE) ratio used for this purpose can be simply expressed as:

$$CE = \frac{C_E - C_P}{LE_E - LE_P}$$

where subscript E is the eptifibatide arm, subscript P is the placebo arm, C is the lifetime cost of each treatment arm, and LE is the life expectancy.

The cost side of this analysis was simplified by the fact that our empirical cost data showed no significant cost difference between the two arms out to 6 mo, so the numerator of the cost-effectiveness ratio consisted only of the cost of the eptifibatide regimen used in PURSUIT. Using the drug's AWP, we estimated this at $1217.

Projecting life expectancy for each treatment arm from the empirical 6-mo PURSUIT clinical data was more complex and was based on a methodology previously developed by us for the GUSTO I study *(26)*. Our method projected an overall life expectancy for the PURSUIT patients of almost 16 yr and an incremental effect of eptifibatide on life expectancy of 0.111 per patient (equivalent to 1 extra survivor per 100 patients shifted to eptifibatide who lives an extra 11.1 yr).

With these two components, the resulting cost-effectiveness ratio was $16,292 per year of life saved (discounted at 3%). Conventional thinking in this field is that any cost-effectiveness ratio smaller than $50,000 per added life year is "economically attractive," whereas a ratio greater than $100,000 is "economically unattractive" *(1)*. By these criteria, use of eptifibatide therapy in acute coronary syndrome patients is quite economically attractive. Furthermore, these results were not sensitive to reasonable variations in the starting parameters of the model.

Studies of Patients with ST-Elevation Myocardial Infarction

Two large-scale trials have tested the addition of GPIIb/IIIa inhibitors to thrombolytic regimens for the treatment of acute ST-elevation MI. GUSTO V compared full-dose reteplase (r-PA) with half-dose r-PA plus full-dose abciximab in 16,588 patients *(27)*. The combination regimen had no significant effect on 30-d mortality but did reduce reinfarction rates. Urgent revascularization was reduced with combination therapy, whereas bleeding was increased. ASSENT 3 compared three regimens in 6095 acute MI patients: tenecteplase (TNK) plus unfractionated heparin, TNK plus enoxaparin, and half-dose TNK plus full-dose abciximab *(28)*. Mortality at 30 d was lowest in the enoxaparin arm, but differences were not significant. Reinfarction rates were 2.7% in the enoxaparin arm, 2.2% in the abciximab arm, and 4.2% in the heparin arm ($p = 0.0001$). Major bleeding was increased in both the enoxaparin and abciximab arms (but not intracranial hemorrhage). A preliminary economic analysis of this trial was presented at the 2002 American Heart Association meeting.

Two trials have also tested the use of abciximab with primary stenting in acute MI *(29, 30)*. To date, neither has reported economic data.

Secondary Prevention

As detailed elsewhere in this text, multiple Phase III trials have failed to show any therapeutic benefit for the use of oral GPIIb/IIIa inhibitors in high-risk atherosclerosis patients.

SUMMARY

GPIIb/IIIa platelet receptor inhibitors represent a major advance in the pharmacotherapy of acute coronary disease, whether occurring spontaneously or following percutaneous intervention. In the percutaneous intervention population, abciximab (EPISTENT) and eptifibatide (ESPRIT) both significantly improved outcomes at an economically attractive price relative to no GPIIb/IIIa use. There are no trials directly comparing these two agents. However, the Do Tirofiban and ReoPro Give Similar Efficacy Trial (TARGET) provides some relevant data on this issue. This trial compared abciximab with tirofiban, a small-molecule inhibitor very similar to eptifibatide *(31)*. In 5308 patients scheduled to undergo elective stenting, the 30-d mortality rate with abciximab was 0.4% vs 0.5% for tirofiban ($p = 0.66$), whereas nonfatal MI occurred in 5.4% and 6.9%, respectively ($p = 0.04$). At 1 yr, mortality in the abciximab group was 1.7% vs 1.9% in the tirofiban group ($p = 0.66$). Furthermore, mortality at 1 yr in the ACS subgroup was virtually identical in the two treatment arms. In short, abciximab provided an incremental 15/1000 reduction in nonfatal MI at 30 d and no incremental mortality benefit at 1 yr compared with tirofiban. Given the approx $1000 incremental cost of abciximab, the TARGET data raise questions about whether abciximab provides enough incremental benefits to make its use in PCI in preference to tirofiban or eptifibatide economically attractive.

The other consideration that has influenced many interventional laboratories is the effect of drug selection on their budgets. For every 1000 patients treated, abciximab would cost the laboratory about $1.4 million, whereas eptifibatide or tirofiban would cost about $500,000. In the absence of compelling evidence of abciximab's clinical superiority, many laboratories now preferentially use one of the small molecules, reserving abciximab for high-risk patients.

In acute coronary syndrome patients, a recent metaanalysis showed that GPIIb/IIIa inhibitors reduced death or MI event rates in patients not routinely scheduled for early revascularization *(32)*. This analysis assumed that all members of the drug class performed equivalently. The PURSUIT economic substudy demonstrates that such use also meets criteria for economic attractiveness.

REFERENCES

1. Mark DB. Medical economics in cardiovascular medicine. In: Topol EJ, ed. Textbook of Cardiovascular Medicine. Lippincott Williams & Wilkins Philadelphia, PA, 2002, pp. 957–979.
2. Fuchs VR. The Health Economy. Harvard University Press, Cambridge, MA, 1986.
3. Feldstein PJ. Health Care Economics, 4th ed. Delmar, Albany, NY, 1993.
4. Drummond MF, O'Brien B, Stoddart GL, Torrance GW. Methods for the Economic Evaluation of Health Care Programmes, 2nd ed. Oxford Medical Publications, Oxford, 1997.
5. Gold MR, Siegel JE, Russell LB, Weinstein MC. Cost-Effectiveness in Health and Medicine. Oxford University Press, New York, 1996.
6. Weinstein MC, Fineberg HV, Elstein AS, et al. Clinical Decision Analysis. WB Saunders, Philadelphia, 1980.
7. Mark DB, Talley JD, Topol EJ, et al. Economic assessment of platelet glycoprotein IIb/IIIa inhibition for prevention of ischemic complications of high risk coronary angioplasty. Circulation 1996;94:629–635.
8. Weintraub WS, Mauldin PD, Becker E, Kosinski AS, King SB. A comparison of the costs of and quality of life after coronary angioplasty or coronary surgery for multivessel coronary disease: results from the Emory Angioplasty Versus Surgery Trial (EAST). Circulation 1995;92:2831–2840.
9. Cohen DJ, Krumholz HM, Sukin CA, et al. In-hospital and one-year economic outcomes after coronary stenting or balloon angioplasty: results from a randomized clinical trial. Circulation 1995;92:2480–2487.
10. Hlatky MA, Rogers WJ, Johnstone I, et al. Medical care costs and quality of life after randomization to coronary angioplasty or coronary bypass surgery. N Engl J Med 1997;336:92–99.
11. Mark DB, Cowper PA, Berkowitz S, et al. Economic assessment of low molecular weight heparin (enoxaparin) versus unfractionated heparin in acute coronary syndrome patients: results from the ESSENCE randomized trial. Circulation 1998;97:1702–1707.
12. The EPIC Investigators. Use of a monoclonal antibody directed against the platelet glycoprotein IIb/IIIa receptor in high-risk coronary angioplasty. The EPIC Investigation. N Engl J Med 1994;330:956–961.
13. Topol EJ, Califf RM, Weisman HF, et al. Randomised trial of coronary intervention with antibody against platelet IIb/IIIa Integrilin for reduction of clinical restenosis: results at six months. Lancet 1994;343:881–886.
14. The EPILOG Investigators. Platelet glycoprotein IIb/IIIa receptor blockade and low-dose heparin during percutaneous coronary revascularization. N Engl J Med 1997;336:1689–1696.

15. Lincoff AM, Mark DB, Tcheng JE, et al. Economic assessment of platelet glycoprotein IIb/IIIa receptor blockade with abciximab and low-dose heparin during percutaneous coronary revascularization: results from the EPILOG randomized trial. Circulation 2000;102:2923–2929.
16. The CAPTURE Investigators. Randomised placebo-controlled trial of abciximab before and during coronary intervention in refractory unstable angina: the CAPTURE study. Lancet 1997;349:1429–1435.
17. The EPISTENT Investigators. Randomised placebo-controlled and balloon-angioplasty-controlled trial to assess safety of coronary stenting with use of platelet glycoprotein IIb/IIIa blockade. Lancet 1998;352: 87–92.
18. Topol EJ, Mark DB, Lincoff AM, et al. Outcomes at 1 year and economic implications of platelet glycoprotein IIb/IIIa blockade in patients undergoing coronary stenting: results from a multicentre randomised trial. Lancet 1999;354:2019–2024.
19. The IMPACT II Investigators. Effects of competitive platelet glycoprotein IIb/IIIa inhibition with Integrilin in reducing complications of percutaneous coronary intervention. Lancet 1997;349:1422–1428.
20. Gibson CM, Cohen DJ, Cohen EA, et al. Effect of eptifibatide on coronary flow reserve following coronary stent implantation (an ESPRIT substudy). Enhanced Suppression of the Platelet IIb/IIIa Receptor with Integrilin Therapy. Am J Cardiol 2001;87:1293–1295.
21. The RESTORE Investigators. Effects of platelet glycoprotein IIb/IIIa blockade with tirofiban on adverse cardiac events in patients with unstable angina or acute myocardial infarction undergoing coronary angioplasty. Circulation 1997;96:1445–1453.
22. Gibson CM, Goel M, Cohen DJ, et al. Six-month angiographic and clinical follow-up of patients prospectively randomized to receive either tirofiban or placebo during angiography in the RESTORE trial. J Am Coll Cardiol 1998;32:28–34.
23. Weintraub WS, Culler S, Boccuzzi SJ, et al. Economic impact of GPIIB/IIIA blockade after high-risk angioplasty: results from the RESTORE trial. J Am Coll Cardiol 1999;34:1061–1066.
24. The PURSUIT Investigators. Inhibition of platelet glycoprotein IIb/IIIa with eptifibatide in patients with acute coronary syndromes without persistent ST-segment elevation. N Engl J Med 1998;339:436–443.
25. Mark DB, Harrington RA, Lincoff AM, et al. Cost effectiveness of platelet glycoprotein IIb/IIIa inhibition with eptifibatide in patients with non-ST elevation acute coronary syndromes. Circulation 2000; 101:366–371.
26. Mark DB, Hlatky MA, Califf RM, et al. Cost effectiveness of thrombolytic therapy with tissue plasminogen activator as compared with streptokinase for acute myocardial infarction. N Engl J Med 1995;332: 1418–1424.
27. Topol EJ. Reperfusion therapy for acute myocardial infarction with fibrinolytic therapy or combination reduced fibrinolytic therapy and platelet glycoprotein IIb/IIIa inhibition: the GUSTO V randomised trial. Lancet 2001;357:1905–1914.
28. Efficacy and safety of tenecteplase in combination with enoxaparin, abciximab, or unfractionated heparin: the ASSENT-3 randomised trial in acute myocardial infarction. Lancet 2001;358:605–613.
29. Stone GW, Grines CL, Cox DA, et al. Comparison of angioplasty with stenting, with or without abciximab, in acute myocardial infarction. N Engl J Med 2002;346:957–966.
30. Montalescot G, Barragan P, Wittenberg O, et al., and for the ADMIRAL Investigators. Platelet glycoprotein IIb/IIIa inhibition with coronary stenting for acute myocardial infarction. N Engl J Med 2001;344: 1895–1903.
31. Topol EJ, Moliterno DJ, Herrmann HC, et al. Comparison of two platelet glycoprotein IIb/IIIa inhibitors, tirofiban and abciximab, for the prevention of ischemic events with percutaneous coronary revascularization. N Engl J Med 2001;344:1888–1894.
32. Boersma E, Harrington RA, Moliterno DJ, et al. Platelet glycoprotein IIb/IIIa inhibitors in acute coronary syndromes: a meta-analysis of all major randomised clinical trials. Lancet 2002;359:189–198.

15

Platelet Monitoring and Interaction of Glycoprotein IIb/IIIa Antagonists with Other Antiplatelet Agents

Steven R. Steinhubl, MD

Contents

Introduction
Platelet Monitoring
Methods of Monitoring of Platelet Inhibition
Interaction of GPIIb/IIIa Antagonists with Other
    Antiplatelet Agents
References

INTRODUCTION

Unlike other available antiplatelet agents, a clear dose-effect relationship for the platelet glycoprotein (GP) IIb/IIIa antagonists was well established in animal models prior to study in humans. Based on these early studies, a specific level of blockade of platelet GPIIb/IIIa receptors was identified as that necessary to prevent intraarterial thrombus formation, and this target level was carried forward into clinical trials. Subsequently, the efficacy of these agents in preventing thrombotic events has been confirmed in placebo-controlled trials involving nearly 50,000 patients (1,2). Despite these overall positive findings with GPIIb/IIIa receptor-blocker therapy, several large individual studies, in specific patient populations or with suboptimal dosing regimens, have found a lack of effect in preventing thrombotic complications (3,4). These results raise the question as to whether a specific dose of a GPIIb/IIIa antagonist, adjusted only by patient weight, can provide the same level of platelet inhibition across all clinical syndromes and across all individuals. If there is interindividual variability in response to standard dosing of GPIIb/IIIa antagonists, monitoring of platelet inhibition would allow for individualization of therapy and might improve the efficacy and safety of these agents.

PLATELET MONITORING

One barrier to the routine monitoring and titrating of GPIIb/IIIa antagonists has been the lack of a convenient, reproducible, clinically relevant measure of platelet function.

From: *Contemporary Cardiology: Platelet Glycoprotein IIb/IIIa
Inhibitors in Cardiovascular Disease, 2nd Edition*
Edited by: A. M. Lincoff © Humana Press Inc., Totowa, NJ

Platelet aggregometry and receptor binding assays, the methods utilized in initial dose-finding studies, require specialized technical expertise, involve substantial time delays, and are unable to be performed in patient care areas. Today, however, there are several simple, whole-blood, point-of-care monitoring devices available, making monitoring of platelet inhibition convenient and clinically relevant.

In this chapter the data demonstrating the clinical relevance of achieving a specific level of platelet function inhibition with GPIIb/IIIa antagonists, and therefore supporting the need for monitoring, are reviewed as well as the multiple monitoring methods available.

Level of Platelet Inhibition to Prevent Thrombotic Events

ANIMAL STUDIES

Early studies performed in animals involving arterial injury and thrombus formation demonstrated a strong correlation between the level of GPIIb/IIIa receptor blockade and prevention of luminal thrombus formation, with a steep dose response. One of the earliest studies to evaluate the clinical dose response of the monoclonal antiplatelet GPIIb/IIIa antibody 7E3 utilized a post-thrombolysis reocclusion dog model *(5)*. Reocclusion was completely prevented in this model with only the highest (0.8 mg/kg) dose of 7E3. At this dose, platelet aggregation induced by 9 µM ADP was completely inhibited, >80% of the GPIIb/IIIa receptors on the platelet surface were blocked, and bleeding time was prolonged to > 30 min in most animals. Lower doses were associated with some reocclusion, but less inhibition of aggregation and shorter prolongations of bleeding time. In a second study, the same monoclonal antibody was evaluated in the less thrombogenic Folts model in the monkey carotid artery *(6)*. In this model, only 0.2 mg/kg of 7E3 was required to inhibit thrombus formation completely, a dose that only rarely prolonged bleeding time beyond 10 min, inhibited ADP-induced aggregation by approx 70%, and blocked approx 70% of GPIIb/IIIa receptors. Although it is possible that the marked difference in doses needed to prevent thrombus formation in these two models may have been related to an interspecies difference in effects of the monoclonal antibody, it is more probable that the disparate results suggest that in the setting of a more thrombogenic stimulus a greater level of receptor blockade is required to prevent the formation of an arterial thrombus (Fig. 1).

Based on the results of these animal models, early dosing of GPIIb/IIIa antagonists was designed to achieve blockade of approx 80% of platelet GPIIb/IIIa receptors and inhibit ADP-induced platelet aggregation to approx 20% of baseline *(7–9)*. This dose was considered necessary to prevent ischemic complications in response to severe thrombotic provocations but was also recognized as being "highly speculative" *(10)*.

INDIRECT DATA FROM CLINICAL TRIALS

Indirect evidence from several placebo-controlled trials of GPIIb/IIIa antagonists in percutaneous coronary intervention (PCI) has suggested the importance of achieving and maintaining a specific level of platelet inhibition in order to minimize thrombotic complications. In the EPIC (Evaluation of 7E3 for the Prevention of Ischemic Complications) trial, patients undergoing a high-risk PCI were randomized to receive either a bolus and infusion of placebo, a bolus of abciximab and an infusion of placebo, or a bolus and infusion of abciximab *(11)*. Patients receiving placebo started to require urgent interventions immediately after the initial percutaneous transluminal coronary angioplasty (PTCA), whereas patients receiving a bolus alone of abciximab were nearly completely protected for the first 4–6 h (during which time receptor blockade was likely to be ≥ 80% in most

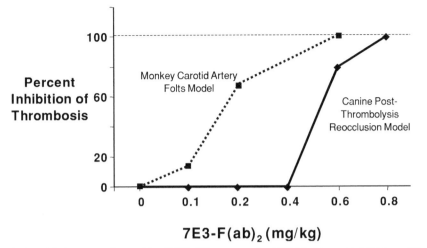

Fig. 1. Relationship between dose of the GPIIb/IIIa antagonist 7E3-F(ab)$_2$ and inhibition of thrombosis formation in two different animal models, suggesting that the correct antithrombotic dose may be dependent on the thrombogenic stimulus (5,6).

patients), and patients treated with a bolus and 12-h infusion of abciximab were protected from ischemic complications almost throughout the infusion period. At 30 d, patients who received a bolus and infusion of abciximab had almost a one-third reduction in ischemic events compared with those treated with a bolus alone. This benefit of a bolus and infusion of abciximab vs a bolus alone was maintained for at least 3 yr (12).

The importance of achieving a high level of receptor blockade with eptifibatide at the time of a PCI is suggested by the discrepant results of two trials utilizing significantly different doses of this agent. In the IMPACT-II (Integrilin to Minimize Platelet Aggregation and Coronary Thrombosis) trial, randomization to a 135 μg/kg bolus and a 0.5 μg/kg/min infusion of eptifibatide at the time of PCI led to an 18% relative decrease in the composite endpoint compared with placebo (9.2% vs 11.4%, $p = 0.063$) (3). Later, this dosing regimen was found to produce only approx 50% receptor blockade (13). In the ESPIRIT (Enhanced Suppression of Platelet Receptor IIb/IIIa Using Integrilin Therapy) trial, a much higher dose of eptifibatide was evaluated, with two 180 μg/kg boluses and a 2 μg/kg/min infusion. In a pilot study, this dose was estimated to provide >90% inhibition of 20 μM ADP-induced aggregation, approx 80% GPIIb/IIIa receptor occupancy, and bleeding times of at least 30 min (14). Clinically, this increased dosing regimen was associated with twice the relative benefit of eptifibatide treatment compared with the results in IMPACT-II, with a 35% reduction in the 30-d composite clinical endpoint of death, myocardial infarction (MI), or urgent revascularization (6.8% vs 10.4%, $p = 0.003$).

DIRECT EVIDENCE CORRELATING THE LEVEL OF PLATELET INHIBITION WITH EFFICACY OUTCOMES FROM CLINICAL TRIALS

Several clinical trials have utilized some measure of platelet inhibition and linked these results with efficacy outcomes. In the PARAGON-A (Platelet IIb/IIIa Antagonism for the Reduction of Acute Coronary Syndrome Events in a Global Organization Network) trial, 2282 patients with a non-ST-elevation acute coronary syndrome were randomized to either a low- or high-dose lamifiban regimen, with or without heparin (15). In an attempt

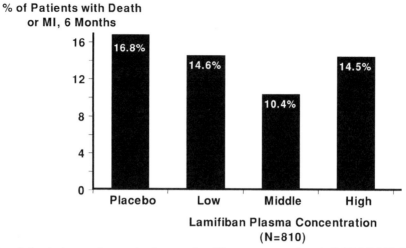

Fig. 2. Correlation between plasma steady-state lamifiban concentrations in PARAGON-A (Platelet IIb/IIIa Antagonism for the Reduction of Acute Coronary Syndrome Events in a Global Organization Network) and the incidence of death and myocardial infarction (MI) at 6 mo in a subgroup of 810 lamifiban-treated patients *(16)*.

to establish a dose-response relationship, steady-state plasma concentrations of lamifiban were determined in a subgroup of 810 lamifiban-treated patients. Interestingly, a U-shaped correlation was found between plasma drug levels and the incidence of death and MI at 6 mo *(16)*. Whereas patients achieving a midrange of concentrations, representing 80–90% GPIIb/IIIa receptor occupancy, realized a 40% relative reduction in death and MI at 30 d, and 38% at 6 mo compared with placebo, higher and lower steady-state plasma levels were associated with no significant benefit over placebo (Fig. 2).

The PARAGON-B trial built on the knowledge gained from the results of the PARAGON-A study by attempting to target drug levels carefully in a similar patient population *(17)*. Of the 5225 patients randomized, steady-state plasma concentrations of lamifiban were available in 1272 patients *(18)*. Interestingly, in contrast to the PARAGON-A results, a U-shaped dose response was not seen, with a trend toward greater benefit with increasing plasma levels in the overall PARAGON-B population (Fig. 3). The importance of achieving an adequate level of inhibition in order to optimize clinical outcomes was highlighted by the results in the subgroup of troponin-positive patients in which patients with low plasma levels derived no benefit compared with patients randomized to placebo, whereas patients with target levels or greater of inhibition experienced a >50% relative decrease in ischemic events (Fig. 3).

The FROST (Fibrinogen Receptor Occupancy Study) study was a Phase II trial evaluating treatment with the oral GPIIb/IIIa antagonist lefradafiban for 1 mo in 531 patients with a non-ST-elevation acute coronary syndrome. The minimum fibrinogen receptor occupancy (FRO) was calculated from up to four plasma concentrations per patient and correlated with clinical outcomes *(19)*. The incidence of the combined endpoint of death, MI, and angina pectoris was found to be directly related to the FRO. Only those patients with an FRO of >70%, correlating with ≥90% inhibition of 20 µM ADP-induced platelet aggregation, achieved outcomes better than the control group.

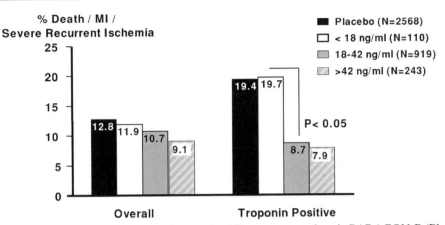

Fig. 3. Correlation between plasma steady-state lamifiban concentrations in PARAGON-B (Platelet IIb/IIIa Antagonism for the Reduction of Acute Coronary Syndrome Events in a Global Organization Network) and the incidence of death, myocardial infarction (MI), and severe recurrent ischemia in 1272 patients *(18)*. A trend toward greater benefit with increasing plasma levels in the overall PARAGON-B population is seen. In the subgroup of troponin-positive patients those with low plasma levels derived no benefit compared with patients randomized to placebo, whereas patients with target levels or greater of inhibition experienced a >50% relative decrease in ischemic events.

The only study to date to evaluate prospectively the level of platelet inhibition achieved with GPIIb/IIIa antagonists and clinical outcomes is the GOLD [AU (Assessing Ultegra)] study *(20)*. In this multicenter study, 500 patients undergoing a PCI with the planned use of a GPIIb/IIIa inhibitor had platelet inhibition measured using the point-of-care Ultegra-Rapid Platelet Function Assay (RPFA) (*see* the RPFA section). The most important finding from this study was that approximately one-fourth of all patients did not achieve ≥95% inhibition 10 min following the bolus and that this lower level of inhibition was associated with a significantly higher incidence of major adverse cardiac events (MACE; 14.4% vs 6.4%, $p = 0.006$). By multivariate analysis, platelet function inhibition ≥95% at 10 min following the start of therapy was associated with a significant decrease in the incidence of a MACE (odds ratio 0.46, 95% confidence interval 0.22–0.96, $p = 0.04$).

Level of Platelet Inhibition and Bleeding Complications

The use of agents that inhibit the platelet GPIIb/IIIa receptor is modeled after the inherited platelet disorder Glanzmann's thrombasthenia, which is characterized by a total deficiency or abnormality in the GPIIb/IIIa receptor. Interestingly, patients with Glanzmann's thrombasthenia, who have essentially infinite bleeding times, only rarely experience spontaneous major bleeding *(21)*. Most serious hemorrhagic problems occur only when associated with either physiologic or pathologic processes that would also cause bleeding in normal individuals. Therefore, it was not surprising that early experience with GPIIb/IIIa antagonists in the setting of PCI was associated with a higher rate of bleeding complications *(11)*. However, later trials, utilizing reduced-dose heparin regimens and earlier arterial sheath removal, led to a marked improvement in major bleeding rates such that they were no different from that of placebo *(22–24)*.

Only a very limited number of clinical studies have attempted to correlate some measure of platelet inhibition and bleeding risk. An early report of bleeding times in two pilot trials investigating the forerunner of abciximab found no correlation between measured template bleeding times and the risk of hemorrhagic events *(25)*. A more recent study, which evaluated bleeding complications among the 500 patients enrolled in the GOLD trial, also found no correlation between the level of platelet inhibition, as measured by the point-of-care Ultegra-RPFA, and major bleeding complications *(26)*. Importantly, the investigators were able to show a significant correlation between major bleeding and increasing procedural activated clotting time (ACT), suggesting that there was adequate power to demonstrate a similar relationship between the level of platelet inhibition and bleeding if one existed.

Presently, no clear threshold level of platelet inhibition with parenteral GPIIb/IIIa antagonists has been established that is associated with an increased risk of major bleeding. However, the ability to ensure a return to normal function in case emergent surgery is required in GPIIb/IIIa antagonist-treated patients, may be an essential role of platelet monitoring.

METHODS OF MONITORING OF PLATELET INHIBITION
Laboratory-Based Assays

TURBIDIMETRIC AGGREGOMETRY

Historically, the most widely used laboratory assay for determining platelet function and response to antiplatelet therapies has been turbidimetric aggregometry. In fact, the current dosing of all available GPIIb/IIIa antagonists was primarily based on turbidimetric aggregation results *(7–9)*. With this technique, platelet-rich plasma (PRP) is stirred while the optical density of the suspension is continuously monitored. An agonist, typically ADP, collagen, epinephrine, or thrombin receptor-activating peptide (TRAP), is then added, causing activation of the platelets in suspension. The degree of platelet activation is dependent on the agonist used and its concentration, as well as platelet-dependent properties. Platelet activation initiates the formation of aggregates, which leads to a decrease in the total number of particles in solution and therefore a decrease in optical density of the PRP. Agents that inhibit platelet activation (such as aspirin and clopidogrel) and platelet aggregation (such as the GPIIb/IIIa antagonists) prevent or diminish this decrease in optical density based, at least in part, on the level of platelet inhibition.

There are a number of limitations to the use of turbidimetric aggregometry that prohibit its routine use for monitoring GPIIb/IIIa antagonist therapy. First, it is a specialized test that requires extensive sample preparation, expensive testing equipment, frequent quality control, and a certain level of operator expertise, all of which make it available only in specialized laboratories in a limited number of hospitals. Besides these practical limitations, certain physiologic limitations also exist. Preparation of PRP creates changes in the milieu and density of platelets, negating the influence of other blood components in thrombus formation. Also, since PRP turbidimetric aggregometry is insensitive to platelet microaggregates, failing to detect aggregates with fewer than approx 100 platelets, clinically important platelet function may remain unmonitored *(27,28)*. Despite these significant limitations, turbidimetric aggregometry remains the gold standard by which other devices are most frequently compared.

ELECTRICAL IMPEDANCE AGGREGOMETRY

Electrical impedance aggregometry is one of the first whole-blood assays developed with the hope of overcoming many of the limitations of turbidimetric aggregometry *(29)*. This technique measures aggregation as an increase in the electrical impedance across two precious metal wires resulting from the accumulation of platelets in response to an agonist. Unlike turbidimetric aggregometry, no cell separation is required, and the sample only needs to be diluted 1:1 with saline followed by a 5-min incubation time prior to the initiation of the assay. Other advantages include a relatively rapid result and a reduced need for lab technician training.

The major disadvantage for this assay in measuring response to GPIIb/IIIa antagonists is the dilution step, which may limit its utility in monitoring the low-molecular-weight agents like tirofiban and eptifibatide with high dissociation constants. Other limitations to its usefulness in routine clinical practice are the need to prepare and pipet reagents and the requirement for frequent, meticulous care of the electrodes. The test is also less reliable at lower hemoglobin concentrations.

Electrical impedance aggregometry has been compared with turbidimetric aggregometry in one study involving 14 patients undergoing a PCI with the use of a standard bolus and infusion of abciximab *(30)*. The investigators found a close correlation between the level of GPIIb/IIIa receptor blockade and platelet inhibition as determined by electrical impedance and turbidimetric aggregometry.

FLOW CYTOMETRY

All other methods of monitoring platelet function discussed in this chapter involve some measurement of actual platelet function in an artificially induced thrombotic environment. In contrast, flow cytometry allows for the direct measurement of the actual in vivo status of the platelet by detecting the expression or configuration of any platelet surface antigen *(31)*. Whole blood flow cytometry allows for the minimization of artifactual platelet activation.

Flow cyotometric analysis begins with the dilution of anticoagulated whole blood in order to minimize platelet aggregate formation *(32)*. The "test" monoclonal antibody (recognizing the antigen to be measured) labeled with a fluorophore is then added at near saturating concentrations. Then the "platelet identifier" monoclonal antibody is added at similar concentrations. An agonist such as TRAP, ADP, collagen, or others can then be added if desired prior to sample stabilization with fixation by paraformaldehyde. Samples are then analyzed by flow cytometry. After the platelets are identified by their characteristic light scatter and by platelet identifier labeling, binding of the test monoclonal antibody is determined by analyzing 5000–10,000 individual platelets.

Flow cytometric methods have been used extensively in the research setting for monitoring GPIIb/IIIa antagonists. Drug receptor occupancy can be measured either directly or indirectly. Examples of direct methods include competitive binding assays and measurement of binding of an antibody directed against the GPIIb/IIIa antagonist being measured *(33,34)*.

A recent investigation utilizing two monoclonal antibodies (MAbs), LYP18 (MAb1) and 4F8 (MAb2), demonstrated the utility of flow cytometry in identifying the difference in binding characteristics of different GPIIb/IIIa antagonists *(35)*. MAb1 binds to the intact GPIIb/IIIa receptor complex, whereas MAb2 binds to a different epitope on the β3 subunit of the GPIIb/IIIa receptor. Abciximab was found to reduce the binding of MAb1 to platelets, probably by occupying the MAb1 binding site on the GPIIb/IIIa receptor but did not alter MAb2 binding. In contrast, the small-molecule GPIIb/IIIa receptor antagonists eptifibatide and xemilofiban did not alter MAb1 binding but displaced MAb2.

The primary limitation of flow cytometry involves the technical sophistication of the technique. The equipment is very specialized and relatively expansive. Also, substantial training and expertise are required to run and interpret results. At present, use of these assays is limited to research purposes.

Point-of-Care Assays

BLEEDING TIME

The bleeding time was initially described in 1901 and first suggested to be a measure of platelet function in 1910 *(36,37)*. The test simply involves a superficial incision, typically with an automated device that creates an incision of controlled dimensions, with serial blotting of the site until bleeding stops and the time is recorded. The most common method is that described by Ivy and coworkers *(38)*, who utilized a blood pressure cuff to the arm to maintain a standard venous pressure and established the site of the superficial incision to the volar aspect of the forearm. The test is labor-intensive and subject to considerable inter- and intraobserver variability.

Although bleeding time has been used for decades for diagnosing platelet-related bleeding disorders, recent reviews have concluded that there is no evidence supporting its use for predicting bleeding or response to antiplatelet therapy *(39)*. As noted above, the one study that specifically evaluated bleeding time in the setting of GPIIb/IIIa antagonist therapy found no correlation with bleeding complications *(25)*.

ULTEGRA-RAPID PLATELET FUNCTION ASSAY (RPFA)

The Ultegra-RPFA (Accumetrics, San Diego, CA), unlike all other methods of measuring platelet function, was specifically designed to be utilized in patients treated with GPIIb/IIIa antagonists. It is an automated, whole-blood, point-of-care assay that allows platelet inhibition to be measured rapidly by patient care providers at the bedside.

The basis of the Ultegra-RPFA assay is that fibrinogen-coated polystyrene microparticles will agglutinate in whole blood in direct proportion to the number of unblocked platelet GPIIb/IIIa receptors. Pharmacologic blockade of GPIIb/IIIa receptors prevents this interaction and therefore diminishes agglutination in proportion to the degree of receptor blockade achieved. Because the speed of bead agglutination is more rapid and reproducible if platelets are activated, a modified thrombin receptor-activating peptide, iso-TRAP [(iso-S)FLLRN] is incorporated into the assay *(40)*. Blood samples are obtained in either a standard citrate blood tube, or PPACK (Phe-Pro-Arg chloromethyl ketone) can be utilized for the anticoagulant instead of citrate. The tube is inserted into a disposable plastic cartridge, and 160 μL of the blood is automatically drawn into two sample channels containing lyophilized iso-TRAP and fibrinogen-coated beads. The reagents are reconstituted so that the final concentration of iso-TRAP is 4 μmol/L, a concentration selected to correlate best with the results obtained with turbidimetric aggregometry using 20 μM ADP as the agonist. The sample is then mixed for 70 s by the movement of a microprocessor-driven steel ball. The light absorbance of the sample is measured 16 times/s by an automated detector. As the platelets interact with the fibrinogen-coated beads, resulting in agglutination, there is a progressive increase in light transmission (Fig. 4). The rate of agglutination is quantified as the slope of the change of absorbance over a fixed time interval and reported

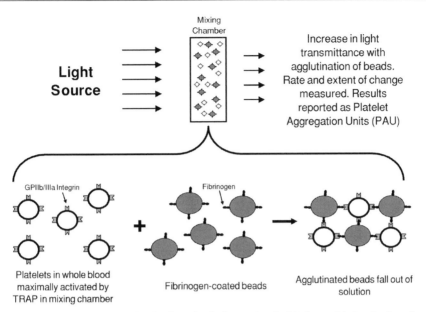

Fig. 4. Diagram representing how platelet function is determined with the rapid platelet function assay. The mixing chamber contains thrombin receptor-activating peptide (TRAP) and the fibrinogen-coated beads. Whole blood is added, and the platelets become activated by the TRAP. The activated GPIIb/IIIa receptors on the platelets bind via the fibrinogen on the beads and cause agglutination of the beads. Light transmittance through the chamber is measured and increases as the agglutinated beads fall out of solution. With blockade of the GPIIb/IIIa receptors, agglutination is much slower, and light transmittance changes much less over time.

as millivolts per 10 s (mV/10 s). This numerical value is reported as platelet aggregation units (PAU). An individual patient's baseline PAU is retained in memory, and all additional specimens are reported as a raw PAU as well as a percentage of the baseline PAU.

Initial evaluations of the automated RPFA found an excellent correlation between the assay and both turbidimetric platelet aggregometry with PRP and radiolabeled receptor binding assays *(40)*. Neither heparin nor aspirin use influenced the results of the assay. To evaluate real-world clinical utility, precision, and reliability of the Ultegra-RPFA, a study involving 192 patients at four centers undergoing PCI with the use of the GPIIb/IIIa inhibitor abciximab was carried out. All patients had platelet function monitored at three time points: (1) baseline, (2) within 1 h of abciximab bolus administration, and (3) at 24 h after the abciximab bolus. Abciximab was administered in the standard bolus and 12 h intravenous infusion. Platelet function was determined at each time point using the Ultegra-RPFA, conventional turbidimetric aggregometry, and [^{125}I]abciximab receptor binding assay. Of the 125 evaluable patients in whom all three methods could be compared, the level of inhibition determined by the Ultegra correlated well with both standard aggregometry ($r = 0.87$) and the receptor binding assay ($r = 0.89$) *(41)*. This level of correlation was similar to that observed in comparisons between the accepted gold standards for determining platelet inhibition—turbidimetric aggregometry and the receptor binding assay ($r = 0.87$).

A number of clinical studies have been carried out using the Ultegra-RPFA. Two early studies performed at The Lindner Center for Research and Education, Cincinnati, Ohio, and at the Cleveland Clinic serially determined platelet function inhibition using the RPFA

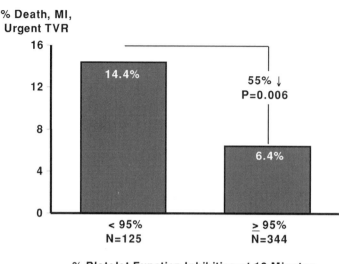

Fig. 5. Incidence of major adverse cardiac events (MACE) in 469 patients undergoing a percutaneous coronary intervention in relation to the level of platelet function inhibition as determined by the Ultegra —Rapid Platelet Function Assay at 10 min following the GPIIb/IIIa inhibitor bolus in the GOLD (AU-Assessing Ultegra) study *(20)*. MI, myocardial infarction; TVR, target vessel revascularization.

in a total of 178 abciximab-treated patients in the setting of PCI *(42,43)*. Both of these studies demonstrated substantial interpatient variability in response to a standard, weight-adjusted infusion of abciximab. Although neither study was designed to evaluate clinical outcomes, the Cleveland Clinic study did find a significant association between the level of platelet inhibition and the occurrence of a peri-PCI MI *(42)*.

Based on these results, the first prospective study designed to correlate the level of platelet inhibition achieved with a GPIIb/IIIa antagonist and clinical outcomes was carried out. The GOLD study serially evaluated platelet function inhibition in 500 patients at 13 centers undergoing a PCI with the use of a GPIIb/IIIa inhibitor *(20)*. Platelet inhibition was measured at 10 min, 1 h, 8 h, and 24 h following the initiation of therapy using the Ultegra-RPFA. MACE (a composite of death, MI, and urgent target vessel revascularization) were prospectively monitored, and their incidence was correlated with the measured level of platelet inhibition at all time points. As noted earlier, one-fourth of all patients did not achieve $\geq 95\%$ inhibition 10 min following the bolus, and these patients experienced a significantly higher incidence of MACE (14.4% vs 6.4%, $p = 0.006$) (Fig. 5). Also, patients whose platelet function was <70% inhibited at 8 h after the start of therapy had a MACE rate of 25% vs 8.1% ($p = 0.009$) compared with those $\geq 70\%$ inhibited.

The observed association between the level of platelet inhibition as determined by the Ultegra-RPFA and clinical outcomes suggests clinical utility of this device; however, further studies are necessary to confirm that titrating GPIIb/IIIa therapy based on measured levels of platelet inhibition will decrease adverse events.

PLATELET FUNCTION ANALYZER (PFA-100)

The PFA-100 (Dade Behring, Miami, FL) is an automated platelet function analyzer that evaluates primary hemostasis in whole blood flowing through high shear conditions.

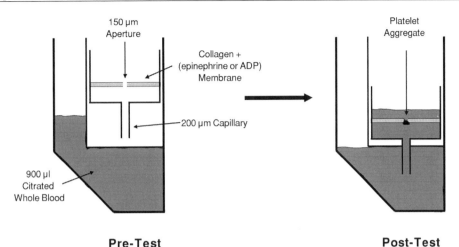

Pre-Test   **Post-Test**

Fig. 6. Schematic of the cartridge of the platelet function analyzer (PFA)-100. The membrane is coated with collagen plus either ADP (50 μg) or epinephrine (10 μg). This instrument provides a constant vacuum that aspirates citrated whole blood through the capillary tube, creating high shear stress, which activates the platelets that then adhere and aggregate at the membrane aperture until it occludes, causing cessation of blood flow.

It is used to screen for von Willebrand's disease and other congenital platelet disorders. It has also been evaluated as a method for monitoring response to aspirin and GPIIb/IIIa antagonists *(44,45)*.

The disposable test cartridge consists of a sample reservoir, capillary, and biochemically active membrane with a central 150-μm aperture (Fig. 6). The membrane is coated with collagen plus either ADP (50 μg) or epinephrine (10 μg). This instrument provides a constant vacuum that apirates citrated whole blood through the capillary tube, where it contacts the membrane. Aspiration through the capillary tube creates high shear stress, which activates the platelets that then adhere and aggregate at the membrane aperture until it occludes, causing cessation of blood flow. The time to cessation of flow is reported as the closure time (CT). The normal range for the CT in a series of 225 patients prior to undergoing PCI was defined as a range of 60–130 s *(45)*. The maximal closure time has been set at 300 s, which represents nonclosure of the aperture after 300 s.

The PFA-100 offers several advantages over laboratory-based methods of measuring platelet function. The testing technique is easy to learn, uses whole blood, and does not require a skilled technician to operate the analyzer. Also, blood is collected into standard Vacutainer tubes and can then be kept at room temperature for up to 4 h before testing. Finally, test results are available in approx 10 min.

The largest study to evaluate the PFA-100 for monitoring GPIIb/IIIa therapy involved 225 patients treated with abciximab in the setting of a PCI, with the results in only 27 patients having been reported to date *(45)*. The CT was compared with turbidimetric aggregometry and receptor occupancy by flow cytometry at 10 min, 4 h, 12 h, and 24 h after the abciximab bolus. The CT was 300 s (maximal) in 96% of patients at 10 min, 100% at 4 h, and 88% at 12 h. At 24 h, 72% of patients had a normal CT (≤130 s). Because virtually all patients achieved maximal CT with abciximab, it was not possible to correlate PFA-100 results with those of the accepted laboratory standards. These results suggest that the

PFA-100 may be too sensitive to detect clinically relevant, high levels of platelet inhibition but that it can rapidly determine when platelet function has returned to normal following treatment.

Cone and Platelet Analyzer

The cone and platelet analyzer (CPA) tests platelet activation in whole blood under flow conditions by monitoring shear-induced platelet deposition onto a surface designed to mimic an extracellular matrix *(46)*. A 200-μL sample of citrated blood is placed in polystyrene wells and circulated at high shear rate (1875 s-1) for 2 min with a rotating Teflon cone. Wells are then washed, stained, and analyzed with an inverted light microscope that is connected to an image analysis system. Results are expressed as the percentage of well surface covered by platelets *(47)*. Determination of both congenital and acquired platelet disorders are determined based on the principle that platelet deposition on polystyrene under flow is dependent on platelet activation and on the presence of fibrinogen, von Willebrand factor, and their receptors. Advantages of this test are that it uses high shear stress to simulate arterial physiology. The test also uses whole blood and does not require a baseline reading.

A recent trial evaluated the CPA, turbidometric aggregometry, and RPFA vs flow cytometry in 10 healthy volunteers *(47)*. The CPA detection of platelet inhibition correlated significantly better with the percentage receptor occupancy by flow cytometry than did turbidimetric aggregometry ($p = 0.0007$), but these measurements were primarily at midlevels of platelet inhibition. Compared with RPFA, CPA was a better predictor of free GPIIb/IIIa receptors when the RPFA data were expressed as absolute values ($p = 0.0015$) but not when RPFA was expressed as a percentage of baseline inhibition. This report also evaluated platelet function in 16 patients who underwent PCI and received abciximab. Platelet function was assessed by the CPA and turbidimetric aggregometry at baseline, 5 min, 4 h, and 1, 3, 7, and 30 d. By turbidometric aggregometry, platelet function remained suppressed for only 1 d after abciximab therapy, whereas CPA-assessed platelet function did not return to normal until between 7 and 30 d. The CPA may therefore have greater sensitivity to detect lower levels of platelet inhibition, but, like the PFA-100, may be too sensitive to monitor the high levels of inhibition required during short-term parenteral GPIIb/IIIa antagonist therapy. Of note, clopidogrel and aspirin therapy in three volunteers did not significantly change CPA values in this study.

Thromboelastography

Thromboelastography (TEG) provides a graphic representation of several aspects of clot formation. Although TEG was used in the past primarily as a means of determining hemostatic derangements in the setting of liver transplant and cardiac surgery, several recent small studies have evaluated its utility in monitoring GPIIb/IIIa therapy *(48)*.

TEG is performed on 0.35 mL of whole blood that is placed in a heated cup. A pin is suspended in the cup from a torsion wire that is transduced to a monitor. The cup oscillates 4° 45' in either direction every 4.5 s. Initially, prior to clotting, the motion of the cup does not affect the suspended pin. When the blood in the cup begins to clot, the motion of the cup is transmitted to the pin, and a tracing is generated. Several parameters of the tracing are routinely measured including the reaction time, which is the latency time between blood being placed in the cup and the start of clotting, and the maximal amplitude, which is the greatest vertical amplitude of the TEG tracing *(48)*.

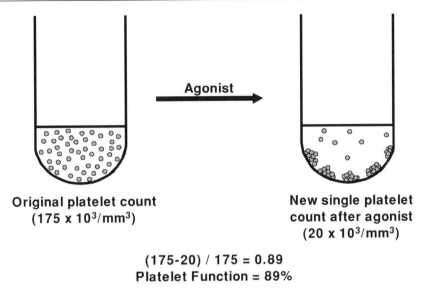

Agonist

Original platelet count
(175 x 10³/mm³)

New single platelet
count after agonist
(20 x 10³/mm³)

(175-20) / 175 = 0.89
Platelet Function = 89%

Fig. 7. Single platelet count ratios are determined by measuring the number of platelets before and after the addition of a specific agonist and then determining the ratio.

A linear dose-dependent reduction in clot strength in response to the in vitro addition of abciximab has been reported using a modified TEG *(49)*. The investigators modified the test by using thrombin as an agonist and found that this allowed the test to be completed in 15 min rather than 1 h. Another modified version of TEG utilizing tissue factor found a differential efficacy among different GPIIb/IIIa antagonists despite equivalent antiaggregatory potency *(50)*.

PLATELET COUNT RATIOS (PLATELETWORKS)

The principle behind the platelet count ratio is that the number of free platelets measured in whole blood is decreased in relation to the number of platelet aggregates that form after an agonist is added (Fig. 7). The Plateletworks (Helena Laboratories, Beaumont, TX) is a point-of-care version of this concept that automatically determines the platelet count ratio between a sample of whole blood in which an agonist such as ADP is added and the same sample in which aggregation is prevented by the addition of a calcium chelating agent *(51)*. The platelet count ratio has been found to correlate well with platelet aggregation measured by turbidometric aggregometry *(52)*, but typically identifies a lower level of inhibition than that determined by turbidimetric aggregometry. This has led some investigators to speculate that whereas turbidimetric aggregometry provides information regarding the inhibition of platelet macroaggregate formation, the platelet count ratio actually measures the inhibition of microaggregation, which might have important implications in terms of the therapeutic effectiveness of GPIIb/IIIa antagonists *(27)*.

Platelet count ratios have an advantage in that the ability to perform platelet counts exists at virtually every hospital, and since samples are fixed following initial preparation, analysis time can be delayed up to 4 h. However, unless the automated Plateletworks device is used, platelet count ratios can only be determined in the laboratory setting with the requirement for sample manipulation.

CLOT SIGNATURE ANALYZER

The Clot Signature Analyzer (CSA; Xylum, Scarsdale, NY) is an automated device designed to mimic vascular injury and provide a measure of both platelet and coagulation function. Nonanticoagulated blood is perfused through two channels. In one channel blood flows through tubing with pressure continuously monitored. The tubing is then pierced by a 0.15-mm needle, causing an immediate drop in pressure. This change in blood flow pattern also leads to a marked increase in shear rate, which initiates platelet activation and aggregation at the punch site. As a platelet aggregate forms at the site, blood flow at the punch site stops, and the measured pressure in the tubing rebounds. As the flow of blood in the tubing continues, the simultaneous activation of the coagulation cascade promotes fibrin generation and the buildup of a fibrin clot that leads to a decrease in flow and pressure. At the same time, in the second channel, blood is perfused at high shear over a collagen fiber. As platelets adhere and aggregate onto this thrombogenic surface, this tubing also occludes, resulting in a decrease in pressure. The changes in pressure in the two channels are monitored and displayed in real time as graphical "signatures" of platelet and coagulation function (53).

The advantages of the CSA are that it is an automated benchtop analyzer and is the only one that does not require the use of anticoagulated blood samples. Also, it has the potential to monitor the effects of both anticoagulant and antiplatelet therapies. Although it can measure the effects of GPIIb/IIIa antagonists, one study involving 36 patients undergoing a PCI with a GPIIb/IIIa antagonist found that CSA results did not correlate with those of turbidimetric aggregometry (54). Also, in many patients only the assay's maximal values were obtained, suggesting that, like the PFA-100 and CPA, the CSA may be overly sensitive to high levels of platelet inhibition.

Special Considerations in Platelet Monitoring

MULTIPLE ANTITHROMBOTIC AGENTS

Patients treated with a GPIIb/IIIa antagonist will almost always also receive at least one and typically several antithrombotic agents including aspirin, clopidogrel, unfractionated heparin, low-molecular-weight heparin, fibrinolytics, or direct thrombin inhibitors. Just monitoring platelet inhibition alone is complicated by the frequent, concomitant use of these antiplatelet agents. An ideal test for monitoring platelet inhibition for the prevention of thrombotic and bleeding events would ideally take into account all antiplatelet therapies a patient is receiving, but such a test does not currently exist.

Although aspirin, clopidogrel, and the GPIIb/IIIa antagonists are all categorized under the umbrella of antiplatelet agents, their very different mechanisms of action have made it difficult to develop a clinically useful test that can distinguish the effects of all three agents. Whereas aspirin and thienopyridines inhibit platelet activation, virtually every test of their antiplatelet effects measures the inhibition of platelet aggregation. The GPIIb/IIIa antagonists so profoundly inhibit platelet aggregation that their effects greatly overwhelm any measured effect on aggregation that aspirin or a thienopyridine might have. The small number of studies that have attempted to measure the additive effects of a thienopyridine and a GPIIb/IIIa antagonist have typically only been able to show an effect of the thienopyridine after treatment with the GPIIb/IIIa antagonists has stopped and its effects diminished (55–58).

ANTICOAGULATION OF SAMPLES

Almost every test of platelet function requires the use of anticoagulated blood. Out of habit and convenience, blood samples for platelet testing in the past most often used citrate, an agent that prevents in vitro clotting by reducing ionized calcium levels, as the anticoagulant. Recently, the importance of physiologic concentrations of calcium for the proper function of the GPIIb/IIIa receptor and its influence on measured levels of platelet inhibition achieved with the various GPIIb/IIIa antagonists has been recognized *(13)*. Although the influence of calcium chelators on artificially inflating the measured level of inhibition are best described for eptifibatide, recent work suggests that the other small molecule, tirofiban, may also be substantially affected, with abciximab to a much lesser extent *(27,59)*.

VARIABLE METHODS OF DETERMINING PLATELET FUNCTION

An 80% level of inhibition is frequently quoted as the goal for therapy with a GPIIb/IIIa antagonist, frequently without stating 80% of what. Although original dosing goals of these agents were targeted for 80% blockade of platelet GPIIb/IIIa receptors, which roughly provided 80% inhibition of 20 μM ADP-induced platelet aggregation as measured by turbidimetric aggregometry, these results cannot be translated into a goal level of inhibition as determined by other methods of measuring platelet function. That is, 80% inhibition of 20 μM ADP-induced turbidimetric aggregometry is not even equivalent to 80% inhibition of platelet function as determined by using another agonist or another concentration of ADP in turbidimetric aggregometry, much less as determined by a point-of-care device or flow cytometry. Therefore, the appropriate level of inhibition needed to optimize outcomes must be determined for each device. Ideally, this would be determined through exploratory clinical trials correlating outcomes with measured levels of platelet function.

Conclusions

Virtually all available data for the GPIIb/IIIa antagonists confirm that the degree of inhibition of the platelet GPIIb/IIIa integrin and platelet aggregation is critical to their clinical effectiveness. Similarly, all studies that have evaluated the level of inhibition achieved with these agents have found substantial interpatient variability. These facts support a compelling theoretical benefit to the monitoring of all patients treated with a GPIIb/IIIa antagonist, coupled with dose adjustment, to optimize their safety and efficacy. In the past, real-time monitoring was not possible owing to the technical constraints of platelet function testing. Today, however, there exist several point-of-care devices that allow for the rapid determination of the effects of a GPIIb/IIIa antagonist at the bedside. At least one of these devices has already been shown to provide clinically relevant results in a large, prospective series. Nevertheless, before platelet monitoring can be routinely recommended for all patients, further studies are needed to prove that dose adjustment is more than just a theoretical benefit. Once the extra effort and expense of platelet monitoring can be justified through the confirmation of improved outcomes, it will probably become a standard component of GPIIb/IIIa antagonist therapy.

INTERACTION OF GPIIb/IIIa
ANTAGONISTS WITH OTHER ANTIPLATELET AGENTS

When a patient is treated with a GPIIb/IIIa antagonist, an additional antiplatelet agent is almost always utilized—in most cases at least aspirin. With recent studies confirming a more widespread and long-term benefit of the ADP receptor antagonist clopidogrel, it is likely that an increasing number of patients who are candidates for treatment with a GPIIb/IIIa antagonist may now be receiving dual antiplatelet therapy with clopidogrel and aspirin.

Because the GPIIb/IIIa antagonists inhibit platelet aggregation caused by all agonists, including thromboxane A_2 and ADP, it might be suspected that any additional antiplatelet effects of aspirin and clopidogrel may be superfluous. This assumption is reinforced by the fact that most routine measures of antiplatelet effects involve some measure of inhibition of in vitro platelet aggregation—a much greater function of GPIIb/IIIa inhibition rather than thromboxane A_2 and ADP inhibition. However, by inhibiting platelet activation rather than aggregation, clopidogrel and aspirin may provide additional important antiplatelet and possibly antiinflammatory effects.

Surprisingly, there are few clinical data regarding the interaction of the currently available antiplatelet agents, even though current guidelines recommend therapy with aspirin, clopidogrel, and a GPIIb/IIIa antagonist in a large proportion of patients with acute coronary syndromes (60). Although randomized trials are currently under way that will help define any potential additive benefits and risks of starting a GPIIb/IIIa antagonist in patients already receiving aspirin and clopidogrel, some observational and nonrandomized data are currently available that provide some evidence of benefit.

GPIIb/IIIa Antagonists and Aspirin

Essentially every clinical trial of the parenteral GPIIb/IIIa antagonists has required concomitant aspirin therapy. There has been one randomized trial in acute coronary syndrome patients that compared aspirin alone with aspirin plus a low dose of the oral GPIIb/IIIa antagonist sibrafiban and a high dose of sibrafiban alone (61). The addition of aspirin to sibrafiban was associated with a nonsignificant trend toward a decrease in the combined primary endpoint of death, MI, or severe refractory ischemia (aspirin plus low-dose sibrafiban 9.2% vs high-dose sibrafiban alone 10.5%). There was also a nonsignificant trend toward increased major bleeding with aspirin plus sibrafiban (5.7%) vs sibrafiban alone (4.6%). However, the many unanswered questions regarding oral agents as well as the different doses of sibrafiban studied make any conclusions regarding the role of aspirin with a GPIIb/IIIa antagonist problematic.

GPIIb/IIIa Antagonists and Thienopyridines

Today, virtually all patients receiving a coronary stent receive a limited course of a thienopyridine, typically clopidogrel, along with aspirin. If the thienopyridine is started after the procedure, there is minimal interaction with any GPIIb/IIIa antagonist utilized owing to the relatively slow (hours for clopidogrel, days for ticlopidine) onset of action of these agents. However, a significant proportion of patients is now being pretreated with a thienopyridine prior to percutaneous coronary intervention because of reports in several studies, none randomized comparisons, of a benefit in decreasing thrombotic complications (62–64). Whether a GPIIb/IIIa antagonist offers additional benefit (or risk) in this patient population is unknown. The results of the EPISTENT analysis suggested that pretreatment was no longer beneficial in reducing adverse events at 30 d when the IIb/IIIa inhibitor abciximab was used, but the duration of pretreatment with the slower onset ticlopidine was unknown and probably short (62) (Fig. 8). On the other hand, the results of the TARGET trial suggested that event rates were lower among patients pretreated with clopidogrel even when all patients received a GPIIb/IIIa antagonist (64) (Fig. 9). However, both the EPISTENT and TARGET trials were not designed to answer the question about the benefit of pretreat-

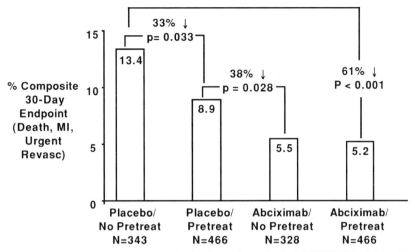

Fig. 8. Incidence of the 30-d composite endpoint in patients in the EPISTENT trial randomized to receive a stent with or without abciximab, who also did or did not receive pretreatment with ticlopidine based on the decision of the treating physician. MI, myocardial infarction.

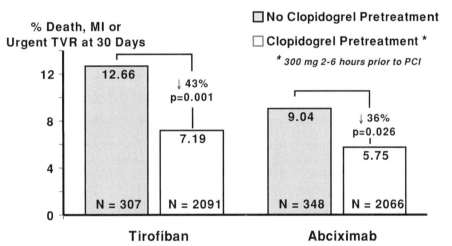

Fig. 9. Incidence of the 30-d composite endpoint in patients in the TARGET trial randomized to the GPIIb/IIIa antagonists abciximab or tirofiban and whether or not they were pretreated with clopidogrel as recommended in the study protocol. MI, myocardial infarction; PCI, percutaneous coronary intervention; TVR, target vessel revascularization.

ment with a thienopyridine among patients receiving a IIb/IIIa inhibitor, and therefore the optimal use of a GPIIb/IIIa antagonist when a patient has already received clopidogrel, or of clopidogrel in a patient already receiving a GPIIb/IIIa antagonist, remains unclear.

Conclusions

Despite current recommendations for greater widespread utilization, the risks and benefits of triple antiplatelet therapy with aspirin, clopidogrel, and a GPIIb/IIIa antagonist remain unknown. The results of future trials will better identify the actual benefit of these regimens and clarify any safety issues.

REFERENCES

1. The GUSTO V Investigators. Reperfusion therapy for acute myocardial infarction with fibrinolytic therapy or combination reduced fibrinolytic therapy and platelet glycoprotein IIb/IIIa inhibition: the GUSTO V randomised trial. Lancet 2001;357:1905–1914.
2. Lincoff AM, Califf R, Topol EJ. Platelet glycoprotein IIb/IIIa receptor blockade in coronary artery disease. J Am Coll Cardiol 2000;35:1103–1115.
3. The IMPACT-II Investigators. Randomised placebo-controlled trial of effect of eptifibatide on complications of percutaneous coronary intervention: IMPACT-II. Lancet 1997;349:1422–1428.
4. The GUSTO IV-ACS Investigators. Effect of glycoprotein IIb/IIIa receptor blocker abcximab on outcome in patients with acute coronary syndromes without early coronary revascularization: the GUSTO IV-ACS randomised trial. Lancet 2001;357:1915–1924.
5. Gold HK, Coller BS, Yasuda T, et al. Rapid and sustained coronary artery recanalization with combined bolus injection of recombinant tissue-type plasminogen activator and monoclonal anti-platelet GPIIb/IIIa antibody in a dog model. Circulation 1988;77:670–677.
6. Coller BS, Folts JD, Smith SR, Scudder LE, Jordan R. Abolition of in vivo platelet thrombus formation in primates with monoclonal antibodies to the platelet GPIIb/IIIa receptor. Correlation with bleeding time, platelet aggregation, and blockade of GPIIb/IIIa receptors. Circulation 1989;80:1766–1774.
7. Tcheng JE, Ellis SG, George BS, et al. Pharmacodynamics of chimeric glycoprotein IIb/IIIa integrin antiplatelet antibody Fab 7E3 in high-risk coronary angioplasty. Circulation 1994;90:1757–1764.
8. Harrington RA, Kleiman NS, Kottke-Marchant K, et al. Immediate and reversible platelet inhibition after intravenous administration of a peptide glycoprotein IIb/IIIa inhibitor during percutaneous coronary intervention. Am J Cardiol 1995;76:1222–1227.
9. Kereiakes DJ, Kleiman NS, Ambrose J, et al. Randomized, double-blind, placebo-controlled dose-ranging study of tirofiban (MK-383) platelet IIb/IIIa blockade in high risk patients undergoing coronary angio-plasty. J Am Coll Cardiol 1996;27:536–542.
10. Coller BS, Scudder LE, Beer J, et al. Monoclonal antibodies to platelet GPIIb/IIIa as antithrombotic agents. Ann NY Acad Sci 1991;614:193–213.
11. The EPIC Investigators. Use of a monoclonal antibody directed against the glycoprotein IIb/IIIa receptor in high-risk coronary angioplasty. N Engl J Med 1994;330:956–961.
12. Topol EJ, Ferguson JJ, Weisman HF, et al., for the EPIC Investigator Group. Long-term protection from myocardial ischemic events in a randomized trial of brief integrin β_3 blockade with percutaneous coronary intervention. JAMA 1997;278:479–484.
13. Phillips DR, Teng W, Arfsten A, et al. Effect of Ca^{2+} on GP IIb-IIIa interactions with Integrilin. Enhanced GP IIb-IIIa binding and inhibition of platelet aggregation by reductions in the concentration of ionized calcium in plasma anticoagulated with citrate. Circulation 1997;96:1488–1494.
14. Gilchrist I, O'Shea J, Kosoglou T, et al. Pharmacodynamics and pharmacokinetics of higher-dose, double-bolus eptifibatide in percutaneous coronary intervention. Circulation 2001;104:406–411.
15. The PARAGON Investigators. International, randomized, controlled trial of lamifiban (a platelet glycoprotein IIb/IIIa inhibitor), heparin, or both in unstable angina. Circulation 1998;97:2386–2395.
16. Steiner B, Wittke B, Harrington RA, Bhapkar MV, Armstrong PW, Moliterno DJ. Plasma level of lamifiban and platelet receptor occupancy best predict clinical outcome in patients with unstable angina: results from PARAGON A (abstract). Circulation 1998;98:I–561.
17. The PARAGON-B Investigators. Randomized, placebo-controlled trial of titrated lamifiban for acute coronary syndromes. Circulation 2002;105:316–321.
18. Dyke C, Mahaffey KW, Berdan LG, et al. Optimal dosing of a glycoprotein IIb/IIIa antagonist with a simplifiede renal-based algorithm: pharmacodynamic and clinical findings from PARAGON-B (abstract). J Am Coll Cardiol 2001:343A.
19. Roth U, Hoffman J, Nehmiz G, et al. Level of inhibition of platelet aggregation predicts outcome of patients treated with the oral glycoprotein IIb/IIIa receptor antagonist lefradafiban: results from the Fibrinogen Receptor Occupancy STudy (FROST) (abstract). Eur Heart J 2000;21:625.
20. Steinhubl S, Talley J, Braden G, et al. Point-of-care measured platelet inhibition correlates with a reduced risk of an adverse cardiac event following percutaneous coronary intervention. Results of the GOLD (AU-Assessing Ultegra) multicenter study. Circulation 2001;103:1403–1409.
21. George J, Caen JP, Nurden A. Glanzmann's thrombasthenia: the spectrum of clinical disease. Blood 1990;175:1383–1395.

22. The EPISTENT Investigators. Randomised placebo-controlled and balloon-angioplasty-controlled trial to assess safety of coronary stenting with use of platelet glycoprotein-IIb/IIIa blockade. Lancet 1998;352: 87–92.

23. The EPILOG Investigators. Platelet glycoprotein IIb/IIIa receptor blockade and low-dose heparin during percutaneous coronary revascularization. N Engl J Med 1997;336:1689–1696.

24. The ESPRIT Investigators. Novel dosing regimen of eptifibatide in planned coronary stent implantation (ESPRIT): a randomised, placebo-controlled trial. Lancet 2000;356:2037–2044.

25. Bernardi MM, Califf RM, Kleiman N, Ellis SG, Topol EJ, for the TAMI Study Group. Lack of usefulness of prolonged bleeding time in predicting hemorrhagic events in patients receiving the 7E3 glycoprotein IIb/IIIa platelet antibody. Am J Cardiol 1993;72:1121–1125.

26. Tamberella M, Bhatt D, Chew D, Kereiakes D, Topol EJ, Steinhubl SR. Relation of platelet inactivation with intravenous glycoprotein IIb/IIIa antagonists to major bleeding (from the GOLD Study). Am J Cardiol 2002;89:1429–1431.

27. Storey R, Wilcox R, Heptinstall S. Differential effects of glycoprotein IIb/IIIa antagonists on platelet microaggregate and macroaggregate formation and effect of anticoagulant on antagonist potency. Implications for assay methology and comparison of different antagonists. Circulation 1998;98:1616–1621.

28. Thompson N, Scrutton M, Wallis R. Particle volume change associated with light transmittance changes in the platelet aggregometer: dependence upon aggregating agent and effectiveness of stimulus. Thromb Res 1986;41:615–626.

29. Cardinal DC, Flower RJ. The electronic aggregometer: a novel device of assessing platelet behavior in blood. J Pharmacol Methods 1980;3:1350–1358.

30. Mascelli MA, Worley S, Veriabo NJ, et al. Rapid assessment of platelet function with a modified whole-blood aggregometer in percutaneous transluminal coronary angioplasty patients receiving anti-GPIIb/IIIa therapy. Circulation 1997;96:3860–3866.

31. Michelson AD. Flow cytometry: a clinical test of platelet function. Blood 1996;87:4925–4936.

32. Michelson AD, Barnard MR, Krueger LA, Frelinger AL, Furman MI. Evaluation of platelet function by flow cytometry. Methods 2000;21:259–270.

33. Gawaz M, Ruf A, Neumann F-J, et al. Effect of glycoprotein IIb/IIa receptor antagonism on platelet membrane glycoproteins after coronary stent placement. Thromb Haemost 1998;80:994–1001.

34. Mascelli MA, Lance ET, Damaraju L, Wagner CL, Weisman HF, Jordan RE. Pharmacodynamic profile of short-term abciximab treatment demonstrates prolonged platelet inhibition with gradual recovery from GP IIb/IIIa receptor blockade. Circulation 1998;97:1680–1688.

35. Quinn M, Deering A, Stewart M, Cox D, Foley B, Fitzgerald D. Quantifying GPIIb/IIIa receptor binding using 2 monoclonal antibodies: discriminating abciximab and small molecular weight antagonists. Circulation 1999;99:2231–2238.

36. Duke W. The relationship of blood platelets to hemorrhagic disease. Description of a method for determining the bleeding time and coagulation time and report of three cases of hemorrhagic disease relieved by transfusions. JAMA 1910;55:1185–1192.

37. Milian MG. Influence de la peau sur la coagulabilité du sang. CR Soc Biol (Paris) 1901;53:576–578.

38. Ivy A, Nelson D, Bucher G. The standardization of certain factors in the cutaneous "venostatsis" bleeding time technique. J Lab Clin Med 1941;26:1812–1822.

39. Channing Rogers RP, Levin J. A critical reappraisal of the bleeding time. Semin Thromb Hemost 1990; 16:1–20.

40. Smith JW, Steinhubl SR, Lincoff AM, et al. The rapid platelet function assay (RPFA): an automated and quantitative cartridge-based method. Circulation 1999;99:620–625.

41. Wheeler G, Braden G, Steinhubl S, et al. The Accumetrics Ultegra RPFA: a study of equivalence to standard platelet function assays in patients undergoing percutaneous coronary intervention with abciximab therapy. Am Heart J 2002;143:602–611.

42. Steinhubl SR, Kottke-Marchant K, Moliterno DJ, et al. Attainment and maintenance of platelet inhibition by standard dosing of abciximab in diabetic and nondiabetic patients undergoing percutaneous coronary intervention. Circulation 1999;100:1977–1982.

43. Kereiakes DJ, Mueller M, Howard W, et al. Efficacy of abciximab induced platelet blockade using a rapid point of care assay. J Thromb Thrombolysis 1999;7:265–275.

44. Gum P, Kottke-Marchant K, Poggio ED, et al. Profile and prevalence of aspirin resistance in patients with cardiovascular disease. Am J Cardiol 2001;88:230–235.

45. Madan M, Berkowitz SD, Christie DJ, et al. Rapid assessment of glycoprotein IIb/IIIa blockade with the platelet function analyzer (PFA-100) during percutaneous coronary intervention. Am Heart J 2001; 141:226–233.
46. Shenkman B, Savion N, Dardik R, Tamarin I, Varon D. Testing of platelet deposition on polystyrene surface under flow conditions by the cone and plate(let) analyzer: role of platelet activation, fibrinogen and von Willebrand factor. Thromb Res 2000;99:353–361.
47. Osende JI, Fuster V, Lev EI, et al. Testing platelet activation with a shear-dependent platelet function test versus aggregation-based tests. Relevance for monitoring long-term glycoprotein IIb/IIIa inhibition. Circulation 2001;103:1488–1491.
48. Salooja N, Perry DJ. Thromboelastography. Blood Coagul Fibrinolysis 2001;12:327–337.
49. Greilich PE, Alving BM, O'Neill KL, Chang AS, Reid TJ. A modified thromboelastographic method of monitoring c7E3 Fab in heparinized patients. Anesth Anal 1997;84:31–38.
50. Mousa SA, Khurana S, Forsythe MS. Comparative in vitro efficacy of different platelet glycoprotein IIb/IIIa antagonists on platelet-mediated clot strength induced by tissue factor with use of thromboelastography. Differentiation among glycoprotein IIb/IIIa antagonists. Arterioscler Thromb Vasc Biol 2000; 20:1162–1167.
51. Lakkis NM, George S, Thomas E, Ali M, Guyer K, Carville D. Use of ICHOR-platelet works to assess platelet function in patients treated with GP IIb/IIIa inhibitors. Cathet Cardiovasc Intervent 2001; 53:346–351.
52. Nicholson NS, Panzer-Knodle SG, Haas NF, et al. Assessment of platelet function assays. Am Heart J 1998;135:S170–S178.
53. Li CKN, Hoffman TJ, Hsieh P-Y, Malik S, Watson WC. The Xylum Clot Signature Analyzer: a dynamic flow system that simulates vascular injury. Thromb Res 1998;92:S67–S77.
54. Simon DI, Liu CB, Ganz P, et al. A comparative study of light transmission aggregometry and automated bedside platelet function assays in patients undergoing percutaneous coronary intervention and receiving abciximab, eptifibatide, or tirofiban. Cathet Cardiovasc Intervent 2001;52:425–432.
55. Fredrickson BJ, Turner NA, Kleiman NS, et al. Effects of abciximab, ticlopidine, and combined abciximab/ticlopidine therapy on platelet and leukocyte function in patients undergoing coronary angioplasty. Circulation 2000;101:1122–1129.
56. Kleiman NS, Graziadei N, Jordan RE, et al. Ticlopidine enhances the platelet inhibitory capacity of abciximab in vitro. J Thromb Thrombolysis 2000;9:29–36.
57. Kleiman NS, Graziadei N, Maresh K, et al. Abciximab, ticlopidine, and comcomitant abciximab-ticlopidine therapy: ex vivo platelet aggregation inhibition profiles in patients undergoing percutaneous coronary interventions. Am Heart J 2000;140:492–501.
58. Klinkhardt U, Kirchmaier CM, Westrup D, et al. Ex vivo-in vitro interaction between aspirin, clopidogrel, and the glycoprotein IIb/IIIa inhibitors abciximab and SR121566A. Clin Pharmacol Ther 2000;67: 305–313.
59. Marciniak SJ Jr, Jordan RE, Mascelli MA. Effect of Ca^{2+} chelation on the platelet inhibitory ability of the GPIIb/IIIa antagonists abciximab, eptifibatide and tirofiban. Thromb Haemost 2001;85:539–543.
60. Braunwald E, Antman E, Beasley J, et al. ACC/AHA guideline update for the management of patients with unstable angina and non-ST-segment elevation myocardial infarction: a report of the American College of Cardiology/American Heart Association Task Force on Practice Guidelines (Committee on the Management of Patients with Unstable Angina). Available at: http://www.acc.org/clinical/guidelines/unstable/unstable.pdf, 2002.
61. Second SYMPHONY Investigators. Randomized trial of aspirin, sibrafiban, or both for secondary prevention after acute coronary syndromes. Circulation 2001;103:1727–1733.
62. Steinhubl SR, Ellis SG, Wolski K, Lincoff AM, Topol EJ. Ticlopidine pretreatment before coronary stenting is associated with sustained decrease in adverse cardiac events: data from the Evaluation of Platelet IIb/IIIa Inhibitor for Stenting (EPISTENT) Trial. Circulation 2001;103:1403–1409.
63. Steinhubl SR, Lauer MS, Mukherjee DP, et al. The duration of pretreatment with ticlopidine prior to stenting is associated with the risk of procedure-related non-Q-wave myocardial infarctions. J Am Coll Cardiol 1998;32:1366–1370.
64. Topol EJ, Moliterno DJ, Herrmann HC, et al., for the Target Investigators. Comparison of two platelet glycoprotein IIb/IIIa inhibitors, tirofiban and abciximab, for the prevention of ischemic events with percutaneous coronary revascularization. N Engl J Med 2001;344:1888–1894.

16

Platelet Glycoprotein IIb/IIIa Antagonists

Their Interaction with Low-Molecular-Weight Heparins and Direct Thrombin Inhibitors

Amol S. Bapat, MD, Naji Yazbek, MD, and Neal S. Kleiman, MD

CONTENTS

INTRODUCTION
PERTINENT BIOLOGY OF THROMBIN AND THROMBIN INHIBITORS
COMBINED GPIIb/IIIa ANTAGONISTS AND ANTITHROMBINS
LOW-MOLECULAR-WEIGHT HEPARIN IN ACUTE CORONARY
   SYNDROMES
LOW-MOLECULAR-WEIGHT HEPARINS IN PERCUTANEOUS
   CORONARY INTERVENTION
GPIIb/IIIa AND LOW-MOLECULAR-WEIGHT HEPARIN
   IN PERCUTANEOUS CORONARY INTERVENTION
GPIIb/IIIa ANTAGONISTS AND LOW-MOLECULAR-WEIGHT
   HEPARIN IN ACUTE CORONARY SYNDROMES AND ACUTE
   MYOCARDIAL INFARCTION
DIRECT THROMBIN INHIBITORS IN ACUTE CORONARY SYNDROMES AND
   MYOCARDIAL INFARCTION
DIRECT THROMBIN INHIBITORS IN PERCUTANEOUS CORONARY
   INTERVENTION
GPIIb/IIIa AND DIRECT THROMBIN INHIBITOR IN PERCUTANEOUS
   CORONARY INTERVENTION
CONCLUSIONS
REFERENCES

INTRODUCTION

The availability of new drugs for the inhibition of platelets and thrombin may alter the strategies used to manage patients with acute coronary syndromes and those undergoing percutaneous coronary interventions. The critical role of the activated platelet in these

From: *Contemporary Cardiology: Platelet Glycoprotein IIb/IIIa
Inhibitors in Cardiovascular Disease, 2nd Edition*
Edited by: A. M. Lincoff © Humana Press Inc., Totowa, NJ

settings has been demonstrated numerous times, and the inhibition of thrombin, one of the most potent naturally occurring platelet agonists, also appears to be necessary to prevent thrombus formation and propagation. Large clinical studies have investigated platelet glycoprotein (GP) IIb/IIIa antagonists in percutaneous coronary intervention, unstable angina, and ST-elevation myocardial infarction. In most of these trials, unfractionated heparin has been used as a concomitant thrombin antagonist, but recent experience now includes low-molecular-weight heparins and direct thrombin antagonists in these settings. It has been argued that event rates for acute coronary syndromes remain unacceptably high, in spite of aggressive care *(1)*.

A time-honored saw has been that as the efficacy of new antithrombotic treatments increases, the risk of bleeding will increase. Although this finding has been true to a certain extent, more sophisticated approaches based on a more thorough understanding of coagulation tend to belie this paradigm. The natural progression of clinical research has led to exploration of the low-molecular-weight heparins and direct thrombin inhibitors as "foundation" anticoagulants for use with GPIIb/IIIa antagonists. Their hypothetical and often established advantages over unfractionated heparin may lead to the evolution of safer and more effective therapies for unstable angina, ST-elevation myocardial infarction, and percutaneous coronary intervention and suggest that they may provide superior platforms on which to use antiplatelet agents. This chapter reviews the extant data concerning these new anticoagulants in combination with GPIIb/IIIa antagonists.

Evidence Favors the Use of GPIIb/IIIa Antagonists

Platelet inhibition in various settings has been exhaustively examined. Although biologic compounds such as thrombin, adenosine diphosphate, thromboxane, collagen, norepinephrine, and serotonin may cause platelet activation, ligation of platelet GPIIb/IIIa by fibrinogen and von Willebrand factor is probably the "final common pathway" for platelet aggregation. GPIIb/IIIa ($\alpha_{IIb}\beta_3$) is a member of the integrin family unique to the platelet *(2)* and is the most expressed receptor on the platelet surface *(3)*. Approximately 80,000 copies of GPIIb/IIIa are expressed on the surface of a quiescent platelet *(4)*, and about 20,000–30,000 more receptors reside in the α-granules and remain in equilibrium with the surface via the open cannicular system *(5)*. Platelet activity plays an important role in ischemic coronary syndromes. Acute coronary syndromes are initiated when the unstable atherosclerotic plaque's fibrous cap is disrupted *(6–9)*. The highly reactive lipid core then acts as a catalyst for platelet activation and thrombosis. Platelets initiate the formation of thrombus at the plaque rupture site and further render the thrombus resistant to clot lysis, delay perfusion, and promote cycles of patency and reocclusion *(10)*. Upon platelet activation, GPIIb/IIIa is expressed on the platelet surface. Findings from animal models that examined the effect of monoclonal antibodies in the setting of thrombosis and reperfusion indicate that approx 80% or more of surface GPIIb/IIIa receptors must be functionally eliminated to achieve clinically significant inhibition of platelet aggregation *(11)*. GPIIb/IIIa antagonists prevent the binding of fibrinogen, which in turn prevents platelets from crosslinking and thereby reduces platelet-induced thrombus formation. Therefore, antagonism of the GPIIb/IIIa receptor is a very tempting target for a host of coronary syndromes.

There are currently three approved GPIIb/IIIa antagonists in the United States: the Fab fragment of chimeric human-murine monoclonal antibody 7E3, abciximab (*ReoPro*), the nonpeptide tirofiban (*Aggrastat*), and the semisynthetic cyclic heptapeptide eptifibatide (*Integrilin*). Abciximab has been approved for use in percutaneous coronary intervention but has also been studied in the acute coronary syndrome and ST-elevation myocardial infarction populations as well; it avidly and irreversibly binds the β-subunit of the GPIIb/IIIa receptor. It has a short plasma half-life but in its bound form has a much longer biologic half-life. After an intravenous bolus, the free drug is rapidly cleared, with an initial half-life of 10 min and a second-phase half-life of 30 min *(2)*: unbound abciximab is cleared by protease degradation. Tirofiban has been approved for use in patients with unstable angina and binds to the RGD motif of GPIIb/IIIa. Tirofiban, in contrast to abciximab, has a less avid binding to its target site but a longer half-life in its unbound form and is renally and hepatically excreted. Eptifibatide has been approved for use in both acute coronary syndromes and percutaneous coronary intervention. It has a sequence specifically targeted for the RGD recognition sequence of GPIIb/IIIa; like tirofiban, has competitive and reversible binding and is also renally excreted. A large number of clinical trials have been performed using these agents in the clinical settings of percutaneous coronary intervention, acute coronary syndromes, and ST-elevation myocardial infarction; these are reviewed extensively in other chapters.

PERTINENT BIOLOGY
OF THROMBIN AND THROMBIN INHIBITORS

Thrombin

Whereas antagonists of platelet GPIIb/IIIa inhibit the "final common pathway" of platelet activation, activation of the soluble coagulation cascade is also important in arterial thrombosis. Thrombin (coagulation factor IIa) acts as a central mediator of clot formation through a variety of related actions. In addition to converting fibrinogen to fibrin, thrombin activates platelets largely through a recently discovered receptor known as protease-activated receptor-1 (PAR-1) *(12)*. The concentrations of thrombin required to activate platelets are considerably lower than those required to convert fibrinogen to fibrin. Even minute concentrations of thrombin are capable of initiating (or amplifying) coagulation by activating platelets, thus permitting assembly of the tenase and prothrombinase complexes that lead to a virtual explosion in the rate of thrombin formation *(13)*. In addition to amplification of its own generation in this fashion, thrombin activates factors VIII and XIII *(14–16)*. The former action is responsible for amplifying the coagulation cascade, whereas the latter leads to crosslinking and clot stabilization.

Human thrombin exists in a "pleated sheet" configuration. Through X-ray crystallographic studies, the structure of this molecule has been elucidated *(17)*. The *active site* of thrombin is responsible for most of the molecule's proteolytic activity. This site is situated within a cleft or "canyon" in the center of the molecule, and access is permitted only to macromolecules with specific configurations. From a teleologic perspective, this structure would seem to confer specificity on thrombin's activity, allowing the cleavage of only a select subgroup of substrates. The exterior surface of thrombin contains several distinct domains including at least two *exosites*. These exosites are of particular clinical importance with regard to antithrombin therapy. The region known as exosite-1 (or the substrate-binding exosite) is responsible for tethering fibrinogen so that the appropriate region of this molecule is exposed to thrombin's active site. Exosite-1 also plays another critically important

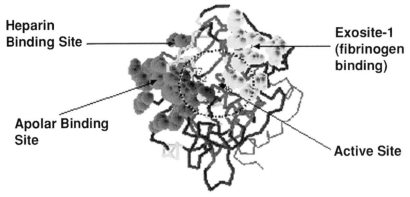

Fig. 1. The thrombin molecule. (From ref. *105*.)

role, as it is the region of thrombin responsible for activating the platelet PAR-1 receptor *(18)*. Additionally, a heparin-binding exosite, exosite-2, has been identified that is responsible for tethering the heparin-antithrombin complex onto the thrombin molecule *(19,20)*. Thrombin molecules are bound to fibrin within the evolving mural coronary thrombus and become exposed during endogenous or exogenous thrombolysis. Thrombolytic agents (and presumably mechanical disruption of a thrombus) can lead to enhanced thrombin generation directly *(21,22)* or indirectly through the activation of plasmin *(23,24)* by prothrombin and factors V and X *(25)*. Enhanced thrombin activity at the site of plaque rupture thus serves as a powerful stimulus for thrombosis and rethrombosis *(19)* (Fig. 1).

The Heparins

The heparins are indirect inhibitors of thrombin. Antithrombin therapy appears to be a necessary adjunct in the therapy of acute coronary syndromes. In a meta-analysis of data from six studies, Oler et al. *(26)* observed a 33% reduction in the rates of death and myocardial infarction among patients with unstable angina when heparin and aspirin were compared with aspirin alone. Studies in which GPIIb/IIIa antagonists have been used to treat acute coronary syndromes without accompanying unfractionated heparin have also suggested that at least some degree of thrombin antagonism may be justified *(27,28)*. Further anecdotal experience suggests that omission of a thrombin antagonist during percutaneous coronary intervention is likely to lead to overt coronary thrombosis.

Unfractionated heparin consists of a mixture of polysaccharide chains of varying lengths, about one-third of which have biologic activity. The heparins must complex with circulating antithrombin (formerly known as antithrombin III) in order to be active. The heparin-antithrombin complex becomes a rapid inactivator of thrombin, factor Xa, and (to a lesser extent) factors XIIa, XIa, and Ixa *(29)*. This activity relies on the presence of a pentasaccharide sequence known as the *essential pentasaccharide* (Fig. 2), which is present in about one-third of the molecules present in pharmaceutical preparations of unfractionated heparin, predominantly in the shorter polysaccharide chains. Anchoring to thrombin requires the presence of an 18-saccharide sequence, found predominantly on higher molecular weight chains within the mixture. Heparin also inhibits thrombin through a complex formed with heparin cofactor-2, although the clinical significance of this interaction is not known

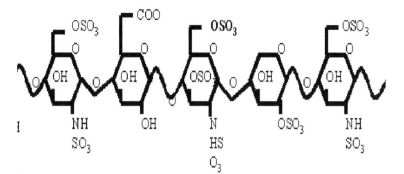

Fig. 2. The structure of the essential heparin pentasaccharide. (Courtesy of Neal Kleiman, MD.)

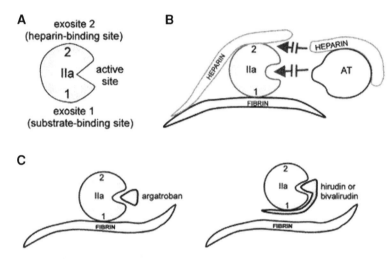

Fig. 3. Thrombin (IIa) interactions with fibrin. (**A**) Thrombin possesses two positively charged exosites; exosite 1 serves as the substrate-binding domain, whereas exosite 2 binds heparin. (**B**) Thrombin binds to fibrin via exosite 1. Heparin bridges thrombin to fibrin, thereby heightening the apparent affinity of thrombin for fibrin and including conformational changes at the active site of the enzyme. Because exosite 2 is occupied by the heparin molecule bridging thrombin to fibrin, antithrombin (AT)-bound heparin cannot bind to thrombin to form a ternary heparin/thrombin/antiithrombin complex. (**C**) Active site-directed inhibitors (such as argatroban) inhibit fibrin-bound thrombin without displacing of the enzyme from fibrin. Bivalent inhibitors (hirudin or bivalirudin) displace thrombin from fibrin during the inactivation process. (From ref. *32*.)

(19,30). The requirement of cofactors for heparin's activity presents a significant limitation to its use. Varying levels of cofactors between patients as well as temporal variations in cofactor concentrations within a patient (particularly in acute coronary syndromes and after recent heparin therapy) render the biologic response to heparin variable *(31)*.

In addition, steric considerations may limit the ability of the heparin-cofactor complexes to inhibit clot-bound thrombin *(31)*. Thrombin binds to fibrin via exosite-1 *(19,20)*, and heparin simultaneously binds to exosite-2 of thrombin and to fibrin. Formation of this ternary heparin/thrombin/fibrin complex actually increases the affinity of the thrombin-fibrin interaction. (Fig. 3) When both thrombin exosites are occupied within this ternary complex, thrombin is relatively protected from inactivation by the heparin-antithrombin complex, and therefore the ternary thrombin/heparin/antithrombin is unable to be formed *(32)*. Other shortcomings of heparin include binding to a variety of circulating "heparin-binding proteins" [many of which are acute-phase reactants *(33)*], which leads to inhibition by plasma proteins and platelet factors (such as platelet factor 4 and thrombospondin) that compete with antithrombin for heparin. Concentrations of these factors vary among patients, resulting in unreliable and unpredictable anticoagulation responses to a given dose of heparin *(31)*. Heparin has also been shown to enhance platelet aggregation *(34)*, possibly through platelet activation *(35)*, or alternatively by promoting agglutination through the platelet surface glycoprotein GPIb/IX/V-von Willebrand factor pathway *(36)*.

Heparin also has several clinically confirmed limitations. The pharmacodynamic response to heparin is nonlinear, and a large proportion of heparin-treated patients have activated partial thromboplastin time (aPTT) values outside the "therapeutic range" despite vigorous attention to dosing considerations. In some studies, this proportion has approached one-half of treated patients *(37–39)*. In addition, a well-demonstrated "rebound" effect of increased thrombotic events has also been described after discontinuing unfractionated heparin therapy *(40,41)*. Finally, heparin-induced thrombocytopenia and thrombosis (HITT) is a well-recognized autoimmune prothrombotic state that is associated with considerable morbidity and precludes the continued use of heparin *(42)*.

Low-Molecular-Weight Heparins

Low-molecular-weight heparins are produced by depolymerization of unfractionated heparin. This process allows elimination of many of the higher weight molecular chains. Although the mixture still contains some of the larger polysaccharide chains, the proportion of lower weight chains is increased, resulting in a mean molecular weight of approx 4000–6000 Daltons *(43)*. Low-molecular-weight heparins retain the critical "essential penta-saccharide" sequence required for the formation of heparin-antithrombin complex. Since most low-molecular-weight heparins consist of <18 saccharide units, fewer chains in the mixture support binding to thrombin. The greater proportion of shortened chain lengths leads to preferential inhibition of factor Xa. An important pharmacologic difference among the low-molecular-weight heparins revolves around the fragment sizes after depolymerization and the resulting Xa/IIa activity ratio *(44)*.

The theoretical advantages of the low-molecular-weight heparins over unfractionated heparin have been described elsewhere and include ease of administration, high biologic availability after subcutaneous injection, less binding to plasma proteins, greater Xa/IIa inhibition ratio (i.e., greater inhibition of thrombin generation), more predictable dose response, and reduced inactivation by platelet factor 4 *(45)*. Clinically reported advantages include a lower incidence of heparin-induced thrombocytopenia *(46)* and the ability to avoid routine monitoring of anti-Xa/IIa activity. However, the superiority of each low-molecular-weight heparin to unfractionated heparin has not been proved in all settings. Potentially, the primary disadvantage of the low-molecular-weight heparins consists of the lack of an easily available, rapid, and reliable measure of antithrombotic activity. Some clinical trials of low-molecular-weight heparins in patients with coronary artery disease have also shown trends toward increased rather than decreased rates of hemorrhage, although most of these bleeding episodes have been classified as "minor" *(47,48)*.

Direct Thrombin Inhibitors

Direct thrombin inhibitors such as hirudin, bivalirudin, and argatroban were initially used as anticoagulants in patients with heparin-induced thrombocytopenia *(49,50)*. The greater predictability of clinical response to these agents has suggested that they may be more useful than unfractionated heparins for routine antithrombotic treatment in patients with acute coronary syndromes and ST-segment elevation myocardial infarction and in those undergoing percutaneous coronary interventions. Direct thrombin inhibitors have several potential advantages. These drugs inhibit protein access to the active site of thrombin without requiring the intermediary molecule antithrombin. They are also able to antagonize clot-bound thrombin more efficiently than can the heparin-antithrombin complex. Finally, they are not affected by plasma proteins or platelet factor 4 *(51)*. Thus, they have a more predictable anticoagulant response than unfractionated heparin on measures of coagulation *(39)*.

Hirudin is the most potent and specific thrombin inhibitor currently known *(52)*. It is a 65-amino acid polypeptide originally isolated from the salivary glands of the medicinal leach *Hirudo medicinalis (53)*. Recombinant hirudin binds tightly to thrombin to form a slowly reversible (essentially irreversible) 1:1 stoichiometric complex *(32,54)*. It inhibits clot-bound thrombin more effectively than heparin *(55)* but is still most active against fluid phase thrombin *(56)*. In individuals with normal renal function, hirudin has a half-life of 40 min after intravenous administration, which increases to 120 min after subcutaneous injection *(57)*. Hirudin binds both the first exosite (N-terminus) and active site (C-terminus) of thrombin and is able to inhibit all proteolytic activity of the molecule. Recombinant hirudin lacks a sulfated tyrosine residue at position 63 and has a 10-fold lower affinity for thrombin than does native hirudin; however, it still remains a potent inhibitor of thrombin *(32)*.

Bivalirudin (originally termed hirulog) is a synthetic 20-amino acid peptide that was designed based on the structure of hirudin. It consists of the amino and carboxy termini of hirudin separated by a "spacer" consisting of four glycine residues *(54,58)*. Like hirudin, bivalirudin attaches to the first exosite of thrombin and blocks access to the molecule's active site. Bivalirudin differs from hirudin in that, once complexed with thrombin, the Arg-Pro bond on the amino-terminal extension is cleaved, converting bivalirudin into a low-affinity (weakly bound) inhibitor of thrombin. Bivalirudin has a plasma half-life of 24 min after intravenous infusion *(59)*, and upon intravenous administration has a linear dose response. Although it is renally excreted, it is also probably degraded by endogenous peptidases to constituent amino acids *(60)*. Robson et al. *(60)* described bivalirudin pharmacokinetics in subjects with normal renal function and in those with varying degrees of renal insufficiency. Patients with normal and mildly impaired renal function had no reduction in bivalirudin clearance rate. Patients with moderate and severe renal insufficiency had bivalirudin clearance rates that were reduced by 45 and 68%, respectively. However, activated clotting time (ACT) values were elevated only in the severely impaired group *(60)*.

Argatroban is a potent inhibitor of thrombin that has been approved in the United States for use in patients with heparin-induced thrombocytopenia *(50,61)*. In Japan it has been approved for treatment of acute ischemic stroke and chronic peripheral arterial obstructive disease *(62)*. Argatroban is a synthetically manufactured derivative of arginine and is a small molecule that reversibly binds soluble and clot-bound thrombin. Unlike hirudin and bivalirudin, argatroban does not bind the first exosite of thrombin but inhibits only the active site. Argatroban also differs from the latter two thrombin antagonists in that it is primarily metabolized in the liver via the CYP3A4/5 microsomal system *(63)*; it has a half-life of 45 min, which is prolonged in patients with hepatic dysfunction *(64)*.

COMBINED GPIIb/IIIa ANTAGONISTS AND ANTITHROMBINS

At a molecular and clinical level, there may be synergistic interactions between inhibitors of thrombin and GPIIb/IIIa antagonists beyond inhibiting thrombosis at different points. Mousa et al. *(65)* used computerized thromboelastography (TEG) to determine the ability of platelets and fibrin to augment human blood clot formation and strength under conditions of maximal platelet activation accelerated by tissue factor in human and dog blood. Platelets were found to enhance clot strength significantly; the GPIIb/IIIa antagonists abciximab and roxifiban effectively inhibited the enhancement of clot strength. The combination of subthreshold doses of tinzaparin (a low-molecular-weight heparin) and roxifiban or abciximab (both GPIIb/IIIa antagonists) resulted in distinct synergy in improving the antiplatelet and anticoagulant efficacy mediated by tissue factor. Pratico et al. *(66)* examined the effect of a direct thrombin inhibitor (napsagatran) alone and in combination with a GPIIb/IIIa antagonist (lamifiban) prior to administration of tissue plasminogen activator in a canine coronary thrombosis model. The direct thrombin inhibitor dramatically reduced time to reperfusion, prevented reocclusion, and demonstrated reduced platelet activity. When subthreshold doses of both drugs were combined, the time to reperfusion was shortened and the time duration of reperfusion was extended.

This potential additive benefit was not observed in a study by Ahmed et al. *(67)*. These investigators exposed blood from normal, healthy volunteers to tissue factor. The blood was incubated with different low-molecular-weight heparins (with adjusted, equivalent anti-Xa inhibition) in combination with tirofiban. Platelet activation status was determined by measuring surface expression of P-selectin (CD62) and generation of platelet aggregates. Of the low-molecular-weight heparins tested, enoxaparin produced the best concentration-dependent inhibition of P-selectin expression and platelet aggregation; enoxaparin at therapeutic concentrations was able to inhibit tissue factor-mediated platelet activation by >70%. Unlike enoxaparin, tirofiban alone produced weak concentration-dependent inhibition of P-selectin and platelet aggregation. Additive effects on inhibition of platelet activation and inhibition between tirofiban and enoxaparin were only noted at lower doses. At therapeutic concentrations of these drugs, the additive effects were no longer present. Although these findings are in large part dependent on the model selected, the assumption that this combination of drugs will necessarily be an improvement over current therapy requires clinical testing.

LOW-MOLECULAR-WEIGHT
HEPARIN IN ACUTE CORONARY SYNDROMES

Studies of low-molecular-weight heparins in patients with acute coronary syndromes have produced varying results. Two trials of the global management of patients with acute coronary syndromes have studied enoxaparin in comparison with unfractionated heparin. The ESSENCE *(48)* (3171 patients) and TIMI 11B *(68)* (3910 patients) trials demonstrated that enoxaparin given as a dose of 1 mg/kg bid (initiated as a 30-mg/kg bolus in TIMI 11B) for 3 d was superior to unfractionated heparin in reducing a composite end-

Table 1
Trials of Low-Molecular-Weight
Heparins vs Unfractionated Heparin in Patients with Acute Coronary Syndromes

| Study | No. of patients | Composite endpoints | Heparin (%) | | p value |
			Unfractionated	Low molecular weight	
ESSENCE (enoxaparin)	3171	14-d endpoint (D, MI, RA)	19.8	16.6	0.019
TIMI 11B (enoxaparin)	3910	8-d endpoint (D, MI, UTVR)	14.5	12.4	0.048
FRIC (dalteparin)	1482	6-d endpoint (D, MI, RA)	7.6	9.3	0.96
FRAXIS (nadroparin)	3468	6-d endpoint (D, MI, RA)	18.1	17.8	0.85

Abbreviations: D, death; MI, myocardial infarction; RA, recurrent angina; RI, recurrent ischemia; UTVR, urgent target vessel revascularization.

point of death, myocardial infarction, and recurrent ischemia. The findings of studies with other low-molecular-weight heparins have been less robust, although it is not clear whether these differences are caused solely by differences in the acuity of patients enrolled in the trials, or by differences between the low-molecular-weight heparins themselves, or by differences in the doses selected (Table 1).

LOW-MOLECULAR-WEIGHT HEPARINS IN PERCUTANEOUS CORONARY INTERVENTION

Hematologic Considerations

The low-molecular-weight heparins are attractive as anticoagulants during percutaneous coronary intervention for several reasons. First, the pharmacodynamic properties of these compounds, as discussed previously, are favorable. Second, the use of low-molecular-weight heparins in patients with acute coronary syndromes is increasing, and logistic considerations would strongly favor their use during percutaneous coronary intervention within the hospital stay. On the other hand, monitoring the level of anticoagulation during treatment with low-molecular weight heparins poses a considerable challenge since the usual measure of anticoagulant response to heparin, the ACT, is relatively insensitive to low-molecular-weight heparins.

No data currently exist to indicate what levels of anticoagulation are optimal when low-molecular-weight heparins are used as anticoagulants during percutaneous coronary intervention. Given the pleiotropic activity of these molecules, it is not at all clear that any single measure will be able to provide a precise indication of antithrombotic activity. Data from animal models of arterial injury indicate that higher concentrations of unfractionated heparin are associated with reduced thrombus deposition on injured arterial surfaces *(69)*. However, the low-molecular-weight heparins in animal models appear to confer an advantage over unfractionated heparin. Reviparine, a low-molecular-weight heparin, was administered in a porcine thrombosis model *(70)*. At low and high shear rates, reviparine significantly reduced fibrinogen deposition at sites of arterial vessel injury compared with unfractionated heparin. In a Folts model, a low dose of enoxaparin (0.5 mg/kg and 5 μg/kg/min infusion) reduced and a higher dose (1.0 mg/kg and 10 μg/kg/min infusion) nearly abolished platelet-dependent cyclic flow reductions. In contrast, unfractionated heparin at doses that increased the aPTT more than 10 times baseline had no effect on platelet-dependent cyclic flow reductions *(71)*.

Maximal plasma concentrations of low-molecular-weight heparins usually occur 1–5 h after a dose, and measurement near its peak (4 h) seems to be more closely related to safety and efficacy than trough levels *(72)*. In recent studies with enoxaparin, the value of anti-Xa activity >0.5–0.6 IU/mL 4 h after administration was selected as a therapeutic target level. This level was chosen in part from research done with low-molecular-weight heparins in deep venous thrombosis. Anti-Xa concentrations >0.8 IU/mL have been associated with higher rates of bleeding *(73)*, but measurement of higher anti-Xa activity has been related to the lower likelihood of recurrent deep venous thrombosis *(74)*. For twice daily administration of low-molecular-weight heparin, anti-Xa levels of 0.6–1.0 IU/mL 4 h after administration have been chosen as target levels for deep venous thrombosis treatment *(72)*. Unfortunately, the utility of these assays is subject to laboratory variability *(75)*. There are few human clinical data that definitively support using these levels in coronary syndromes, other than inference from studies using similar dosing regimens in patients with deep venous thrombosis.

Observational data from a variety of sources indicate that when unfractionated heparin is used as the foundation anticoagulant during percutaneous coronary intervention, increasing levels of ACT are associated with decreases in the risk of abrupt vessel closure, myocardial infarction, and other ischemic complications *(76–78)*. However the ACT appears to be considerably more sensitive to anti-IIa than anti-Xa activity. Several experimental models of vascular injury provide some evidence of a dose-response relationship between levels of direct Xa antagonists and thrombus deposition. Schaffer et al. *(79)* examined the use of recombinant antistasin (rATS), a potent inhibitor of factor Xa, in a baboon model of high-shear platelet-dependent vascular graft thrombosis and demonstrated that rATS dose-dependently decreased platelet and fibrinogen adherence to the vascular graft. Although higher anti-Xa levels seem to reduce thrombosis in this model, the ACT remains unaffected and negates this measurement as a tool in the cardiac catheterization laboratory. The relationship between these findings and the effects of low-molecular-weight heparins is less clear because of the other anticoagulant effects (anti-IIa) the low-molecular-weight heparins possess.

Consequently, low-molecular-weight heparins, which have high anti-Xa/anti-IIa levels, may have profound antithrombotic effects but little effect on the ACT *(80)*. The marker most likely to be useful in dose determination when using low-molecular-weight heparins is anti-Xa activity. In the TIMI 11A trial (a multicenter, dose-ranging trial to assess the safety of subcutaneous enoxaparin in patients with an acute coronary syndrome), ACT and anti-Xa levels were measured at peak (mean 4.3 h after enoxaparin) and trough (mean 11.5 h after enoxaparin) levels *(81)*. There was very little change in ACT levels of the enoxaparin peak (127 ± 9 s) and trough (127 ± 21 s) serum levels with the Hemotec device and no correlation between the ACT and anti-Xa activity. Peak anti-Xa activity was 1.3 ± 0.40 and trough activity was 0.51 ± 0.28 ($p < 0.0001$ peak vs trough) *(80)*.

Clinical Studies

A potential advantage of low-molecular-weight heparins as anticoagulation during percutaneous coronary intervention is the fact that patients with an acute coronary syndrome are often treated with a low-molecular-weight heparin and may already be anticoagulated when they enter the cardiac catheterization laboratory. Collet and colleagues *(82)* studied 451 consecutive patients who were treated with subcutaneous enoxaparin for at least 48 h for an acute coronary syndrome. A total of 293 patients underwent a coronary angiogram within 8 h of the morning enoxaparin dose, and 132 patients had immediate percutaneous coronary intervention without any additional dose of low-molecular-weight heparin or unfractionated heparin. These investigators selected a cutoff value of 0.5 IU/L as an indication of therapeutic efficacy. When patients had received a minimum of 48 h of dosing, 97.6% of patients had anti-Xa levels exceeding 0.5 IU/mL at the time of coronary angiography; moreover, during the 8-h window prior to catheterization, anti-Xa levels remained at a consistently therapeutic level. (The mean time between last enoxaparin administration and catheterization was 5.3 h ± 1.8 h.) The rate of myocardial infarction and death at 30 d following this procedure was 3.0%.

Martin et al. *(83)* examined the pharmacokinetics of enoxaparin given subcutaneously 8–12 h prior to percutaneous coronary intervention, with a supplemental 0.3 mg/kg bolus intravenously at the start of the percutaneous coronary intervention. Almost all patients who had received the initial enoxaparin dose 8–11 h prior to the percutaneous coronary intervention had anti-Xa levels >0.6 IU/mL, and this remained true at 2 h postprocedure. Furthermore, 98% of patients' actual anti-Xa levels fell within minimum and maximum predicted values, 2–8 h after subcutaneous enoxaparin administration. However, among the group that had received enoxaparin 11–12 h prior to PCI, very few patients had anti-Xa levels >0.6 IU/mL, and even after the enoxaparin bolus, several patients remained below this level. Thus, although effective anticoagulation can be achieved with enoxaparin, guidelines for time to administration must be developed. A number of point-of-care assays of anti-Xa activity are now being developed for this purpose *(84,85)*.

Intravenous Low-Molecular-Weight Heparins

The data from Collet and Martin are supported by observations made by the National Investigators Collaborating on Enoxaparin (NICE 1) *(86)* registry. In this registry, 828 patients received enoxaparin 1 mg/kg intravenously at the time of percutaneous coronary intervention. Four hours after receiving enoxaparin, measured anti-Xa activity was 0.8 ± 0.3 IU/mL. Interpretation of these data is confounded by the relatively large number of patients who had been on intravenous heparin prior to enrollment. Rates of major and minor bleeding were 1.0% and 2.5%, respectively. The composite of death, myocardial infarction, and urgent revascularization was observed in 6.2% of patients in hospital and 7.7% at 30 d.

Reviparin was studied in the percutaneous coronary intervention population by Karsch et al. *(87)*. A total of 625 patients undergoing percutaneous coronary transluminal angioplasty were randomized to either receive reviparin bolus/infusion followed by subcutaneous injection for 28 d or unfractionated heparin bolus/infusion and then subcutaneous placebo for 28 d. There was no difference between the two groups in the primary endpoint (death, myocardial infarction or revascularization: 33.3% reviparin arm, 32% control arm; $p = 0.7$) or in late luminal loss. However, events during or immediately after the procedure in the two groups were significantly different, with emergency stent implantation more frequent in the unfractionated heparin group [21 patients in control arm, 6 patients in the reviparin arm; relative risk (RR) = 0.29, 95% confidence interval (CI) 0.13–0.66, p = 0.003].

GPIIb/IIIa AND LOW-MOLECULAR-WEIGHT HEPARIN IN PERCUTANEOUS CORONARY INTERVENTION

The logical extension of these investigations is to test low-molecular-weight heparins in combination with antagonists of GPIIb/IIIa. Information concerning this combination, as of early 2002, is derived from a number of registries and small randomized clinical trials. The NICE trial examined the safety, dosing, and efficacy of enoxaparin with different GPIIb/IIIa antagonists. The NICE 3 and NICE 4 registries (86) included patients referred for elective or urgent percutaneous coronary intervention. NICE 4 enrollees (n = 818) received intravenous enoxaparin 0.75 mg/kg 5 min prior to a standard dose of abciximab (0.25 mg/kg) bolus and infusion (0.125 µg/kg/min) immediately preceding percutaneous coronary intervention. The incidence of major hemorrhage was 0.4%, and the secondary combined endpoint of death, myocardial infarction, and urgent revascularization was 6.5% during hospitalization, and 6.8% at 30 d.

The NICE 3 (88) investigators examined the use of enoxaparin in combination with GPIIb/IIIa antagonists in patients with an acute coronary syndromes. In this study, 645 patients were administered subcutaneous enoxaparin 1 mg/kg twice daily and a GPIIb/IIIa inhibitor (eptifibatide, n = 272; tirofiban, n = 229; abciximab, n = 144). If percutaneous coronary intervention was required, combination therapy was continued through the procedure; if the last dose of enoxaparin was given >8 h prior to the percutaneous coronary intervention, an additional dose of 0.3 mg/kg of enoxaparin was given intravenously periprocedurally. The overall major bleeding rate was 1.9%. Secondary outcomes included a mortality of 0.9%, myocardial infarction in 3.4%, and urgent target vessel revascularization of 2.6%, which were comparable to historical controls.

Kereiakes at al. (89) studied the combination of dalteparin and abciximab during percutaneous coronary intervention. The original design of the registry specified that all patients were to receive abciximab and then be randomized to intravenous bolus doses of either 40 or 60 IU/kg of dalteparin. Early in the course of the investigation, it was noted that patients who received low-dose dalteparin (40 IU/kg) developed thrombus in the guiding catheters and on the guidewires, indicating an inadequate level of anticoagulation, and this arm was terminated; all patients then received 60 IU/kg of dalteparin. Levels of anti-Xa activity were more consistently >0.6 IU/mL for patients receiving 60 IU/kg in comparison with the 40-IU/kg dose. Of interest is the rise of the ACT in the 60-IU/kg group 30 min post percutaneous coronary intervention (180 ± 38 s, median 238 s) vs the 40-IU/kg group (166 ± 28 s, median 168 s). The increase in ACT value is greater than that generally seen with other low-molecular-weight heparins and may be owing to dalteparin's greater anti-IIa activity compared to enoxaparin (Tables 2 and 3).

Cohen et al. (90) studied 525 patients with an acute coronary syndrome who were treated with tirofiban and then randomized to receive either intravenous unfractionated heparin or subcutaneous enoxaparin. Coronary angiography followed by percutaneous coronary intervention was allowed after 24 h of treatment, but at least 8 h after the last dose of enoxaparin. The primary endpoint was bleeding up to 24 h after discontinuation of anticoagulation. There was no difference between the two arms (4.7% tirofiban and enoxaparin

Table 2
Low-Molecular-Weight Heparins
and GPIIb/IIIa Antagonists in Percutaneous Coronary Intervention (%)

Endpoint	NICE 1[a] (n = 828)	NICE 3[b] (n = 645)	NICE 4[c] (n = 818)	Kereiakes[d] (n = 76)
Bleeding				
Major	1.0	1.9	0.4	2.6
Minor	2.5	n/a	2.9	4.0
Death	0.8	0.9	0.4	1.3
Myocardial infarction	5.7	3.4	6.2	3.9
Urgent revascularization	2.5	2.6	0.6	1.3

[a] Enoxaparin (1.0 mg/kg iv).
[b] Enoxaparin (>8 h after last dose, 0.3 mg/kg iv) and abciximab (n = 144) (0.25 mg/kg bolus then 0.125 µg/kg/min) or eptifibatide (n = 272) (180 µg/kg bolus then 2 µg/kg/min infusion) or tirofiban (n = 229) (0.4 µg/kg bolus, then 0.1 µg/kg infusion).
[c] Enoxaparin (0.75 mg/kg iv) and abciximab (0.25 mg/kg bolus, then 0.125 µg/kg/min).
[d] Dalteparin (60 IU/kg) and abciximab (0.25 mg/kg bolus then 0.125 µg/kg/min).

Table 3
Dalteparin in Percutaneous Coronary Intervention

	Dalteparin 60 IU/kg (n = 76)
ACT (s)	
Pre-PCI	
Mean ± SD	128 ± 22
Median (range)	131 (91–212)
30 min	
Mean ± SD	180 ± 38
Median (range)	238 (89–238)
4 h	
Mean ± SD	128 ± 15
Median (range)	130 (106–155)
Anti-Xa activity (IU/mL)	
Pre-PCI	
Mean ± SD	0.1 ± 0.22
Median (range)	(0.0–1.5)
30 min	
Mean ± SD	0.9 ± 0.30
Median (range)	0.8 (0.4–2.5)
4 h	
Mean ± SD	0.2 ± 0.14
Median (range)	0.3 (0.1–1.0)

Abbreviations: PCI, percutaneous coronary intervention; ACT, activated clotting time.
From ref. 89.

Table 4
ACUTE II: The Antithrombotic
Combination Using Tirofiban and Enoxaparin

Endpoint	Tirofiban plus enoxaparin (n = 315)	Tirofiban plus unfractionated heparin (n = 210)
Safety endpoints (%)		
Any TIMI bleeding	4.7	5.2
TIMI major bleeding	0.6	0.5
Cutaneous bleeding	19.4	21
Requiring transfusions	2.2	2.9
Thrombocytopenia	0.3	0.5
Thirty-day event rates (%)		
Death	2.2	2.4
Myocardial infarction	7.0	7.6
Stroke	0.3	1.4
Rehospitalization for unstable angina	2.5	6.6*
Revascularization	12.1	18.1**

*$p = 0.026$.
**$p = 0.058$.
From ref. 90.

vs 5.2% tirofiban and unfractionated heparin). However, at 30 d, the trend of the secondary endpoint of total ischemic events (death, myocardial infarction, recurrent angina, and ischemic cerebrovascular accident) was toward fewer events with enoxaparin (11.7% vs 16.7%). Also there was a trend toward fewer revascularizations in the enoxaparin group (12.1 vs 18.1%, $p = 0.058$) and a significant difference in rehospitalization for unstable angina (2.5% vs 6.6%, $p = 0.026$) (Table 4).

GPIIb/IIIa ANTAGONISTS AND LOW-MOLECULAR-WEIGHT HEPARIN IN ACUTE CORONARY SYNDROMES AND ACUTE MYOCARDIAL INFARCTION

Combination therapy in the acute coronary syndrome population has a firm basis in theory and practical use. Individually the GPIIb/IIIa antagonists and low-molecular-weight heparins have had solid data backing their use in this population. Furthermore, low-molecular-weight heparin in acute coronary syndromes has been shown to be cost-effective (91), easier to use, and less variable in anticoagulant effect than unfractionated heparin. Goodman (92) studied 746 high-risk acute coronary syndrome patients, all of whom received eptifibatide and were randomized to intravenous unfractionated heparin (70 U/kg bolus and then 15 U/kg/h titrated to an aPTT of 1.5–2 times standard) or subcutaneous enoxaparin (1 mg/kg) every 12 h for a minimum of 4 doses. Major bleeding at 48 and 96 h was significantly reduced in the enoxaparin arm (4.6% vs 1.8%, $p = 0.03$). Furthermore, secondary endpoints of death and myocardial infarction were also lowered (9% vs 5%, $p = 0.031$). Minor bleeding was increased in the enoxaparin arm, but this was

Table 5
INTERACT: Integrilin and Enoxaparin
Randomized Assessment of Acute Coronary Syndromes Treatment

	UFH (%)	Enoxaparin (%)	p value
Rate of major bleeds			
Major bleeding at 48 h	3.8	1.1	0.014
Minor bleeding at 96 h	24.9	32.5	0.024
Major bleeding at 96 h	4.6	1.8	0.03
Ischemic episodes as measured by ECG recording			
0–48 h	25.1	14.1	0.0002
48–96 h	25.9	12.7	0.0001
30-d events			
Death/myocardial infarction	9	5	0.031
Death/myocardial infarction/ recurrent ischemia	16.2	13.5	0.30
Death/myocardial infarction/ recurrent ischemia with ischemic ECG changes	12.6	8.4	0.064

Abbreviations: UFH, unfractionated heparin.
From ref. *92.*

attributed to bleeding at the injection site. These data support the supposition that low-molecular-weight heparin can safely and effectively be used in the acute coronary syndrome population (Table 5).

Tirofiban will be studied in combination with the low-molecular-weight heparin enoxaparin in the acute myocardial infarction setting in the TETAMI trial (safety and efficacy of subcutaneous enoxaparin vs intravenous unfractionated heparin and of tirofiban in the treatment of acute myocardial infarction for patients who have not been given thrombolytics) *(93)*. The goal of the study is to examine the treatment outlined above for patients otherwise not eligible for early reperfusion therapy. A broader randomized clinical trial of enoxaparin in patients treated with GPIIb/IIIa antagonists in acute coronary syndromes (SYNERGY) is now under way. This trial will include 8000 high-risk patients, a substantial proportion of whom are expected to undergo percutaneous coronary intervention.

DIRECT THROMBIN INHIBITORS IN ACUTE CORONARY SYNDROMES AND MYOCARDIAL INFARCTION

Hirudin was one of the first direct thrombin inhibitors to be studied in the acute coronary syndrome population. Several of the early hirudin trials were terminated prematurely because of increased bleeding. This finding may stem from some drawbacks of hirudin, including its narrow therapeutic window, irreversible binding, and dependence on renal excretion. The Global Use of Strategies to Open Occluded Arteries (GUSTO) IIa *(38)* trial (unfractionated heparin adjusted to aPTT of 60–90 s vs hirudin 0.6 mg/kg bolus and then 0.2 mg/kg infusion without aPTT adjustment) intended to enroll 12,000 patients with an acute coronary syndrome but was terminated early because of a higher incidence of hemorrhagic stroke. Similarly, the TIMI 9a Trial *(94)* examined heparin vs hirudin with thrombolytics in acute myocardial infarction and was terminated prematurely because of excessive bleeding in the hirudin arm.

Subsequently, in the GUSTO IIb *(39)* trial, 12,142 patients with acute coronary syndromes (including ST-elevation myocardial infarction) were randomized to heparin and reduced dose of hirudin (0.1 mg/kg bolus followed by infusion of 0.1 mg/kg/h). At 30 d, there was no significant difference between the two treatment arms, but there was no increase in serious bleeding complications in the hirudin group. The TIMI 9b *(95)* trial randomized patients with acute myocardial infarction to the same reduced dose of hirudin or unfractionated heparin, in combination with thrombolytics. There was no difference in primary endpoint (death, nonfatal myocardial infarction, or cardiogenic shock at 30 d) or bleeding between the two arms. The Organization to Assess Strategies for Ischemic Syndromes-2 (OASIS-2) *(96)* demonstrated evidence of superiority of hirudin (0.4 mg/kg bolus and then 0.15 mg/kg/h infusion) over unfractionated heparin (5000 U bolus and then 15 U/kg/h infusion) in 10,141 patients with an acute coronary syndrome. Combined primary and secondary endpoints were significantly in favor of hirudin, but hirudin was also associated with a greater incidence of major bleeding.

Bivalirudin's consistent anticoagulant effect, shorter half-life, its ability to bind reversibly to free circulating and fibrin-bound thrombin, and pharmokinetic profile may contribute to its improved efficacy. Bivalirudin was studied in 17,073 patients with acute myocardial infarction in the HERO-2 trial *(97)*. There was no statistically significant difference between the heparin and bivalirudin groups for the primary endpoint of mortality, but the secondary endpoint of reinfarction at 96 h demonstrated a significant reduction in the bivalirudin group (1.6% vs 3.2%, $p = 0.001$) at the cost of significantly higher rates of moderate and mild bleeding. The Argatroban in Acute Myocardial Infraction (ARGAMI) *(98)* pilot study randomized 127 patients to heparin or argatroban as an adjunct to accelerated tissue plasminogen factor; there was no difference in angiographic patency vs heparin. ARGAMI-2, which had low- and high-dose arms of argatroban, showed no difference in efficacy or bleeding endpoints.

DIRECT THROMBIN INHIBITORS
IN PERCUTANEOUS CORONARY INTERVENTION

Because the dose-response curve for direct thrombin antagonists is more easily titratable than heparin, they possess the theoretical advantage of being less likely to result in bleeding complications. In the HELVETICA trial, 1141 patients with unstable angina who were scheduled for angioplasty were randomized into three groups: heparin bolus and infusion for 24 h followed by placebo subcutaneous injection for 3 d, hirudin bolus and infusion for 24 h followed by placebo subcutaneous injection for 3 d, and hirudin bolus and infusion for 24 h followed by hirudin subcutaneous injection twice daily for 3 d. The primary endpoint was event-free survival at 7 mo, and secondary endpoints included early cardiac events (within 96 h), bleeding, and angiographic measurements of coronary diameter at 6-mo follow-up. At the 6-mo follow-up, there was no difference in the primary endpoint or in coronary lumen diameters; however, cardiac events within the first 96 h were significantly reduced in the hirudin groups, which occurred in 11.0, 7.9, and 5.6% of

Table 6
Bivalirudin Angioplasty Trial

	Bivalirudin (n = 2161)	Heparin (n = 2151)	Odds ratio (95% CI)	p value
Clinical ischemic endpoints in hospital through 7 d by treatment group				
All patients				
Death, myocardial infarction, revascularization (%)	135 (6.2)	169 (7.9)	0.78 (0.62–0.99)	0.039
Death (%)	5 (0.2)	5 (0.2)	0.99 (0.28–3.46)	0.987
Myocardial infarction (%)	71 (3.3)	90 (4.2)	0.78 (0.57–1.07)	0.126
Revascularization (%)	91 (4.2)	121 (5.6)	0.74 (0.56-0.97)	0.030
Postinfarction angina cohort	(n = 369)	(n = 372)		
Death, myocardial infarction, or revascularization (%)	18 (4.9)	37 (9.9)	0.47 (0.26–0.84)	0.009
Death (%)	0 (0.0)	2 (0.5)	—	0.118
Myocardial infarction (%)	11 (3.0)	21 (5.6)	0.51 (0.24–1.07)	0.068
Revascularization (%)	11 (3.0)	23 (6.2)	0.47 (0.22–0.98)	0.038
Bleeding endpoints in hospital up to 7 d by treatment group				
All patients				
Clinically significant bleeding (%)	76 (3.5)	199 (9.3)	0.34 (0.26–0.45)	<0.001
Intracranial hemorrhage (%)	1 (0.04)	2 (0.09)	0.50 (0.05–5.23)	0.624
Retroperitoneal bleeding (%)	5 (0.2)	15 (0.7)	0.33 (0.13–0.87)	0.026
Red blood cell transfusion 2 U (%)	43 (2.0)	123 (5.7)	0.34 (0.24–0.47)	<0.001
With >3 g/dL fall in hemoglobin (%)	41 (1.9)	124 (5.8)	0.33 (0.24–0.46)	<0.001
With >5 g/dL fall in hemoglobin (%)	14 (0.6)	47 (2.2)	0.29 (0.17–0.51)	<0.001

From ref. *100.*

patients in the respective groups (combined relative risk with hirudin, 0.61; 95% CI 0.41–0.90; $p = 0.023$) *(99).*

Bivalirudin was compared with unfractionated heparin in 4312 patients undergoing coronary balloon angioplasty for unstable angina. The primary endpoint of this trial was a composite of death, myocardial infarction, and repeat target vessel revascularization at 7 d. This endpoint was reduced in the bivalirudin group (6.2% vs 7.9%, $p = 0.039$). This advantage remained at 90 d ($p = 0.12$). It is quite important to note that, there was a marked reduction in bleeding events in the bivalirudin group (3.5% vs 9.3%, $p < 0.001$) *(100)* (Table 6).

A recent meta-analysis by the Direct Thrombin Inhibitor Trialists' Collaborative Group *(101)* examined trials that involved at least 200 patients with either an acute coronary syndrome or undergoing a percutaneous coronary intervention who were randomized to receive either hirudin, bivalirudin, argatroban, efegatran, or inogatran vs heparin. Trials that used "excessive" doses of anticoagulation were excluded. In the 35,970 patients who were analyzed, the direct thrombin inhibitors were associated with a significantly lower risk of death or myocardial infarction at the end of treatment (4.3% vs 5.1%, $p = 0.001$) and at 30 d (7.4% vs 8.2%, $p = 0.02$). These findings were attributed to reductions seen with hirudin and bivalirudin, but not with the other agents. Bivalirudin was found to have decreased bleeding, in contrast to hirudin, which was associated with more frequent bleeding compared with heparin.

GPIIb/IIIa AND DIRECT THROMBIN
INHIBITOR IN PERCUTANEOUS CORONARY INTERVENTION

The first combination study of a direct thrombin antagonist and a GPIIb/IIIa antagonist was the Comparison of Abciximab Complications with Hirulog (Bivalirudin) Events Trial (CACHET) pilot study *(102)*. In an initial phase (phase A) of this study, 60 patients undergoing elective percutaneous coronary intervention received abciximab and were randomized to receive either unfractionated heparin given as 70 U/kg or bivalirudin 1.0 mg/kg bolus followed by an infusion of 2.5 mg/kg/h for 4 h. (The bivalirudin dose was that used in the prior Hirulog Angioplasty Trial.) No overt increases in bleeding were noted during this phase of the trial, although the median ACT value in the bivalirudin-treated patients was 443 ± 117 s.

The next two phases of this pilot study were designed to test whether bivalirudin could be used as part of a GP IIb/IIIa-sparing strategy, since such a strategy might have both economic and safety advantages. Patients were randomized in a 2:1 or 3:1 ratio to receive either heparin with abciximab or bivalirudin with abciximab added in a "provisional use strategy," that is, for intraprocedural treatment of an unsatisfactory or threatening angiographic result. In phase B, bivalirudin was administered as a bolus of 0.5 mg/kg, with an infusion of 1.75 mg/kg/h for the procedure duration. In phase C, a bolus of 0.75 mg/kg was given, with an infusion of 1.75 mg/kg/h. Abciximab was used in 24% of patients in the bivalirudin/provisional abciximab arms of phases B and C. The composite clinical endpoint of death, myocardial infarction, repeat revascularization, or major bleeding by 7 d occurred in 5.9, 0.0, and 10.6% of patients in the bivalirudin phase B, bivalirudin phase C, and heparin plus planned abciximab arms, respectively ($p = 0.018$ for the pooled bivalirudin groups versus the heparin group).

A recent open-label study examined the safety and effect on several markers of thrombosis with the combination of bivalirudin and eptifibatide during percutaneous coronary intervention *(103)*. Forty-two patients undergoing elective percutaneous coronary intervention were randomized to receive bivalirudin 1.0 mg/kg bolus followed by a 4-h infusion at 2.5 mg/kg/h; or bivalirudin 0.75 mg/kg bolus followed by a 4-h infusion at 1.75 mg/kg; or a heparin 60 U/kg bolus. All patients also received aspirin and eptifibatide given as two sequential boluses of 180 µg/kg, followed by a 2 µg/kg/min infusion for 18–24 h. After the bolus dose of study drug, turbidimetric platelet aggregation in response to 5 µM ADP increased in patients assigned to heparin but not bivalirudin. After eptifibatide, platelet aggregation was eliminated in all three treatment groups. The effects of either drug on the formation of thrombin antithrombin complexes and prothrombin fragment 1.2 were comparable. Neither agent affected the formation of platelet-monocyte complexes or expression of CD63 lysosomal antigen. There were no major bleeding events, and a single non-Q-wave myocardial infarction occurred in a patient treated with bivalirudin. Although the study clearly did not have adequate statistical power to detect realistic differences between patients treated with bivalirudin and those receiving heparin, it did provide preliminary support for the notion that thrombin antagonism with bivalirudin can be performed safely at the profound levels of platelet inhibition that are achieved with eptifibatide.

The Randomized Evaluation in PCI Linking Angiomax to Reduced Clinical Events (REPLACE-1) *(104)* study was an open-labeled randomized pilot trial of bivalirudin com-

Table 7
Clinical Events at 48 Hours in the REPLACE-1 Trial

48-h events	Heparin (n = 524)	Bivalirudin (n = 532)	OR (95% CI)
All patients			
Death/myocardial infarction/ revascularization/major bleeding (%)	49 (9.4)	40 (7.5)	0.79 (0.51–1.22)
Death/myocardial infarction/ revascularization (%)	36 (6.9)	30 (5.6)	0.81 (0.49–1.34)
Death/myocardial infarction (%)	28 (5.3)	26 (4.9)	0.91 (0.53–1.57)
TIMI major/minor/transfusion	18 (3.4)	15 (2.8)	0.82 (0.41–1.64)
48-h events	Heparin (n = 377)	Bivalirudin (n = 375)	OR (95% CI)
REPLACE-1 GPIIb/IIIa antagonist-treated patients			
Death/myocardial infarction/ revascularization/major bleeding (%)	39 (10.3)	33 (8.8)	0.84 (0.51–1.36)
Death/myocardial infarction/ revascularization (%)	27 (7.2)	23 (6.1)	0.85 (0.48–1.51)
Death/myocardial infarction (%)	24 (6.4)	21 (5.6)	0.87 (0.48–1.59)
TIMI major/minor/transfusion	16 (4.2)	13 (3.5)	0.81 (0.38–1.71)

From ref. *104*.

pared with heparin in 1056 patients undergoing percutaneous coronary intervention, enrolled from 77 centers within the United States. Bivalirudin was administered as a 0.75 mg/kg bolus and then given as a 1.75/mg/kg/h infusion. Pretreatment with a thienopyridine was encouraged, but the use of a stent or GPIIb/IIIa inhibitor was left to the investigator's discretion. GPIIb/IIIa antagonists were used on a provisional basis by the investigator rather than protocol specified. Approximately 71% of patients in both arms received a GPIIb/IIIa antagonist. Stents were implanted in 85% of the procedures. The mean ACT was 304 ± 88 s in the unfractionated heparin group and 370 ± 102 s in the bivalirudin group. The quadruple endpoint of death, myocardial infarction, urgent revascularization, and bleeding was 7.5% in the bivalirudin arm and 9.4% in the unfractionated heparin arm. In the patients treated with a GPIIb/IIIa antagonist, the quadruple endpoint occurred in 8.8 and 10.3%, respectively. There was a 39% reduction in major bleeding and 35% reduction in clinically significant bleeding in the bivalirudin arm. Although there was a trend toward improved outcomes for the quadruple endpoint in both the GPIIb/IIIa antagonist treated and untreated arms, there was no statistically significant difference between the two arms (Table 7).

The study was designed to gain further experience with the combinations and to provide an estimate of event rates for the design of the large-scale REPLACE-2 study and was not meant to be statistically conclusive. REPLACE-2 will compare unfractionated heparin and GPIIb/IIIa inhibitor vs bivalirudin alone, with a GPIIb/IIIa antagonist used on provisional basis. A total of 6000 patients will be enrolled with a quadruple endpoint of death, myocardial infarction, revascularization, and clinically significant bleeding at 30 d and follow-up in 1 yr. Enrollment is expected to be complete by 2002.

CONCLUSIONS

Thrombin's central role in platelet activation, thrombus formation, and propagation is abundantly clear from numerous animal and human studies. Although unfractionated heparin has been instrumental in reducing events in many cardiac settings, its practical and theoretical limitations have become more evident. Low-molecular-weight heparins and direct thrombin inhibitors, which have theoretical and practical advantages over unfractionated heparin, have shown favorable outcomes when used in a variety of cardiac settings. In combination with a GPIIb/IIIa antagonist, preliminary data have provided evidence of safety and efficacy. New randomized clinical trials are under way to determine whether combination therapy may be the next standard of care in modern practice.

REFERENCES

1. White HD. Improved efficacy and less bleeding: further evidence of a unique uncoupling of benefit and risk with bivalirudin. Am Heart J 2002;143:189–192.
2. Frishman WH, Burns B, Atac B, et al. Novel antiplatelet therapies for treatment of patients with ischemic heart disease: inhibitors of the platelet glycoprotein IIb/IIIa integrin receptor. Am Heart J 1995;130: 877–892.
3. Hynes RO. Integrins: a family of cell surface receptors. Cell 1987;48:549–554.
4. Wagner CL, Mascelli MA, Neblock DS, et al. Analysis of GPIIb/IIIa receptor number by quantification of 7E3 binding to human platelets. Blood 1996;88:907–914.
5. van Willigen G, Akkerman JW. Regulation of glycoprotein IIB/IIIA exposure on platelets stimulated with alpha-thrombin. Blood 1992;79:82–90.
6. Fuster V, Stein B, Ambrose JA, et al. Atherosclerotic plaque rupture and thrombosis. Evolving concepts. Circulation 1990;82:II47–II59.
7. Ambrose JA, Weinrauch M. Thrombosis in ischemic heart disease. Arch Intern Med 1996;156:1382–1394.
8. Fuster V, Badimon JJ, Badimon L. Clinical-pathological correlations of coronary disease progression and regression. Circulation 1992;86:III1–III11.
9. Fuster V, Badimon L, Badimon JJ, et al. The pathogenesis of coronary artery disease and the acute coronary syndromes. N Engl J Med 1992;326:242–250.
10. Lincoff AM. GUSTO IV: expanding therapeutic options in acute coronary syndromes. Am Heart J 2000; 140:S103–S114.
11. Mazur W, Kaluza G, Kleiman NS. Antiplatelet therapy for treatment of acute coronary syndromes. Cardiol Clin 1999;17:345–357.
12. Kahn ML, Zheng YW, Huang W, et al. A dual thrombin receptor system for platelet activation. Nature 1998;394:690–694.
13. Lawson JH, Kalafatis M, Stram S, et al. A model for the tissue factor pathway to thrombin. I. An empirical study. J Biol Chem 1994;269:23,357–23,366.
14. Fuster V, Lewis A. Conner Memorial Lecture. Mechanisms leading to myocardial infarction: insights from studies of vascular biology. Circulation 1994;90:2126–2146.
15. Stein B, Fuster V, Halperin JL, et al. Antithrombotic therapy in cardiac disease. An emerging approach based on pathogenesis and risk. Circulation 1989;80:1501–1513.
16. Fuster V. Elucidation of the role of plaque instability and rupture in acute coronary events. Am J Cardiol 1995;76:24C–33C.
17. Bode W, Mayr I, Baumann U, et al. The refined 1.9 A crystal structure of human alpha-thrombin: interaction with D-Phe-Pro-Arg chloromethylketone and significance of the Tyr-Pro-Pro-Trp insertion segment. EMBO J 1989;8:3467–3475.
18. Dery O, Corvera CU, Steinhoff M, et al. Proteinase-activated receptors: novel mechanisms of signaling by serine proteases. Am J Physiol 1998;274:C1429–C1452.
19. Liaw PC, Becker DL, Stafford AR, et al. Molecular basis for the susceptibility of fibrin-bound thrombin to inactivation by heparin cofactor ii in the presence of dermatan sulfate but not heparin. J Biol Chem 2001;276:20,959–20,965.

20. Hogg PJ, Bock PE. Modulation of thrombin and heparin activities by fibrin. Thromb Haemost 1997;77: 424–433.
21. Eisenberg PR, Sobel BE, Jaffe AS. Activation of prothrombin accompanying thrombolysis with recombinant tissue-type plasminogen activator. J Am Coll Cardiol 1992;19:1065–1069.
22. Winters KJ, Santoro SA, Miletich JP, et al. Relative importance of thrombin compared with plasmin-mediated platelet activation in response to plasminogen activation with streptokinase. Circulation 1991; 84:1552–1560.
23. Helft G, Abdelouahed M, Vacheron A, et al. [Effects of thrombolysis on platelets and coagulation]. Ann Cardiol Angeiol (Paris) 1995;44:354–360.
24. Becker R. Dynamics of coronary thrombolysis and reocclusion. Clin Cardiol 1997;20:III2–III5.
25. Aronson DL, Chang P, Kessler CM. Platelet-dependent thrombin generation after in vitro fibrinolytic treatment. Circulation 1992;85:1706–1712.
26. Oler A, Whooley MA, Oler J, et al. Adding heparin to aspirin reduces the incidence of myocardial infarction and death in patients with unstable angina. A meta-analysis. JAMA 1996;276:811–815.
27. Inhibition of the platelet glycoprotein IIb/IIIa receptor with tirofiban in unstable angina and non-Q-wave myocardial infarction. Platelet Receptor Inhibition in Ischemic Syndrome Management in Patients Limited by Unstable Signs and Symptoms (PRISM-PLUS) Study Investigators. N Engl J Med 1998; 338:1488–1497.
28. International, randomized, controlled trial of lamifiban (a platelet glycoprotein IIb/IIIa inhibitor), heparin, or both in unstable angina. The PARAGON Investigators. Platelet IIb/IIIa Antagonism for the Reduction of Acute coronary syndrome events in a Global Organization Network. Circulation 1998; 97:2386–2395.
29. Olson ST, Bjork I. Regulation of thrombin activity by antithrombin and heparin. Semin Thromb Hemost 1994;20:373–409.
30. He L, Vicente CP, Westrick RJ, et al. Heparin cofactor II inhibits arterial thrombosis after endothelial injury. J Clin Invest 2002;109:213–219.
31. Hirsh J. Heparin. N Engl J Med 1991;324:1565–1574.
32. Weitz JI, Buller HR. Direct thrombin inhibitors in acute coronary syndromes: present and future. Circulation 2002;105:1004–1011.
33. Hirsh J, Warkentin TE, Shaughnessy SG, et al. Heparin and low-molecular-weight heparin: mechanisms of action, pharmacokinetics, dosing, monitoring, efficacy, and safety. Chest 2001;119:64S–94S.
34. Mascelli MA, Kleiman NS, Marciniak SJ Jr, et al. Therapeutic heparin concentrations augment platelet reactivity: implications for the pharmacologic assessment of the glycoprotein IIb/IIIa antagonist abciximab. Am Heart J 2000;139:696–703.
35. Xiao Z, Theroux P. Platelet activation with unfractionated heparin at therapeutic concentrations and comparisons with a low-molecular-weight heparin and with a direct thrombin inhibitor. Circulation 1998;97:251–256.
36. Poletti LF, Bird KE, Marques D, et al. Structural aspects of heparin responsible for interactions with von Willebrand factor. Arterioscler Thromb Vasc Biol 1997;17:925–931.
37. An international randomized trial comparing four thrombolytic strategies for acute myocardial infarction. The GUSTO investigators. N Engl J Med 1993;329:673–682.
38. Randomized trial of intravenous heparin versus recombinant hirudin for acute coronary syndromes. The Global Use of Strategies to Open Occluded Coronary Arteries (GUSTO) IIa Investigators. Circulation 1994;90:1631–1637.
39. A comparison of recombinant hirudin with heparin for the treatment of acute coronary syndromes. The Global Use of Strategies to Open Occluded Coronary Arteries (GUSTO) IIb investigators. N Engl J Med 1996;335:775–782.
40. Theroux P, Ouimet H, McCans J, et al. Aspirin, heparin, or both to treat acute unstable angina. N Engl J Med 1988;319:1105–1111.
41. Bahit MC, Topol EJ, Califf RM, et al. Reactivation of ischemic events in acute coronary syndromes: results from GUSTO-IIb. Gobal Use of Strategies To Open occluded arteries in acute coronary syndromes. J Am Coll Cardiol 2001;37:1001–1007.
42. Warkentin TE, Levine MN, Hirsh J, et al. Heparin-induced thrombocytopenia in patients treated with low-molecular-weight heparin or unfractionated heparin. N Engl J Med 1995;332:1330–1335.
43. Kaplan KL, Francis CW. Heparin-induced thrombocytopenia. Blood Rev 1999;13:1–7.
44. Antman EM, Cohen M. Newer antithrombin agents in acute coronary syndromes. Am Heart J 1999; 138:S563–S569.

45. Padilla A, Gray E, Pepper DS, et al. Inhibition of thrombin generation by heparin and low molecular weight (LMW) heparins in the absence and presence of platelet factor 4 (PF4). Br J Haematol 1992;82:406–413.

46. Cohen M. Heparin-induced thrombocytopenia and the clinical use of low molecular weight heparins in acute coronary syndromes. Semin Hematol 1999;36:33–36.

47. Comparison of two treatment durations (6 d and 14 d) of a low molecular weight heparin with a 6-d treatment of unfractionated heparin in the initial management of unstable angina or non-Q wave myocardial infarction: FRAX.I.S. (FRAxiparine in Ischaemic Syndrome). Eur Heart J 1999;20:1553–1562.

48. Cohen M, Demers C, Gurfinkel EP, et al. Low-molecular-weight heparins in non-ST-segment elevation ischemia: the ESSENCE trial. Efficacy and safety of subcutaneous enoxaparin versus intravenous unfractionated heparin, in non-Q-wave coronary events. Am J Cardiol 1998;82:19L–24L.

49. Greinacher A, Volpel H, Janssens U, et al. Recombinant hirudin (lepirudin) provides safe and effective anticoagulation in patients with heparin-induced thrombocytopenia: a prospective study. Circulation 1999;99:73–80.

50. Lewis BE, Walenga JM, Wallis DE. Anticoagulation with Novastan (argatroban) in patients with heparin- induced thrombocytopenia and heparin-induced thrombocytopenia and thrombosis syndrome. Semin Thromb Hemost 1997;23:197–202.

51. Bates SM, Weitz JI. The mechanism of action of thrombin inhibitors. J Invasive Cardiol 2000;12(Suppl F):27F–32F.

52. Levy JH. Novel intravenous antithrombins. Am Heart J 2001;141:1043–1047.

53. Wallis RB. Hirudins: from leeches to man. Semin Thromb Hemost 1996;22:185–196.

54. Hirsh J. New anticoagulants. Am Heart J 2001;142:S3–S8.

55. Weitz JI, Hudoba M, Massel D, et al. Clot-bound thrombin is protected from inhibition by heparin-antithrombin III but is susceptible to inactivation by antithrombin III-independent inhibitors. J Clin Invest 1990;86:385–391.

56. Visentin GP, Ford SE, Scott JP, et al. Antibodies from patients with heparin-induced thrombocytopenia/thrombosis are specific for platelet factor 4 complexed with heparin or bound to endothelial cells. J Clin Invest 1994;93:81–88.

57. Weitz JI, Hirsh J. New antithrombotic agents. Chest 1998;114:715S–727S.

58. Kelly AB, Maraganore JM, Bourdon P, et al. Antithrombotic effects of synthetic peptides targeting various functional domains of thrombin. Proc Natl Acad Sci USA 1992;89:6040–6044.

59. Fox I, Dawson A, Loynds P, et al. Anticoagulant activity of Hirulog, a direct thrombin inhibitor, in humans. Thromb Haemost 1993;69:157–163.

60. Robson R. The use of bivalirudin in patients with renal impairment. J Invasive Cardiol 2000;12(Suppl F): 33F–36F.

61. Lewis BE, Wallis DE, Berkowitz SD, et al. Argatroban anticoagulant therapy in patients with heparin-induced thrombocytopenia. Circulation 2001;103:1838–1843.

62. Matsuo T, Koide M, Kario K. Development of argatroban, a direct thrombin inhibitor, and its clinical application. Semin Thromb Hemost 1997;23:517–522.

63. Tran JQ, Di Cicco RA, Sheth SB, et al. Assessment of the potential pharmacokinetic and pharmacodynamic interactions between erythromycin and argatroban. J Clin Pharmacol 1999;39:513–519.

64. Swan SK, Hursting MJ. The pharmacokinetics and pharmacodynamics of argatroban: effects of age, gender, and hepatic or renal dysfunction. Pharmacotherapy 2000;20:318–329.

65. Mousa SA. Comparative efficacy of different low-molecular-weight heparins (LMWHs) and drug interactions with LMWH: implications for management of vascular disorders. Semin Thromb Hemost 2000; 26(Suppl 1):39–46.

66. Pratico D, Murphy NP, Fitzgerald DJ. Interaction of a thrombin inhibitor and a platelet GP IIb/IIIa antagonist in vivo: evidence that thrombin mediates platelet aggregation and subsequent thromboxane A2 formation during coronary thrombolysis. J Pharmacol Exp Ther 1997;281:1178–1185.

67. Ahmad S, Jeske WP, Ma Q, et al. Inhibition of tissue factor-activated platelets by low-molecular-weight heparins and glycoprotein IIb/IIIa receptor antagonist. Thromb Res 2001;102:143–151.

68. Antman EM, McCabe CH, Gurfinkel EP, et al. Enoxaparin prevents death and cardiac ischemic events in unstable angina/non-Q-wave myocardial infarction. Results of the thrombolysis in myocardial infarction (TIMI) 11B trial. Circulation 1999;100:1593–1601.

69. Heras M, Chesebro JH, Penny WJ, et al. Effects of thrombin inhibition on the development of acute platelet-thrombus deposition during angioplasty in pigs. Heparin versus recombinant hirudin, a specific thrombin inhibitor. Circulation 1989;79:657–665.

70. Roque M, Rauch U, Reis ED, et al. Comparative study of antithrombotic effect of a low molecular weight heparin and unfractionated heparin in an ex vivo model of deep arterial injury. Thromb Res 2000;98:499–505.
71. Leadley RJ Jr, Kasiewski CJ, Bostwick JS, et al. Inhibition of repetitive thrombus formation in the stenosed canine coronary artery by enoxaparin, but not by unfractionated heparin. Arterioscler Thromb Vasc Biol 1998;18:908–914.
72. Laposata M, Green D, Van Cott EM, et al. College of American Pathologists Conference XXXI on laboratory monitoring of anticoagulant therapy: the clinical use and laboratory monitoring of low-molecular-weight heparin, danaparoid, hirudin and related compounds, and argatroban. Arch Pathol Lab Med 1998;122:799–807.
73. Nieuwenhuis HK, Albada J, Banga JD, et al. Identification of risk factors for bleeding during treatment of acute venous thromboembolism with heparin or low molecular weight heparin. Blood 1991;78:2337–2343.
74. Levine MN, Planes A, Hirsh J, et al. The relationship between anti-factor Xa level and clinical outcome in patients receiving enoxaparine low molecular weight heparin to prevent deep vein thrombosis after hip replacement. Thromb Haemost 1989;62:940–944.
75. College of American Pathologists. Coagulation (Comprehensive) Survey. Set CG2-B. College of American Pathologists, Northfield, IL, 1999.
76. Narins CR, Hillegass WB Jr, Nelson CL, et al. Relation between activated clotting time during angioplasty and abrupt closure. Circulation 1996;93:667–671.
77. Chew DP, Bhatt DL, Lincoff AM, et al. Defining the optimal activated clotting time during percutaneous coronary intervention: aggregate results from 6 randomized, controlled trials. Circulation 2001;103:961–966.
78. Ferguson JJ, Dougherty KG, Gaos CM, et al. Relation between procedural activated coagulation time and outcome after percutaneous transluminal coronary angioplasty. J Am Coll Cardiol 1994;23:1061–1065.
79. Schaffer LW, Davidson JT, Vlasuk GP, et al. Selective factor Xa inhibition by recombinant antistasin prevents vascular graft thrombosis in baboons. Arterioscler Thromb 1992;12:879–885.
80. Henry TD, Satran D, Knox LL, et al. Are activated clotting times helpful in the management of anticoagulation with subcutaneous low-molecular-weight heparin? Am Heart J 2001;142:590–593.
81. Dose-ranging trial of enoxaparin for unstable angina: results of TIMI 11A. The Thrombolysis in Myocardial Infarction (TIMI) 11A Trial Investigators. J Am Coll Cardiol 1997;29:1474–1482.
82. Collet JP, Montalescot G, Lison L, et al. Percutaneous coronary intervention after subcutaneous enoxaparin pretreatment in patients with unstable angina pectoris. Circulation 2001;103:658–663.
83. Martin J, et al. Eur Heart J 2002;22(abstract Suppl):14.
84. Hansen R, Koster A, Kukucka M, et al. A quick anti-Xa-activity-based whole blood coagulation assay for monitoring unfractionated heparin during cardiopulmonary bypass: a pilot investigation. Anesth Analg 2000;91:533–538.
85. Holmes MB, Schneider DJ, Hayes MG, et al. Novel, bedside, tissue factor-dependent clotting assay permits improved assessment of combination antithrombotic and antiplatelet therapy. Circulation 2000;102:2051–2057.
86. Kereiakes DJ, Grines C, Fry E, et al. Enoxaparin and abciximab adjunctive pharmacotherapy during percutaneous coronary intervention. J Invasive Cardiol 2001;13:272–278.
87. Karsch KR, Preisack MB, Baildon R, et al. Low molecular weight heparin (reviparin) in percutaneous transluminal coronary angioplasty. Results of a randomized, double-blind, unfractionated heparin and placebo-controlled, multicenter trial (REDUCE trial). Reduction of Restenosis after PTCA, Early Administration of Reviparin in a Double-Blind Unfractionated Heparin and Placebo-Controlled Evaluation. J Am Coll Cardiol 1996;28:1437–1443.
88. Ferguson J. NICE 3 Preliminary Results. Theheart.org cybersession. Available from: URL: http://dev.cybersessions.com/conference/06nov01/. Website accessed 5/16/2002.
89. Kereiakes DJ, Kleiman NS, Fry E, et al. Dalteparin in combination with abciximab during percutaneous coronary intervention. Am Heart J 2001;141:348–352.
90. Cohen M, Theroux P, Borzak S, et al. Randomized double-blind safety study of enoxaparin versus unfractionated heparin in patients with non-ST-segment elevation acute coronary syndromes treated with tirofiban and aspirin: The ACUTE II study. Am Heart J 2002;144:470–477.
91. Detournay B, Huet X, Fagnani F, et al. Economic evaluation of enoxaparin sodium versus heparin in unstable angina. A French sub-study of the ESSENCE trial. Pharmacoeconomics 2000;18:83–89.

92. Goodman S. Integrilin and Enoxaparin Randomized assessment of Acute Coronary Syndromes Treatment (INTERACT). Late breaking session, American College of Cardiology, 2002.
93. Cohen M, Maritz F, Gensini GF, et al. The TETAMI trial: the safety and efficacy of subcutaneous enoxaparin versus intravenous unfractionated heparin and of tirofiban versus placebo in the treatment of acute myocardial infarction for patients not thrombolyzed: methods and design. J Thromb Thrombolysis 2000;10:241–246.
94. Antman EM. Hirudin in acute myocardial infarction. Safety report from the Thrombolysis and Thrombin Inhibition in Myocardial Infarction (TIMI) 9A trial. Circulation 1994;90:1624–1630.
95. Antman EM. Hirudin in acute myocardial infarction. Thrombolysis and Thrombin Inhibition in Myocardial Infarction (TIMI) 9B trial. Circulation 1996;94:911–921.
96. Yusuf S. Design, baseline characteristics, and preliminary clinical results of the Organization to Assess Strategies for Ischemic Syndromes-2 (OASIS- 2) trial. Am J Cardiol 1999;84:20M–25M.
97. White H. Thrombin-specific anticoagulation with bivalirudin versus heparin in patients receiving fibrinolytic therapy for acute myocardial infarction: the HERO-2 randomised trial. Lancet 2001;358:1855–1863.
98. Vermeer F, Vahanian A, Fels PW, et al. Argatroban and alteplase in patients with acute myocardial infarction: the ARGAMI Study. J Thromb Thrombolysis 2000;10:233–240.
99. Serruys PW, Herrman JP, Simon R, et al. A comparison of hirudin with heparin in the prevention of restenosis after coronary angioplasty. Helvetica investigators. N Engl J Med 1995;333:757–763.
100. Bittl JA, Chaitman BR, Feit F, et al. Bivalirudin versus heparin during coronary angioplasty for unstable or postinfarction angina: final report reanalysis of the Bivalirudin Angioplasty Study. Am Heart J 2001; 142:952–959.
101. Direct thrombin inhibitors in acute coronary syndromes: principal results of a meta-analysis based on individual patients' data. Lancet 2002;359:294–302.
102. Lincoff AM, Kleiman N, Kottke-Marchant K, et al. Bivalirudin with planned or provisional abciximab versus low-dose heparin and abciximab during percutaneous coronary revascularization: results of the Comparison of Abciximab Complications with Hirulog for Ischemic Events Trial (CACHET). Am Heart J 2002;143:847–853.
103. Kleiman NS, Klem J, Fernandes LS, et al. Pharmacodynamic profile of the direct thrombin antagonist bivalirudin given in combination with the glycoprotein IIb/IIIa antagonist eptifibatide. Am Heart J 2002; 143:585–593.
104. Lincoff AM, Bittl JA, Kleiman N, et al. The REPLACE 1 Trial: a pilot study of bivalirudin versus heparin during percutaneous coronary intervention with stenting and GP IIb/IIIa blockade. J Am Coll Cardiol 2002;39(Suppl A):1053–1053 (abstract).
105. Bode W, Turk D, Karshikov A. The refined 1.9-angstrom X-ray crystal structure of D-Phe-Pro-Arg chloromethylketone-inhibited human alpha-thrombin: structure analysis, overall structure, electrostatic properties, detailed active-site geometry, and structure-function relationships. Protein Sci 1992; 1:426–471.

17   Oral Agents

L. Kristin Newby, MD

CONTENTS

INTRODUCTION
THE ORAL GLYCOPROTEIN IIb/IIIa INHIBITORS
THE ORAL AGENTS IN PHASE II STUDIES
THE ORAL AGENTS IN PHASE III TRIALS
SYSTEMATIC OVERVIEWS OF PHASE III TRIALS
THE FAILURE OF THE ORAL AGENTS: WHAT WENT WRONG?
REFERENCES

INTRODUCTION

As discussed in previous chapters, platelets play a central role in the pathogenesis of thrombosis and acute coronary events. Thus, antiplatelet therapy is a cornerstone of treatment for patients with atherosclerotic coronary artery disease. Despite the effectiveness of intravenous inhibitors of the platelet glycoprotein (GP) IIb/IIIa receptor in patients with acute coronary syndromes or undergoing percutaneous coronary intervention (PCI), little additional benefit is realized beyond the termination of therapy, and 30-d death or myocardial infarction rates remain in the 7–13% range *(1,2)*.

Aspirin, a weak inhibitor of platelet activation and aggregation via inhibition of the cyclooxygenase-1 enzyme and thromboxane A_2 production, is effective for long-term secondary prevention of vascular events *(3,4)*. However, many patients have ischemic coronary events while taking aspirin, suggesting resistance to its antiplatelet effects, and outcomes among these patients are worse than for patients not taking aspirin when they have an event *(5)*. Furthermore, in vitro studies have demonstrated that as many as 9.5% of patients have platelets that are resistant to the antiaggregatory effects of aspirin *(6)*. As shown in Fig. 1, in a small study of stroke patients who were defined as "nonresponders" to aspirin, based on in vitro platelet function assessment, the rate of death, myocardial infarction, or recurrent stroke at 2 yr was 40% compared with 5% among "responders" *(7)*. For these reasons, more potent, long-term inhibition of the final common pathway to platelet aggregation with orally administered GPIIb/IIIa receptor inhibitors similar to the successful intravenous compounds appeared attractive.

From: *Contemporary Cardiology: Platelet Glycoprotein IIb/IIIa
Inhibitors in Cardiovascular Disease, 2nd Edition*
Edited by: A. M. Lincoff © Humana Press Inc., Totowa, NJ

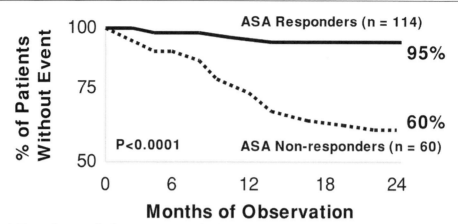

Fig. 1. Event-free survival among "responders" and "nonresponders" to the antiplatelet effects of aspirin. (Adapted from ref. 7.)

Unfortunately, despite more potent antiplatelet effect than aspirin, none of the oral agents that have been tested have succeeded in improving outcomes in cardiovascular disease secondary prevention. In fact, each agent tested in Phase III trials has resulted in increased mortality relative to aspirin-treated patients that in aggregate is statistically significant. This chapter discusses the oral class of GPIIb/IIIa inhibitors and the unexpected results of the large-scale trials designed to evaluate their effect in secondary prevention.

THE ORAL GLYCOPROTEIN IIb/IIIa INHIBITORS

Shown in Table 1 are the intrinsic pharmacokinetic and pharmacodynamic properties of the oral GPIIb/IIIa inhibitors that have been tested in Phase II and III studies *(8–11)*. All are synthetic, small-molecule inhibitors that competitively and reversibly bind the platelet GPIIb/IIIa receptor via an RGD binding sequence mimicking that of fibrinogen. Sibrafiban, lefradafiban, Klerval, and roxifiban were selective for $\alpha_{IIb}\beta_3$, whereas xemilofiban, lotrafiban, and orbofiban also could bind $\alpha_v\beta_3$. Xemilofiban, orbofiban, sibrafiban, Klerval, and lefradafiban were considered first-generation agents, characterized by shorter half-lives and twice-daily to three times a day dosing, weaker receptor binding, and more rapid dissociation from the receptor than roxifiban, a newer agent considered the prototypical second-generation compound. Although lotrafiban had a short half-life and high peak/trough ratio similar to other first-generation agents, its affinity for the $\alpha_{IIb}\beta_3$ receptor (K_d = 2.5 nM) approached that for roxifiban (K_d = 1–2 nM). All first-generation agents except Klerval were exclusively renally eliminated. Lotrafiban and Klerval were both active in the orally administered form, which for Klerval was the same as the available intravenous form, allowing consideration of intravenous to oral treatment transition.

Of these agents, xemilofiban, orbofiban, sibrafiban, lotrafiban, and roxifiban were tested in large-scale Phase III effectiveness trials. Klerval was not taken to Phase III testing, partly because of the expense of preparing the compound, the low bioavailability, and the necessity for multiple daily dosing. Lefradafiban was successfully tested in Phase II trials and provided some potentially interesting insights into mechanisms of the oral agents, but it was not taken into Phase III testing after the failures of orbofiban, xemilofiban, and sibrafiban in four large-scale Phase III trials. Phase III trials of lotrafiban in coronary and

Table 1
Overview of Oral Glycoprotein IIb/IIIa Inhibitors

Drug	Oral form	Bioavailability (%)	Receptor affinity (nM)	Half-life (h)	Dosing	Peak/ trough ratio	Excretion	Phase II studies	Phase III studies
Xemilofiban	Prodrug	13	20.7	4–6	tid	4.5	Renal	ORBIT	EXCITE
Orbofiban	Prodrug	9	52	16–18	bid	2.7	Renal	SOAR	OPUS- TIMI 16
Sibrafiban	Prodrug	38	20	11–12	bid	2.0	Renal	TIMI 12	SYMPHONY 2nd SYMPHONY
Lefradafiban	Prodrug	25	35	11–13	bid	2.0-2.4	Renal	FROST	NA
Klerval	Active drug	2.3	16 106	4–5	tid	1.4-2.7	Renal/ nonrenal	TIMI 15 A/B	NA
Lotrafiban	Active drug	NA	2.5	6–8	bid	NA	Renal	APLAUD	BRAVO
Roxifiban	Prodrug	21	1-2	5 d	qd	1.8	Nonrenal	ROCKET	PURPOSE

cerebrovascular disease and roxifiban in peripheral vascular disease were stopped early after the unfavorable results of the trials of orbofiban, xemilofiban, and sibrafiban, and Phase III testing of roxifiban for coronary disease secondary prevention was not initiated.

THE ORAL AGENTS IN PHASE II STUDIES

Seven oral GPIIb/IIIa receptor inhibitors have been evaluated in Phase II studies (Table 2) *(12–18)*. The primary concern of these studies was further investigation of the pharmacokinetics, pharmacodynamics, and safety of these agents in patients with cardiovascular disease, as well as dose finding for Phase III investigation. The largest of these studies enrolled only 614 patients.

As expected, for each agent there was dose-dependent inhibition of platelet aggregation, and each study established dose ranges associated with acceptable safety and tolerability as measured primarily by bleeding, which was also increased in a dose-dependent fashion. Of importance, the Thrombolysis In Myocardial Infarction (TIMI) 12 investigators noted an association among dose, renal function, and bleeding, which led to renal function-based dosing in Phase III investigation *(14)*. No concerns regarding thrombocytopenia were raised in Phase II investigations, but, unlike other agents, lefradafiban administration was associated with an increased incidence of neutropenia, 5.2% overall compared with 1.5% in the placebo group *(15)*.

Phase II studies of the oral agents were not powered to study the effect of these drugs on efficacy endpoints. However, no concerns were raised of increased ischemic events in any of the Phase II studies. In fact, several studies suggested trends toward reductions in efficacy composites that were driven largely by reductions in measures of recurrent ischemia *(12,15,18)*. Deaths were few, and there was no pattern with respect to treatment. Of interest, after the failed Phase III trials of xemilofiban, orbofiban, and sibrafiban, the Fibrinogen Receptor Occupancy Study (FROST) investigators noted that at minimum fibrinogen receptor occupancy levels <50%, there was a tendency toward increased thrombotic events in patients treated with lefradafiban compared with aspirin control group patients *(15)*. Rates of the composite of death, myocardial infarction (MI), or recurrent angina were lowest when minimum fibrinogen receptor occupancy levels were >70%. Furthermore, the FROST investigators noted a trend toward benefit on their efficacy composite among patients who were troponin-positive at presentation *(15)*, a finding similar to the enhanced benefit shown for the intravenous agents lamifiban and tirofiban among troponin-positive patients *(19,20)*. However, with the mounting evidence of harm associated with similar agents in Phase III testing and concerns about neutropenia, these interesting observations were never tested in further studies.

THE ORAL AGENTS IN PHASE III TRIALS

Based on favorable safety and tolerability profiles in Phase II testing, five agents were tested further in large-scale Phase III clinical outcomes trials: xemilofiban, orbofiban, sibrafiban, lotrafiban, and roxifiban.

Study Design

The key features of five Phase III trials of four oral GPIIb/IIIa inhibitors (xemilofiban, orbofiban, sibrafiban, and lotrafiban) are reviewed in Table 3 *(21–26)*. In these studies, the agents were tested in four clinical indications: PCI, Evaluation of Xemilofiban in

Table 2
Phase II Studies of Oral Agents

Study	Sample size	Agent studied	Population	Treatment duration	Major findings
ORBIT	549	Xemilofiban	PCI	4 wk	Dose-dependent platelet inhibition; trend toward reduction in composite cardiovascular endpoint
SOAR	279	Orbofiban	Post-ACS	Up to 3 mo	Dose-dependent platelet inhibition
TIMI-12	329	Sibrafiban	Post-ACS	28 d	Dose-dependent platelet inhibition; relationship among plasma concentration, renal function, and bleeding; high incidence of minor bleeding
TIMI 15A/B	89 (A)	Klerval	ACS	1 mo	Dose-dependent platelet inhibition; iv to oral transition feasible
FROST	531	Lefradafiban	ACS/Post-ACS	1 mo	Dose-dependent platelet inhibition; excess bleeding at highest dose; leukopenia/neutropenia with all doses; benefit on composite endpoint in troponin-positive patients; increased thrombotic events at fibrinogen receptor occupancy <50%
APLAUD	444	Lotrafiban	Post-ACS/CVA/TIA	12 wk	Dose-dependent platelet inhibition; high incidence of minor bleeding (highest dose arm stopped owing to bleeding)
ROCKET	614	Roxifiban	High-risk stable CAD	6 mo	Major bleeding and thrombocytopenia within acceptable limits at each of two doses; trend toward benefit on a composite clinical endpoint

Abbreviations: ACS, acute coronary syndrome; CAD, coronary artery disease; CVA, cerebrovascular accident; PCI, percutaneous coronary intervention; TIA, transient ischemic attack.

Controlling Thrombotic Events, (EXCITE); postacute coronary syndromes, Orbofiban in Patients with Unstable Coronary Syndromes (OPUS-TIMI 16), Sibrafiban Versus Aspirin to Yield Maximum Protection from Ischemic Heart Events Post Acute Coronary Syndromes (SYMPHONY), and 2nd SYMPHONY; and secondary prevention, Blockade of the Receptor Against Vascular Occlusion (BRAVO). A sixth Phase III trial called PURPOSE (Peripheral Arterial Disease Utilization of Roxifiban to Prevent Outcomes of Ischemic Events) was initiated to study the effects of roxifiban in noncoronary vascular disease—specifically, patients with peripheral arterial disease. This study was stopped early, but details of the study design and outcomes have not been published to date.

From data in Phase II studies, moderate levels of platelet aggregation inhibition in 20 μM ADP were targeted, ranging from a minimum of at least 25% inhibition with low-dose sibrafiban to as high as 55–80% with the 50-mg twice-daily regimen of orbofiban in OPUS-TIMI 16 and 60–90% with the 20-mg three times a day regimen in EXCITE. Systematic measurement of platelet aggregation inhibition was not performed in Phase III, and only SYMPHONY measured plasma concentrations of study drug. In that study >90% of patients were within the target concentration range using dosing based on weight and serum creatinine *(23,24)*.

EXCITE

The EXCITE trial was the only Phase III study of the oral GPIIb/IIIa inhibitors specifically for patients undergoing PCI *(21)*. A total of 7232 patients undergoing elective PCI were randomized in the EXCITE trial to one of two dose regimens of xemilofiban or aspirin. Patients randomized to the xemilofiban arms received 20 mg of oral xemilofiban 30–90 min prior to the interventional procedure and then either 10 mg three times a day or 20 mg three times a day for 6 mo. All patients in the xemilofiban arms received background aspirin therapy, and use of ticlopidine (250 mg twice-daily) was allowed for patients receiving a coronary stent during the interventional procedure. The primary endpoint was a composite of death, myocardial infarction, or revascularization at 6 mo.

OPUS-TIMI 16

OPUS-TIMI 16 randomized 10,302 patients within 72-h of presentation with an acute coronary syndrome to either aspirin or one of two dose regimens of orbofiban with background aspirin therapy *(22)*. Patients did not have to be stabilized from their acute presentation prior to randomization. Patients in both orbofiban treatment arms received orbofiban 50 mg twice daily for 30 d. Patients randomized to the 50/50 arm then received 50 mg twice daily for the remainder of the study treatment period (planned 1 yr), and those randomized to the 50/30 arm received 30 mg twice daily for the remainder of the treatment period. No dose adjustments were made for renal function. Although planned for 1-yr follow-up, the study was terminated early at 10 mo. The primary endpoint was a composite of death, MI, ischemia leading to urgent revascularization, ischemia leading to rehospitalization, or stroke and was reported at both 30 d and 10 mo.

SYMPHONY AND 2ND SYMPHONY

SYMPHONY and 2nd SYMPHONY were part of a development plan designed to test the hypothesis that the more potent long-term platelet aggregation inhibition with an oral inhibitor of the GPIIb/IIIa receptor would be more effective and better tolerated in secondary prevention than long-term treatment with aspirin *(23–25)*. As a proof of concept, the SYMPHONY trial randomized 9233 high-risk acute coronary syndrome patients between

Table 3
Phase III trials of Oral Glycoprotein IIb/IIIa Inhibitors

	Randomized (no.)	Efficacy analysis (no.)	Agent[a]	Indication	Enrollment	Target effect[b] (%)	Treatment duration	Primary endpoint
EXCITE	7232	7232	Xemilofiban 10 mg tid 20 mg tid	Elective percutaneous coronary intervention	30–90 min before percutaneous coronary intervention	40–70 60–90	6 mo	Death, myocardial infarction, revascularization
OPUS-TIMI 16	10,302	10,288	Orbofiban 50/30 50/50	Post-acute coronary syndrome	Within 72 h	45–65 55–80	Planned 1 yr	Death, myocardial infarction, urgent revascularization, rehospitalization, stroke
SYMPHONY	9233	9169	Sibrafiban Low dose High dose	Post-acute coronary syndrome	12 h to 7 d	≥25 ≥50	90 d	Death, myocardial infarction, severe recurrent ischemia
2nd SYMPHONY	6671	6637	Sibrafiban Low dose High dose	Post-acute coronary syndrome	12 h to 7 d	≥25 ≥50	Planned 12–18 mo	Death, myocardial infarction, severe recurrent ischemia
BRAVO[c]	9198	NA	Lotrafiban	Secondary prevention	>14 d (myocardial infarction) >30 d (stroke)	60–70	Event driven; ≥6 mo	Death, myocardial infarction, stroke, recurrent ischemia, urgent revascularization
PURPOSE	NA	NA	Roxifiban	Peripheral vascular disease	NA	NA	NA	NA

[a] Background aspirin in all studies except SYMPHONY; only in low-dose arm of 2nd SYMPHONY.
[b] Platelet aggregation inhibition, 20 μM ADP.
[c] Study terminated early by Data and Safety Monitoring Committee.
(Adapted from ref. 41.)

12 h and 7 d after presentation with either ST-segment elevation or non-ST-segment elevation MI or unstable angina with documented ST-segment depression to either aspirin 80 mg twice daily or one of two dose regimens of sibrafiban (low- or high-dose) twice daily without background aspirin therapy for 90 d *(23,24)*.

A unique feature of the SYMPHONY trial was the requirement that patients be stable without ongoing ischemia or hemodynamic instability and with Killip class <2 for at least 12 h prior to randomization. Furthermore, SYMPHONY was the first of the oral GPIIb/IIIa inhibitor trials to assign treatment on the basis of estimated renal function. Patients randomized in the low-dose arm received either 3, 4.5, or 6 mg of sibrafiban twice daily based on weight and serum creatinine to achieve a target plasma concentration that would yield at least 25% steady-state platelet aggregation inhibition with 20 µM ADP stimulation. Similarly, patients in the high-dose arm received one of these same dose regimens, but weight and serum creatinine were used to achieve at least 50% platelet aggregation inhibition based on Phase II work. The primary endpoint of SYMPHONY was the 90-d incidence of a composite of death, MI, or severe recurrent ischemia leading to unplanned or unscheduled revascularization.

2nd SYMPHONY was designed to assess the effects of sibrafiban compared with aspirin at longer treatment duration (12–18 mo) and also to allow an assessment of sibrafiban with background aspirin vs aspirin alone and high-dose sibrafiban alone *(25)*. Planned enrollment was 8400 patients randomly assigned one of three arms: aspirin 80 mg twice daily, aspirin 80 mg twice daily plus low-dose sibrafiban twice daily based on weight and renal function, or high-dose sibrafiban twice daily based on weight and renal function. After the results of SYMPHONY were known, 2nd SYMPHONY was terminated early after enrolling 6671 patients with moderate- to high-risk ACS, stable for at least 12 h and within 7 d of presentation. Median treatment duration was 90 (36, 139) d, and median duration of follow-up was 95 (65, 158) d. The primary endpoint was the time to a composite of death, MI, or severe recurrent ischemia leading to unplanned or unscheduled revascularization.

BRAVO

The BRAVO trial was unique in testing an oral GPIIb/IIIa inhibitor in a true long-term secondary prevention study *(26)*. Furthermore, patients could be entered after either neurologic (stroke or transient ischemic attack) or cardiac vascular events, or if they had documented multibed vascular disease (peripheral vascular disease with at least one of either cerebrovascular disease or coronary artery disease). Patients had to have been stable for at least 14 d after an ACS or 30 d after a stroke or transient ischemic attack. Prior to early termination, a total of 9198 patients were randomized to either aspirin or lotrafiban [30 or 50 mg based on renal function *(27)* twice daily for a planned treatment duration of at least 6 mo in all patients. The primary endpoint was the time to a composite of death, MI, stroke, recurrent ischemia, or urgent revascularization.

Results

The primary efficacy and bleeding results of the published Phase III trials of oral GPIIb/IIIa inhibitors are summarized in Figs. 2 and 3, respectively *(21,22,24,25)*. Overall, no trial revealed a benefit of the oral GPIIb/IIIa inhibitor compared with aspirin on its primary composite endpoint. However, in each trial bleeding was increased in a dose-dependent fashion among patients treated with the GPIIb/IIIa inhibitor, suggesting that an increased antiplatelet effect was achieved. A brief summary of key results of individual studies follows.

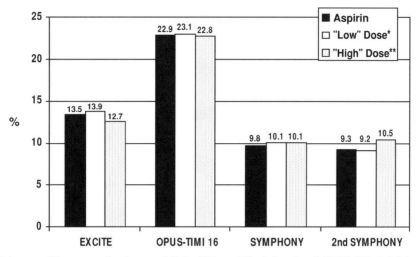

Fig. 2. Primary efficacy results from published Phase III trials of oral GPIIb/IIIa inhibitor trials. *, Low-dose refers to the arm containing the lower of the two doses of oral agent, as outlined in Table 3. **, High-dose refers to the arm containing the higher dose of the oral agent. Primary composite endpoints for each trial are listed in Table 3.

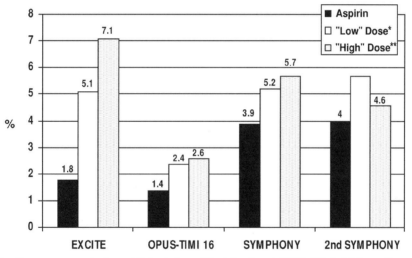

Fig. 3. Bleeding outcomes in the published phase III trials of oral GPIIb/IIIa inhibitors. For asterisks, *see* Fig. 2 legend.

EXCITE

In EXCITE, there were no significant differences between treatment groups in the 6-mo primary death, MI, or urgent revascularization composite endpoint *(21)*. However, the patterns of the component outcomes shown in Fig. 4 were interesting. Although the overall event rate was low, among patients treated with xemilofiban 10 mg, mortality was significantly increased at 6 mo compared with aspirin-treated patients (1.7% vs 1.0%, *p* = 0.04) but was not increased among patients treated with xemilofiban 20 mg (1.1% vs 1.0%, *p* = 0.68) *(21)*. Similar to trials of intravenous GPIIb/IIIa inhibitors used for PCI, there was a significant reduction in MI within 24 h post-PCI in both xemilofiban-treated groups

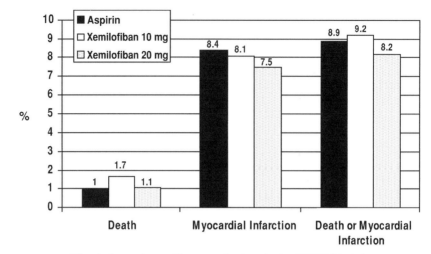

Fig. 4. Secondary efficacy endpoints in the EXCITE trial.

compared with aspirin (Fig. 5) *(21)*. However, at 6 mo, the MI rates were similar between the groups (aspirin, 8.4%; xemilofiban 10 mg, 8.1%; and xemilofiban 20 mg, 7.5%), suggesting that the rates of MI in the xemilofiban groups during longer term treatment were higher than in the aspirin group.

The EXCITE results raised questions about the administration of an oral agent with a time to peak antiaggregatory effect of 4 h only 60–90 min prior to PCI. However, the reduction in MI in the immediate postprocedure period suggests that even for the low-dose arm this cannot be the full explanation for the failure to realize a treatment benefit from long-term administration of xemilofiban. The short half-life of xemilofiban and need for frequent multiple doses coupled with a high peak/trough ratio may, however, have left receptors unoccupied and vulnerable to fibrinogen binding, particularly at the end of a dosing interval or in situations of missed doses. Subsequent studies have also suggested that xemilofiban has intrinsic activating properties that could be either proinflammatory, prothrombotic, or both *(28–33)*. These findings are not consistently reproducible, however, and a recent study has suggested that even though xemilofiban does possess receptor activating properties, under conditions more closely approximating physiologic, increased platelet aggregation does not result *(34)*.

OPUS-TIMI 16

As in EXCITE, within the overall neutral result on the primary endpoint was a finding of increased mortality, both at 30 d and at 10 mo *(22)*. In fact, the excess mortality observed in the 50/30 arm (which was statistically significant) resulted in early termination of enrollment in OPUS-TIMI 16 and ultimately early termination of the treatment and follow-up for all enrolled patients. Final data revealed significantly higher mortality in both orbofiban-treated groups compared with aspirin-only patients (orbofiban 50/30, 5.1%; orbofiban 50/50, 4.5%; aspirin alone, 3.7%) (Fig. 6). A blinded cause-of-death analysis identified an excess of death classified as owing to new thrombotic events among both orbofiban groups compared with the aspirin-only group. Although the data were not statistically significant, MI alone and death or MI rates were also higher among orbofiban-treated patients (Fig. 6).

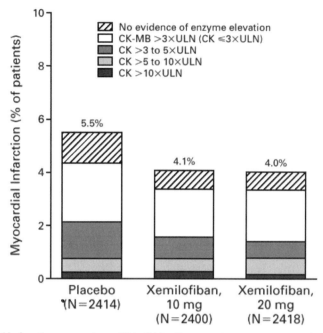

Fig. 5. Myocardial infarction occurring within 24 h after percutaneous coronary intervention by randomized treatment assignment in the EXCITE trial. (From ref. *21*, with permission.)

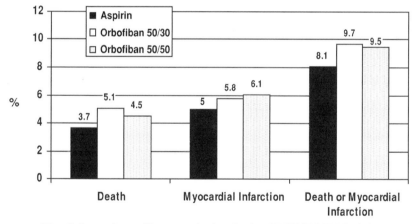

Fig. 6. Secondary efficacy endpoints in the OPUS-TIMI 16 trial.

A number of subgroup analyses were performed in an attempt to understand the lack of treatment benefit overall and increased mortality observed among orbofiban-treated patients in OPUS-TIMI 16 *(22)*. The only subgroup in which there was an associated treatment benefit for orbofiban was the group of patients who underwent PCI for the index ACS event while on study drug. Patients with particularly adverse effects of treatment included those with creatinine clearance ≤100 mL/min and those who were more unstable at entry, including Killip class ≥II. These findings raised questions about trial design such as not adjusting dose for renal function despite orbofiban's renal elimination. Finally, the need for concomitant antithrombin therapy in conjunction with oral GPIIb/IIIa inhibitor therapy was raised by the observation that patients who received either low-molecular-weight heparin or unfractionated heparin with orbofiban had fewer recurrent ischemic events during the first 2 d of treatment than those who did not. This finding was not observed in the SYMPHONY or 2nd SYMPHONY databases, however (Newby, unpublished data).

As with all first-generation agents, the pharmacokinetic and pharmacodynamic properties of orbofiban may have contributed to the observed results of the OPUS-TIMI 16 trial by potentially leaving activated receptors unoccupied and vulnerable to fibrinogen binding at trough concentrations at the end of dosing intervals. Furthermore, like xemilofiban, orbofiban has also been shown in some studies, but not all, to have partial activating properties that could be prothrombotic and/or proinflammatory and contribute to increased thrombotic events over the course of therapy (28–33,35,36).

Preliminary reports of genotyping for the Pl^{A2} polymorphism of the GPIIIa receptor subunit among a subset of OPUS-TIMI 16 patients suggest that patients carrying the Pl^{A2} allele may be less responsive to treatment, whereas $Pl^{A1/A1}$ homozygotes have lower event rates with orbofiban treatment (Fitzgerald, Leuven Symposium, 2000). Finally, in vitro data in cultured rat cardiomyocytes suggest that orbofiban (and xemilofiban) may have direct toxic effects resulting from binding proteins other than the GPIIb/IIIa receptor, in this case procaspase-3, with resultant activation to caspase-3, leading to induction of apoptosis (37, 38). Such an effect could help to explain the observation of greater increases in mortality than in MI and other ischemic events among patients treated with these agents.

SYMPHONY AND 2ND SYMPHONY

In SYMPHONY, the effect of sibrafiban at low and high dose (without background aspirin therapy) on the 90-d composite endpoint of death, MI, or severe recurrent ischemia was similar to that of aspirin (24). In this study death was only slightly higher in the sibrafiban-treated groups (2.0% for both the low- and high-dose sibrafiban groups) compared with aspirin-treated patients (1.8%). However, there was a nonsignificant, but dose-dependent increase in the MI and the death or MI composite (Fig. 7). Unlike OPUS-TIMI 16, multiple subgroup analyses revealed no subgroups for which there was a statistically significant treatment interaction.

The major criticism of the SYMPHONY trial design before the results of OPUS-TIMI 16 and EXCITE were known was the lack of background aspirin therapy in the sibrafiban treatment arms. Although aspirin is a weak antiplatelet agent, it is possible that its inhibition of platelet activation as well as its antiinflammatory properties could be important even as background therapy with a more potent aggregation inhibitor. Furthermore, even though weak, its antiaggregatory effect during periods of low sibrafiban concentration at the end of dosing intervals or with treatment interruptions could have been important. Ultimately, the results were similar to those for orbofiban and xemilofiban administered with aspirin, as would also be shown in 2nd SYMPHONY. Furthermore, the SYMPHONY trial in which background aspirin was not used, in conjunction with 2nd SYMPHONY, supports the notion that no adverse treatment interaction between aspirin and the oral GPIIb/IIIa inhibitors contributed to the unexpected findings of OPUS-TIMI 16 and EXCITE. Fewer data are available regarding proinflammatory or prothrombotic properties of sibrafiban, but no such evidence has been published to date (39).

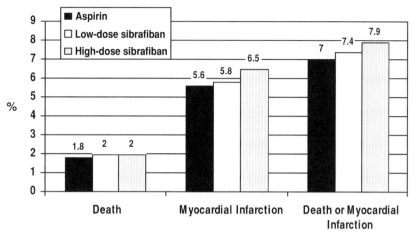

Fig. 7. Secondary efficacy endpoints in the SYMPHONY trial.

Despite the addition of aspirin to the low-dose sibrafiban arm of 2nd SYMPHONY, the results of the study were similar to all previous studies of the oral GPIIb/IIIa inhibitors *(25)*. There was no effect of sibrafiban therapy at low or high dose on the time to or incidence of the primary triple composite endpoint of death, MI, or severe recurrent ischemia. Mortality was increased significantly in the high-dose arm relative to aspirin alone [2.4% vs 1.3%, odds ratio (OR) 1.83 (1.17–2.88)] and nonsignificantly by 31% in the low-dose arm (1.7%) compared with the aspirin arm (1.3%). Blinded cause-of-death review revealed an excess of ischemic event and sudden deaths among high-dose patients. As shown in Fig. 8, MI was similar in the low-dose sibrafiban and aspirin arms but significantly higher in the high-dose sibrafiban arm. The composite of death or MI increased in a dose-dependent fashion, significantly so in the high-dose arm. These results suggest that there was no additive effect of aspirin with sibrafiban across the spectrum of treatment duration in 2nd SYMPHONY.

In 2nd SYMPHONY, there was the opportunity to observe event rates after the withdrawal of study drug at the early termination of the trial *(25)*. No differences in 30-d posttreatment rates of death, MI, or their composite were observed to suggest rebound events at treatment interruption.

BRAVO

After the results of the four previous trials were known, BRAVO continued to enroll patients under the close scrutiny of its Data and Safety Monitoring Committee (DSMC) for any unfavorable effects on mortality or other thrombotic events. After enrolling 9198 patients, the trial was stopped by its DSMC in December of 2000 when an increase in mortality of a magnitude similar to that in the other oral agent trials was observed. At the point of early termination, preliminary data revealed an increase in mortality in the lotrafiban arm (2.7%) relative to placebo (2.0%) that was statistically significant ($p = 0.022$) *(40)*. Similar to previous trials, bleeding was also significantly increased in lotrafiban-treated patients. Although not observed with xemilofiban, orbofiban, or sibrafiban, these preliminary results also suggested that lotrafiban treatment was associated with significantly more thrombocytopenia. Because the adverse effects were not offset by any beneficial effects,

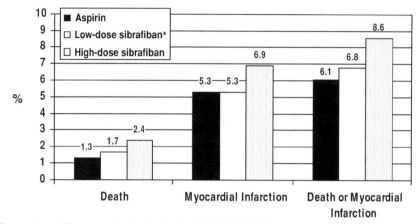

Fig. 8. Secondary efficacy endpoints in the 2nd SYMPHONY trial. *, Low-dose sibrafiban patients received background aspirin therapy.

the DSMC recommended early termination, which followed. In the preliminary report, there were no differences in treatment effect in patients enrolled after an ACS or with stroke or transient ischemic attack. Data collection was completed, and publication of the final results is expected.

The preliminary BRAVO results do help to dispel some of the trial design concerns raised by previous trials. As in the SYMPHONY studies, despite dosing based on renal function and the requirement for stabilization prior to enrollment, there was no overall treatment effect in preliminary analysis, and, similarly, higher mortality was observed in lotrafiban-treated patients as in the GPIIb/IIIa inhibitor-treated groups in the earlier studies. Additional review of the final data may offer further insights into the failure of these agents.

SYSTEMATIC OVERVIEWS OF PHASE III TRIALS

Odds ratios with 95% confidence intervals for mortality for the combined oral GPIIb/IIIa treatment arms compared with aspirin during the primary treatment period in each oral GPIIb/IIIa inhibitor trial are shown in Fig. 9. As previously noted, mortality was low overall. In both OPUS and 2nd SYMPHONY, mortality was significantly increased relative to aspirin control. In EXCITE and SYMPHONY, the point estimates of the odds ratios favored aspirin treatment but were not statistically significant. Pooled, the odds ratio for mortality for patients treated with GPIIb/IIIa inhibitors relative to aspirin control was 1.31 (1.12–1.53), $p = 0.0001$ *(41)*. The pattern of results was not different after stratifying by background aspirin therapy: for GPIIb/IIIa inhibitor alone vs aspirin (SYMPHONY and high-dose arm of 2nd SYMPHONY), the pooled odds ratio for mortality was 1.37 (1.00–1.86), and for GPIIb/IIIa inhibitor plus aspirin vs aspirin it was 1.38 (1.15–1.86) *(41)*. Blinded cause-of-death reviews were performed in both OPUS and 2nd SYMPHONY and suggested that much of this mortality excess may have been accounted for by more ische-mic/thrombotic event deaths in oral GPIIb/IIIa inhibitor-treated patients *(22,25)*.

In another metaanalysis using a uniform 30-d endpoint for analysis, mortality was similarly increased in GPIIb/IIIa inhibitor-treated patients compared with aspirin-treated

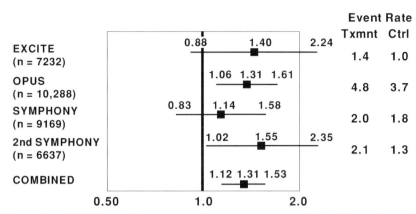

Fig. 9. Odds ratios with 95% confidence intervals for mortality in published Phase III studies of oral GPIIb/IIIa antagonists and for a combined analysis of these results. Event rates (%) are shown for treatment and control arms.

patients *(42)*. Although the association of oral GPIIb/IIIa inhibitor treatment with increased mortality is highly consistent, the relationship of treatment with MI is dependent on timing and what trials are included *(41,42)*. As discussed, MI within the first 24 h after PCI in EXCITE was associated with lower rates of MI in both xemilofiban treatment arms. Driven by inclusion of these endpoint data, a meta-analysis including xemilofiban and assessing at a 30-d time point reveals no increase in MI associated with treatment with the oral agents *(42)*. However, in an analysis limited to the post-ACS trial results and using their longer follow-up periods, a significant increase in MI is observed [OR 1.16 (1.03–1.29)] *(41)*.

The relationship of oral GPIIb/IIIa inhibitor treatment with recurrent ischemia is interesting. When recurrent ischemia is defined by symptoms associated with revascularization, as it was in EXCITE, SYMPHONY, and 2nd SYMPHONY, treatment with an oral GPIIb/IIIa inhibitor appears to have a favorable effect on this endpoint relative to aspirin *(21–23)*. This pattern is also seen in the subset of recurrent ischemia in OPUS that is defined by its association with a revascularization procedure *(22)*. However, when recurrent ischemia is defined by other criteria (including rehospitalization or electrocardiographic changes), a pattern of increased events associated with treatment with these agents relative to aspirin, and similar to that observed for mortality and MI, is observed *(22,24,25)*. The pathophysiologic rationale for this dichotomy of findings is not clear, but these findings tend to argue against simply a direct toxic effect of these agents as the sole explanation and suggest a complexity that goes beyond physiologic constructs. It also highlights the pitfalls of depending on surrogate endpoints alone or as a part of a composite in both Phase II and Phase III clinical trials.

THE FAILURE OF THE ORAL AGENTS: WHAT WENT WRONG?

Despite more potent platelet aggregation inhibition than aspirin, use of the oral GPIIb/IIIa inhibitors in Phase III trials has resulted in unexpected excess mortality relative to aspirin: pooled OR 1.31 (1.12–1.53) *(41)*. Although a number of potential mechanisms have been postulated to explain the failure of the oral GPIIb/IIIa inhibitors, no single explanation is completely satisfactory. Furthermore, the favorable results of the recently completed

Clopidogrel in Unstable Angina to Prevent Recurrent Events (CURE) trial provide evidence that the concept of prolonged antiplatelet therapy at moderate levels of platelet aggregation inhibition in secondary prevention can lead to improved outcomes with acceptable increases in bleeding *(43)*.

Although in retrospect issues were raised with trial design in each of the published Phase III studies, it is unlikely, given the consistency of the findings across studies, that trial design in and of itself can account for the observed results. Furthermore, the rapid development of these compounds and limited Phase II experience have been criticized. Although greater Phase II experience may have allowed more detailed pharmacokinetic and pharmacodynamic assessment of these compounds, at the low event rates observed, even larger Phase II studies of 2000–3000 patients would have been unlikely to detect the increases in events, particularly mortality, that became apparent in the large Phase III trials and in pooled analyses.

Pharmacokinetic and pharmacodynamic characteristics are probably strong contributors and may explain some of the dichotomy between outcomes with oral and intravenous agents. Studies of both the oral and intravenous inhibitors have revealed partial agonist activity and potential prothrombotic and proinflammatory properties of these agents. Such proinflammatory and prothrombotic tendencies of GPIIb/IIIa inhibitors on a background of fluctuating plasma levels, interpatient variability in response, and rapidly reversible receptor inhibition may be particularly problematic in long-term oral administration, for which platelet activation may be more important than aggregation. Clopidogrel and aspirin, which inhibit platelet activation rather than the receptor itself, may avoid these complications. The potential role of genetics and concepts such as apoptosis or unintended targets are less clear, but they warrant further investigation. Particularly in the development of new oral agents, careful scrutiny for each putative mechanism is indicated.

The quest to understand the failure of oral GPIIb/IIIa antagonists will undoubtedly advance our understanding of platelet physiology and the complex pathophysiology of acute and chronic coronary artery disease. To that end, developing an understanding of the causes of their failure provides a tremendous opportunity for advances in the care of patients with coronary artery disease.

REFERENCES

1. Kong DF, Califf RM, Miller DP, et al. Clinical outcomes of therapeutic agents that block the platelet glycoprotein IIb/IIIa integrin in ischemic heart disease. Circulation 1998;98:2829–2835.
2. Chew DP, Moliterno DJ. A critical appraisal of platelet glycoprotein IIb/IIIa inhibition. J Am Coll Cardiol 2000;36:2028–2035.
3. Patrono C. Drug therapy: aspirin as an antiplatelet drug. N Engl J Med 1994;330:1287–1294.
4. Antiplatelet Trialists Collaboration. Collaborative overview of randomised trials of antiplatelet therapy— I: Prevention of death, myocardial infarction, and stroke by prolonged antiplatelet therapy in various categories of patients. BMJ 1994;308:81–106.
5. Alexander JH, Harrington RA, Tuttle RH, et al. Prior aspirin use predicts worse outcomes in patients with non-ST-elevation acute coronary syndromes. Am J Cardiol 1999;83:1147–1151.
6. Gum PA, Kottke-Marchant K, Poggio ED, et al. Profile and prevalence of aspirin resistance among patients with cardiovascular disease. Am J Cardiol 2001;88:230–235.
7. Grotemeyer KH, Scharafinski HW, Husstedt IW. Two-year follow-up of aspirin responder and aspirin non-responders. A pilot-study including 180 post-stroke patients. Thromb Res 1993;71:397–403.
8. Verstraete M. Synthetic inhibitors of platelet glycoprotein IIb/IIIa in clinical development. Circulation 2000;101:76–80.

9. Leebeek FWG, Boersma E, Cannon CP, Van de Werf FJJ, Simoons ML. Oral glycoprotein IIB/IIIA receptor inhibitors in patients with cardiovascular disease: why were the results so unfavourable? Eur Heart J 2002;23:444–457.

10. Scarborough RM, Kleiman NS, Phillips DR. Platelet glycoprotein IIb/IIIa antagonists: what are the relevant issues concerning their pharmacology and clinical use? Circulation 1999;100:437–444.

11. Mousa S, Kapil R, Mu D-X. Intravenous and oral antithrombotic efficacy of the novel platelet GPIIb/IIIa antagonist roxifiban (DMP754) and its free acid form, XV459. Arterioscler Thromb Vasc Biol 1999; 19:2535–2541.

12. Kereiakes DJ, Kleiman NS, Ferguson JJ, et al. Pharmacodynamic efficacy, clinical safety, and outcomes after prolonged platelet glycoprotein IIb/IIIa receptor blockade with oral xemilofiban: results of a multi-center, placebo-controlled, randomized trial. Circulation 1998;98:1268–1278.

13. Ferguson JJ, Deewania PC, Kereiakes DJ, et al. Sustained platelet GP IIb/IIIa blockade with oral orbo-fiban: interim pharmacodynamic results of the SOAR study. J Am Coll Cardiol 1998;31:185A (abstract).

14. Cannon CP, McCabe CH, Borzak, et al. Randomized trial of an oral platelet glycoprotein IIb/IIIa antag-onist, sibrafiban in patients after an acute coronary syndrome: results of the TIMI 12 Trial. Circulation 1998;97:340–349.

15. Akkerhuis KM, Neuhaus KL, Wilcox RG, et al. Safety and preliminary efficacy of one month glycopro-tein IIb/IIIa inhibition with lefradafiban in patients with acute coronary syndromes without ST-elevation. Eur Heart J 2000;21:2042–2055.

16. Harrington RA, Armstrong PW, Graffignino C, et al, for the Anti-PLAtelet Useful Dose (APLAUD) Study Investigators. Dose-finding, safety, and tolerability of an oral platelet glycoprotein IIb/IIIa inhibitor, lotrafiban, in patients with coronary or cerebral atherosclerotic disease. Circulation 2000;102:728–735.

17. Jennings L, Wise K, Ramsey M, et al. Comparison of platelet aggregation response and receptor occu-pancy of RPR 109891 administered intravenously in patients with recent acute recent acute coronary syndromes (TIMI 15A). J Am Coll Cardiol 1998;31:353A (abstract).

18. Langer A, Goodman SG, Reilly TM, et al. Second generation oral IIb/IIIa receptor blockade: phase II experience with roxifiban. J Am Coll Cardiol 2000;35:308A (abstract).

19. Newby LK, Ohman EM, Christenson RH, et al., for the PARAGON B Investigators. Benefit of glyco-protein IIb/IIIa inhibition in patients with acute coronary syndromes and troponin T-positive status: the PARAGON B Troponin T Substudy. Circulation 2001;103:2891–2896.

20. Heeshcen C, Hamm CW, Goldmann B, et al. Troponin concentrations for stratification of patients with acute coronary syndromes in relation to therapeutic efficacy of tirofiban. Lancet 1999;354:1757–1762.

21. O'Neill WW, Serruys P, Knudtson M, et al. Long-term treatment with a platelet glycoprotein-receptor antagonist after percutaneous coronary revascularization. N Engl J Med 2000;342:1316–1324.

22. Cannon CP, McCabe CH, Wilcox RG, et al. Oral glycoprotein IIb/IIIa inhibition with orbofiban in patients with unstable coronary syndromes (OPUS-TIMI 16) trial. Circulation 2000;102:149–156.

23. Newby LK. Long-term oral platelet glycoprotein IIb/IIIa receptor antagonism with sibrafiban after acute coronary syndromes: study design of the SYMPHONY trial. Am Heart J 1999;138:210–218.

24. The SYMPHONY Investigators. Comparison of sibrafiban with aspirin for prevention of cardiovascu-lar events after acute coronary syndromes: a randomised trial. Lancet 2000;355:337–345.

25. The 2nd SYMPHONY Investigators. Randomized trial of aspirin, sibrafiban, or both for secondary pre-vention after acute coronary syndromes. Circulation 2001;103:1727–1733.

26. Topol EJ, Easton JD, Amarenco P, et al. Design of the Blockade of the glycoprotein IIb/IIIa Receptor to Avoid Vascular Occlusion (BRAVO) trial. Am Heart J 2000;139:927–933.

27. Mould D, Chapelsky M, Aluri J, Swagzdis J, Samuels R, Granett J. A population pharmacokinetic-phar-macodynamic and logistic regression analysis of lotrafiban in patients. Clin Pharmacol Ther 2001;69: 210–222.

28. Cox D, Smith R, Quinn M, Theroux P, Crean P, Fitzgerald DJ. Evidence of platelet activation during treatment with a GPIIb/IIIa antagonist in patients presenting with acute coronary syndromes. J Am Coll Cardiol 2000;36:1514–1519.

29. Quinn MJ, Cox D, Foley JB, Fitzgerald DJ. Glycoprotein IIb/IIIa receptor number and occupancy dur-ing chronic administration of an oral antagonist. JPET 2000;295:670–676.

30. Quinn M, Deering A, Stewart M, Cox D, Foley B, Fitzgerald D. Quantifying GPIIb/IIIa receptor binding using 2 monoclonal antibodies: discriminating abciximab and small molecular weight antagonists. Circulation 1999;99:2231–2238.

31. Schneider DJ, Taatjes DJ, Sobel BE. Paradoxical inhibition of fibrinogen binding and potentiation of α-granule release by specific types of inhibitors of glycoprotein IIb-IIIa. Cardiovasc Res 2000;45:437–446.

32. Jennings LK, White MM. Expression of ligand-induced binding sites on glycoprotein IIb/IIIa complexes and the effect of various inhibitors. Am Heart J 1998;135:S179–S183.
33. Jennings LK, White MM, Mandrell TD. Interspecies comparison of platelet aggregation, LIBS expression and clot retraction: observed differences in GPIIb/IIIa functional activity. Thromb Haemost 1995; 74:1551–1556.
34. Frelinger AL, Furman MI, Krueger LA, Barnard MR, Michelson AD. Dissociation of glycoprotein IIb/ IIIa antagonists from platelets does not result in fibrinogen binding or platelet aggregation. Circulation 2001;104:1374–1379.
35. Holmes MB, Sobel BE, Cannon CP, et al. Increased platelet reactivity in patients given orbofiban after an acute coronary syndrome: an OPUS-TIMI 16 substudy. Am J Cardiol 2000;85:491–493.
36. Serrano CV, Venturinelli M, Ramires JAF, Cannon CP, Nicolau JC. Role of oral blockade of platelet glycoprotein IIb/IIIa on neutrophil-platelet interactions in patients with acute coronary syndromes. J Am Coll Cardiol 2000;35:343A (abstract).
37. Adderly SR, Fitzgerald DJ. Glycoprotein IIb/IIIa antagonists induce apoptosis in rat cardiomyocytes by caspase-3 activation. J Biol Chem 2000;275:5760–5766.
38. Buckley CD, Pilling D, Henriquez NV, et al. RGD peptides induce apoptosis by direct caspase-3 activation. Nature 1999;397:534–539.
39. Ault KA, Cannon CP, Mitchell J, et al. Platelet activation in patients after an acute coronary syndrome: results from the TIMI-12 trial. J Am Coll Cardiol 1999;33:634–639.
40. Hughes S. BRAVO trial stopped: lotrafiban increases mortality. TheHeart.org.
41. Newby LK, Califf RM, White HD, et al. The failure of orally administered glycoprotein IIb/IIIa inhibitors to prevent recurrent cardiac events. Am J Med 2002;112:647–658.
42. Chew DP, Bhatt DL, Sapp S, Topol EJ. Increased mortality with oral platelet glycoprotein IIb/IIIa antagonists: a meta-analysis of phase III multicenter randomized trials. Circulation 2001;103:201–206.
43. The Clopidogrel in Unstable angina to prevent Recurrent Events Trial Investigators. Effects of clopidogrel in addition to aspirin in patients with acute coronary syndromes without ST-segment elevation. N Engl J Med 2001;345:494–502.

18 Platelet Glycoprotein IIb/IIIa Inhibitors

Effects Beyond the Platelet

Dean J. Kereiakes, MD
and Pascal J. Goldschmidt-Clermont, MD

CONTENTS

INTRODUCTION
DIFFERENTIAL RECEPTOR AFFINITY
DURABILITY AND REDISTRIBUTION
THE PARADIGM SHIFT: DISCONNECTING EARLY AND LATE EVENTS
INFLAMMATION: THE UNIFYING HYPOTHESIS
PREDICTING LATE SURVIVAL
CONCLUSIONS
REFERENCES

INTRODUCTION

Adjunctive blockade of platelet glycoprotein (GP) IIb/IIIa during percutaneous coronary intervention (PCI) or in patients who present with acute coronary syndromes has been effective in reducing platelet-mediated adverse ischemic clinical outcomes *(1–6)*. Although this class of therapeutic agents has been defined by a shared common affinity for the GPIIb/IIIa integrin receptor, the three agents that are currently US Food and Drug Administration (FDA)-approved differ markedly in pharmacodynamic and pharmacokinetic profile as well as receptor affinity. Separate specific and distinct binding sites on the GPIIb/IIIa receptor complex have been delineated for abciximab and the small-molecule GPIIb/IIIa inhibitors (eptifibatide, tirofiban) by means of differential displacement of site-specific monoclonal antibodies, including MAb1 (LYP18) and MAb2 (4F8) *(7)*. Abciximab has been demonstrated to bind a specific complex recognition site, whereas the small-molecule antagonists bind directly to the RGD component on the β_3 subunit of the receptor. Furthermore, abciximab is unique by demonstrating cross-affinity for additional integrin receptors, $\alpha_v\beta_3$ (vitronectin) *(8–10)*, and CD11b/18 (Mac1) *(11,12)*, which are found predominantly on white blood cells, smooth muscle cells, and endothelial cells. These additional integrin receptors modulate multiple functions distinct from platelet aggregation

From: *Contemporary Cardiology: Platelet Glycoprotein IIb/IIIa*
Inhibitors in Cardiovascular Disease, 2nd Edition
Edited by: A. M. Lincoff © Humana Press Inc., Totowa, NJ

and could confer differential clinical benefit for abciximab in addition to its platelet-inhibitory effects. With increasing interest in these "non-platelet-receptor" effects, spawned by observations that platelet inhibition alone may not fully explain the magnitude of clinical benefit attributable to abciximab, particularly with respect to long-term survival *(13,14)*, it is appropriate to review new developments in this field.

DIFFERENTIAL RECEPTOR AFFINITY

Although the single defining characteristic common to this class of therapeutic agents is an affinity for the platelet GPIIb/IIIa receptor, only abciximab demonstrates affinity for the CD11b/18 and $\alpha_v\beta_3$ receptors *(12)*. For example, abciximab binds to an activated confirmation of the CD11b/18 ($\alpha_m\beta_2$) or Mac1 receptor, which is found on granulocytes, monocytes, and natural killer cells *(10,12)*. CD11b/18 undergoes a conformational change in response to white cell stimulation by a variety of agonists including adenosine diphosphate. CD11b/18 contributes to the process of neutrophil adhesion, leukocyte transmigration across endothelium or epithelium, neutrophil aggregation, chemotaxis, and phagocytosis, as well as leukocyte-platelet interactions *(10–15)*. White cell surface expression of CD11b/18 is increased in patients with active coronary heart disease and following PCI *(11,17–20)*. Recent data suggest not only that CD11b/18 is upregulated following PCI but also it appears to be more so following coronary stent deployment than balloon angioplasty alone *(21)*. This observation may reflect the exaggerated proinflammatory stimulus of stenting owing to a greater propensity for atherothrombosis following stent deployment. Furthermore, the response to stent vessel injury includes a localized inflammatory infiltrate predominating in neutrophils (early) and lymphocyte-macrophages (late) *(22,23)*. White cell adhesion to the site of stent deployment or balloon-vessel injury is significantly reduced by abciximab *(10,24)*.

In addition, white cell-platelet interactions contribute to atherogenesis, restenosis, and reperfusion injury. In vitro experiments have shown that both tirofiban and eptifibatide, but not abciximab, may promote leukocyte-platelet aggregation in whole blood *(15)*. Indeed, a significant reduction in circulating monocyte and neutrophil-platelet aggregates has been observed following abciximab administration to patients undergoing PCI *(25)*. Recent data have also suggested the involvement of CD11b/18 in the process of restenosis following PCI *(26)*. Patients react with varying degrees of expression of CD11b/18 following catheter-based interventions, and higher levels of expression appear to augment the risk of restenosis *(17–20)*. In this respect, it is noteworthy that progressively lower rates of binary restenosis following coronary stent deployment have been associated with the prevalence of T-alleles (polymorphism) on the CD18 gene in a gene-dose-dependent manner (genotype CC 38.1%, CT 31.7%, TT 26.0%: $p = 0.004$) *(26)*. Abciximab crossreactivity for binding to the CD11b/18 receptor has been demonstrated for another human monoclonal antibody, CD18, which is in clinical development specifically to limit reperfusion injury and reduce restenosis.

Abciximab (but not tirofiban or eptifibatide) also demonstrates affinity for the $\alpha_v\beta_3$ (vitronectin) receptor, which shares the same β_3 subunit with the GPIIb/IIIa receptor *(8, 10)*. Although approx 80,000 GPIIb/IIIa receptors may be found on the surface of each platelet, $\alpha_v\beta_3$ receptors on the platelet surface usually number ≤500 *(10,12)*. The $\alpha_v\beta_3$ receptor is expressed at high density on osteoclasts and certain tumor cells and in variable density on endothelial and smooth muscle cells as well as monocytes, polymorphonuclear leukocytes, and T-lymphocytes *(8,9,27,28)*. Endothelial cells from different vascular beds may vary in their expression of $\alpha_v\beta_3$, whereas those endothelial cells overlying atherosclerotic plaque or involved in plaque neovascularization show a high degree of $\alpha_v\beta_3$ expression *(27–29)*. Furthermore, vascular smooth muscle cells may dramatically increase $\alpha_v\beta_3$ receptor expression following vascular injury *(9,30)*. $\alpha v\beta 3$ receptors present on smooth muscle cells have been implicated in the process of neointimal hyperplasia that follows vascular injury and that contributes to the process of "restenosis" after PCI.

Animal models have demonstrated that specific blockade of the $\alpha_v\beta_3$ receptor with abciximab, LM609 (a specific monoclonal antibody to $\alpha_v\beta_3$) *(9,30)*, or XT199 (a synthetic small-molecule antagonist of $\alpha_v\beta_3$) *(31)* can limit neointimal hyperplasia and late-vessel lumen loss following balloon angioplasty or stent deployment. This application appears to require protracted high-dose exposure, as yet not employed in humans. In fact, currently available data do not support the presence of a clinically demonstrable antiproliferative effect of abciximab when infused at currently recommended doses for 12–24 h in humans. Although the evaluation of 7E3 for prevention of ischemic complications (EPIC trial) demonstrated a 27% reduction in "clinical restenosis" (target vessel revascularization) in favor of abciximab (vs placebo) following balloon angioplasty *(1)*, other trials have not confirmed an effect of abciximab on restenosis. For example, in the Evaluation of ReoPro And Stenting to Eliminate Restenosis (ERASER) trial, quantitative coronary angiography and intravascular ultrasound measurements were used to assess the antiproliferative effect of abciximab infused for either 12 or 24 h following coronary stent deployment *(32)*. No significant differences in angiographic stenosis or ultrasound volume of neointimal obstruction was demonstrated for either infusion duration (vs placebo).

More recently, the Evaluation of IIb/IIIa Platelet Inhibitor for Stenting (EPISTENT) trial demonstrated an 18% reduction in target vessel revascularization to 6 mo for patients who were administered abciximab bolus and 12-h infusion (vs placebo) following coronary stent deployment *(33)*. This result primarily reflected a 51% reduction ($p = 0.02$ abciximab vs placebo) in target vessel revascularization for the diabetic cohort. This clinical observation was substantiated by reduction in late coronary lumen loss by quantitative coronary angiography in the cohort of diabetics included in the EPISTENT angiographic substudy and raised the possibility that abciximab may preferentially reduce stent-related neointimal hyperplasia in diabetic patients *(33)*. Noteworthy in this respect was the extremely small number of diabetic patients ($n = 19$) included in the previously described ERASER study, which precluded meaningful analysis of this diabetic subgroup *(32)*.

The observation of selective late clinical benefit from abciximab in diabetic patients was again made from the French Abciximab Before Direct Angioplasty and Stenting in Myocardial Infarction Regarding Acute and Long Term Follow-up (ADMIRAL) trial *(34)*. In ADMIRAL, abciximab (vs placebo) was administered to patients undergoing coronary stent deployment for evolving acute myocardial infarction. At 6-mo follow-up, a 61% reduction in target vessel revascularization for diabetics who received abciximab (vs placebo) was observed *(34)*. This clinical benefit was, however, not substantiated by a quantitative reduction in lumen diameter obstruction on late (6-mo) coronary angiography *(35)*. Although isolated GPIIb/IIIa receptor inhibition could be responsible for this benefit by reducing mural thrombus formation and the subsequent release of platelet-derived smooth muscle growth factors, other studies using prolonged GPIIb/IIIa receptor inhibition following PCI have not demonstrated benefit for either clinical or angiographic restenosis *(36)*.

Although few in number, $\alpha_v\beta_3$ receptors on activated platelets have been implicated in platelet adhesion to osteopontin present in atherosclerotic plaque and for platelet-supported thrombin generation *(37)*. "Dual" receptor blockade of the GPIIb/IIIa and $\alpha_v\beta_3$ receptors by abciximab provides greater inhibition of platelet-supported thrombin generation than mono-receptor blockade of either GPIIb/IIIa or $\alpha_v\beta_3$ with specific monoclonal antibodies (10E5 or LM 609, respectively) or their combination *(38)*. This observation may be explained by the fact that abciximab appears to interfere with binding of factor V/Va to the platelet surface and thus with assembly of the platelet prothombinase complex *(39)*.

DURABILITY AND REDISTRIBUTION

The currently available GPIIb/IIIa inhibitors differ remarkedly in pharmacokinetic and pharmacodynamic profiles, as exemplified by the phenomenon of *gradual redistribution* following abciximab administration *(40)*. Recovery in platelet aggregability is gradual and smoothly transitioned after abciximab discontinuation vs rapid following eptifibatide or tirofiban termination *(40,41)*. The durable presence of abciximab far exceeds the usual lifespan of the platelet (7–9 d) such that GPIIb/IIIa receptor occupancy exceeds 30% at 8 d and 10% at 15 d after discontinuing therapy *(41)*. Prolonged receptor occupancy by abciximab in effect "transforms" the platelet into a "drug delivery" system. This phenomenon is not solely explained by low K_d (high-affinity) GPIIb/IIIa receptor binding. For instance, at equilibrium binding, K_d is equal to the product of the free (unbound) drug concentration and the free platelet receptor concentration divided by the concentration of the drug-receptor complex. Thus, to achieve the same level of receptor occupancy, drugs that have a high K_d (low affinity) will have a large, unbound concentration at steady state, whereas drugs with a low K_d (high affinity) are predominantly receptor bound, with little unbound drug present in the plasma *(42)*. Abciximab is a low K_d (high-affinity) agent with a very short plasma half-life and a prolonged duration of action at the platelet target receptor. Eptifibatide and tirofiban are high K_d (low-affinity) agents with a relatively long plasma half-life and a short duration of action on the platelet receptor. The durability of abciximab presence might also be explained, at least in part, by gradual "migration" across receptor types. Thus, abciximab present at 2 wk or more following discontinuation of treatment may have spent variable periods of time attached to white cells (CD11b/18), smooth muscle cells, or endothelial cells ($\alpha_v\beta_3$) as well as platelets.

THE PARADIGM SHIFT:
DISCONNECTING EARLY AND LATE EVENTS

A recent metanalysis of eight placebo randomized trials of abciximab administration during PCI in more than 9000 patients demonstrates a highly significant ($p = 0.003$) approx 30% reduction of late mortality in favor of abciximab (13). Furthermore, divergence in the mortality curves between abciximab vs placebo over time was observed (Fig. 1). In addition, a completed 3-yr follow-up with patients enrolled in the EPIC, EPILOG, and EPISTENT trials has demonstrated a 22% relative and 1.3% absolute reduction in mortality (6.3% placebo, 5.0% abciximab; $p = 0.03$) to 3 yr following abciximab therapy (Fig. 2) *(14)*. Interestingly, the major portion (75%) of this significant reduction in mortality favoring abciximab cannot be explained by a concomitant reduction in early platelet-mediated major adverse cardiac events (MACE), which include death, myocardial

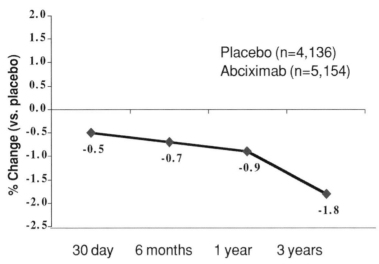

Fig. 1. Percent reduction in mortality (abciximab vs placebo) over time from meta-analysis of eight placebo-controlled randomized trials of abciximab for PCI. (Data abstracted from ref. *13*.)

infarction [defined as creatine kinase (CK) or CK-MB exceeding 3 × upper limit of normal or new Q waves], and the requirement for urgent revascularization (Fig. 3) *(13,43,44)*. Although the focus of therapy with GPIIb/IIIa inhibitors for PCI has been a reduction in these early MACE events, particularly periprocedural myocardial infarction (defined as CK or CK-MB >3 × upper limit of normal), approx 75% of patients who were dead by 3-yr follow-up had no detectable MACE to 48 h postprocedure (Fig. 3) *(44,44a)*. The suppression of periprocedural CPK elevation by platelet GPIIb/IIIa inhibition has been, in theory, linked mechanistically to improvement in late survival. Recent observations that the survival advantage, which has been demonstrated for abciximab and which is directionally consistent across clinical trials, increases progressively over time and is not explained by suppression of periprocedural myocardial necrosis have spawned controversy over potential underlying mechanisms.

INFLAMMATION: THE UNIFYING HYPOTHESIS

Much data exist in support of the contention that PCI, particularly stenting, provokes an inflammatory response owing to both distal atheroembolism and local stent-vessel injury. Inflammatory markers including interleukin-6 (IL-6) and C-reactive protein (CRP) are markedly increased over 48–72 h following coronary stent deployment *(45–47)*. Elevated levels of CRP late (≥72 h) following stent deployment have been correlated with subsequent coronary restenosis and with diminished late cardiac event-free survival *(46, 47)*. Likewise, IL-6 has proved to be a prognostic indicator for the future occurrence of death or myocardial infarction *(48–50)*. Recent data also suggest that physiologic concentrations of CRP may have proinflammatory effects on intercellular adhesion molecule (ICAM), vascular cell adhesion molecule (VCAM) *(51)*, and monocyte chemoattractant protein 1 (MCP1) *(52)* expression. Abciximab has demonstrated a potent and sustained suppressive effect on IL-6 and CRP levels following PCI *(53)*. Interestingly, although a

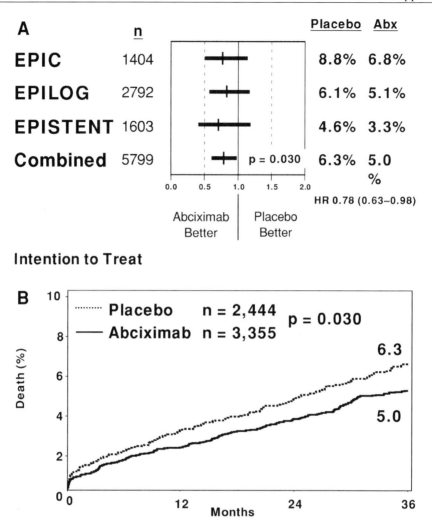

Fig. 2. Pooled analysis of EPIC, EPILOG, and EPISTENT patient cohorts. (**A**) Odds ratio and 95% confidence intervals for mortality to 3 yr by pharmacologic treatment strategy (intention to treat) and by individual trial. Data are 96.2% complete follow-up to 3 yr. (**B**) Kaplan-Meier curves for mortality by pharmacologic treatment regimen (intention to treat). (Reproduced with permission from ref. *44a*.)

reduction in CRP levels accompanied infusion of eptifibatide for coronary stent deployment, a substantial increase in CRP followed termination of the eptifibatide infusion *(54)*. These observations are consistent with an inflammatory response following coronary stent deployment and a sustained antiinflammatory effect of abciximab.

Multiple pathologic and histologic observations have also incriminated an inflammatory process in atherosclerotic plaque instability *(55,56)*. For example, plaques prone to rupture, which cause sudden cardiac death or myocardial infarction and which have ulcerative or thrombotic characteristics, frequently have monocyte-macrophage infiltration of the plaque fibrous cap and diminished smooth muscle content in both the cap and plaque periphery *(55)*. In addition, the degree of plaque inflammation with macrophages and T-lymphocytes has been correlated with the occurrence of symptomatic restenosis in the

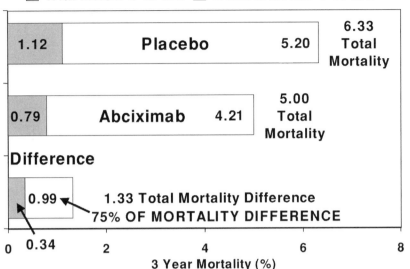

Fig. 3. Mortality to 3 yr by pharmacologic treatment regimen (intention to treat) and MACE status. The greatest proportion of mortality reduction (75%) was observed in patients with no MACE to 48 h post-PCI.

year following directional atherectomy *(57)*. Macrophage infiltration of plaque has also been correlated with restenosis following PCI *(58)*, atherosclerotic disease activity (unstable syndromes) *(56)*, and the presence of diabetes *(59)*.

Clinically, blood levels of monocyte colony-stimulating factor (MCSF) are elevated (in patients) in direct proportion to the severity of coronary disease activity (particularly unstable angina, non-ST-elevation myocardial infarction) *(60,61)*. In vitro incubation of vascular smooth muscle cells (VSMCs) with monocytes in the presence of MCSF results in VSMC death (apoptosis) *(62)*. Interestingly, VSMC killing requires MCSF and can be inhibited by CD18, the human monoclonal antibody to the CD11b/18 receptor. Abciximab (but not eptifibatide or tirofiban) in physiologic concentrations provides a similar degree of VSMC protection/preservation as does CD18 (Fig. 4) *(63)*. These observations suggest that antiinflammatory effects of abciximab, mediated at least in part by its affinity for the CD11b/18 receptor, provide "cytoprotection" for VSMCs that could confer long-term clinical stability.

This proposed mechanism could explain a number of previous observations, including why: (1) periprocedural CPK elevations are poorly correlated with late mortality, (2) both MCSF and macrophage infiltration of plaque correlate with coronary disease activity, and, (3) plaques prone to rupture are depleted in VSMCs. This theory proposes that quiescent myocardial cell death (apoptosis) is mediated by the inflammatory response to PCI, particularly stent deployment. This hypothesis represents a drastic divergence from the traditional concept of myocardial infarction and invokes silent (asymptomatic) late cell death (apoptosis) as the underlying mechanism for late divergence in mortality curves between abciximab and placebo. Indeed, PCI triggers a vicious cycle of molecular reactions, particularly with stent placement: the first step requires the recruitment and activation of platelets (Fig. 5). Local production of platelet agonists by the damaged vessel

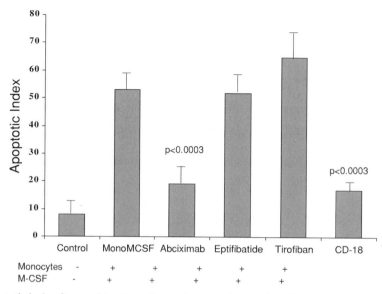

Fig. 4. Apoptotic index for combination of vascular smooth muscle cells, monocytes, and monocyte colony-stimulating factor (mono-MCSF) and with addition of ReoPro (abciximab), eptifibatide, tiro-fiban, or the human monoclonal antibody to CD11b/18, CD18. Both ReoPro and CD18 provide protection (reduction in vascular smooth muscle cell death) in physiologic concentrations.

wall, such as adenosine diphosphate, thrombin, and collagen, contributes to the activation and aggregation of platelets at the stented site.

All parenteral GPIIb/IIIa antagonists (abciximab and small-molecule blockers) have the ability to suppress platelet recruitment and thereby consequent steps of the cycle. Activated platelets display on their surface CD40 ligand (CD154), which in turn stimulates neighboring vascular cells, thus provoking the production of cytokines like IL-1, IL-6, and MCSF and chemokines like MCP-1. MCSF induces the maturation and activation of macrophages recruited by MCP-1 and other proinflammatory chemokines and enables the activated macrophages to kill smooth muscle cells (SMCs), a key step in the process of plaque destabilization. MCSF binding to its receptor on macrophages appears to function as a "final common pathway" in the induction of SMC death by activated macrophages, as many cytokines can induce SMC killing by macrophages, but in a process that requires the production of MCSF by cytokine-stimulated macrophages.

Such killing of SMCs by activated macrophages is a two-step process mediated through activation of programmed cell death within SMCs (apoptosis) and requires a functional CD11b/18 (Mac1), and the death receptor Fas (CD95) on the surface of SMCs. First, CD11b/18 on the surface of activated macrophages establishes a firm contact with its adhesive ligands (ICAM1) on the surface of target SMCs. Second, the Fas death pathway of SMCs is activated by crosslinking of Fas-ligand (CD95-ligand) displayed by macrophages. The loss of SMCs triggers a series of reactions, which in turns disturbs the homeostasis of extracellular matrix proteins, the production of metalloproteinases, growth factors like platelet-derived growth factor (PDGF), and transforming growth factor-β (TGF-β). The migration and proliferation of residual SMCs are then triggered, resulting in substantial remodeling of the vascular wall. Abciximab, with its blocking activity toward CD11b/18 and $\alpha_v\beta_3$, can affect the vicious cycle at two additional strategic points (Fig. 3). Such

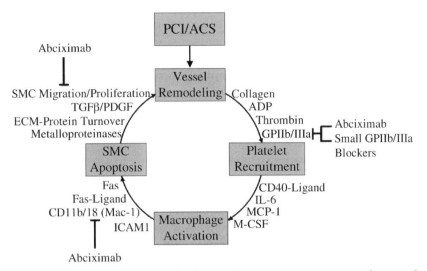

Fig. 5. Cycle of thrombosis and inflammation induced by percutaneous coronary intervention (PCI) and acute coronary syndrome (ACS). Spontaneous or induced (PCI) disruption of coronary plaque triggers a cascade of molecular reactions that culminate with the recruitment of platelets, activation of macrophages, death or smooth muscle cells (SMCs), and remodeling of the vessel wall. Parenteral GPIIb/IIIa blockers (eptifibatide, tirofiban, HCl, and abciximab) suppress the platelet contribution to this cycle. As a consequence of thrombosis and inflammation, cytokines and chemokines are produced [interleukin-1 (IL-1), IL-6, and monocyte chemoattractant protein-1 (MCP-1)]. Monocytes and macrophages secrete macrophage colony stimulating factor (M-CSF), which enables macrophages to bind SMCs, via their CD11b/18 (Mac1) receptor, and to induce apoptosis through the Fas cell death pathway. Abciximab can impact on this cycle at the binding of macrophage Mac1 to adhesive ligands on SMCs [such as intercellular adhesion molecule (ICAM1)] and on the migration of SMCs, which requires the activity of the $\alpha_V\beta_3$ receptor. ECM, extracellular matrix; PDGF, platelet-derived growth factor; TGFβ, transforming growth factor β.

a pleiotropic effect of abciximab on the vicious cycle may explain its superior impact on survival post PCI, compared with small-molecule inhibitors of GPIIb/IIIa.

The non-GPIIb/IIIa receptor-mediated antiinflammatory, cytoprotective effects of abciximab could thus confer late clinical stability.

PREDICTING LATE SURVIVAL

As stated previously, the completed pooled analysis of the EPIC, EPILOG, and EPISTENT trials demonstrated a statistically significant 22% reduction in mortality at 3 yr following PCI in those patients who received abciximab (vs placebo). A multivariate proportional hazards model was developed using a step-down procedure on available baseline clinical characteristics from patients included in this pooled analysis to identify factors associated with increased risk of death to 3-yr follow-up. The minimum *p* value required for retention of individual variables in the model was 0.05. Variables found to be statistically significantly associated with risk of death in late follow-up included age, diabetes mellitus, history of congestive heart failure, history of prior coronary artery bypass grafting, history of smoking (defined as current smoker or quit <1 yr), history of hypertension, history of clinical peripheral vascular disease, creatinine, and history of prior myocardial infarction

Table 1
Multivariate Regression for Variables Associated with Mortality to 3 Years

Variable analyzed	Coefficient	SD	p value
Diabetes mellitus	0.426	0.086	<0.001
Age	0.049	0.004	<0.001
History of congestive heart failure	0.859	0.104	<0.001
Previous coronary artery bypass graft	0.570	0.094	<0.001
Smoker	0.460	0.094	<0.001
History of hypertension	0.246	0.085	0.002
History of peripheral vascular disease	0.290	0.113	0.007
Previous myocardial infarction	0.200	0.082	0.010
Creatinine	0.236	0.080	0.007

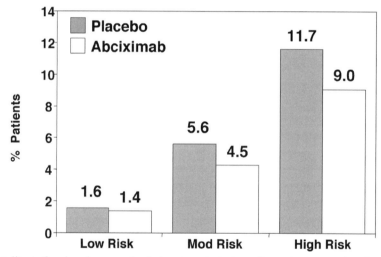

Fig. 6. Mortality to 3 yr by pharmacologic treatment strategy (intention to treat) and tertile of risk profile using multivariate regression model.

(Table 1). Patients were stratified into tertiles of risk using the simple arithmetic sum of coefficients for those clinical variables found to be associated with mortality to 3-yr follow-up. Using simple tertiles, those patients at lowest risk had a coefficient sum of <3.5, those at moderate risk had a sum of 3.5–4.1, and those in the highest risk tertile had sums >4.1. Mortality at 3 yr by risk tertile using this model is depicted in Fig. 6.

No survival advantage is demonstrated for abciximab in the lowest risk tertile. Patients in the moderate risk tertile manifest a 1.1% (absolute) reduction in mortality, and those in the highest risk tertile were observed to have a 2.7% (absolute) reduction in mortality to 3 yr. Again, the lack of correlation between early platelet-mediated MACE ischemic

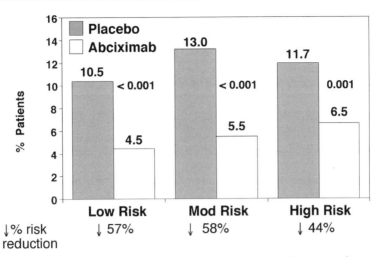

Fig. 7. Composite clinical primary endpoint (death, myocardial infarction, or requirement for urgent coronary revascularization) by pharmacologic treatment regimen (intention to treat) and tertile of risk profile. Patients in the lowest risk tertile manifest the greatest relative reduction in early (30-d) primary endpoint events despite absence of a survival advantage in favor of abciximab, as noted previously (Fig. 5).

outcomes and late survival is illustrated by the relationship between the similar primary composite clinical endpoint for each trial (death, myocardial infarction, and urgent revascularization to 30 d) by randomly allocated pharmacologic treatment regimen and risk tertile (Fig. 7). Those patients in the lowest risk tertile who derived no survival benefit to 3 yr from abciximab administration demonstrated the greatest relative magnitude of reduction (57%) in primary endpoint events, whereas those patients in the highest risk tertile who derived the greatest magnitude of reduction in mortality to 3-yr follow-up had the least magnitude (44%) reduction in the same primary endpoint events at 30 d. This relationship (between early MACE and late survival) again underscores the fact that late survival benefit was not accurately reflected in the magnitude of early primary endpoint reduction.

CONCLUSIONS

Although this class of new therapeutic agents has been simplistically defined by a common affinity for the platelet GPIIb/IIIa receptor, important differences exist between members of this class with respect to pharmacokinetic and pharmacodynamic profiles, specific binding sites on the GPIIb/IIIa receptor, and differential receptor affinities *(40)*. The affinity of abciximab for the $\alpha_v\beta_3$ and CD11b/18 receptors coupled with the phenomenon of pharmacodynamic gradual redistribution may contribute to a profound and sustained antiinflammatory effect of this agent. Late myocardial cell death (apoptosis) engendered by the inflammatory response that follows PCI and that appears to be mediated by MCSF and macrophages may be prevented by the specific affinity of abciximab for the CD11b/18 receptor. These non-GPIIb/IIIa receptor activities of abciximab are distinct from its platelet-inhibitory effects and yet probably contribute to specific and preferential plaque stabilization and enhanced late survival following administration of this agent.

REFERENCES

1. The EPIC investigators. Use of a monoclonal antibody directed against the platelet glycoprotein IIb/IIIa receptor in high risk coronary angioplasty. N Engl J Med 1994;330:956–961.
2. The EPILOG Investigators. Platelet glycoprotein IIb/IIIa receptor blockade and low-dose heparin during percutaneous coronary revascularization. N Engl J Med 1997;336:1689–1696.
3. Lincoff AM, Califf RM, Moliterno DJ, et al., for the Evaluation of Platelet IIb/IIIa Inhibition in Stenting Investigators. Complementary clinical benefits of coronary-artery stenting and blockade of platelet glycoprotein IIb/IIIa receptors. N Engl J Med 1999;341:319–327.
4. RESTORE Investigators. Effects of platelet glycoprotein IIb/IIIa blockade with tirofiban on adverse cardiac events in patients with unstable angina or acute myocardial infarction undergoing coronary angioplasty. Circulation 1997;96:1445–1453.
5. The Platelet Receptor Inhibition in Ischemic Syndrome Management (PRISM) Study Investigators. A comparison of aspirin plus tirofiban with aspirin plus heparin for unstable angina. N Engl J Med 1998; 338:1498–1505.
6. Inhibition of platelet glycoprotein IIb/IIIa with eptifibatide in patients with acute coronary syndromes. The PURSUIT trial investigators. Platelet glycoprotein IIb/IIIa in unstable angina: receptor suppression using integrilin therapy. N Engl J Med 1998;339:436–443.
7. Quinn M, Deering A, Stewart M, Cox D, Foley B, Fitzgerald D. Quantifying GPIIb/IIIa receptor binding using 2 monoclonal antibodies. Circulation 1999;99:2231–2238.
8. Tam SH, Sassoli PM, Jordan RE, Nakada MT. Abciximab (ReoPro, chimeric 7E3 Fab) demonstrates equivalent affinity and functional blockade of glycoprotein IIb/IIIa and alpha(v)beta3 integrins. Circulation 1998;98:1085–1091.
9. Stouffer GA, Hu Z, Sajid M, et al. Beta3 integrins are upregulated after vascular injury and modulate thrombospondin- and thrombin-induced proliferation of cultured smooth muscle cells. Circulation 1998;97: 907–915.
10. Coller BS. Binding of abciximab to $\alpha V\beta 3$ and activated $\alpha M\beta 2$ receptors: with a review of platelet-leukocyte interactions. Thromb Haemost 1999;82:326–335.
11. Mickelson JK, Ali MN, Kleiman NS, et al. Chimeric 7E3 Fab (ReoPro) decreases detectable CD11b on neutrophils from patients undergoing coronary angioplasty. J Am Coll Cardiol 1999;33:97–106.
12. Coller BS. Potential non-glycoprotein IIb/IIIa effects of abciximab. Am Heart J (Suppl) 1999;138:S1–S5.
13. Anderson KM, Califf RM, Stone GW, et al. Long-term mortality benefit with abciximab in patients undergoing percutaneous coronary intervention. J Am Coll Cardiol 2001;37:2059–2065.
14. Quinn MJ, Lincoff, AM, Kereiakes DJ, et al. Long-term mortality benefit of abciximab in percutaneous intervention. Circulation 2001;104:II–387 (abstract).
15. Furman MI, Krueger LA, Frelinger AL, et al. Tirofiban and eptifibatide, but not abciximab, induce leukocyte-platelet aggregation. Circulation 1999;100:I–681 (abstract).
16. Kassirer M, Zeltser D, Prochorov V, et al. Increased expression of the CD11b/CD18 antigen on the surface of peripheral white blood cells in patients with ischemic heart disease: further evidence for smoldering inflammation in patients with atherosclerosis. Am Heart J 1999;138:555–559.
17. Neumann FJ, Ott I, Gawaz M, Puchner G, Schomig A. Neutrophil and platelet activation at balloon-injured coronary artery plaque in patients undergoing angioplasty. J Am Coll Cardiol 1996;27: 819–824.
18. Serrano CV Jr, Ramires JA, Venturinelli M, et al. Coronary angioplasty results in leukocyte and platelet activation with adhesion molecule expression. Evidence of inflammatory responses in coronary angioplasty. J Am Coll Cardiol 1997;29:1276–1283.
19. Inoue T, Sakai Y, Morooka S, Hayashi T, Takayanagi K, Takabatake Y. Expression of polymorphonuclear leukocyte adhesion molecules and its clinical significance in patients treated with percutaneous transluminal coronary angioplasty. J Am Coll Cardiol 1996;28:1127–1133.
20. Inoue T, Sakai Y, Hoshi K, Yaguchi I, Fujito T, Morooka S. Lower expression of neutrophil adhesion molecule indicates less vessel wall injury and might explain lower restenosis rate after cutting balloon angioplasty. Circulation 1998;97:2511–2518.
21. Inoue T, Sohma R, Miyazaki T, Iwasaki Y, Yaguchi I, Morooka S. Comparison of activation process of platelets and neutrophils after coronary stent implantation versus balloon angioplasty for stable angina pectoris. Am J Cardiol 2000;86:1057–1062.
22. Farb A, Sangiorgi G, Carter AJ, et al. Pathology of acute and chronic coronary stenting in humans. Circulation 1999;99:44–52.

23. Grewe PH, Deneke T, Machraoui A, Barmeyer J, Muller KM. Acute and chronic tissue response to coronary stent implantation: pathologic findings in human specimen. J Am Coll Cardiol 2000;35:157–163.
24. Palmerini T, Nedelman MA, Scudder LE, et al. Effects of abciximab on the acute pathology of blood vessels after arterial stenting in non human primates. J Am Coll Cardiol 1999;100:I–857 (abstract).
25. Furman MI, Kereiakes DJ, Krueger LA, et al. Leukocyte-platelet aggregation and platelet P-selectin and GP IIIa expression following percutaneous coronary intervention: effects of dalteparin or unfractionated heparin in combination with abciximab. Am Heart J 2001;142:790–798.
26. Koch W, Bottiger C, Mehilli J, et al. Association of a CD18 gene polymorphism with a reduced risk of restenosis after coronary stenting. Am J Cardiol 2001;88:1120–1124.
27. Byzova TV, Rabbani R, D'Souza SE, Plow EF. Role of integrin alpha(v)beta3 in vascular biology. Thromb Haemost 1998;80:726–734.
28. Hoshiga M, Alpers CE Smith LL, Giachelli CM, Schwartz SM. Alpha-v beta-3 integrin expression in normal and atherosclerotic artery. Circ Res 1995;77:1129–1135.
29. Brooks PC, Clark RA, Cheresh DA. Requirement of vascular integrin alpha v beta 3 for angiogenesis. Science 1994;264:569–571.
30. Srivatsa SS, Fitzpatrick LA, Tsao PW, et al. Selective αVβ3 integrin blockade potently limits neointimal hyperplasia and lumen stenosis following deep coronary arterial stent injury: evidence for the functional importance of integrin αVβ3 and osteopontin expression during neointima formation. Cardiovasc Res 1997;36:408–428.
31. Bishop GG, McPherson JA, Sanders JM, et al. Selective alpha beta 3 receptor blockade reduces macrophage infiltration and restenosis after balloon angioplasty in the atherosclerotic rabbit. Circulation 2001; 103:1906–1911.
32. The ERASER Investigators. Acute platelet inhibition with abciximab does not reduce in-stent restenosis (ERASER study). Circulation 1999;100:799–806.
33. Lincoff AM, Moliterno DJ, Ellis SG, et al. Six month angiographic outcome with abciximab and stents: the EPISTENT angiographic substudy. Circulation 1998;98:I:768 (abstract).
34. Montalescot G, Barragan P, Wittenberg O, et al. Platelet glycoprotein IIb/IIIa inhibition with coronary stenting for acute myocardial infarction. N Engl J Med 2001;344:1895–1903.
35. Montalescot G, Barragan P, Wittemberg O, et al. Abciximab reduces clinical restenosis in diabetic patients undergoing primary stenting for acute myocardial infarction (the ADMIRAL trial). Circulation 2001; 104:II–386 (abstract).
36. Gibson CM, Goel M, Cohen D, et al. Six-month angiographic and clinical follow-up of patients prospectively randomized to receive either tirofiban or placebo during angioplasty in the RESTORE trial. J Am Coll Cardiol 1998;32:28–34.
37. Byzova TV, Plow EF. Activation of alphaVbeta3 on vascular cells controls recognition of prothrombin. J Cell Biol 1998;143:2081–2092.
38. Reverter JC, Beguin S, Kessels H, Dumar R, Hember HC, Coller BS. Inhibition of platelet-mediated, tissue factor-induced, thrombin generation by the mouse/human chimeric 7E3 antibody: potential implications for the effect of c7E3 Fab treatment on acute thrombosis and "clinical restenosis". J Clin Invest 1996;98:863–874
39. Furman MI, Krueger LA, Frelinger AL III, Barnard MR, Mascelli MA, Nakada MT. GP IIb/IIIa antagonist-induced reduction in platelet surface von Willebrand factor binding and phosphatidylserine expression in whole blood. Thromb Haemost 2000;84:492–498.
40. Kereiakes DJ, Runyon JP, Broderick TM, Shimshak TM. IIb's are not IIb's. Am J Cardiol 2000;85: 23C–31C.
41. Mascelli MA, Lance ET, Damaraju L, Wagner CL, Weisman HF, Jordan RE. Pharmacodynamic profile of short-term abciximab treatment demonstrates prolonged platelet inhibition with gradual recovery from GP IIb/IIia receptor blockade. Circulation 1998;97:1680–1688.
42. Scarborough RM, Kleiman NS, Phillips DR. Platelet glycoproteins IIb/IIIa antagonists. What are the relevant issues concerning their pharmacology and clinical use? Circulation 1999;100:437–444.
43. Kereiakes DJ, Anderson KM, Achenbach RE, Melsheimer RM, Kurz MA, Barnathan E. Abciximab survival advantage is not explained by reduction in early major cardiac events: EPIC, EPILOG and EPISTENT 3 year analysis. Circulation 2001;104:II–87 (abstract).
44. Kereiakes DJ, Lincoff AM, Anderson KM, et al., on behalf of the EPIC, EPILOG, and EPISTENT Investigators. Abciximab survival advantage following percutaneous coronary intervention is predicted by clinical risk profile. Am J Cardiol 2002;90:628–630.

44a. Topol EJ, Lincoff AM, Kereiakes DJ, et al. for the EPIC, EPILOG, and EPISTENT Investigators. Multi-year follow-up of abciximab therapy in three randomized, placebo-controlled trials of percutaneous coronary revascularization. Am J Med 2002;113:1–6.

45. Heeschen C, Hamm CW, Bruemmer J, Simmoons ML. Predictive value of C-reactive protein and troponin T in patients with unstable angina: a comparative analysis. CAPTURE investigators. Chimeric c7E3 AntiPlatelet Therapy in Unstable angina Refractory to standard treatment trial. J Am Coll Cardiol 2000; 35:1535–1542

46. Gaspardone A, Crea F, Versaci F, et al. Predictive value of C-reactive protein after successful coronary-artery stenting in patients with unstable angina. Am J Cardiol 1998;82:515–518.

47. Gottsauner-Wolf M, Zasmeta G, Hornykewycz S, et al. Plasma levels of C-reactive protein after coronary stent implantation. Eur Heart J 2000;21:1152–1158.

48. Ridker PM, Rifai NA, Stampfer MJ, Hennekens CH. Plasma concentrations of interleukin-6 and the risk of future myocardial infarction among apparently healthy men. Circulation 2000;101:1767–1772.

49. Harris TB, Ferrucci L, Tracy RP, et al. Associations of elevated interleukin-6 and C-reactive protein levels with mortality in the elderly. Am J Med 1999;106:506–512.

50. Lindmark E, Diderholm E, Wallentin L, Siegbahn A. Relationship between interleukin 6 and mortality in patients with unstable coronary artery disease—effects of an early invasive or noninvasive strategy. JAMA 2001;286:2107–2113.

51. Pasceri V, Willerson JT, Yeh ET. Direct proinflammatory effect of C-reactive protein on human endothelial cells. Circulation 2000;102:2165–2168.

52. Pasceri V, Cheng JS, Willerson JT, Yeh ET, Chang J. Modulation of C-reactive protein-mediated monocyte chemoattractant protein-1 induction in human endothelial cells by anti-atherosclerosis drugs. Circulation 2001;103:2531–2534.

53. Lincoff AM, Kereiakes DJ, Mascelli MA, et al. Abciximab suppresses the rise in levels of circulating inflammatory markers after percutaneous coronary revascularization. Circulation 2001;104:163–167.

54. Merino A, Artaiz M, Vidal B, et al. Eptifibatide blocks the increase in C-reactive protein concentrations induced by coronary angioplasty. Circulation 2001;104:II–56 (abstract)

55. Davies MJ, Richardson PD, Woolf N, Katz DR, Mann J. Risk of thrombosis in human atherosclerotic plaques: role of extracellular lipid, macrophage, and smooth muscle cell content. Br Heart J 1993:69:377–381.

56. Moreno PR, Falk E, Palacios IF, Newell JB, Fuster V, Fallon JT. Macrophage infiltration in acute coronary syndromes. Implications for plaque rupture. Circulation 1994;90:775–779.

57. Meuwissen M. Piek JJ, van der Wal AC, et al. Recurrent unstable angina after directional coronary atherectomy is related to the extent of initial coronary plaque inflammation. J Am Coll Cardiol 2001;37:1271–1276

58. Moreno PR, Bernardi VH, Lopez-Cuellar J, et al. Macrophage infiltration predicts restenosis after coronary intervention in patients with unstable angina Circulation 1996;94:3098–3102.

59. Moreno PR, Murcia AM, Palacios IF, et al. Coronary composition and macrophage infiltration in atherectomy specimens from patients with diabetes mellitus. Circulation 2000;102:2180–2184.

60. Saitoh T, Kishida H, Tsukada Y, et al. Clinical significance of increased plasma concentration of macrophage colony-stimulating factor in patients with angina pectoris. J Am Coll Cardiol 2000;35:655–665.

61. Ikonomidis I, Andreotti F, Eonomou E, Stefanadis C, Toutouzas P, Nihoyannopoulos P. Increased proinflammatory cytokines in patients with chronic Circulation 1999;100:793–799.

62. Seshiah PV, Kereiakes DJ, Shanker SS, Lopes N, Goldschmidt-Clermont PJ. Activated monocytes induce smooth muscle cell death—role of M-CSF in coronary plaque instability: molecular mechanisms in vitro. J Am Coll Cardiol 2001;37:501A (abstract).

63. Seshiah PN, Kereiakes DJ, Vasudevan SS, et al. Activated monocytes induce smooth muscle cell death —role of M-CSF and abciximab. Circulation 2002;105:174–180.

19

Cerebrovascular Interventions

Leslie Cho, MD and Jay S. Yadav, MD

CONTENTS

INTRODUCTION
CAROTID STENTING
ADJUNCTIVE THERAPY: ASPIRIN AND THIENOPYRIDINES
ADJUNCTIVE THERAPY: GPIIb/IIIa INHIBITORS
EMBOLI PROTECTION DEVICES
CONCLUSIONS
REFERENCES

INTRODUCTION

Carotid angioplasty was first proposed by Mathias in 1997 *(1)*, and in 1980 both Kerber et al. *(2)* and Mullan et al. *(3)* published case reports of successful carotid angioplasty during carotid endarterectomy. A percutaneous carotid intervention offers several advantages to surgery. It eliminates the potential risk of general anesthesia and surgical complications of endarterectomy, such as neck hematoma, infection, cervical strain, and cranial nerve damage. Also, high-risk patients such as those with previous ipsilateral carotid endarterectomy, previous radiation therapy to the neck or previous neck surgery, contralateral carotid occlusion, lesions above the mandible or below the clavicle, or neurologic instability, with coexistent coronary or pulmonary disease may be treated *(4)*. Although percutaneous transcatheter techniques have been widely accepted in other vascular areas, they have met with tempered enthusiasm in the carotid arteries owing to the fear of cerebral embolism. However, the recent rapid growth of new technologic advances has aroused greater interest in the endovascular procedures.

CAROTID STENTING (TABLE 1)

In 1987, Theron et al. *(5)* published the first small series of internal carotid angioplasties. With the advent of the stent, multiple reports of carotid stenting have been published (Table 1).

From: *Contemporary Cardiology: Platelet Glycoprotein IIb/IIIa
Inhibitors in Cardiovascular Disease, 2nd Edition*
Edited by: A. M. Lincoff © Humana Press Inc., Totowa, NJ

Table 1
Carotid Stent Studies

Study	Lesion	Success	30-d stroke (%)	30-d MI (%)	30-d death (%)	Follow-up (mo)	Stroke after 30 d (%)	Emboli protection
Diethrich et al. (7)	117	116	8.3	0.0	0.9	7.6	2 (no.)	None
Henry et al. (9)	174	173	2.9	0.0	0.0	12.7	0.0	None
Laborde (26)	87	87	5.3	0.0	1.1	8.7	1.1	None
Wholey et al. (10)	114	108	3.5	0.9	1.9	6	0.0	None
Shawl (25)	96	96	3.1	0.0	0.0	8	0.0	None
Yadav et al. (6)	126	126	6.3	0.0	0.8	6	0.0	None
Global Exp (10)	3129	3091	3.9		2.0	6	0.0	None
Roubin et al. (11)	604	592	5.8		1.3	36	0.7	None
CAVATAS (12)	251	213	8.0		2	36	0.6	None
Henry et al. (21)	270		1.5		0.0	6		PercuSurge
Tubler et al. (22)	58	58	5.2		0.0			PercuSurge
Reimer et al. (24)	88	86	1.2	2.3	0.0			Filter
CAFÉ-USA (27)	212	207	2.4		1.4			Distal balloon

Yadav et al. *(6)* published their initial experience of carotid stenting in 107 consecutive patients. There was a 100% procedural success rate. Periprocedural complications included one stent thrombosis, six minor strokes, and one major stroke. The incidence of combined endpoint of all strokes and death was 7.9%, with 1.6% ipsilateral major stroke and death. Of 107 patients, 76% underwent repeat angiography or ultrasound evaluation at 6 mo following stenting. There was 4.9% asymptomatic restenosis. At 6 mo, there were no additional strokes or deaths from cerebrovascular disease. These initial carotid stents were performed in a high-risk cohort and represent the early learning curve years for percutaneous carotid intervention.

Diethrich et al. *(7)* have also reported their experience in 110 patients with severe carotid stenosis. They reported a 99% procedural success rate with 6.4% stroke (two major and five minor), 4.5% transient ischemic attack (TIA), and two asymptomatic stent occlusion in the first 30 d. During 7.6-mo follow-up, no additional neurologic events were reported.

Wholey et al. *(8)* reported on their carotid stenting experience in 114 lesions in 108 consecutive patients with severe stenosis. The total stroke or death rate at 30 d was 5.3%. There were no neurologic sequelae, cranial nerve palsies, or cases of stent or vessel thrombosis at follow-up. However, there was one case of restenosis owing to stent compression. In addition, Henry et al. *(9)* have published their experience of 174 carotid stenting procedures. Unlike other studies, a small portion of the patients in this study had a cerebral emboli protection device. There was a 99.4% procedural success rate with a 4.6% (eight patients) periprocedural neurologic complication rate. Of these, three were TIAs, two were minor strokes, and three were major strokes. Two major complications were seen in the patients with emboli protection devices. Over a 1-yr follow-up, there was a 2.3% restenosis rate with no ipsilateral neurologic complications.

Wholey et al. *(10)* published the global experience of carotid stent placement. They surveyed 36 centers that performed 5210 procedures in 2757 patients. Even though comparative analysis of these centers is made difficult by the different patient populations, lesion characteristics, endovascular techniques, and follow-up data, this review underscores the safety of carotid stenting in the hands of experienced operators. They reported a 98.4% procedural success rate, with technical success defined as <30% residual stenosis covering a region longer than the original lesion without any alteration of intracranial arterial anatomy. Various different stents were used depending on the availability and operator preferences. In most of these patients, no emboli protection device was used. There were 2.8% reported TIAs. Minor strokes were defined as new neurologic events that resulted in functional impairment that either completely resolved within 7 d or caused an increase in the National Institutes of Health (NIH) stroke scale of <4. Minor stroke rate was 2.7%. A major stroke was defined as a new neurologic deficit that persisted after 7 d and increased the NIH stroke scale by 4 or more. Major stroke rates were 1.5%, and procedure-related mortality at 3 d was 0.96%. There was a restenosis rate of 2.3% and a stent deformation rate of 2.5%.

Recently, Roubin et al. *(11)* reported a 5-yr prospective analysis of immediate and late clinical outcomes in carotid artery stenting in patients with symptomatic and asymptomatic carotid artery stenosis. In 528 consecutive patients undergoing percutaneous carotid intervention, they reported a procedural success rate of 98%, with a 0.6% fatal stroke rate and a 1% nonstroke death rate at 30 d *(11)*. In this study, 83% patients were ineligible for carotid endarterectomy according to the NASCET trial. The major stroke rate was 1% and the minor stroke rate was 4.8%. The overall 3-d stroke and death rate was 7.4%. After the 30-d period, the incidence of fatal and nonfatal stroke was 3.2%. The 3-yr freedom from ipsilateral or fatal stroke was 92%. Of note, their minor stroke rate decreased significantly after their first year of carotid interventions. This large series suggests that carotid stenting is not only safe but also durable.

The only randomized study to date, the Carotid and Vertebral Artery Transluminal Angioplasty Study (CAVATAS), compared carotid angioplasty vs carotid endarterectomy in 504 symptomatic patients *(12)*. This trial demonstrated a similar death or stroke rate at 30 d (10% in the angioplasty group vs 10% in the surgery group). The periprocedural disabling stroke and nondisabling stroke rates were similar between the two groups. Moreover, there was no substantial difference in the rate of ipsilateral stroke at 3 yr between the two groups [odds ratio (OR) 1.04, 95% confidence interval (CI) 0.63–1.70, $p = 0.9$]. Local complications were lower for the PTA group than the surgery group. This trial has been criticized by both carotid interventionalists and surgeons. In this study, only 25% had stent use and there was no emboli protection used. These devices were not widely accepted or used during the enrollment time of CAVATAS. Also, the surgical stroke and death rates were higher than those reported by the NASCET investigators. The stroke and death rate was 5.8% in that trial compared with 9.9% in CAVATAS *(12,13)*. CAVATAS II will enroll patients to carotid stent vs endarterectomy using stents and emboli protection device. As of now, the current indication for carotid stenting is reserved for high-risk carotid endarterectomy patients. From all these studies, carotid stenting appears safe and feasible. The next 2 yr will bring much data from many randomized trials currently enrolling patients.

ADJUNCTIVE THERAPY: ASPIRIN AND THIENOPYRIDINES

The role of aspirin and thienopyridines for percutaneous carotid intervention has not been well studied. Aspirin monotherapy has not been tested in percutaneous carotid intervention. Ticlopidine with aspirin has been tested as adjuvant therapy for carotid angioplasty and stenting in patients with contralateral occlusion or post-carotid endarterectomy restenosis. These types of patients typically have higher complication rates after procedure. In 31 patients who underwent elective carotid stenting in the presence of contralateral occlusion, there were no neurologic events during a mean follow-up of 16 mo. Because of serious hematologic side effects with ticlopidine, clopidogrel has become the preferred thienopyridine. To date, there has been only one study comparing ticlopidine with clopidogrel in carotid stenting. Bhatt et al. published a single center experience of 162 patients undergoing carotid stenting. The cumulative rate of 30-d death, stroke, TIA, or myocardial infarction (MI) was 13% in the ticlopidine group compared with 4.3% in the clopidogrel group ($p = 0.001$) and 5.6% in the overall cohort *(13a)*.

ADJUNCTIVE THERAPY: GPIIb/IIIa INHIBITORS

The role of glycoprotein (GP) IIb/IIIa inhibitors has been established in coronary interventions. These agents decrease periprocedural ischemic complications in patients undergoing both emergent and elective coronary interventions. However, there have been few studies using these agents in carotid interventions. In a small study, 22 patients undergoing carotid intervention involving visible thrombus, total occlusion, or acute stroke were given abciximab *(14)*. The preliminary data from these high-risk patients suggested higher bleeding complications, with two patients having central nervous system bleeding, one patient with hemorrhagic transformation of a previously ischemic stroke, and one patient having subarachnoid hemorrhage from a ruptured aneurysm. Another small study reported outcomes of 13 internal carotid, 4 vertebral, and two basilar artery angioplasty and stenting procedure using abciximab *(15)*. Two patients experienced transient ischemic attacks during and immediately after the procedure. Major or minor bleeding was not experienced in any patient. Schneiderman et al. *(16)* published a 16-patient study using abciximab in patients undergoing carotid stenting for recurrent internal carotid artery stenosis. They found no neurologic ischemic events during and following the procedure and no greater increase in bleeding rates.

In a much larger study, Kapadia et al. *(17)* have studied the safety and efficacy of abciximab in 151 consecutive patients at high surgical risk undergoing carotid stenting. In this study 128 high surgical risk patients received adjuvant therapy with abciximab (0.25 mg/kg bolus before the lesion was crossed with guidewire and 0.125 µg/kg/min infusion for 12 h) with 50 U/kg of heparin at the time of carotid stenting; 23 patients were used as controls. An activated clotting time was maintained between 250 and 300 s. All patients received aspirin and thienopyridine. The primary endpoints of stroke (major or minor), intracranial hemorrhage, and neurologic death within 30 d were more frequent in the control group (8% vs 1.6%, $p = 0.05$) (Table 2). At 30-d follow-up, one patient presented with delayed intracranial hemorrhage in the abciximab group. This study demonstrated that abciximab appears to be safe, with no increase in the risk of intracranial hemorrhage and a lowering of the ischemic stroke risk.

GPIIb/IIIa inhibitors may play a role in stroke patients. In an experimental stroke model, studies have shown that marked sparing of brain infarction and relief of microvascular obstruction using a platelet GPIIb/IIIa inhibitor *(17a,17b)*. Initial experience with GPIIb/IIIa inhibitors in acute stroke management appeared to be safe and showed a trend toward improved outcome in stroke patients treated up to 24 h after symptom onset in a joint US European clinical trial *(17c)*. This study randomized 74 patients in a 1:3 ratio to placebo or to one of four doses of abciximab bolus: (1) 0.15 mg/kg or 0.20 mg/kg (2) 0.20 mg/kg or 0.25 mg/kg followed by 0.125 µg/kg/min infusion for 12 h. The primary safety endpoint was the presence or absence of major intracerebral hemorrhage on d 5 accompanied by neurologic worsening. No patient had intracranial hemorrhage associated with neurologic worsening. The 3-mo follow-up showed that 10 of 54 abciximab patients had asymptomatic hemorrhagic transformation compared with 1 of 20 placebo patients. Abciximab-treated patients showed a trend toward improved outcome. Global recovery was measured by Rankin score, which showed that 35% of abciximab patients had minimal or no deficit at 3 mo compared with 20% of placebo patients. On the Barthel index of daily activities, 50% of abciximab patients had a score of 95 or higher compared with 40% of placebo patients. Also, stroke progression occurred in 11% of abciximab patients and 15% of the placebo group, and the stroke recurrence occurred in 2% of the abciximab patient compared with 5% of the placebo group. A large clinical trial is needed to assess the role of abciximab further in stroke.

In coronary interventions, periprocedural ischemic complications are easier to quantify, whereas in carotid interventions small embolic phenomenon may be more difficult to detect. Embolization detection with transcranial Doppler (TCD) during carotid intervention may better assess the effectiveness of GPIIb/IIIa inhibitors. However, to date, no study has been done using TCD and GPIIb/IIIa inhibitors. Although it may be safe to use GPIIb/IIIa

Table 2
Procedural Event Rates Using Abciximab

Event (%)	Control (n = 23)	Abciximab (n = 128)
Major stroke	4	0
Minor stroke	0	1
Retinal infarct	0	1
Intracerebral hemorrhage	0	0
Death	1	0

inhibitors in carotid interventions, its role may be less important now that mechanical strategies for emboli protection have emerged.

EMBOLI PROTECTION DEVICES

A major cause of neurologic complications during carotid endarterectomy and percutaneous carotid intervention is microembolization of plaque debris. This leads to release of platelet and thrombin aggregates into the cerebral circulation. TCD monitoring, a noninvasive method to detect microemboli, has demonstrated frequent embolization with both endarterectomy and stenting (18–20). There appears to be some correlation between the number of emboli and neurologic outcome. Currently, there are several mechanical devices for emboli protection under investigation. The first approach is the use of distal occlusion balloon to occlude the outflow temporarily from the distal internal carotid artery. The PercuSurge Guard Wire has a low crossing profile and flexibility and provides occlusion of the distal internal carotid artery (Fig. 1). However, because of the complete occlusion of flow, patients are exposed to a prolonged ischemic time. Although this is well tolerated by many, it may be risky in patients with contralateral occlusions or an incomplete circle of Willis. Also, the inability to perform angiograms is problematic. Finally, there is a potential for particles to embolize via the patent external carotid artery.

The second method is the filter wire device placed distal to the lesion (AngioGuard or AccuNet) (Fig. 2). The advantages of this system are preservation of flow, ability to perform angiograms during the procedure, and ease of use of the device. However, these filter wire devices may allow larger particles to pass through than the balloon occlusion devices. The third type of embolism protection devices occludes the inflow to the brain by using a proximal occlusion balloon in the common carotid artery (ArteriA PAEC). Unlike the other two, the proximal occlusion system protects the brain prior to manipulating the lesion, captures particle of all sizes, can use the guidewire of choice, and allows the operators to treat tight and tortuous lesions. However, like PercuSurge, they do occlude flow and require larger puncture sites in the groin. Also, like all the devices, they may cause spasm and dissection of the artery.

To date there have been several reports of carotid interventions using these emboli protection devices. Henry et al. (21) have reported 58 carotid stent procedures using a distal occlusion balloon protection device and compared the results with 212 other patients treated without emboli protection device. In this study, there were two major strokes with the

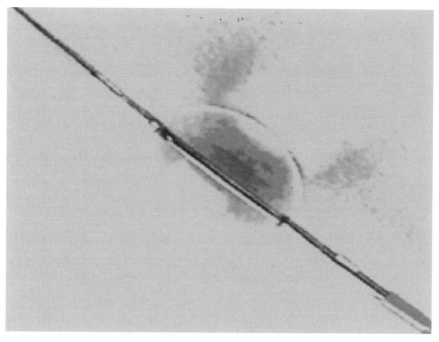

Fig. 1. PercuSurge, a balloon occlusion emboli protection device.

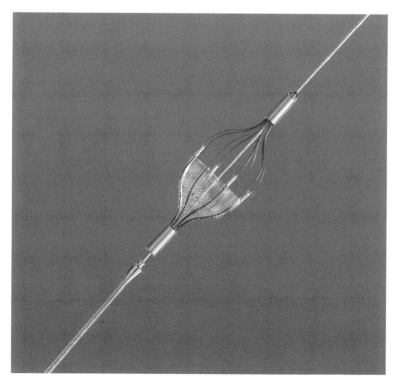

Fig. 2. Angioguard, a filter wire emboli protection device.

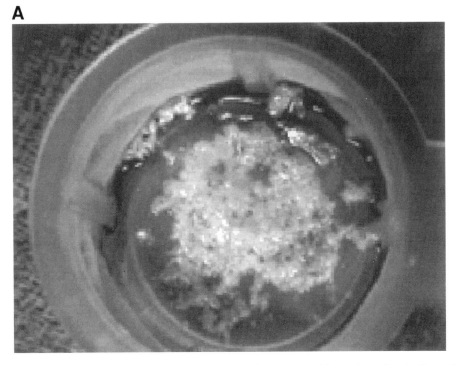

Fig. 3. (**A**) Aspirated particles from a patient who underwent carotid stenting with the PercuSurge emboli protection device.

cerebral protection balloon catheter and one major stroke, one minor stroke, and three TIAs without its use.

Tubler et al. *(22)* reported a multicenter, Phase I trial of 54 patients undergoing carotid stenting using the PercuSurge Guard Wire system. They reported one prolonged reversible ischemic deficit that resolved in less than 48 h, one stroke, and one TIA. They found particles with areas >10,000 μm^2 in 83% of the patients (Fig. 3).

Al-Mubarak et al. *(23)* have reported the effect of a distal balloon protection system on microembolization during carotid stenting. They used TCD studies to demonstrate microembolization. They found that microembolization was significantly decreased by the use of a distal balloon protection device (164 ± 108 vs 68 ± 83, $p = 0002$) in patients undergoing percutaneous carotid intervention. Also, Reimer et al. *(24)* have reported on their feasibility and safety study using three types of filter wire emboli protection devices. They reported 96.5% procedural success rate in placing the filter device. They were unable to place the filter in 3.5% of the cases owing to the inability of the filter to cross the lesion. In 6.9% of the patients, they predilated with 2.0-mm balloons prior to placing the filter device. They reported a 3.6% rate of vessel spasm requiring nitroglycerin and no case of dissection. However, in 7.2% of patients, the filter did cause flow impairment owing to heavy emboli burden. They retrieved macroscopic evidence of emboli in 53% of these patients. At 30 d, they found one case of minor stroke and two cases of MI.

The largest study to date is the Carotid Artery Intervention Free of Emboli (CAFÉ-USA), which used a distal balloon protection device in 212 patients undergoing carotid stenting. The device was successfully deployed in 98.1% of patients, and 92.3% patients

B

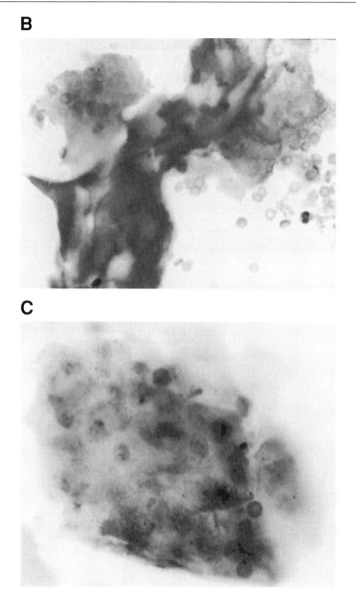

C

Fig. 3. (B,C) Microscopic view of a particle retrieved from a PercuSurge emboli protection device.

were able to tolerate the complete occlusion. There were 3 deaths, 2 of which were neurologic deaths from hemorrhagic stroke, 12 ipsilateral strokes, 5 TIAs, and no major strokes. In both hemorrhagic stroke cases, GPIIb/IIIa inhibitors were used. These initial trials point to the safety and feasibility of using these devices in high-risk patients undergoing carotid stenting.

There are two important trials currently under way comparing carotid artery stenting with endarterectomy using emboli protection devices. The Stenting and Angioplasty with Protection in Patients at High Risk for Endarterectomy (SAPPHIRE) trial will randomize patients at high surgical risk to carotid endarterectomy or carotid artery stenting using the Cordis nitinol carotid stent and Cordis Angioguard, a filter-type emboli protection device. The high-risk patient population is defined as patients with severe cardiac comorbidities (severe congestive heart failure, valvular heart disease, or unstable angina), previous neck radiation or neck dissection, and restenosis after endarterectomy or presence of contralateral occlusion. Both de novo and restenotic lesions will be treated in symptomatic (>70% stenosis) or asymptomatic (>80% stenosis) patients. A total of 720 patients at 24 sites will be enrolled, and parallel registries for both percutaneous intervention and surgery will be maintained for randomized patients. The primary endpoint is a 30-d composite of any stroke, death, or MI. The secondary endpoint is the 1-yr ipsilateral stroke and death rate. The Carotid Revascularization Endarterectomy versus Stent Trial (CREST) will randomize patients who are at low surgical risk to stenting or surgery. The primary endpoints for this trial are any stroke, MI, or death within 30 d and ipsilateral stroke after 30 d. This trial is planning to recruit 2500 patients and will use Guidant AccuLink and Guidant AccuNet, another filter-type emboli protection device.

CONCLUSIONS

Much has been learned about antiplatelet therapy in coronary intervention in the last two decades. Although the role of aspirin and thienopyridine has been solidified in percutaneous carotid interventions, the role of GPIIb/IIIa inhibitors is uncertain with the advent of emboli protection devices. Promising preliminary studies have been performed in acute stroke patients using GPIIb/IIIa inhibitors. Further large, randomized studies are warranted.

REFERENCES

1. Mathias K. [A new catheter system for percutaneous transluminal angioplasty (PTA) of carotid artery stenoses]. Fortschr Med 1977;95:1007–1011.
2. Kerber CW, Cromwell LD, Loehden OL. Catheter dilatation of proximal carotid stenosis during distal bifurcation endarterectomy. AJNR Am J Neuroradiol 1980;1:348–349.
3. Mullan S, Duda EE, Patronas NJ. Some examples of balloon technology in neurosurgery. J Neurosurg 1980;52:321–329.
4. Mukherjee D, Yadav JS. Carotid and cerebrovascular disease. Cardiol Rev 2000;8:322–332.
5. Theron J, Raymond J, Casasco A, Courtheoux F. Percutaneous angioplasty of atherosclerotic and postsurgical stenosis of carotid arteries. AJNR Am J Neuroradiol 1987;8:495–500.
6. Yadav JS, Roubin GS, King P, Iyer S, Vitek J. Angioplasty and stenting for restenosis after carotid endarterectomy. Initial experience. Stroke 1996;27:2075–2079.
7. Diethrich EB, Ndiaye M, Reid DB. Stenting in the carotid artery: initial experience in 110 patients. J Endovasc Surg 1996;3:42–62.
8. Wholey MH, Jarmolowski CR, Eles G, Levy D, Buecthel J. Endovascular stents for carotid artery occlusive disease. J Endovasc Surg 1997;4:326–338.
9. Henry M, Amor M, Masson I, Henry I, Tzvetanov KV, Chati Z, Khanna N. Angioplasty and stenting of the extracranial carotid arteries. J Endovasc Surg 1998;5:293–304.
10. Wholey MH, Wholey M, Mathias K, et al. Global experience in cervical carotid artery stent placement. Catheter Cardiovasc Interv 2000;50:160–167.
11. Roubin GS, New G, Iyer SS, et al. Immediate and late clinical outcomes of carotid artery stenting in patients with symptomatic and asymptomatic carotid artery stenosis: a 5-year prospective analysis. Circulation 2001;103:532–537.
12. CAVATAS Investigators. Endovascular versus surgical treatment in patients with carotid stenosis in the Carotid and Vertebral Artery Transluminal Angioplasty Study (CAVATAS): a randomized trial. Lancet 2001;357:1729–1737.
13. Beneficial effect of carotid endarterectomy in symptomatic patients with high-grade carotid stenosis. North American Symptomatic Carotid Endarterectomy Trial Collaborators. N Engl J Med 1991;325:445–453.

13a. Bhatt DL, Kapadia SR, Bajzer CT, et al. Dual antiplatelet therapy with clopidogrel and aspirin after carotid artery stenting. J Inv Cardiol 2001;13:767–771.

14. Chastain HD, Wong PM, Mathur A. Does abciximab reduce complications of cerebral vascular stenting in high risk patients? Circulation 1997;96:I283 (abstract).

15. Qureshi AI, Suri MF, Khan J, Fessler RD, Guterman LR, Hopkins LN. Abciximab as an adjunct to high-risk carotid or vertebrobasilar angioplasty: preliminary experience. Neurosurgery 2000;46:1316–1324; discussion 1324–1325.

16. Schneiderman J, Morag B, Gerniak A, et al. Abciximab in carotid stenting for postsurgical carotid restenosis: intermediate results. J Endovasc Ther 2000;7:263–272.

17. Kapadia SR, Bajzer CT, Ziada KM, et al. Initial experience of platelet glycoprotein IIb/IIIa inhibition with abciximab during carotid stenting: a safe and effective adjunctive therapy. Stroke 2001;32:2328–2332.

17a. Abumiya T, Fitridge R, Mazur C, et al. Integrin alpha(IIb)beta(3) inhibitor preserves microvascular patency in experimental acute focal cerebral ischemia. Stroke 2000;31:1402–1409.

17b. Nishimura H, Naritomi H, Iwamoto Y, Tachibana H, Sugita M. In vivo evaluation of antiplatelet agents in gerbil model of carotid artery thrombosis. Stroke 1996;27:1099–1103.

17c. The Abciximab in Ischemic Stroke Investigators. Abciximab in acute ischemic stroke: a randomized, double-blind, placebo-controlled, dose-escalation study. Stroke 2000;31:601–609.

18. McCleary AJ, Nelson M, Dearden NM, Calvey TA, Gough MJ. Cerebral haemodynamics and embolization during carotid angioplasty in high-risk patients. Br J Surg 1998;85:771–774.

19. Markus HS, Clifton A, Buckenham T, Brown MM. Carotid angioplasty. Detection of embolic signals during and after the procedure. Stroke 1994;25:2403–2406.

20. Gaunt ME, Martin PJ, Smith JL, et al. Clinical relevance of intraoperative embolization detected by transcranial Doppler ultrasonography during carotid endarterectomy: a prospective study of 100 patients. Br J Surg 1994;81:1435–1439.

21. Henry M, Amor M, Henry I, et al. Carotid stenting with cerebral protection: the first clinical experience using the PercuSurge GuardWire system. J Endovasc Surg 1999;6:321–331.

22. Tubler T, Schluter M, Dirsch O, et al. Balloon-protected carotid artery stenting: relationship of periprocedural neurological complications with the size of particulate debris. Circulation 2001;104:2791–2796.

23. Al-Mubarak N, Roubin GS, Vitek JJ, Iyer SS, New G, Leon MB. Effect of the distal-balloon protection system on microembolization during carotid stenting. Circulation 2001;104:1999–2002.

24. Reimer B, Corvaja N, Moshiri S, et al. Cerebral protection with filter devices during carotid artery stenting. Circulation 2001;104:12–15.

25. Shawl F, Kadro W, Domanski MJ, et al. Safety and efficacy of elective carotid artery stenting in high-risk patients. J Am Coll Cardiol 2000;35:1721–1728.

26. Wholey MH, Wholey M, Bergeron P, et al. Current global status of carotid artery stent placement. Catheter Cardiovasc Diag 1998;44:1–6.

27. CAFÉ-USA Investigators. Presented at AHA Association 72nd Scientific Sessions, 1999.

20

Cerebrovascular Aspects of Glycoprotein IIb/IIIa Receptor Inhibitors

Cathy A. Sila, MD

CONTENTS

INTRODUCTION
TREATMENTS FOR CARDIAC DISEASE
TREATMENTS FOR CEREBROVASCULAR DISEASE
CONCLUSIONS
REFERENCES

INTRODUCTION

Ischemic and hemorrhagic subtypes of stroke are important complications of treatments for cardiac disease, as they impact significantly on patient management and outcome. Their frequency varies with the characteristics of the patient population under study, the procedures involved, and the combination and intensity of antiplatelet, antithrombotic, and fibrinolytic strategies employed. Understanding the mechanisms contributing to the various stroke subtypes is important, not only to improve the overall outcome for patients with cardiac disease, but also to translate similar strategies to patients with cerebrovascular disease, for whom the risk-to-benefit ratio is more acute.

TREATMENTS FOR CARDIAC DISEASE

Ischemic Stroke Complicating Coronary Artery Disease and Treatment

In the prethrombolytic era, stroke occurred in 0.8–5.5% of patients with acute myocardial infarction (AMI) and was largely ischemic in nature *(1)*. Features typical of cerebral embolism include predominantly middle cerebral artery territory involvement, the relationship to cardiac rhythm and ventricular function, and declining risk over time. With the introduction of thrombolysis for AMI, the risk of ischemic stroke declined to 0.1–1.3% within the first month, with one-third occurring within the first day, one-third within the first week, and the remaining one-third clustered within the second week *(1,2)*. Risk factors for stroke include advanced age, higher heart rate, history of prior stroke, diabetes mellitus, previous angina, hypertension, worse Kilip class, coronary angiography, bypass surgery,

From: *Contemporary Cardiology: Platelet Glycoprotein IIb/IIIa
Inhibitors in Cardiovascular Disease, 2nd Edition*
Edited by: A. M. Lincoff © Humana Press Inc., Totowa, NJ

and atrial fibrillation or flutter *(3)*. The complicating stroke morbidity of 40–60% impacts in turn on the aggressiveness of treatment for the underlying cardiac disease and translates into a stroke-related mortality of 15–20% *(4)*.

The risk of stroke in patients with acute coronary syndromes (ACS) not managed with thrombolysis or glycoprotein (GP) IIb/IIIa receptor antagonists is approx 0.6–0.8%, is largely ischemic in nature, and occurs at a median of 6.5 d. Risk factors for stroke with ACS are similar to those in the setting of AMI and include advanced age, prior anterior myocardial infarction, female gender, lower body weight, higher heart rate, history of prior stroke, hypertension, diabetes mellitus, hypercholesterolemia, history of prior myocardial infarction, and prior coronary bypass surgery. Stroke victims experience more in-hospital complications of atrial fibrillation, hypotension, congestive heart failure, cardiogenic shock, and coronary bypass surgery, and at 1 mo, half are dead or disabled *(5–7)*.

Cardiac catheterization, for purposes of diagnosis or therapeutic intervention, is complicated by ischemic stroke in 0.1–1.0%, and half of the cases resolve within 48 h *(8)*. There is a vertebrobasilar predominance, with 60–70% presenting as confusion, visual field defects, and brainstem signs and 30–40% with carotid distribution symptoms of hemiparesis, hemisensory deficits, dysphasia, and retinal ischemia *(9)*. As the confusional states can mimic medication effects and metabolic encephalopathy, the true incidence may be underestimated *(10)*. The mechanism is attributed to cerebral embolism of particulate matter or air during catheter manipulation or flushing, and as the posterior circulation predominance persists regardless of the method of arterial access, it is likely to be related to the catheter position within the aorta *(11)*.

The risk of stroke during percutaneous coronary intervention (PCI) is similar to that of diagnostic angiography. A combined analysis of four trials (EPIC, EPILOG, CAPTURE, and EPISTENT) assessing the risk of stroke in 8555 patients undergoing PCI with abciximab vs placebo as well as aspirin and heparin demonstrated no significant difference in the rate of both hemorrhagic and ischemic stroke between those assigned to placebo (9/3079, 0.29%) vs any abciximab dose (22/5476, 0.40%; $p = 0.46$) or abciximab bolus plus infusion (15/4680, 0.32%) (Table 1) *(12)*. The numbers of patients with ischemic stroke were small but not significantly different between the two groups (0.17% vs 0.2%) overall. The challenge of finding the optimum combination of antithrombotic therapies is highlighted by the interesting observation that although overall bleeding complications were greater in abciximab-treated patients, the rate of ischemic stroke was less in those who received the standard heparin dose vs the low-dose heparin regimen (0.09% vs 0.24%; $p = 0.3$).

Hemorrhagic Stroke Complicating Coronary Artery Disease and Treatment

The risk of any intracranial bleeding increases with the aggressiveness of antithrombotic and antifibrinolytic therapies, particularly with higher dosages and combination therapies *(13)*. Intracranial hemorrhage following aspirin or heparin therapy for AMI is typically caused by a delayed hemorrhagic transformation of an ischemic stroke. Risk factors for hemorrhagic transformation of an ischemic stroke include advanced age, hypertension, embolic mechanism, volume of cerebral infarct by neuroimaging or severity of clinical deficit, early anticoagulant therapy of large ischemic stroke, use of bolus dosing of heparin, higher heparin dosages, and excessive prolongation of the activated partial thromboplastin time *(14–16)*.

The risk of stroke with platelet GPIIb/IIIa inhibition for PCI was not increased in patients receiving abciximab vs placebo with aspirin and heparin in a combined analysis of 8555

Table 1
Stroke Risk (%) with Glycoprotein IIb/IIIa Inhibitors in Cardiac Trials[a]

| | | | Heparin | |
	Abciximab *(n = 5476)*	*Control* *(n = 3079)*	*Standard*	*Low-dose*
Percutaneous interventions				
(8555 patients from EPIC, CAPTURE, EPILOG, and EPISTENT)				
All stroke	0.4	0.29 ($p = 0.46$)		
Ischemic	0.17	0.20		
Hemorrhagic	0.15	0.10	0.27	0.04 ($p = 0.057$)

	Various	*Control*		
Acute coronary syndromes				
(31,402 patients from PRISM, PRISM-PLUS, PARAGON-A, PARAGON-B, PURSUIT, and GUSTO-IV ACS)				
Hemorrhagic	0.09	0.06 ($p = 0.40$)		

	Abciximab + heparin *(n = 8328)*	*Heparin from GUSTO-V* *(n = 8260)*		
Acute MI: combination therapy with thrombolysis				
All stroke	1.0	0.9 ($p = 0.37$)		
Ischemic	0.3	0.3		
Hemorrhagic	0.7	0.6		

	Abciximab + heparin *(n = 2017)*	*Heparin* *(n = 2038)*	*LMWH* *(n = 2040)* *from ASSENT-3*
All stroke	1.49	1.52	1.62 ($p = 0.94$)
Ischemic	0.35	0.54	0.59
Hemorrhagic	1.14	0.98	1.08

Abbreviations: LMWH, low-molecular-weight heparin; MI, myocardial infarction.
[a]Hemorrhagic stroke includes intracranial hemorrhage, hemorrhagic conversion of ischemic stroke, and unknown type.

patients from four trials *(12)*. There was no significant difference in the rate of hemorrhagic stroke (0.15% vs 0.1%) between abciximab-treated patients vs controls. However, the rate of hemorrhagic stroke was greater in patients who received abciximab with standard-dose heparin at 0.27% vs low-dose, weight-adjusted heparin at 0.04% ($p = 0.057$), and mortality after hemorrhagic stroke was greater in abciximab-treated patients, supporting the recommendations for the use of low-dose, weight-adjusted heparin when patients receive abciximab for PCI.

The risk of stroke with platelet GPIIb/IIIa inhibition for ACS was prospectively addressed in the PURSUIT trial, which compared two doses of eptifibatide in addition to aspirin and recommended heparin *(6)*. There was no significant difference between eptifibatide and control in the rate of all stroke (0.6% vs 0.8%) or hemorrhagic stroke (0.13% vs 0.11%, including intracranial hemorrhage, hemorrhagic conversion of infarction, and uncertain type). In a meta-analysis of GPIIb/IIIa inhibitors in ACS combining these data with data from PRISM, PRISM-PLUS, PARAGON-A and B, and GUSTO-IV ACS, although overall bleeding complications were significantly more frequent, there was no significant increase in the rate of intracranial bleeding (0.09% vs 0.06%, $p = 0.40$) *(17)*.

Although the overall rate of stroke with AMI is reduced with thrombolytic therapy, the rate of hemorrhagic stroke is significantly increased at 0.3–1.5% and includes spontaneous intracerebral, subdural, subarachnoid, and intraventricular hemorrhage as well as hemorrhagic transformation of cerebral infarcts *(1,18)*. Hemorrhagic transformation complicates 30% of ischemic strokes and is severe enough to produce symptoms of neurologic deterioration in two-thirds *(2)*. Intracranial hemorrhage after thrombolysis for AMI is usually caused by a solitary intracerebral hemorrhage involving the deep lobar white matter. However, there is substantial variability in the size and nature of intracranial hemorrhages, with multifocality, bizarre-appearing hemorrhages, and blood-fluid levels or a mottled appearance typical of an underlying coagulopathy *(18)*. Many are recognized during the infusion as a subacute but rapidly progressive headache with nausea, vomiting, and focal neurologic signs, and most occur within 24 h, but the risk of persists for days. The fear of stroke complicating cardiac interventions emanates from the dismal outcome of patients with intracranial hemorrhage, as 60% die and an additional 25% remain disabled *(4,19)*. Risk factors for intracranial hemorrhage after thrombolysis for AMI include advanced age, hypertension, and prior neurologic disease, as well as the intensity of the coagulopathy induced by the type, dosage, and concomitant therapies administered *(20)*. Amyloid angiopathy is the most common substrate in surgical or autopsy specimens and probably explains the important relationship between advanced age and risk of cerebral hemorrhage *(21)*.

The reduction in the rate of cardiac complications after AMI treated with combination therapy with thrombolytics, GPIIb/IIIa inhibitors, and heparin comes at the price of an increase in overall bleeding complications, particularly in those over 75 yr or when streptokinase is used. Small, nonpivotal trials had rates of intracranial hemorrhage similar to that seen with thrombolysis alone *(22)*. In GUSTO-V, the rates of all stroke (1.0% vs 0.9%, $p = 0.37$), ischemic stroke (0.3% vs 0.3%), and hemorrhagic stroke (0.7% vs 0.6%) were quite low overall and were no different with abciximab and reduced-dose reteplase over standard-dose reteplase *(23)*. Similarly, in ASSENT-3, the rates of all stroke were low and not significantly different among those who received tenecteplase with abciximab and heparin vs heparin vs enoxaparin (1.49% vs 1.52% vs 1.62%, $p = 0.94$) *(24)*. Although the events were few and <15% of patients were over 75 yr, there was a suggestion that the combination of abciximab with heparin had a somewhat lower rate of ischemic stroke and higher rate of hemorrhagic stroke (including hemorrhagic transformations and unknown type) compared with heparins alone. The differential risk of ischemic vs hemorrhagic stroke may warrant tailoring combination therapy to special at-risk patients with AMI and will be particularly important as these combinations are explored for patients with acute ischemic stroke (AIS).

TREATMENTS FOR CEREBROVASCULAR DISEASE

Risks and Benefits of Antiplatelet Therapy for the Prevention of Recurrent Ischemic Stroke

Although aspirin remains the standard preventive therapy for patients at risk for stroke, the effect, operating through inhibition of thromboxane A_2, is modest and calls for improvement. Despite numerous metaanalyses, there is no consensus on the optimum dose of aspirin for prevention of ischemic stroke, and most physicians now use low to medium doses

(50–325 mg/d). Establishing superior preventive efficacy has been the goal of development of other antiplatelet agents that target platelet surface glycoproteins, ADP receptors, or platelet-dependent thrombin generation in the hopes that combination therapy will provide synergistic effects. Although the orally active platelet GPIIb/IIIa inhibitor lotrafiban was felt to be safe and well tolerated in combination with aspirin in a preliminary trial, the pivotal trial including patients with cerebrovascular disease was prematurely terminated owing to an excess of adverse events *(25)*.

The antiplatelet effect achieved by the inhibition of ADP binding to its platelet receptor with ticlopidine and clopidogrel has been compared with that of aspirin in two trials of stroke prevention. The Ticlopidine Aspirin Stroke Study (TASS) compared ticlopidine (250 mg twice daily) with high-dose aspirin (650 mg twice daily) in 3069 patients with transient ischemic attacks (TIAs) or minor stroke *(26)*. Ticlopidine reduced the risk of stroke by 21% over high-dose aspirin, but with small numbers of other events, the 9% reduction in the combined endpoint of stroke, myocardial infarction, or vascular death did not reach significance. In the Clopidigrel versus Aspirin in Patients at Risk of Ischemic Events (CAPRIE) study, clopidogrel (75 mg once daily) reduced the annual risk of the combined endpoint of stroke, myocardial infarction, or vascular death by 9% (5.32% vs 5.83%, $p = 0.043$) over aspirin 325 mg daily in 19,185 patients with various manifestations of vascular disease *(27)*. As the study was designed to detect an overall relative risk reduction of 12–13%, the 7.3% reduction in recurrent events, mostly stroke, for the stroke subset of 6431 patients did not reach significance (7.15% vs 7.71%, $p = 0.26$). Hematologic side effects include neutropenia in <2% of ticlopidine-treated patients and thrombotic thrombocytopenic purpura (TTP) in 200–625/million ticlopidine-treated and 3.7/million clopidogrel-treated patients *(28)*. Only ticlopidine warrants hematologic monitoring every 2 wk for the first 3 mo to screen for neutropenia, but as 80% of TTP cases appeared within the first few weeks of therapy, hematologic monitoring is not reliable for surveillance of this condition. Given the similar efficacy and superior safety, clopidogrel has essentially replaced ticlopidine as an aspirin alternative.

Combination antiplatelet therapy with aspirin and dipyridamole has been studied in various dosing schedules in five clinical trials. The combination of aspirin (330 mg tid) and dipyridamole (75 mg tid) reduced stroke by 38% and the combined endpoint of stroke, myocardial infarction, or vascular death by 31% over placebo but smaller trials did not demonstrate efficacy over high-dose aspirin alone *(29–31)*. The Second European Stroke Prevention Study (EPSP-2) compared the combination of low-dose aspirin (50 mg daily) and modified-release dipyridamole (400 mg daily) with each agent alone and placebo. The combination reduced stroke by 23.1% ($p = 0.006$) over low-dose aspirin alone, and comparisons suggested a synergistic effect *(32)*. None of the treatments reduced mortality, and there were too few endpoints to demonstrate any effect on fatal stroke or myocardial infarction. EPSP-2 prompted the ACCP guidelines for lower doses of aspirin, 50–325 mg daily, for secondary stroke prevention.

Combination therapy with clopidogrel (75 mg daily) and aspirin (75 mg daily) for secondary stroke prevention is currently being studied in 7600 high-risk patients with recent TIA or ischemic stroke, with results anticipated by 2004.

Complications of Endovascular Therapy for Cerebrovascular Disease

Endovascular treatment of cerebrovascular disease began in the 1980s with primary angioplasty of extracranial vessels. By 1995, stents dedicated to the extracranial carotid artery were available and were followed shortly by numerous emboli protection devices. Although case series report results that are comparable to those of carotid endarterectomy, this has not been confirmed by randomized clinical trials. Between 1992 and 1997, the Carotid and Vertebral Artery Transluminal Angioplasty Study (CAVATAS) trial randomized 560 patients (most with symptomatic >80% carotid stenosis) to angioplasty, surgery, or medical therapy if patients were not appropriate candidates for surgery (33). The 30-d rate of stroke and death was high, 9.9% for the 253 patients who underwent carotid endarterectomy and 10% for the 251 patients who underwent angioplasty, 26% with stenting. At 1-yr follow-up, restenosis of >70% was rare in endartectomy patients but was present in 21% with endovascular therapy. The Schneider trial randomized 223 patients with >60% symptomatic carotid stenosis to carotid stenting with aspirin and ticlopidine vs endarterectomy (34). Statistically designed as an equivalency analysis, stenting was determined not to be equivalent or better to endarterectomy based on the 12% vs 3.5% rate in the primary endpoint of ipsilateral stroke, periprocedural death, or vascular death at 1 yr.

Currently, there are numerous uncontrolled registry-based studies investigating different stents and emboli protection devices as well as two randomized trials. The NIH-funded Carotid Revascularization: Endarterectomy vs Stent Trial (CREST) is randomizing patients with symptomatic >50% extracranial carotid stenosis who are eligible for either procedure. The Stenting and Angioplasty for Patients at High Risk for Endarterectomy (SAPPHIRE) trial employs both a randomized trial and registry approach to patients with symptomatic >50% and asymptomatic >80% extracranial carotid stenosis who are at high risk for treatment. Antiplatelet and antithrombotic regimens vary, but many specify aspirin 325 mg and clopidogrel 75 mg for 72 h before and 4 wk after the procedure and periprocedural heparin therapy titrated to a target activated clotting time (ACT) of 200–250 s.

The safety of adding GPIIb/IIIa receptor inhibition in carotid stenting has been explored in several case series with no bleeding complications reported in bolus and infusion regimens of 10 patients receiving eptifibatide and 15 patients receiving abciximab for carotid interventions (35,36). In the largest series, 151 patients at high risk for carotid endarterectomy underwent carotid angioplasty and stenting with heparin, aspirin, and ticlopidine or clopidogrel (37). The initial 23 patients served as historical controls for the subsequent 128 patients (134 arteries), who also received an abciximab bolus and 12 h infusion. In the abciximab group, one patient developed a minor hemorrhagic transformation of a prior stroke 4 d after the procedure. In the control group, 1 patient died of an intracranial hemorrhage, but this occurred in the setting of intraarterial thrombolysis for a procedural embolic stroke. Although the numbers are small, no other significant bleeding complications were reported with this approach.

Endovascular techniques now offer a therapeutic option for patients with intracranial atherosclerosis Angioplasty, with or without stenting, of intracranial carotid, middle cerebral artery, or vertebrobasilar stenoses with variable antithrombotic regimens has been described in multiple case reports and small series to be now technically feasible in >80% but associated with periprocedural risks of 5–15%. The largest reported prospective registry of endovascular therapy of intracranial atherosclerosis included 42 patients with symptomatic intracranial stenosis, primarily involving the internal carotid or basilar arteries, and 19 patients with vertebral ostial stenosis. All received combination antiplatelet therapy with GPIIb/IIIa inhibitors and heparin at the discretion of the investigator. They reported a 6.6% risk of stroke at 30 d, restenosis of >50% at 6 mo, and 11.5% risk of ipsilateral stroke at 1 yr (38). In a series of eight patients with stent-assisted angioplasty

Table 2
Hemorrhagic Stroke Complicating Therapy of Acute Ischemic Stroke

	Increased absolute risk (%)		
Therapy	Symptomatic	Asymptomatic	Reference
Aspirin 160–300 mg/d (IST, CAST)	0.1–0.2		40,41
Heparin 10,000–25,000 U/d (IST)	0.8		41
IV tPA (NINDS protocol)	5.8		22
IA prourokinase (PROACT-2)	8.4		45
Abciximab (AbESTT pilot)	0	13	47

of symptomatic vertebrobasilar stenosis with abciximab bolus and 12 h infusion, heparin during the procedure, aspirin and ticlopidine or clopidogrel, one patient died after a dissection-related subarachnoid hemorrhage, and two had other serious bleeding *(39)*.

Hemorrhagic Stroke Complicating Therapy for Acute Ischemic Stroke

When administered within 48 h of acute AIS, 160–300 mg of aspirin significantly reduced absolute recurrent ischemic stroke by 0.5–1.1% and early mortality by 0.5–0.6% while increasing the risk of symptomatic hemorrhagic stroke by a nonsignificant 0.1–0.2% (Table 2) *(40,41)*. The International Stroke Trial also evaluated combination therapy with subcutaneous heparin (10,000 or 25,000 U/d) with or without aspirin 300 mg/d, and placebo. Heparin was not effective in reducing overall stroke, as the early reduction in recurrent ischemic stroke in patients allocated to heparin compared with those without heparin (2.9% vs 3.8%) was negated by a delayed increase in the rate of hemorrhagic stroke (1.2% vs 0.4%) *(41)*.

Thrombolysis for AIS is complicated by an increased risk of intracranial hemorrhage related to petechial or confluent hemorrhagic transformation of the infarct. The NINDS trial of weight-adjusted tissue plasminogen activator (tPA) given intravenously within 3 h of symptom onset, without any concomitant antiplatelet or antithrombotic agent for the first 24 h, is the only Food and Drug Administration-approved thrombolytic regimen for AIS *(12)*. Thrombolytic therapy significantly increased the rate of excellent neurologic outcome at 3 mo by an absolute 11–13%, but the risk of symptomatic and fatal intracranial hemorrhage was increased 10-fold from 0.6 to 6.4%, and mortality was unchanged. However, the benefit-to-risk ratio was marginal for patients with severe stroke (NIH Stroke Scale Score >22) or over 77 yr of age, who were at increased risk for intracranial hemorrhage. Excessive rates of symptomatic and fatal intracranial hemorrhage in numerous trials have thus far resulted in the abandonment of streptokinase, streptokinase with aspirin, and tPA after 3 h of symptom onset but agents with greater fibrin selectivity, like desmetoplase, are in Phase I trials *(42–44)*.

Intraarterial thrombolysis for AIS owing to middle cerebral artery occlusion was studied in a randomized controlled trial of 180 patients who received heparin, 2000 U bolus and 500 U/h for 4 h, with or without prourokinase within 6 h of symptom onset *(46)*. No adjunctive antithrombotic agents were then allowed until after 24 h of treatment. Thrombolytic therapy increased the chance of a good neurologic outcome by an absolute 15%, but the absolute risk of symptomatic intracranial hemorrhage was increased 8.3% over heparin alone at 24 h. At 10 d, however, evidence of any intracranial bleeding was present in 50.4%

of those who received prourokinase and heparin vs 44.1% with heparin alone, and overall mortality was unchanged.

Risk factors for intracranial hemorrhage after thrombolysis for AIS include the presence of early infarct signs on brain computed tomography (CT), stroke severity, hyperglycemia at time of presentation, history of diabetes, advanced age, and use of high-dose heparin *(47)*.

Given the limited applicability of thrombolysis in AIS dictated by the narrow margin between reperfusion benefit and hemorrhagic risk, it is hoped that GPIIb/IIIa receptor antagonists, alone or with reduced doses of thrombolytics, can expand therapy to more patients with AIS and beyond the 3-h window. Abciximab was demonstrated to be safe when administered within 24 h of AIS in a small, randomized, double-blind, placebo-controlled, dose-escalation trial. No patient had a major intracranial hemorrhage. Asymptomatic parenchymal hemorrhagic transformation was noted on surveillance brain CT scans in 7% (4/54) of abciximab-treated patients and 5% (1/20) of controls at 24–36 h. An additional six abciximab-treated patients had an asymptomatic hemorrhagic transformation during follow-up for a total rate of 18% *(48)*. Anecdotally, however, symptomatic parenchymal hemorrhagic transformation can complicate abciximab therapy after acute ischemic stroke (Figs. 1 and 2). Safety and perhaps efficacy data will be available in late 2002 with the results of AbESTT, the follow-up randomized, placebo-controlled clinical trial of abciximab in AIS of <6 h duration.

Asymptomatic hemorrhagic transformation was also noted in one-third of 18 patients who received weight-adjusted intravenous tirofiban for a mean period of 46 h in the setting of progressing ischemic stroke *(48)*.

Abciximab has been used in several case reports as rescue therapy in the treatment of acute ischemic stroke failing other chemical and mechanical reperfusion strategies as well as for reocclusion after initially successful cerebral reperfusion (Figs. 3–8) *(50,51)*. Of a consecutive series of 49 patients evaluated for intraarterial thrombolysis, 37 patients were treated with intraarterial tPA, and 24 of them also received eptifibatide in a reduced regimen of 90 µg/kg bolus and 0.5–2.0 µg/kg/min infusion. The small series suggested that the combination showed a trend toward improved reperfusion (58% vs 31% TIMI 2+3) and could rescue resistant reocclusion without an apparent increase in the rate of symptomatic or asymptomatic intracranial bleeding *(52)*.

CONCLUSIONS

The challenge of treating coronary artery disease and stroke is often one of maximizing reperfusion while limiting hemorrhagic complications. The risk of ischemic stoke, largely cardioembolic in nature, is lessened with those strategies that improve myocardial outcome while bleeding complications, including hemorrhagic stroke from transformation of ischemic stroke or primary intracranial hemorrhages, limit the aggressiveness of the therapies. This complex interplay is illustrated in the shifting risks of stroke subtypes since the introduction of thrombolysis for AMI.

GPIIb/IIIa receptor inhibitors in combination with aspirin and heparin and even reduced-dose thrombolytics for coronary interventions appear to be safe, with low rates of stroke. However, the reported rare cases of intracranial hemorrhage are similar to those seen with a coagulopathy. At present, there are no reliable means of prospectively identifying those patients at increased risk for intracranial hemorrhage, although amyloid angiopathy, common in the very elderly and cognitively impaired, is probably a major determinant (Fig. 9).

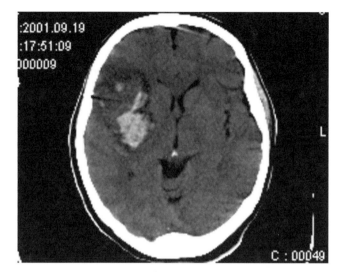

Fig. 1. Hemorrhagic transformation of acute ischemic stroke associated with abciximab therapy.

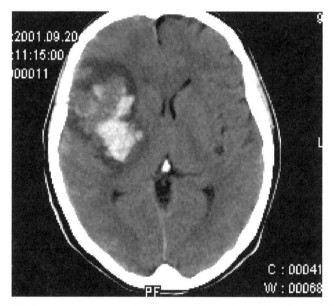

Fig. 2. Expansion of hemorrhagic transformation within the first 18 h.

Although hemorrhagic transformation of acute ischemic stroke occurs in the absence of any antiplatelet, anthrombotic, or antifibrinolytic therapy, it is progressively enhanced with the aggressiveness of such therapies and reduces the risk-to-benefit ratio to a critical margin. Interventional neurologists will continue to follow in the footsteps of the interventional cardiologists in considering data on stroke risk from large clinical trials of patients with heart disease and translating them cautiously to smaller clinical trials of patients with threatened or evolving ischemic stroke.

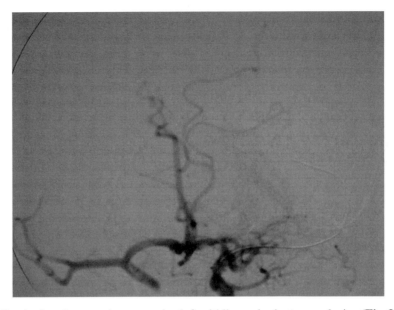

Figs. 3–8. Cerebral angiograms demonstrating left middle cerebral artery occlusion (**Fig. 3**) with partial reperfusion of perforating lenticulostriate vessels (left, **Fig. 4**; *see* below) and middle cerebral artery branches (right, **Fig. 4**) after intraarterial infusion of tPA; reocclusion occurred minutes later (**Fig. 5**; *see* opposite page). Reperfusion was finally established after intraarterial abciximab (**Fig. 6**; *see* opposite page and **Fig. 7**; *see* p. 420). Vessel patency was documented by CT angiography the following day (**Fig. 8**; *see* p. 420).

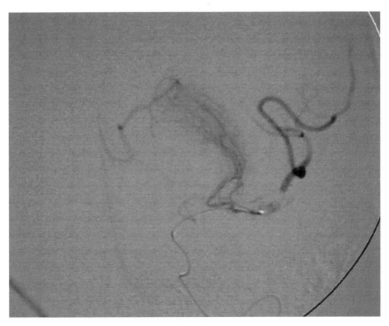

Fig. 4.

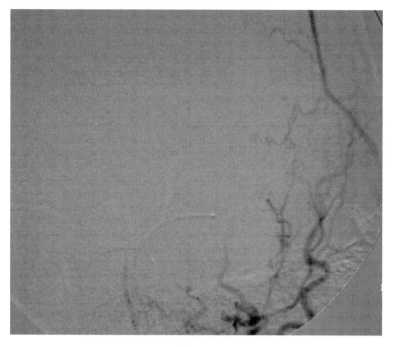

Fig. 5.

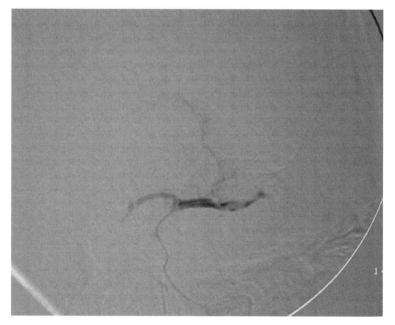

Fig. 6.

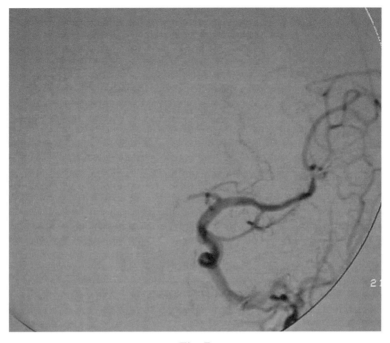

Fig. 7.

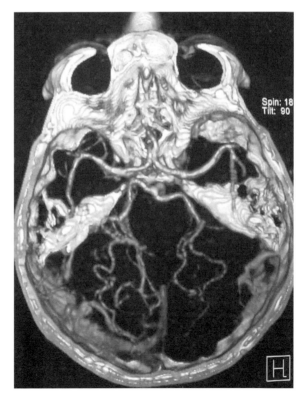

Fig. 8.

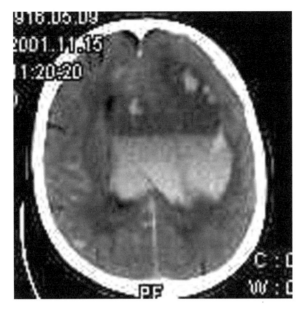

Fig. 9. Thrombolysis-related hemorrhagic stroke related to unsuspected underlying amyloid angiopathy.

REFERENCES

1. Longstreth WT, Litwin PE, Weaver WD. Myocardial infarction, thrombolytic therapy, and stroke. Stroke 1993;24:587–590.
2. Sloan MA, Price TR, Terrin ML, et al. Ischemic cerebral infarction after rt-PA and heparin therapy for acute myocardial infarction. The TIMI-II pilot and randomized clinical trial combined experience. Stroke 1997;28:1107–1114.
3. Mahaffey KW, Granger CB, Sloan MA, et al. Risk factors for in-hospital nonhemorrhagic stroke in patients with acute myocardial infarction treated with thrombolysis: results from GUSTO-I. Circulation 1998;97:757–764.
4. Gore JM, Granger CB, Simoons ML, et al. Stroke after thrombolysis. Mortality and functional outcomes in the GUSTO-I trial. Circulation 1995;92:2811-2818.
5. The GUSTO IIb Investigators. A comparison of recombinant hirudin with heparin for the treatment of acute coronary syndromes. N Engl J Med 1996;335:775–782.
6. Mahaffey KW, Harrington RA, Simoons ML, et al. Stroke in patients with acute coronary syndromes: incidence and outcomes in the Platelet Glycoprotein IIb/IIIa in Unstable Angina: Receptor Suppression Using Integrilin Therapy (PURSUIT) trial. Circulation 1999;99:2371–2377.
7. The TIMI IIIB Investigators. Effects of tissue plasminogen activator and a comparison of early invasive and conservative strategies in unstable angina and non-Q-wave myocardial infarction: results of the TIMI IIIB Trial. Circulation 1994;89:1545–1556.
8. Sila CA. Neurologic complications of vascular surgery. Neurol Clin North Am 1998;16:9–20.
9. Dawson DM, Fischer EG. Neurologic complications of cardiac catheterization. Neurology 1977;27: 496–497.
10. Kosmorsky G, Hanson MR, Tomsak RL. Neuro-ophthalmologic complications of cardiac catheterization. Neurology 1988;38:483–485.
11. Galbreath C, Salgado ED, Furlan AJ, Hollman J. Central nervous system complications of percutaneous transluminal coronary angioplasty. Stroke 1986;17:616–619.
12. Akkerhuis KM, Deckers JW, Lincoff AM, et al. Risk of stroke associated with abciximab among patients undergoing percutaneous coronary intervention. JAMA 2001;286:78–82.

13. The Gusto Investigators. An international randomized trial comparing four thrombolytic strategies for acute myocardial infarction. N Engl J Med 1993;329:673–682.
14. Babikian VL, Kase CS, Pessin MS, Norrving B, Gorelick PB. Intracerebral hemorrhage in stroke patients anticoagulated with heparin. Stroke 1989;20:1500–1503.
15. Cerebral Embolism Study Group. Cardiogenic stroke, early anticoagulation, and brain hemorrhage. Arch Intern Med 1987;147:636–639.
16. Shields RW Jr, Laureno R, Lachman T, Victor M. Anticoagulant-related hemorrhage in acute cerebral embolism. Stroke 1984;15:426–437.
17. Boersma E, Harrington RA, Moliterno DJ, et al. Platelet glycoprotein IIb/IIIa inhibitors in acute coronary syndromes: a meta-analysis of all major randomized clinical trials. Lancet 2002;359:189–198.
18. Gebel J, Sila CA, Sloan MA, et al. Thrombolysis-related intracranial hemorrhage. A radiographic analysis of 244 cases from the GUSTO-I trial with clinical correlation. Stroke 1998;29:563–569.
19. Vaitkus PT, Berlin JA, Schwartz JS, Barnathan ES. Stroke complicating acute myocardial infarction—a meta-analysis of risk modification by anticoagulation and thrombolytic therapy. Arch Intern Med 1992; 152:2020–2024.
20. Sloan MA, Sila CA, Mahaffey KW, et al. Prediction of 30-d mortality among patients with thrombolysis-related intracranial hemorrhage. Circulation 1998;14:1376–1382.
21. Widjicks EFM, Jack C. Intracerebral hemorrhage after fibrinolytic therapy for acute myocardial infarction. Stroke 1993;24:554–557.
22. Ohman EM, Kleiman NS, Gacioch G, et al. Combined accelerated tissue-plasminogen activator and platelet glycoprotein IIb/IIIa integrin receptor blockade with integrilin in acute myocardial infarction. Circulation 1997;95:846–854.
23. Topol EJ, for the GUSTO V Investigators. Reperfusion therapy for acute myocardial infarction with fibrinolytic therapy or combination reduced fibrinolytic therapy and platelet glycoprotein IIb/IIIa inhibition: the GUSTO V randomized trial. Lancet 2001;357:1898–1899.
24. The ASSENT-3 Investigators. Efficacy and safety of tenecteplase in combination with enoxaparin, abciximab, or unfractionated heparin: the ASSENT-3 randomised trial in acute myocardial infarction. Lancet 2001;358:605–613.
25. SoRelle R. SmithKline Beecham halts tests of lotrafiban, an oral glycoprotein IIb/IIIa inhibitor. Circulation 2001;103:E9001–E9002.
26. Hass WK, Easton JD, Adams HP, et al., for the Ticlopidine Aspirin Stroke Study Group. A randomized trial comparing ticlopidine hydrochloride with aspirin for the prevention of stroke in high risk patients. N Engl J Med 1989;321:501–507.
27. CAPRIE Steering Committee. A randomized, blinded, trial of clopidogrel versus aspirin in patients at risk of ischaemic events (CAPRIE). Lancet 1996;348:1329–1339.
28. Bennett CL, Weinberg PD, Rozenberg-Ben-Dror K, Yarnold PR, Kwaan HC, Green D. Thrombotic thrombocytopenic purpura associated with ticlopidine. A review of 60 cases. Ann Intern Med 1998;128: 541–544.
29. American-Canadian Co-operative Study Group. Persantin aspirin trial in cerebral ischemia. Part II. Endpoint results. Stroke 1983;16:406–415.
30. Bousser MG, Eschwege E, Hagenaah M, et al. AICLA controlled trial of aspirin and diypridamole in the secondary prevention of athero-thrombotic cerebral ischemia. Stroke 1983;14:5–14.
31. ESPS Group. European Stroke Prevention Study. Stroke 1990;21:1122–1130.
32. Diener HC, Cunha L, Forbes C, Sivenius J, Smets P, Lowenthal A. European Stroke Prevention Study 2. Dipyridamole and acetylsalicylic acid in the secondary prevention of stroke. J Neurol Sci 1996;143:1–13.
33. CAVATAS Investigators. Endovascular vs surgical treatment in patients with carotid stenosis in the Carotid and Vertebral Artery Transluminal Angioplasty Study: a randomized trial. Lancet 2001;357:1729–1737.
34. Alberts MJ (for the Publications Committee). Results of a multicenter prospective randomized trial of carotid artery stenting vs carotid endarterectomy. Stroke 2001;32:325 (abstract).
35. Qureshi AI, Ali Z, Suri MF, et al. Open-label phase I clinical study to assess the safety of intravenous eptifibatide in patients undergoing internal carotid artery angioplasty and stent placement. Neurosurgery 2001;48:998–1005.
36. Schneiderman J, Morag B, Gerniak A, et al. Abciximab in carotid stenting for postsurgical carotid restenosis: immediate results. J Endovasc Ther 2000;7:263–272.
37. Kapadia SR, Bajzer CT, Ziada KM, et al. Initial experience with platelet glycoprotein IIb/IIIa inhibition with abciximab during carotid stenting: a safe and effective adjunctive therapy. Stroke 2001;32: 2328–2332.

38. Hopkins LN for the SSYLVIA Trial Investigators, American Society of Interventional and Therapeutic Neuroradiology Meeting, February, 2002.

39. Rasmussen PA, Perl J, Barr JD, et al. Stent-assisted angioplasty of intracranial vertebrobasilar atherosclerosis: an initial experience. J Neurosurg 2000;92:771–778.

40. Chinese Acute Stroke Trial Collaborative Group. Randomised placebo-controlled trial of early aspirin use in 20,000 patients with acute ischemic stroke. Lancet 1997;349:1641–1649.

41. International Stroke Trial Collaborative Group. The International Stroke Trial (IST): a randomised trial of aspirin, subcutaneous heparin, both, or neither among 19,435 patients with acute ischemic stroke. Lancet 1997;349:1569–1581.

42. The National Institute of Neurological Disorders and Stroke rt-PA Stroke Study Group. Tissue plasminogen activator for acute ischemic stroke. N Engl J Med 1995;333:1581–1587.

43. Donnan GA, Davis SM, Chambers BR, et al. Streptokinase for acute ischemic stroke with relationship to time of administration. JAMA 1996;276:961–966.

44. The Multicentre Acute Stroke Trial-Europe Group. Thrombolytic therapy with streptokinase in acute ischemic stroke. N Engl J Med 1996;335:145–150.

45. Multicentre Acute Stroke Trial—Italy (MAST-I) Group. Randomised controlled trial of streptokinase, aspirin, and combination of both in treatment of acute ischemic stroke. Lancet 1995;346:1509–1514.

46. delZoppo GJ, Higashida RT, Furlan AJ, Pessin MS, Rowley HA, Gent M. Proact: a phase II randomized trial of recombinant pro-urokinase by direct arterial delivery in acute middle cerebral artery stroke. Stroke 1998;29:4–11.

47. Kase CS, Furlan AJ, Wechsler LR, et al. Symptomatic intracerebral hemorrhage after intra-arterial thrombolysis with prourokinase in acute ischemic stroke: the PROACT II trial. Neurology 2001;57:1603–1610.

48. Abciximab in Ischemic Stroke Investigators. Abciximab in acute ischemic stroke: a randomized, double-blind, placebo-controlled, dose-escalation study. Stroke 2000;31:2526–2527.

49. Junghans U, Seitz RJ, Aulich A, Freund HJ, Siebler M. Bleeding risk of tirofiban, a nonpeptide GP IIb/IIIa platelet receptor antagonist in progressive stroke: an open pilot study. Cerebrovasc Dis 2001;12:308–312.

50. Lee KY, Heo JH, Lee SI, Yoon PH. Rescue treatment with abciximab in acute ischemic stroke. Neurology 2001;56:1585–1587.

51. Wallace RC, Furlan AJ, Moliterno DJ, Stevens GHJ, Masaryk TJ, Perl J. Basilar artery rethrombosis: successful treatment with platelet glycoprotein IIb/IIIa receptor inhibitor. AJNR 1997;18:1257–1260.

52. Koroshetz W, et al. Intra-arterial thrombolysis: combined GIIb/IIIa antagonist with rt-PA. Stroke 2002 (abstract).

21 Evolution of Drug Development in Evidence-Based Medicine

Summary and the Future

David E. Kandzari, MD,
David F. Kong, MD,
and Robert M. Califf, MD

CONTENTS

INTRODUCTION
PATHOPHYSIOLOGY OF UNSTABLE ATHEROSCLEROTIC PLAQUES
    AND THERAPEUTIC TARGETS
CONTEMPORARY CLINICAL TRIALS OF GPIIb/IIIa INHIBITION IN ACS
PROGRESSION AND REGRESSION: DEVELOPMENT AND FAILURE
    OF ORAL GPIIb/IIIa INHIBITORS
ALTERNATIVE ANTIPLATELET AND ANTITHROMBOTIC THERAPIES
FUTURE DIRECTIONS
CONCLUSIONS
REFERENCES

INTRODUCTION

Clinical medicine has entered a new era, characterized by dramatic advances in the understanding of disease biology and a new focus on the organization of medical practice. Identification of receptors, agonists, and antagonists permits development of therapies targeted against specific biologic processes. Development of new therapies has consumed substantial resources from government and industry. The estimated cost to develop and market a new prescription drug averaged $802 million for the year 2000, three times higher than estimates from a decade ago *(1)*. Despite these daunting costs, the world will accrue long-standing benefit from these huge investments in biomedical research as the number of medical treatments for chronic diseases increases exponentially.

Shortly after investigators clarified the role of the glycoprotein (GP) IIb/IIIa receptor in thrombosis, they rapidly turned their attention from its physiologic function to its therapeutic potential. As a result, several promising molecular targets have been identified.

From: *Contemporary Cardiology: Platelet Glycoprotein IIb/IIIa*
Inhibitors in Cardiovascular Disease, 2nd Edition
Edited by: A. M. Lincoff © Humana Press Inc., Totowa, NJ

Table 1
Pharmacologic Properties
of Food and Drug Administration (FDA)-Approved Platelet GPIIb/IIIa Inhibitors

	Abciximab	Eptifibatide	Tirofiban
Chemical nature	Antibody	Peptide	Nonpeptide
Size	Large (48 kDa)	Small (1 kDa)	Small (<1 kDa)
Onset of effect	Rapid	Rapid	Rapid
Reversibility	Slow	Rapid	Rapid
Binds other integrins?	Yes	No	No
Antibody response?	Yes	No	No

Recent discoveries have provided insight into the influence of genetic variants on the development of atherosclerotic disease and arterial thrombosis, enhancing our understanding of ischemic heart disease. Unprecedented efforts are under way to identify variations of single nucleotides and complex polymorphisms. Ongoing translational research seeks to establish the genotypic and phenotypic bases for ischemic heart disease susceptibility and drug response. Many therapeutic agents will be derived from the Human Genome Project and computer simulations of receptors, genes, and gene products. Sophisticated receptor models allow synthesis of agonists and antagonists even before their biologic functions are known. Before clinicians and scientists are led astray by technology that outpaces the application of proven therapies, however, the GPIIb/IIIa receptor experience should serve as an educational template for this more complex future.

The continuing rigorous evaluation of the safety and efficacy of GPIIb/IIIa inhibitors reflects the clinical and scientific communities' changing approach to new cardiovascular therapies. Before therapies such as fibrinolytics or GPIIb/IIIa inhibitors were scrutinized in large, randomized clinical trials, health care providers would have embraced any major therapeutic advance after studies of a relatively few patients and would have eagerly applied it to various indications. Today, regulatory authorities apply immensely higher standards for proof of safety and efficacy, requiring definitive evidence that a new agent does not cause potential harm in trials involving thousands of patients. Furthermore, health care systems are concerned about not only the potential benefits of a new therapy but also the incremental costs. Compared with aspirin, possibly the most effective and yet inexpensive therapy for ischemic heart disease, these new antiplatelet therapies face a challenging standard. As an example, although investigations of GPIIb/IIIa inhibitors now have randomized over 60,000 patients, only a few agents have been approved and marketed (Table 1).

PATHOPHYSIOLOGY OF UNSTABLE
ATHEROSCLEROTIC PLAQUES AND THERAPEUTIC TARGETS

Our understanding of the pathophysiology, therapeutic applications, and clinical outcomes of patients with acute coronary syndromes (ACS) continues to evolve. Envisaging the future of GPIIb/IIIa antagonists requires an understanding of the rationale for their application and the measures of their clinical effects.

Role of the GPIIb/IIIa Receptor in ACS

The pathophysiology of ACS is defined by atherosclerotic plaque rupture, platelet activation, and resultant thrombus formation *(2,3)*. In atherosclerotic coronary vessels, plaque rupture exposes the subendothelium, precipitating clot formation. Platelets first adhere to the subendothelium by binding to class I glycoproteins. The presence of thrombin or other agonists such as adenosine or epinephrine activates platelets, causing a conformational change in the GPIIb/IIIa receptor and platelet degranulation. These changes cause the release of serotonin, adenosine diphosphate (ADP), and other vasoactive substances, which stimulate further platelet activation and recruitment. The conformational change in the GPIIb/IIIa receptor allows crossbinding of fibrinogen and von Willebrand factor with other platelets, resulting in platelet aggregation and thrombus formation. The associated clinical presentation depends on whether the clot is occlusive, subocclusive, or nonobstructive and is influenced by collateral flow, baseline left ventricular function, amount of jeopardized myocardium, diabetes, and other factors. Patients therefore may have severe angina with ST-segment elevation, mild angina, or no symptoms at all.

The role of the GPIIb/IIIa receptor as the final common pathway for platelet aggregation made its inhibition a pivotal transition from bench work to clinical practice *(4,5)*. In 1983, Coller and coworkers *(6)* first reported a murine monoclonal antibody that blocked this receptor. These findings led to the engineering of a chimeric monoclonal antibody, abciximab (ReoPro™), which was first studied in patients undergoing high-risk percutaneous coronary intervention (PCI) (Table 1) *(7)*. Since then, several other inhibitors that mimic the arginine-glycine-aspartic acid (RGD) binding sequences of the GPIIb/IIIa receptor have undergone extensive clinical investigation. These include the synthetic cyclic heptapeptide eptifibatide (Integrilin®) as well as peptidomimetics such as tirofiban (Aggrastat®) and lamifiban (Ro 44-9883) (Table 1). Despite differences in pharmacodynamics, the common mechanism of these drugs is to inhibit platelet aggregation by occupying the fibrinogen binding site.

CONTEMPORARY
CLINICAL TRIALS OF GPIIb/IIIa INHIBITION IN ACS

GPIIb/IIIa Inhibition in PCI

For the past 30 years, the animal model for atherosclerosis was predicated on mechanical abrasion of the arterial endothelial surface, coupled with a high-cholesterol diet. Balloon dilation and mechanical debulking cause similar biologic reactions, creating a human model for cellular proliferation and thrombotic vascular occlusion. Platelets often provide a protective barrier in response to vascular injury, but when this process becomes excessive, vessel occlusion or embolism can result. Therefore, the acute thrombotic reaction to PCI creates an ideal opportunity for platelet inhibitors. Prevention of platelet aggregation during and after intentional vessel injury reduced clinical complications by antagonizing a molecular target.

In the past decade, advances in interventional drugs and devices have improved outcomes significantly for patients undergoing elective PCI. Stenting has reduced the incidence of abrupt vessel closure to <0.5% and the need for repeat revascularization by 30–50% *(8–10)*. In addition, several randomized trials have shown that GPIIb/IIIa inhi-

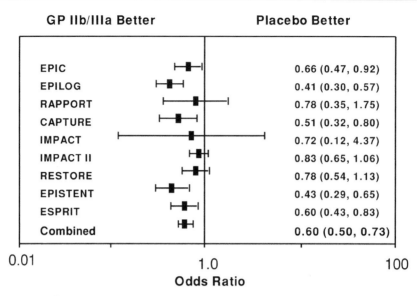

Fig. 1. Odds ratios for death or MI at 30 d with GPIIb/IIIa inhibition vs placebo; all published trials in routine PCI (12–16).

bition during elective PCI reduces the composite incidence of death, nonfatal myocardial infarction (MI), or target-vessel revascularization (TVR) at both 30 d and 6 mo *(7,11)*. The synergy between PCI and GPIIb/IIIa blockade is especially prominent for patients with ACS without ST-segment elevation, although similar clinical benefit has been observed for patients with acute ST-elevation MI.

GPIIb/IIIa INHIBITION AND PCI IN NON-ST-ELEVATION ACS

The application of GPIIb/IIIa inhibitors as adjuncts to PCI has been modeled after an initial series of large, randomized, placebo-controlled trials (Fig. 1) *(12–16)*. A systematic overview of these trials has shown a highly significant reduction in the endpoint of death, nonfatal MI, or urgent revascularization at 48–96 h ($p < 0.001$), 30 d ($p < 0.001$), and 6 mo ($p < 0.003$) *(11)*. Furthermore, the addition of GPIIb/IIIa antagonists to coronary stenting is supported by the significant reduction in 30-d death, MI, or urgent revascularization observed in the EPISTENT *(17)* trial (5.3% in the stent-plus-abciximab group versus 10.8% in the stent-only group; $p < 0.001$) (*see* Appendix for definitions of all trials).

The recent ESPRIT trial not only confirmed that treatment with a GPIIb/IIIa inhibitor before stenting was the superior approach but also showed improved outcomes among low-risk patients treated with more modern stenting techniques, thereby broadening the applicability of the therapy to nearly all patients undergoing PCI *(18)*. In the ESPRIT trial, the control arm was "rescue" or "bailout" GPIIb/IIIa blockade therapy. Among 2064 patients undergoing elective (nonurgent) angioplasty with stenting, treatment with double-bolus eptifibatide was associated with a 37% relative reduction in the composite rate of death, MI, urgent revascularization, or "bailout" GPIIb/IIIa inhibitor therapy at 48 h ($p = 0.0015$). The benefit of preprocedural eptifibatide was consistent across all components of the primary endpoint and was maintained at 30-d and 6-mo follow-up *(18,19)*. At 1 yr, the eptifibatide group showed continued benefit, with a significantly lower rate of death or MI (8.0% vs 12.4% with placebo; $p = 0.001$) (20).

For patients undergoing PCI, a large portion of the benefit of GPIIb/IIIa inhibition reflects a reduction in periprocedural MI. New angiographic techniques, including the Thrombolysis In Myocardial Infarction (TIMI) myocardial blush score, and noninvasive diagnostic tests (e.g., continuous ST-segment monitoring) have shown that epicardial TIMI grade 3 flow may be an incomplete measure of reperfusion success (21). Depending on the clinical setting, up to 40% of patients develop myocardial necrosis with elevation of creatine kinase-MB (CK-MB). Although most of these events can be identified by angiography, a substantial number of "angiographically silent" events occur at the cellular level of myocardial perfusion. Despite epicardial vessel patency, disrupted microvascular function and inadequate myocardial perfusion often result from thromboembolic debris. Use of balloon occlusion and filter devices to prevent distal embolization during high-risk PCI has reduced the occurrence of periprocedural MI in recent studies. To date, these devices have not been systematically compared with GPIIb/IIIa inhibition. Although elevated cardiac enzymes clearly reflect myocardial injury and necrosis, the clinical significance of periprocedural myocardial necrosis has been debated. The relative contribution of myocardial necrosis to mortality has been difficult to discern, given the confounding fact that patients with more severe disease are more likely to have such necrosis.

Collectively, these investigations have shown markedly improved outcomes with a variety of GPIIb/IIIa inhibitors in thousands of patients undergoing PCI and in an array of clinical settings. Whether GPIIb/IIIa inhibitors improve survival after elective intervention remains a topic of great debate (22), although the inability of GPIIb/IIIa inhibition to influence restenosis appears more certain. By 6 mo after initial PCI, restenosis, unimpeded by GPIIb/IIIa inhibition, accounts for most repeat procedures. Thus, clinical events accrue equally after 6 mo independent of earlier GPIIb/IIIa inhibition, and the relative difference between groups diminishes (23–25).

Further uncertainty exists about the selection of adjunctive GPIIb/IIIa inhibition in PCI. Despite a lack of interest from industry, additional comparative studies are needed. In the only comparative trial of GPIIb/IIIa inhibition in PCI to date, the TARGET study showed a significant 26% reduction in the composite of death, MI, or urgent revascularization at 30 d with abciximab compared with tirofiban (6.01% vs 7.55%; $p = 0.038$) (Fig. 2) (26). Although this difference deserves further exploration, one potential explanation is inadequate platelet inhibition with the tirofiban regimen used (see Dosing and Intensity of Platelet Inhibition section). Other continuing uncertainties for GPIIb/IIIa inhibitors in PCI include optimal dosing and monitoring (27), immunogenicity (28), and selection of patients based on underlying risk, to optimize the economic outlay relative to benefits achieved (29).

GPIIb/IIIa Inhibition and PCI in ST-Elevation MI

Recent trials have established evidence supporting GPIIb/IIIa inhibition for acute ST-segment elevation MI. Given the abundant platelet-rich thrombus present in almost all patients with acute MI, it is intuitive that these agents might be effective in this syndrome. Furthermore, a "reperfusion ceiling" has been reached, given that no more than 55% of patients achieve TIMI grade 3 flow after fibrinolytic monotherapy (Fig. 3). Addition of GPIIb/IIIa inhibition to PCI for ST-elevation MI has substantially reduced recurrent ischemic events and improved early survival, ventricular function, and vessel patency.

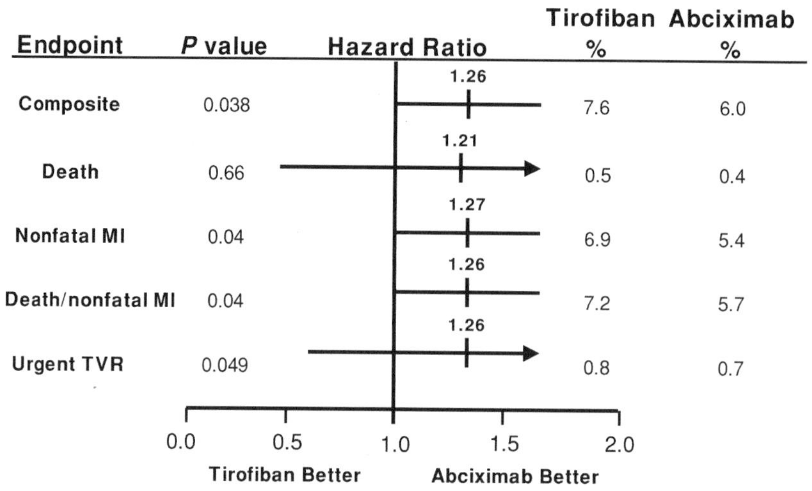

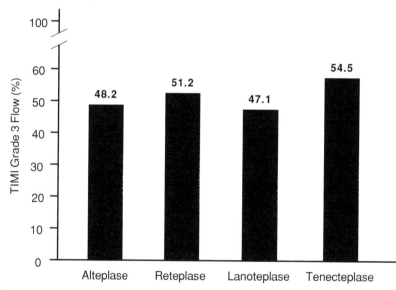

Endpoint
P value
Hazard Ratio
Tirofiban %
Abciximab %
Composite
0.038
1.26
7.6
6.0
Death
0.66
1.21
0.5
0.4
Nonfatal MI
0.04
1.27
6.9
5.4
Death/nonfatal MI
0.04
1.26
7.2
5.7
Urgent TVR
0.049
1.26
0.8
0.7
0.0
0.5
1.0
1.5
2.0
Tirofiban Better
Abciximab Better

Fig. 2. Hazard ratios for 30-d clinical endpoints with tirofiban vs placebo in the TARGET trial. MI, myocardial infarction; TVR, target vessel revascularization. (From ref. *26*, with permission.) Copyright ©2001 Massachusetts Medical Society. All rights reserved.

TIMI Grade 3 Flow (%)
100
60
50
40
30
20
10
0
48.2
51.2
47.1
54.5
Alteplase
Reteplase
Lanoteplase
Tenecteplase

Fig. 3. Sixty-minute angiographic TIMI grade 3 flow rates with contemporary fibrinolytic agents in patients with acute MI *(44–46)*.

In the RAPPORT trial, patients with acute MI given abciximab before primary angioplasty had a >70% relative reduction in the primary endpoint of death, reinfarction, or revascularization (5.6% vs 11.2% at 30 d; $p = 0.03$) *(30)*. In the single-center, open-label, randomized STOP-AMI trial, the combination of stenting plus abciximab was shown to enhance myocardial salvage and markedly improve event-free survival at 30 d and 1 yr compared with accelerated alteplase *(31)*. These investigators also explored the benefits of adding abciximab to early stenting in MI in the ISAR-2 trial *(32)*. In that study, 200 patients within 48 h of onset of acute MI in whom primary or rescue stenting was planned were randomized to receive a bolus and 12-h infusion of abciximab, or control. Patients

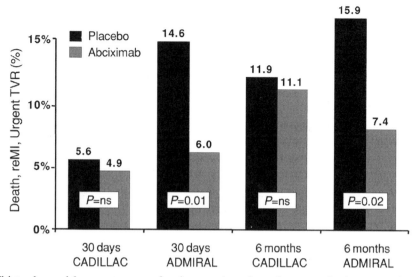

Fig. 4. Thirty-day and 6-mo outcomes of patients undergoing primary angioplasty, stenting, or both in the CADILLAC (33) and ADMIRAL (34) trials. reMI, reinfarction; TVR, target vessel revascularization.

treated with abciximab had a lower composite rate of in-hospital death, reinfarction, or urgent TVR (9.2% vs 2.0%; $p < 0.05$). Regional wall motion, global left ventricular function, and peak coronary blood flow velocity by Doppler angiography were better in abciximab-treated patients, consistent with improved distal microcirculatory function, presumably owing to reduced distal thromboemboli or capillary plugging. The rate of clinical events or angiographic restenosis did not differ at 6 mo, however (24).

The ADMIRAL study showed that abciximab was associated with a higher rate of early TIMI grade 3 flow (95.1% vs 86.7% for placebo, $p = 0.04$), greater left ventricular ejection fractions (57.0 ± 10.4% vs 53.9 ± 10.4%; $p < 0.05$), and a significantly lower rate of the primary composite endpoint of death, reinfarction, and urgent TVR at 30 d after enrollment (14.6% vs 6.0%; $p = 0.01$; Fig. 4) (33). In the CADILLAC trial (Fig. 4), 2081 patients with acute ST-segment elevation MI were randomized to receive one of four treatment strategies: (1) balloon angioplasty alone, (2) balloon angioplasty plus abciximab, (3) stenting alone, or (4) stenting plus abciximab (34). Although TIMI grade 3 flow was not significantly improved in the abciximab group compared with the stenting-alone group, abciximab administration was associated with significant reductions in recurrent ischemia, subacute thrombosis, and length of hospitalization.

Facilitated Fibrinolysis: GPIIb/IIIa Inhibitors in ST-Elevation MI

In addition to their antiplatelet effects, GPIIb/IIIa inhibitors also augment intrinsic fibrinolysis, creating a dual rationale for their application in acute MI. GPIIb/IIIa inhibitors independently exhibit some intrinsic clot-dissolving activity (35). Early animal studies showed the benefit of combining GPIIb/IIIa blockade with heparin and fibrinolytic therapy in acute coronary occlusion (36,37). Theoretical advantages of "facilitated fibrinolysis" include a reduction in plasminogen activator-mediated platelet aggregability, earlier infarct-vessel patency, increased safety, and less reocclusion.

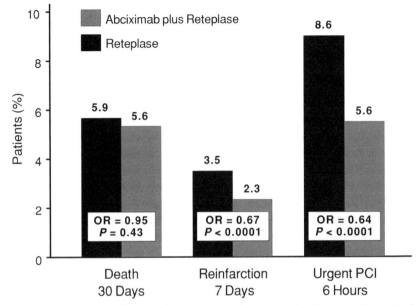

Fig. 5. Death and ischemic complications in patients receiving abciximab or reteplase plus abciximab for acute MI in the GUSTO V trial *(45)*. PCI, percutaneous coronary intervention.

Contemporary trials combining GPIIb/IIIa blockade with reduced-dose fibrinolytic therapy have shown a higher rate of TIMI grade 3 flow with acceptable bleeding risk *(38–43)*. In the ASSENT-3 trial, two new therapies were compared with unfractionated heparin and full-dose fibrinolytic therapy *(44)*. The experimental arms consisted of (1) low-molecular-weight heparin (enoxaparin) plus full-dose tenecteplase and (2) reduced-dose tenecteplase, abciximab, and unfractionated heparin. Among 6095 patients, the incidence of 30-d mortality, in-hospital reinfarction, or in-hospital recurrent ischemia was 11.2% in the enoxaparin group, 11.4% in the abciximab group, and 15.4% in the full-dose tenecteplase plus unfractionated heparin group (*p* = 0.0001).

In the largest trial of "facilitated fibrinolysis" to date, the GUSTO-V study compared standard-dose reteplase alone with half-dose reteplase plus full-dose abciximab in 16,588 patients with acute MI (Fig. 5) *(45)*. For the primary endpoint of 30-d survival, combined treatment with reteplase and abciximab offered no significant advantage over reteplase alone (5.9% with reteplase vs 5.6% with combined therapy; *p* = 0.43). Combination therapy was associated with fewer nonfatal ischemic complications (28.6% vs 31.7% for any complication; *p* < 0.0001) but also significantly greater bleeding complications (4.6% vs 2.3%; *p* < 0.0001 for moderate and severe nonintracranial bleeding). The rate of stroke (both ischemic and hemorrhagic) did not differ significantly between the groups. In a subgroup analysis, elderly patients receiving combination therapy tended to have more intracranial hemorrhages (2.1% with combination therapy vs 1.1% with alteplase alone; *p* = 0.069) compared with younger patients. The INTRO-AMI trial likewise showed a 3% intracranial hemorrhage rate among patients receiving the higher-dose eptifibatide regimen *(46)*. Before combination therapy is adopted into routine clinical practice, the reduction in post-MI complications must be balanced against the increased risk of bleeding, complexity of dosing, and potentially higher costs.

GPIIb/IIIa Inhibition in Non-ST Elevation ACS

In the United States, non-ST-elevation (NSTE) ACS remains a leading cause of cardio-vascular-related hospitalizations, accounting for more than 750,000 annual admissions *(47)*. More than one-third of admissions for acute MI are related to NSTE infarctions *(48)*. Although NSTE-ACS manifests as heterogeneous combinations of clinical symptoms, electrocardiographic changes, and biochemical markers of myocardial injury, treatment remains directed at the common underlying event of platelet activation and thrombus formation.

In the past decade, patients with NSTE-ACS were at substantial risk for adverse clinical outcome events even after intensive in-hospital treatment. Among such patients enrolled in the TIMI-IIIB trial, 6.2% died or had an MI by 42 d, and more than half required revascularization *(49)*. In addition, in the GUSTO-IIb study, 9.8% of patients had an MI or died within 30 d *(50)*.

The substantial benefit with adjunctive GPIIb/IIIa blockade for PCI has been established for several years. More recently, the importance of GPIIb/IIIa antagonism for patients presenting with ACS has also become clear. Unlike coronary intervention, in which the presence of coronary artery disease and the timing of intentional intimal injury are both known, the broad treatment of patients presenting with chest pain symptoms is less certain. Unstable angina remains a clinical diagnosis, relying on patient symptoms that may be atypical and electrocardiographic changes and serum cardiac markers that may be inconsistent. Extending the application of GPIIb/IIIa inhibitors to patients based on imprecise initial symptoms may not provide the same benefit as administration before PCI of a known coronary lesion. Despite these challenges, large randomized trials have shown the efficacy of GPIIb/IIIa antagonists for patients with NSTE-ACS (Fig. 6).

The PRISM trial, the first large trial of GPIIb/IIIa inhibitors, randomly assigned 3232 patients with ACS to intravenous tirofiban or heparin for 48 h *(51)*. At 48 h, the primary composite endpoint of death, MI, or refractory ischemia was reduced in the tirofiban group (3.8% vs 5.9%; $p = 0.014$). This benefit did not persist at 30 d, however (12.8% vs 13.9%; $p = $ ns) despite an unexpected, significant reduction in mortality (2.3% vs 3.6%; $p = 0.02$). Among troponin I-positive patients, treatment with tirofiban was also associated with significant reductions in the composite of death or MI and length of hospitalization compared with heparin treatment alone *(46)*.

The PRISM-PLUS trial enrolled 1915 high-risk patients with ACS to test tirofiban as part of a comprehensive strategy of standard therapy with heparin and aspirin and the selective use of PCI *(52)*. As part of the study design, PRISM-PLUS examined an aggressive strategy with angiography performed in 90% of patients and revascularization in 54%, typically after at least 48 h of study drug treatment. Patients received heparin, tirofiban plus heparin, or tirofiban alone for a mean of 71 h. Notably, the tirofiban monotherapy arm was stopped prematurely because of excess mortality at 7 d (4.6% vs 1.1%; $p = 0.012$). At 7 d, tirofiban plus heparin reduced the primary composite endpoint of death, MI, or refractory angina compared with heparin alone (12.9% vs 17.9%; $p = 0.004$). The benefit of combination therapy persisted at both 30 d (22.3% vs 18.5%; $p = 0.03$) and 6 mo (32.1% vs 27.7%; $p = 0.02$).

The PARAGON-A *(53)* trial was a dose-ranging pilot study of lamifiban in NSTE-ACS. Nearly 2300 patients were treated with one of two doses of lamifiban, with or without heparin, or heparin alone. All patients received aspirin. At 30 d, the composite endpoint of

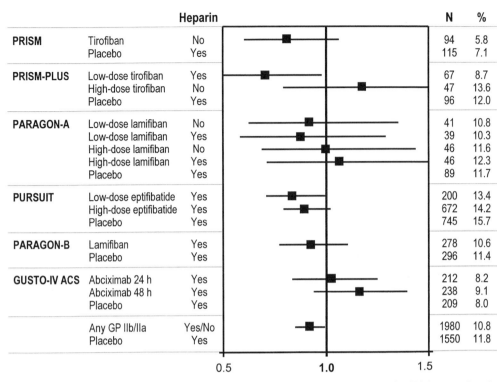

	Heparin			N	%
PRISM	Tirofiban	No		94	5.8
	Placebo	Yes		115	7.1
PRISM-PLUS	Low-dose tirofiban	Yes		67	8.7
	High-dose tirofiban	No		47	13.6
	Placebo	Yes		96	12.0
PARAGON-A	Low-dose lamifiban	No		41	10.8
	Low-dose lamifiban	Yes		39	10.3
	High-dose lamifiban	No		46	11.6
	High-dose lamifiban	Yes		46	12.3
	Placebo	Yes		89	11.7
PURSUIT	Low-dose eptifibatide	Yes		200	13.4
	High-dose eptifibatide	Yes		672	14.2
	Placebo	Yes		745	15.7
PARAGON-B	Lamifiban	Yes		278	10.6
	Placebo	Yes		296	11.4
GUSTO-IV ACS	Abciximab 24 h	Yes		212	8.2
	Abciximab 48 h	Yes		238	9.1
	Placebo	Yes		209	8.0
	Any GP IIb/IIIa	Yes/No		1980	10.8
	Placebo	Yes		1550	11.8

0.5   1.0   1.5

Fig. 6. Odds ratios for death or MI at 30 d; contemporary trials of GPIIb/IIIa inhibition vs placebo for NSTE-ACS. (Data from ref. *61*.)

death or nonfatal MI was not reduced with either dose of lamifiban therapy. By 6 mo, patients assigned to low-dose lamifiban showed a lower incidence of death or MI than those treated with heparin alone (12.6% vs 17.9%; $p = 0.025$). High-dose lamifiban therapy, however, did not confer any advantage with regard to ischemic events and, when combined with heparin, was associated with more bleeding. No clear explanation exists for the lack of benefit and potential harm of high-dose therapy, particularly because a much smaller study preceding PARAGON-A reported greater platelet inhibition and lower 30-d event rates with higher doses *(54)*.

Retrospective analyses of patients enrolled in PARAGON-A indicated improved outcomes among patients with plasma levels of lamifiban between 18 and 42 ng/mL *(55)*. The effect of optimally dosed lamifiban (based on renal function) and concomitant heparin therapy therefore was assessed in the placebo-controlled PARAGON-B trial *(56)*. Unlike previous trials of GPIIb/IIIa inhibition in NSTE-ACS, PARAGON-B was powered to detect a more ambitious 25% relative reduction in the primary endpoint of death, MI, or urgent revascularization at 30 d. A total of 5225 patients with NSTE-ACS were randomized to receive either placebo or dose-adjusted lamifiban. GP IIb/IIa inhibition with intravenous lamifiban was associated with an approximate 10% relative reduction in the primary endpoint, but this difference was not statistically significant (11.8% with lamifiban vs 12.8% with placebo; $p = 0.329$). In a prespecified substudy of 1160 patients with elevated troponin T levels, lamifiban was associated with a significant reduction in death or MI at

30 d compared with placebo (11.0% vs 19.4%; $p = 0.018$), reaffirming that GPIIb/IIIa inhibition improves the outcomes of high-risk patients *(57)*.

In the largest investigation of GPIIb/IIIa antagonists in ACS, the PURSUIT trial, 10,948 patients in 28 countries were randomly assigned to receive eptifibatide or placebo with adjunctive heparin and aspirin therapy *(58)*. Entry criteria included either dynamic ST-segment shift or enzyme evidence of myocardial injury, establishing the study population as a relatively high-risk group. Previous experience with eptifibatide showed a reduction in the frequency and duration of ischemic events detected by Holter monitoring *(59)*. In PURSUIT, eptifibatide was associated with an absolute 1.5% reduction in the primary endpoint of death or MI at 30 d (14.2% vs 15.7%; $p = 0.04$). The benefit was apparent by 96 h and persisted through the 30-d follow-up. Bleeding was more common in patients assigned eptifibatide, but there was no increase in hemorrhagic stroke.

In contrast to previous trials showing a benefit with intravenous GPIIb/IIIa inhibition in NSTE-ACS, the GUSTO-IV trial showed no clinical advantage in treating such patients with abciximab compared with placebo *(60)*. Specifically, 7800 patients were randomly assigned to treatment with placebo, a 24-h abciximab infusion, or a 48-h abciximab infusion. The primary endpoint of 30-d death or MI occurred in 8.0, 8.2, and 9.1% of patients, respectively ($p =$ ns). Only 1.6% of patients underwent revascularization within the 48-h treatment period. In contrast to PARAGON-B, GUSTO-IV did not detect a particular benefit from GPIIb/IIIa inhibition among patients with elevated troponin levels. The reasons for this discrepancy are unclear, but they may relate to paradoxical platelet activation with abciximab, a lower risk study population, or heterogeneity in platelet inhibition among patients treated over a period of days. Another explanation may be the absence of early revascularization. A modest but distinct clinical benefit of early or "upstream" treatment with GPIIb/IIIa inhibitors before PCI has been established in ACS trials, however, such that the benefit of an invasive strategy is not strictly because of PCI alone. More likely, GUSTO-IV did not have adequate statistical power to detect a realistic effect of GPIIb/IIIa inhibition as medical therapy alone—10% relative reduction in death or MI, consonant with GPIIb/IIIa inhibition as medical therapy in previous studies, vs the intended 20% event-rate reduction.

Compared with previous studies, patients in the GUSTO-IV trial also were at lower risk, having the lowest incidence of death or MI at 30 d. Furthermore, GUSTO-IV enrolled more women (38%). Whether this observation relates to a sex-related difference in treatment response or the fact that troponin-positive patients in trials are more often male requires further study. Factors such as being younger and male have consistently been associated with greater treatment effects in ACS patients, however, and a systematic overview of GPIIb/IIIa inhibition in NSTE-ACS has shown consistently reduced ischemic events among troponin-positive patients (Fig. 7) *(61)*. Alternatively, abciximab may promote an inflammatory reaction by aiding P-selectin-mediated leukocyte adhesion *(62)*, although studies of abciximab therapy for PCI suggest early, but nonsustained, suppression of C-reactive protein, tumor necrosis factor, and interleukin-6 *(63)*.

PROGRESSION AND REGRESSION: DEVELOPMENT AND FAILURE OF ORAL GPIIb/IIIa INHIBITORS

Prevention of recurrent events after patients are admitted for ACS poses a continuing challenge. Activation of the coagulation system and inflammation within the coronary

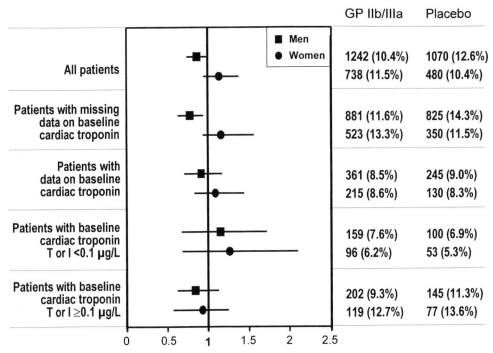

Fig. 7. Odds ratios for death or myocardial infarction at 30 d by sex and troponin status; contemporary trials of GPIIb/IIIa inhibition in NSTE. (Data from ref. *61*.)

artery plaque may persist up to several months after the initial event *(64,65)*. Clinical experience supports these observations with high rates of recurrent cardiac events in this population. For example, in the GUSTO-IIb study, >6% of patients with NSTE-ACS died, >10% had an MI, and >45% were readmitted by 6-mo follow-up *(66)*. Although the absolute benefit of eptifibatide in the PURSUIT trial was preserved at 6 mo, there were no additional reductions in death or infarction between 1 and 6 mo. This suggests that most of the benefit occurs in the early phase of treatment, with no further effect after the drug infusion ends *(67)*.

Several studies have examined both the safety and clinical benefit of sustained platelet suppression with oral GPIIb/IIIa antagonists for secondary prevention after a cardiac event. In the TIMI-12 study, major bleeding occurred among those treated with oral sibrafiban to nearly the same extent as those receiving aspirin alone *(68)*. Minor bleeding, however, particularly mucocutaneous bleeding, was more common with increasing doses of sibrafiban. The safety profile and risk for bleeding appeared to be largely determined by total daily dose, renal function, and daily dosing frequency. Other trials of oral GPIIb/IIIa inhibition after PCI also seemed promising at first. The ORBIT investigators reported effective long-term suppression of platelet aggregation with xemilofiban after angioplasty, with a trend toward fewer cardiovascular events at early (3-mo) follow-up *(69)*. Clinical development of xemilofiban was discontinued, however, after publication of the EXCITE trial results *(70)*. Among 7232 patients undergoing PCI and randomized to receive one of two doses of xemilofiban or placebo for 6 mo, the incidence of death or MI did not differ significantly, although bleeding rates were higher with both low- and high-dose xemilofiban.

Development of other oral GPIIb/IIIa inhibitors has been abandoned because of lack of efficacy and potential harm. Results of the SYMPHONY and 2nd SYMPHONY trials evaluating sibrafiban alone and with aspirin showed no clinical benefit and significantly higher rates of ischemic events with high-dose sibrafiban (71,72). The OPUS-TIMI 16 study was terminated early because of an unexpectedly higher mortality among patients treated with orbofiban (73). Finally, the BRAVO trial (74) was stopped early for significant increases in death, serious thrombocytopenia, and major bleeding associated with lotrafiban use. In a systematic overview of four randomized trials of oral GPIIb/IIIa inhibition enrolling more than 33,000 patients, treatment with oral GPIIb/IIIa agents was associated with a 31% increase in mortality (odds ratio, 1.31; 95% confidence interval, 1.12–1.53; $p = 0.0001$) (75). Results were similar whether the agent was added to or substituted for aspirin. Ischemic events or sudden death tended to be increased (odds ratio, 1.22; 95% confidence interval, 0.91–1.63), and among patients with ACS, the incidence of MI was increased (odds ratio, 1.16; 95% confidence interval, 1.03–1.29).

Although many potential explanations exist for the poorer clinical outcomes associated with oral GPIIb/IIIa inhibition, a prothrombotic effect most likely contributes to the observed higher rate of ischemic events (75,76). Oral GPIIb/IIIa inhibitors may paradoxically activate platelets, enhance fibrinogen binding, or potentiate inflammation (76–78). In contrast to intravenous agents given at doses that achieve sustained levels of receptor occupancy, oral agents are used at lower doses, and plasma levels may vary considerably between doses (78,79). Supporting this theory, the Phase II FROST trial showed that clinical outcomes with the oral GPIIb/IIIa antagonist lefradafiban related directly to the degree of platelet inhibition, suggesting that longer-acting drugs with more effective platelet inhibition may offer clinical benefit (80). Finally, based on the association of oral GPIIb/IIIa inhibitors with increased mortality despite a reduction in urgent revascularization, a direct toxic effect of these agents also been has suggested (75).

ALTERNATIVE ANTIPLATELET AND ANTITHROMBOTIC THERAPIES

Antiplatelet Therapies

ASPIRIN

Aspirin is the "wonder drug" of cardiovascular medicine. Introduced as a medicine over 100 years ago, this drug has a significant beneficial effect—reducing ischemic events in patients with atherosclerosis—at a cost of less than a penny a day. Aside from its effect on platelet aggregation, aspirin's antiinflammatory effects also may contribute to its observed reduction in ischemic events.

Aspirin has a dramatic effect on the risk of vascular events in patients with known atherosclerosis. The Antiplatelet Trialists' Collaboration showed a 20–40% reduction in the risk of death, MI, or stroke (81). This benefit is clear for patients with primary disease in the coronary and cerebrovascular beds and for patients after MI, unstable angina, transient ischemic attacks, or stroke. More recently, aspirin has been associated with lower all-cause mortality over the long term. Among 6174 patients undergoing stress echocardiography to evaluate known or suspected coronary artery disease, aspirin therapy was associated with reduced all-cause mortality over an approximate 3-yr follow-up period (hazard ratio, 0.67; 95% confidence interval, 0.51–0.87; $p = 0.002$). After adjusting for the propensity for using aspirin, as well as other possible interactions, aspirin use remained associated with a lower risk of death (hazard ratio, 0.56; 95% confidence interval, 0.40–0.78; $p < 0.001$). Although this multicenter observational study cannot be definitive, its findings are consistent with data from randomized trials.

Recent analyses also have stressed the benefit of aspirin in primary prevention. Both the HOT Trial *(82)* and the Primary Prevention Project *(83)* showed that relatively low doses of aspirin (80–100 mg/d) were effective in preventing cardiovascular events in patients with at least one risk factor but no overt coronary disease. In the Physicians' Health Study, primary prevention with 325 mg every other day resulted in a significant reduction in MI but no overall reduction in cardiovascular mortality *(84)*. A recent review of aspirin therapy in primary prevention trials involving more than 50,000 patients showed a reduction in the relative risk of ischemic adverse events in all trials except one *(85)*.

Despite dozens of clinical trials involving over 100,000 patients, the most effective aspirin dose has not been identified. A broad clinical consensus has developed, nonetheless, with recommendations for aspirin dosing between 75 and 325 mg/d in patients with coronary disease. Overall, this practice has been primarily driven by simplicity, commercial availability, physician preference, and concerns about the adverse effects such as abdominal discomfort and gastrointestinal bleeding associated with higher doses. Although this dose range has developed empirically over time, evaluation of the optimal dose for aspirin therapy (balancing clinical benefit with adverse effects) has largely resulted from indirect comparisons among multiple trials performed in various clinical settings.

Varied results from previous trials addressing aspirin dosing have underscored the uncertainty with regard to aspirin dosing in reducing secondary vascular events. In the largest experience to date, the Antiplatelet Trialists' Collaboration performed a systematic overview of 11 trials of antiplatelet therapy, suggesting no dose relationship of aspirin in the secondary prevention of cardiovascular events *(80)*. Alternatively, a recent analysis of aspirin dosing in the CURE trial (S. Mehta, personal communication) showed the lowest rates of bleeding and ischemic events among patients taking <100 mg/d of aspirin. For patients receiving combined aspirin and clopidogrel (75 mg/d), adverse events were lowest among those patients taking <100 mg/d of aspirin compared with 100–200 mg/d and >200 mg/d, such that the benefit of combination therapy was largely owing to the reduction in ischemic events compared with aspirin alone at doses >100 mg/d. Similarly, two recent systematic overviews of aspirin trials showed a greater benefit of lower doses of aspirin in reducing ischemic adverse events in ACS *(86;* D. Kong, personal communication).

Accordingly, there is a clear need to define the optimal dose of aspirin therapy in an adequately powered, randomized controlled trial with reference to prevention of both ischemic vascular events and excess bleeding. Despite its widespread availability and low cost, identifying the optimal dose of aspirin will have major effects, considering the potential reduction in both ischemic and bleeding events. Bleeding is slightly but significantly increased with 75 mg of aspirin per day compared with placebo, but gastric bleeding is doubled with 300 mg/d and increased fivefold with 1.8–2.4 g/d *(87)*. Potential implications of aspirin dosing underscore the need for a large, randomized clinical trial.

THIENOPYRIDINES: TICLOPIDINE AND CLOPIDOGREL

Thienopyridine platelet inhibitors have been in clinical use for over a decade. Ticlopidine, the prototype, was shown in a series of clinical trials to reduce ischemic events compared with placebo *(88,89)*, to be marginally superior to aspirin in one trial of cerebrovascular disease *(90)*, and to provide additive benefit to aspirin in PCI *(91)*. Clopidogrel is structurally similar to ticlopidine but is associated with a much lower rate of adverse events. Most notably, ticlopidine treatment carries troublesome rates of neutropenia, thrombocytopenia, and thrombotic thrombocytopenic purpura *(92)*. In comparison, these events have not been identified with clopidogrel in large clinical trials.

The first major study with clopidogrel was the CAPRIE trial, which showed a modest benefit over aspirin (relative reduction, 8.7%; $p = 0.043$) in the secondary prevention of ischemic stroke, MI, or vascular death among patients with vascular disease *(93)*. These results were important in providing substantial evidence that aspirin-intolerant patients could take clopidogrel with at least equal clinical benefit. The substantially higher cost of clopidogrel, however, has inhibited most health care providers from substituting clopidogrel for aspirin in routine secondary prevention.

Recently, the CURE trial compared the combination of aspirin and clopidogrel with aspirin alone in patients with ACS *(94)*. The trial showed a 22% relative reduction in the composite endpoint of death, MI, or stroke with combined aspirin and clopidogrel therapy (9.3% with clopidogrel and aspirin vs 11.4% with aspirin alone; $p < 0.001$). Although major bleeding occurred significantly more often with combined therapy (3.7% with aspirin and clopidogrel vs 2.7% with aspirin alone; $p = 0.001$), there was no difference in major bleeding after 30 d. This relationship suggests that most of the hemorrhagic risk occurred with revascularization procedures.

As a result of these findings, contemporary guidelines for the treatment of non-ST-elevation ACS emphasize prompt administration of clopidogrel and aspirin for patients in whom a noninvasive strategy is planned and for patients scheduled to undergo PCI. Because of an increased risk of perioperative bleeding, clopidogrel should be discontinued a minimum of 5 d before elective bypass surgery *(47)*. Although CURE was not designed as a long-term prevention study (follow-up period of 1 yr), it might be reasonable to continue clopidogrel beyond this period.

Thrombin Inhibitors

UNFRACTIONATED AND LOW-MOLECULAR-WEIGHT HEPARINS

A mainstay of conventional therapy in ACS patients has been adjunctive antithrombin treatment. In clinical trials, however, the addition of heparin or direct thrombin inhibitors has conferred only a modest benefit with regard to clinical outcomes. Oler and colleagues performed a systematic overview of six trials of aspirin alone vs aspirin and unfractionated heparin (UFH). No individual trial reached statistical significance, and the pooled risk of MI or death was reduced by a relative 33% ($p = 0.06$) in patients with unstable angina given aspirin alone *(95)*.

Even though UFH appears to provide a benefit in ACS, event rates increase when it is discontinued, although GPIIb/IIIa inhibition appears to attenuate this rebound effect *(96)*. Heparin is also associated with thrombocytopenia and the potential to cause malignant thrombosis. Finally, it is difficult to titrate heparin dosing within a therapeutic range, and both insufficient and excessive doses are associated with worse clinical outcomes.

Low-molecular-weight heparins (LMWHs) offer several conceptual advantages over UFH. First, through preferential inhibition of factor Xa over thrombin, LMWHs produce more effective anticoagulation earlier in the coagulation cascade. They also are less likely to cause heparin-induced thrombocytopenia, and current standards do not require therapeutic monitoring. In several direct comparative trials of patients with NSTE-ACS and ST-elevation ACS, the LMWHs have been at least as effective, if not superior to, UFH *(44,*

97). A prospectively defined metaanalysis of the two enoxaparin trials, ESSENCE and TIMI-11B, showed consistent reductions in the composite endpoints of death, MI, or urgent revascularization and death or MI in favor of enoxaparin over UFH through 43 d *(98)*. The benefits of enoxaparin reflected similar, proportionate reductions in each element of the composite endpoints, indicating that the results were not driven by any individual event. At 1 yr, the rate of death, MI, or urgent revascularization remained significantly lower in enoxaparin-treated patients (23.3% vs 25.8%; $p = 0.008$). In contrast to enoxaparin, greater efficacy with dalteparin and fraxiparine compared with UFH has not been confirmed *(99,100)*. Possible reasons for the benefit of enoxaparin include more selective anti-Xa/anti-IIa activity and inactivation of platelet-released von Willebrand factor.

Clinical experience with combined LMWH and GPIIb/IIIa inhibition is limited. Results from the ongoing SYNERGY and A to Z trials in patients with NSTE-ACS and PCI should help delineate the safety and efficacy of this combination. The need for therapeutic monitoring of LMWH activity during PCI also remains controversial. Standard measurements of anticoagulation during PCI (e.g., activated clotting time) are unreliable with LMWHs, and devices that measure factor Xa activity directly may be a solution for those who believe therapeutic monitoring is indicated.

WARFARIN

Like unfractionated heparin, warfarin treatment requires laboratory monitoring to remain within a therapeutic window. Although initial studies of warfarin showed a reduction in recurrent cardiac ischemia and embolic cerebrovascular events, the long-term benefit of warfarin with aspirin appears limited. The CARS trial compared aspirin alone with a combined regimen of aspirin and fixed, low-dose warfarin in 8803 patients after MI *(101)*. Fixed-dose warfarin (1 or 3 mg) combined with low-dose aspirin (80 mg) did not surpass the efficacy achieved with 160 mg aspirin alone (8.6% with aspirin vs 8.8% with 3 mg warfarin/80 mg aspirin for the composite endpoint of reinfarction, nonfatal ischemic stroke, or cardiovascular death; $p = $ ns). Similarly, the CHAMP study randomized 5059 patients to low-dose warfarin (mean international normalized ratio [INR], 1.8) plus 81 mg aspirin or aspirin 162 mg monotherapy within 14 d after MI *(102)*. At a median 2.7 yr of follow-up, the rates of death, MI, or stroke were nearly identical, with significantly more major bleeding events in the combination-therapy group (1.28 vs 0.72 events per 100 person-years; $p < 0.001$).

These findings were further supported by the OASIS study in unstable angina, in which treatment with moderate-dose warfarin and aspirin was associated with a small, nonsignificant reduction in recurrent ischemic events (7.6% with warfarin and aspirin vs 8.3% with aspirin alone; $p = $ ns) at the expense of significantly greater bleeding (2.7% vs 1.3%, respectively; $p < 0.05$) *(103)*. On the other hand, the WARIS-II study showed a significant reduction in cardiac and cerebrovascular events among patients randomized to receive warfarin plus aspirin after MI vs aspirin alone *(104)*. Given the increased risk of bleeding and need for monitoring, warfarin is unlikely to become routine therapy for patients with ischemic heart disease. Like warfarin, combined antiplatelet therapy with aspirin and clopidogrel has been associated with reduced ischemic outcomes but greater bleeding risk *(94)*. Future studies should determine the most appropriate balance between safety and efficacy.

DIRECT THROMBIN INHIBITORS

Direct antithrombins have several advantages over UFH for use in ACS or PCI. These include (1) high specificity and potency for thrombin inhibition, (2) a lack of dependence on antithrombin III for anticoagulant activity, (3) the ability to inactivate both clot-bound and free thrombin, and (4) a lack of aggregatory effects on platelets. Pooled data from the GUSTO-IIb and TIMI-9B studies comparing hirudin with UFH as an adjunct to fibrinolytic therapy showed no significant reduction in mortality and a nonsignificant 14% reduction in recurrent infarction at 30 d *(105)*. In the recent HERO-2 trial of UFH vs bivalirudin as adjunctive therapy to streptokinase for acute MI, 30-d mortality was not significantly reduced with bivalirudin (10.5% with bivalirudin vs 10.9% with heparin; $p = 0.46$), although reinfarction was significantly reduced by 30% (1.6% vs 2.3%; $p = 0.001$) *(106)*.

Compared with UFH, significantly fewer bleeding and ischemic adverse events have been observed among patients undergoing angioplasty with adjunctive bivalirudin *(107)*. In a systematic overview of four trials comparing bivalirudin with UFH in PCI or ACS, bivalirudin was associated with a significant reduction in the composite of death or infarction (odds ratio, 0.73; 95% confidence interval, 0.57–0.95; $p = 0.02$) at 30–50 d, or 14 fewer events per 1000 patients treated *(108)*. There also was a significant reduction in major hemorrhage for the same trials (odds ratio, 0.41; 95% confidence interval, 0.32–0.52; $p < 0.001$, or 58 fewer events per 1000 patients treated). In a systematic overview of 11 randomized trials involving nearly 36,000 patients, direct thrombin inhibitors were associated with a lower risk of death or MI at 30 d compared with UFH (7.4% vs 8.2%; $p = 0.02$) *(109)*. Subgroup analyses indicated a benefit with direct thrombin inhibitors in both ACS and PCI. Of note, there was an apparent reduction in ischemic events with bivalirudin and hirudin, but not with univalent agents. More recent studies of bivalirudin in PCI have suggested reduced ischemic adverse events compared with UFH and GPIIb/IIIa inhibition with the potential for equivalent outcomes without the use of GPIIb/IIIa inhibitors. Results from the REPLACE-2 trial, comparing UFH plus mandatory GPIIb/IIIa inhibition with bivalirudin plus provisional GPIIb/IIIa inhibitors in PCI, are eagerly awaited.

FACTOR Xa INHIBITORS

Molecules that directly inhibit factor Xa are in development, and early clinical results appear promising. Fondaparinux is a synthetic, highly sulfated pentasaccharide that mimics the biologically active region of heparin but specifically inhibits factor Xa. Early studies of patients at high risk for developing deep-vein thrombosis showed the superiority of fondaparinux over enoxaparin *(110)*. In a dose-finding study among patients with ACS, fondaparinux was associated with fewer early adverse ischemic events compared with enoxaparin *(111)*. Although bleeding was not significantly increased with fondaparinux therapy, no dose response was observed for ischemic outcomes, suggesting that further studies to characterize its effects are required.

In a Phase I trial of patients with ST-elevation MI, adjunctive administration of SR9010A/ORG31540, a synthetic pentasaccharide that selectively inhibits factor Xa, with standard fibrinolytic therapy resulted in no excess bleeding and similar rates of TIMI grade 3 flow at 90 min and 6 d compared with UFH, with trends toward less reocclusion and urgent revascularization *(57)*. Results from ongoing evaluations of other factor Xa inhibitors performed in various clinical settings are forthcoming.

INHIBITORS OF THE TISSUE FACTOR PATHWAY

Considering the central role of tissue factor in initiating the coagulation cascade at sites of vascular injury, interest has arisen in the possible clinical effects of its inhibition. Adenoviral gene transfer of recombinant tissue factor pathway inhibitor (TFPI) in animals has been shown to prevent local arterial thrombus formation and the neointimal response after balloon-induced injury without impairing hemostasis *(112)*. At present, however, no studies of TFPI have been performed in patients with cardiovascular disease.

FUTURE DIRECTIONS

Pharmacodynamics and Monitoring of Therapy

DOSING AND INTENSITY OF PLATELET INHIBITION

Despite more recent attention to the relationship between the pharmacodynamics of GPIIb/IIIa inhibition and clinical outcomes, the most effective intensity of platelet inhibition remains unknown. In the GOLD trial evaluating the intensity of platelet inhibition with GPIIb/IIIa therapy in patients undergoing PCI, <70% platelet inhibition after steady-state drug infusion was associated with a higher incidence of ischemic adverse events *(113)*. More adverse events likewise occurred among the 25% of patients who did not achieve >95% inhibition within 10 min of administration. Based on preclinical studies with abciximab, at least 80% receptor occupancy was required to maintain continuous arterial perfusion. Notably, the use of a calcium-chelating anticoagulant (such as citrate) in ex vivo platelet aggregation studies overestimates the in vivo inhibitory effects of GPIIb/IIIa inhibitors. This phenomenon confounded the search for optimal dosing of eptifibatide and tirofiban. Doses of eptifibatide used in the IMPACT-II study *(15)* achieved 50–60% inhibition by standard platelet aggregometry. This finding led to higher dosing in the PURSUIT and ESPRIT trials and may partly explain the larger clinical benefit observed in these studies compared with IMPACT-II.

Similarly, variable platelet inhibition may have contributed to the negative findings of the TARGET *(26)* and RESTORE *(16)* trials of tirofiban and the GUSTO-IV study of abciximab *(60)*. In the COMPARE trial, serial platelet aggregometry was performed in 73 patients randomized to receive either abciximab, eptifibatide, or tirofiban using doses established in contemporary ACS trials (W. Batchelor, personal communication). Platelet aggregation in the first 30 min after administration was reduced least with tirofiban (RESTORE dose regimen). The greatest variability in platelet aggregation was observed with abciximab during late infusion (≥4 h). In contrast, the most consistent inhibition of platelet aggregation occurred with the eptifibatide regimen (PURSUIT dose regimen). Although the RESTORE-tirofiban dosing regimen provided platelet inhibition comparable with that of eptifibatide and abciximab with extended infusion, it did not produce a similar degree of platelet inhibition during immediate PCI. Consistent platelet inhibition after several hours of continued infusion may account for the efficacy observed when PCI is delayed 4–48 h after administration, as in the PRISM-PLUS and TACTICS-TIMI 18 *(114)* studies. Alternatively, the finding of platelet recovery (i.e., reduced platelet inhibition) after several hours of abciximab therapy may in part explain the negative findings with abciximab in the GUSTO-IV trial, which discouraged early revascularization.

Further studies in ACS and PCI are required to determine how pharmacodynamic differences may influence the efficacy of GPIIb/IIIa antagonists. In addition, reasons for interpatient variability in response to GPIIb/IIIa inhibition need to be clarified. Potential contributing factors include individual cardiovascular risk profiles (e.g., diabetes, age), resistance to adjunctive antiplatelet therapies (e.g., aspirin), or inherited genetic polymorphisms regarding platelets. Moreover, there is a need for standardized, accurate methods of determining platelet inhibition, because current measures of platelet inhibition are imprecise

(115). Based on these findings, however, potent platelet inhibition at the time of intentional vessel injury probably determines benefit during PCI, whereas a more prolonged and consistent reduction in platelet aggregation may be required for ACS applications.

Monitoring

The relationship between GPIIb/IIIa receptor occupancy and physiologic measures of platelet function varies. Platelet aggregometry has been the accepted standard for determining the intensity of antiplatelet therapies, but this technique is limited by intra- and interindividual variation, the need for fresh samples, and excessive time and cost to complete the assay. Moreover, this method does not specifically measure GPIIb/IIIa binding activity but rather global platelet function.

Newer assays such as the Ultegra Rapid Platelet Function Assay (RPFA, Accumetrics, Inc.) have provided a more rapid and specific assessment of GPIIb/IIIa receptor occupancy. By measuring the interaction between GPIIb/IIIa and fibrinogen-coated beads, the RPFA offers an efficient, bedside method for determining the specific receptor inhibition with GPIIb/IIIa blockade. Interpretation of RPFA results differs from that of aggregometry results, creating a need to reconcile the disparate results before a uniform method is adopted. Clinicians accustomed to giving antiplatelet therapy without monitoring may be slow to adopt routine platelet assays during PCI. For these reasons, routine platelet monitoring will probably be used to support clinical trial results, but routine clinical use is unlikely.

Whether other measures of platelet function yield more consistent results than aggregometry has not been well studied. Studies examining the effects of GPIIb/IIIa antagonists on inflammation—for example, inhibition of the $\alpha_v\beta_3$ or Mac-1 integrin receptors—may instead provide more reliable and yet clinically relevant assessments of platelet activity. As an antagonist of both GPIIb/IIIa and $\alpha_v\beta_3$ with equal affinity, abciximab may provide additional benefit in preventing $\alpha_v\beta_3$-mediated thrombin generation and smooth muscle cell migration *(116)*, Mac-1-regulated platelet-leukocyte interaction, or both *(117)*.

Bleeding and Thrombocytopenia

Although further studies are needed to clarify the relationship between ischemic events and the level of platelet inhibition with GPIIb/IIIa blockade, the likelihood of bleeding complications correlates more directly with the level of impaired platelet activity. In the EPILOG study, a nonsignificantly lower bleeding rate was observed with abciximab and low-dose heparin vs standard heparin *(13)*, and bleeding may even be further reduced with thrombin inhibitors such as bivalirudin.

All GPIIb/IIIa inhibitors are associated with some risk of thrombocytopenia, which occurs in 0.4–4% of patients. The precise mechanism and optimal treatment remain unknown, and treatment is usually limited to platelet transfusions. Thrombocytopenia is associated with not only a greater risk of hemorrhage but also a paradoxically greater likelihood of ischemic adverse events *(118)*. Pseudothrombocytopenia, or artifactual platelet clumping in vitro owing to autologous antibodies, may occur in up to 1% of patients receiving abciximab but does not affect clinical outcome *(119)*.

Except for abciximab, readministration of GPIIb/IIIa antagonists remains uncertain. In the ReoPro Readministration Study *(28)*, overall rates of thrombocytopenia with abciximab were similar to rates for first-time administration, yet there appeared to be a greater incidence of profound thrombocytopenia as well as delayed presentations of thrombocytopenia after hospital discharge. Despite the development of human antichimeric antibodies in a small number of patients after initial exposure to abciximab, neither hypersensitivity reactions nor neutralization of the abciximab effect were observed.

For most patients, the risk of thrombocytopenia will not preclude the use of a GPIIb/IIIa inhibitor. Instead, the uncertainty about which patients will develop thrombocytopenia and our inability to prevent it should reinforce the need for vigilant periprocedural monitoring of platelet counts. Advanced age and lower body weight are associated with a greater likelihood of thrombocytopenia, although no risk factor has been established with any certainty to preclude GPIIb/IIIa inhibitor administration. Importantly, the ReoPro Readministration Study did not include patients who developed thrombocytopenia with initial therapy, such that potential risks from readministration to this particular subgroup are not well understood. Although it is customary among patients with abciximab-associated thrombocytopenia to avoid GPIIb/IIIa inhibition altogether or substitute a small-molecule inhibitor, there are few prospective data to support this practice.

New Strategies for NSTE-ACS: "Upstream" Therapy

Recent trials have supported the idea that the optimal management strategy for patients with ACS involves a combination of pharmacologic therapy and PCI. Despite earlier studies (TIMI-IIIB *[49]*, VANQWISH *[120]*) that failed to show a clinical benefit with the routine use of an early invasive strategy vs a more conservative approach that involved noninvasive testing, more recent trials of GPIIb/IIIa inhibitors with early revascularization have supported a combined approach to reduce ischemic adverse events. Whether the mechanism of benefit with early GPIIb/IIIa inhibition is passivation of an unstable plaque, improved microvascular function, or greater epicardial patency, recent trials of early GPIIb/IIIa inhibition followed by PCI have fueled enthusiasm for this complementary approach.

The clinical benefit of GPIIb/IIIa inhibitors before revascularization is not because of PCI alone. In recent trials of patients with NSTE-ACS, most MIs have not been related to revascularization procedures, underscoring the benefit of GPIIb/IIIa inhibition beyond the catheterization laboratory *(121)*. A consistent reduction in death or MI with GPIIb/IIIa inhibition exists, regardless of management with an early invasive strategy or early conservative approach *(61)*.

In the TACTICS-TIMI 18 study, upfront administration of tirofiban coupled with an early invasive strategy resulted in lower rates of death and MI (4.7% with early invasive strategy vs 7.0% with conservative management at 30 d; $p = 0.02$) *(114)*. The highest-risk patients (e.g., troponin-positive, ST-segment depression) derived the greatest benefit from the early invasive strategy combined with GPIIb/IIIa inhibition. An important limitation of this study, however, is that all patients received tirofiban, precluding comparisons with early revascularization without GPIIb/IIIa inhibition.

Alternative early revascularization strategies might be considered before advance therapy with GPIIb/IIIa inhibition becomes common. In the FRISC-II trial, an early invasive approach, similar to that taken in TACTICS-TIMI 18, showed a lower incidence of death or MI among patients randomized to early revascularization and treatment with dalteparin. Six-month rates of death or MI were 9.4% for the early invasive approach vs 12.1% for the conservative strategy ($p = 0.03$). The results were independent of dalteparin treatment *(122)*. In the observational PCI-CURE trial, treatment with clopidogrel an average 6 d before PCI followed by long-term clopidogrel therapy was associated with a significant reduction in the rate of cardiovascular death, MI, or revascularization at 30 d (relative risk, 0.70; $p = 0.03$) *(123)*. In this study, use of GPIIb/IIIa inhibitors was infrequent, and the apparent benefit of early combined aspirin and clopidogrel has advanced the notion that GPIIb/IIIa inhibitors may not be warranted in some cases. Still, the PCI-CURE strategy has not been prospectively tested against the use of GPIIb/IIIa inhibitors in a randomized fashion, and current evidence suggests that the two therapies appear more complementary than exclusionary in contemporary practice. Although clinicians may favor prescribing a GPIIb/IIIa inhibitor without early clopidogrel treatment, the available evidence supports the use of a GPIIb/IIIa inhibitor during PCI with both aspirin and a thienopyridine. A trial that measures the clinical and economic outcomes of early aspirin/clopidogrel treatment and aspirin/GPIIb/IIIa inhibitor treatment is required to clarify this important issue. Remaining issues for advance therapy include identifying which patients benefit most from GPIIb/IIIa inhibition and early revascularization and the interaction of GPIIb/IIIa inhibitor pharmacodynamics with timing of revascularization.

New Strategies for ST-Elevation MI: "Facilitated PCI"

Facilitated PCI, or the strategy of planned early PCI after pharmacologic reperfusion therapy, fuses the best aspects of fibrinolysis and primary angioplasty in the management of ST-elevation MI. On the one hand, fibrinolysis can result in TIMI grade 3 flow as early as 60 min after administration. On the other hand, primary angioplasty achieves higher rates of normal epicardial artery blood flow but generally at later times. As a combined approach, facilitated PCI may provide the best outcomes based on TIMI flow and clinical events.

In the ADMIRAL trial, nearly one-fourth of patients received early administration of abciximab in either the emergency room or the ambulance *(33)*. Baseline TIMI grade 3 flow was significantly more common among patients receiving abciximab both immediately before and after revascularization (Fig. 8), a finding consonant with prior studies showing a 25–35% rate of TIMI grade 3 flow with abciximab when given 60–90 min before angiography *(41,42)*. These data are also consistent with (1) a previous report from 2507 patients in the PAMI trials, in which early and late mortality were strikingly reduced for patients with spontaneously recovery of TIMI 3 flow before the procedure, independent of the final TIMI flow grade (Fig. 8) *(124)*; (2) the randomized PACT trial, in which early reperfusion with reduced-dose alteplase resulted in greater early recovery of left ventricular function *(125)*; and (3) a metaanalysis showing that mortality is reduced when thrombolytic therapy is started before arrival at the hospital rather than in the emergency room *(126)*. In comparison, abciximab was given only in the catheterization laboratory to patients in the CADILLAC trial, which may account for the lack of improvement in epicardial flow. Although some of the marked benefit in the early-treatment group in ADMIRAL may reflect the play of chance, resulting in an inexplicably high rate of adverse events in the placebo-treated patients, these data support ongoing trials of pharmacologic reperfusion before mechanical revascularization.

The GUSTO IV SPEED investigators described the outcomes of 323 patients who underwent PCI about 1 h after reperfusion therapy and compared them with a similar cohort who did not undergo early revascularization *(127)*. For the facilitated-therapy group, procedural success was 88%, and the 30-d composite endpoint of death, reinfarction, or urgent TVR occurred in 5.6% of patients (Fig. 9). Although these findings are more descriptive than comparative, they are encouraging, because earlier trials consistently showed lower immediate procedural success rates, higher mortality, and higher rates of reinfarction, bypass

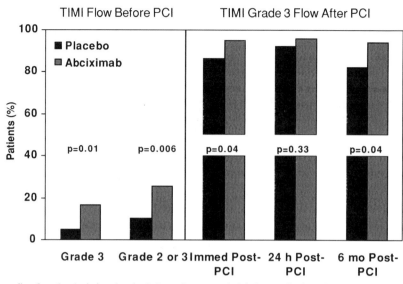

Fig. 8. Benefit of early abciximab administration as an initial reperfusion therapy in the ADMIRAL trial. PCI, percutaneous coronary intervention. (Adapted from ref. *33*.)

surgery, and bleeding than with a conservative approach. With a greater likelihood for epicardial artery patency, facilitated PCI may also improve patient stability and reduce periinfarction complications such as shock. Still more trials are under way, including the ADVANCE MI trial (with eptifibatide/tenecteplase followed by early PCI) and the FINESSE trial (abciximab/reteplase followed by early PCI).

Targeting Patient Populations

As the approach to treating ACS patients with GPIIb/IIIa inhibitors becomes further refined, so does our understanding of which patients benefit from therapy most. For example, several studies have suggested that troponin-positive patients who are at higher risk for death and myocardial (re)infarction may show an enhanced treatment effect with GPIIb/IIIa inhibitors. In the CAPTURE study, the incidence of death or nonfatal MI at 6 mo was reduced by 60% among abciximab-treated patients who were troponin-positive at randomization, whereas troponin-negative patients showed no treatment effect of abciximab *(128)*. In a recent systematic overview of GPIIb/IIIa inhibition in NSTE-ACS trials (including the GUSTO-IV study), patients with elevated baseline troponin levels showed a consistent reduction in ischemic events (Fig. 7) *(60)*. These findings were supported in the PRISM *(129)* and PARAGON-B *(57)* trials, which not only reaffirmed the higher clinical risk associated with elevated troponin levels but also showed that treatment with GPIIb/IIIa inhibitors in such patients appeared to reduce adverse outcomes to a rate nearly identical to that of troponin-negative patients.

Further investigations should define the interactions of other clinical characteristics with GPIIb/IIIa administration. In a systematic overview of GPIIb/IIIa therapies in patients with NSTE-ACS, for example, features such as younger age and male sex were consistently associated with a greater treatment effect *(61)*. Whether this latter observation is related to sex-related differences in treatment response or whether troponin-positive patients in trials are more likely to be male will require further study. Similarly, the magnitude of

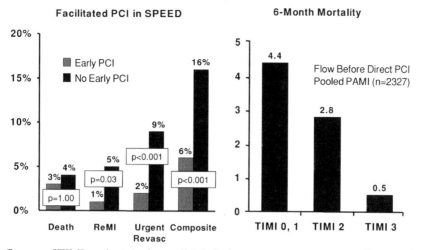

Fig. 9. Influence of TIMI grade status immediately before percutaneous coronary intervention (PCI) for acute MI and the reduction in clinical events observed with facilitated PCI in the SPEED (GUSTO-IV Pilot) trial *(43,127)*. ReMI, reinfarction.

benefit from treatment with eptifibatide in the PURSUIT trial was greater in the United States than elsewhere in the world *(130)*. In the absence of dedicated, prospective randomized trials, however, the certainty of these results is limited by the possibility of chance findings when multiple comparisons are performed.

New Indications

CEREBROVASCULAR DISEASE

Fibrinolytic therapy is approved for the treatment of acute ischemic stroke, yet few patients are eligible for treatment. Although efficacious, the practical use of fibrinolytic therapy is confined by a short treatment window of 3 h from stroke onset and the risk of intracranial hemorrhage, which can occur in nearly 10% of patients. Recent trials suggesting a clinical benefit of aspirin therapy given within 48 h of stroke onset raise the possibility of improved efficacy with more potent platelet inhibitors *(131)*. Further support of safety with GPIIb/IIIa inhibition is derived from the low risk of intracranial hemorrhage (approx 0.15%) in the PCI setting. Treatment of ischemic cerebrovascular events with GPIIb/IIIa inhibitors, alone or combined with reduced-dose fibrinolytic therapy, therefore may improve reperfusion, reduce the risk of intracranial hemorrhage, and extend the time frame for therapeutic benefit. Among 74 patients arriving within 24 h of symptom onset, randomization to abciximab resulted in a trend toward lesser disability with no cases of major intracranial hemorrhage *(132)*. Patients did not receive adjunctive aspirin or heparin, however. Although preliminary, these findings are encouraging, considering the paucity of effective therapies for acute ischemic stroke.

HEART FAILURE

Heart failure remains an important public health concern in the United States, accounting for over 1 million hospitalizations each year. Although considerable attention has been given to the contribution of neurohormonal activation and loading conditions to ventricular dysfunction, the role of atherosclerotic disease should not be underestimated, since acute myocardial ischemia or infarction contributes to 30–50% of sudden-death events in patients with heart failure *(133)*. Up to one-third of patients with heart failure who suffered a sudden death and who had significant coronary disease on autopsy were misdiagnosed as having "nonischemic" cardiomyopathy in life *(134)*. These findings suggest that acute coronary thrombosis and the accompanying ischemia are important contributors to sudden cardiac death and that these events often are unrecognized during life among patients with advanced heart failure.

Aside from the reduction in ischemic events by treatment with angiotensin-converting enzyme inhibitors and β-blockers, evidence supports a neurohormonal mechanism of platelet activation in heart failure. In addition, chronic aspirin use is associated with a reduced risk of hospital admission and all-cause mortality, regardless of the etiology of cardiomyopathy *(135)*. As a result, platelet activation and resultant myocardial ischemia may contribute to elevated levels of cardiac troponin T observed in patients with worsening heart failure *(136)*. Not only may elevations of markers of myocardial injury identify a population of patients who may specifically benefit from antiplatelet therapy, but the use of GPIIb/IIIa inhibitors may reduce ischemic complications, thereby possibly reducing the risk of sudden death. Forthcoming trials of GPIIb/IIIa inhibition in patients with advanced heart failure should clarify potential applications for these agents.

PERIPHERAL ARTERIAL DISEASE

The relative risk of cardiovascular death for patients with peripheral arterial disease (PAD) alone approximates that of patients with known coronary or cerebrovascular disease *(137)*. The severity of PAD is closely associated with the risk of MI, ischemic stroke, and death from vascular causes. The lower the ankle-brachial index, the greater the likelihood for cardiovascular events, such that patients with critical limb ischemia have an annual mortality rate of nearly 25%.

Clinical experience with GPIIb/IIIa inhibition in patients with PAD is limited. Studies of these agents in catheter-based carotid interventions, although showing some benefit, are restricted by their lack of randomized design and small sample sizes *(138)*. Considering the lower incidence of periprocedural ischemic events relative to PCI, definitive randomized trials are unlikely to be performed because their design would require substantial numbers of patients. Alternatively, randomized trials of GPIIb/IIIa inhibition may be possible if limited to high-risk patients with a greater likelihood of ischemic events, such as those with critical limb ischemia. Roxifiban, an oral agent with a longer half-life and greater receptor affinity, has shown an acceptable safety profile with reduced ischemic events *(139)*, yet its evaluation in PAD patients was halted based on the general negative findings with other oral GPIIb/IIIa inhibitors.

CORONARY ARTERY BYPASS GRAFTING

An increasing number of patients have undergone bypass surgery after treatment with GPIIb/IIIa inhibitors. To date, there appears to be no major increase in the risk of bleeding, although many patients have received perioperative platelet transfusions. Formal randomized trials are needed to investigate whether GPIIb/IIIa inhibitors reduce platelet consumption during cardiopulmonary bypass and whether these drugs ameliorate the effect of platelet activation on systemic outcomes.

Despite recent advances in the medical stabilization of patients with recent ACS, those who require bypass surgery during the initial admission have increased perioperative morbidity and mortality. Pretreatment with GPIIb/IIIa inhibition may attenuate some risk, however. In the PURSUIT trial, for example, eptifibatide administration in patients with ACS undergoing bypass surgery during the index hospitalization resulted in both early and late reductions in the occurrence of death or MI (32.7% with placebo vs 27.6% with eptifibatide for the composite of death or MI at 6 mo; $p = 0.029$) *(140)*.

Effect of Genetics on Dosing

The role of platelets in unstable coronary syndromes and adverse events after coronary intervention are typical examples of the interplay between genetic and environmental factors. A number of genetic polymorphisms within the subunits of platelet receptors may induce gain or loss of function, thereby predisposing some individuals to thrombotic events. Platelet function may reflect variations that either encode a missense mutation (the resulting codon changes the amino acid) or modify the level of expression of the gene product.

The Pl[A2] polymorphism of the GPIIIa is the first genetic variant that has been shown to modify the platelet response to antiplatelet therapy. Pl[A2] does not destroy the activity of GPIIb/IIIa but can affect its properties, thereby affecting the responsiveness and adhesive properties of platelets *(140,141)*. Compared with Pl[A1,A1] platelets (wild type), Pl[A2]-positive platelets express significantly more P-selectin, GP IIb/IIIa-bound fibrinogen, and activated GPIIb/IIIa in vitro in response to platelet agonists *(142)*.

Pl[A2] has been implicated in arterial thrombosis and the development of unstable coronary syndromes. Specifically, a high prevalence of the Pl[A2] allele has been reported in patients with unstable angina or MI and in siblings of patients with a history of premature ischemic heart disease *(143,144)*. Mikkelson et al. *(145)* reported a higher prevalence of Pl[A2] among victims of sudden cardiac death whose coronary arteries contained thrombus. The Pl[A2] polymorphism has also been related to a higher incidence of adverse ischemic events after catheter-based procedures, in particular subacute stent thrombosis *(146–148)*. The Pl[A2] polymorphism may thus represent a major risk for the development of coronary thrombosis in susceptible individuals.

Because many case-control studies have reported varied findings about the clinical relevance of the Pl[A2] polymorphism, further studies are needed to define prospectively the effect of this genetic variant on clinical outcomes and response to drug therapies. Recent studies examining the effect of GPIIb/IIIa inhibition on Pl[A2]-positive platelets with various agonists have yielded conflicting results *(141,149)*. Incorporation of mechanistic studies, such as genotyping and platelet function, should further define clinical outcomes data and enable specific antithrombotic regimens to be tailored to individual patients.

CONCLUSIONS

Alone and combined with other pharmacologic and mechanical interventions, the use of GPIIb/IIIa inhibitors reflects considerable progress in the treatment of patients with ACS. From early benchwork and clinical development to primary indications for therapy, GPIIb/IIIa inhibitors are transitioning from an era of rapid growth (e.g., adoption into routine therapy) to maturity (e.g., novel indications, new trials). Prescription of GPIIb/IIIa inhibitors remains surprisingly infrequent despite established benefit and cost effectiveness in various clinical settings. Between 50 and 75% of the patients who would derive a benefit from GPIIb/IIIa inhibitors do not receive this therapy. The limited efficacy of "standard" antithrombotic and anticoagulant therapy with aspirin and heparin alone should remind clinicians of the continued need to apply therapies with proven benefit. Based on

Table 2
Authors' Recommendations for Evidence-Based Selection of GPIIb/IIIa Antagonist

Clinical indication	GPIIb/IIIa antagonist
Non-ST-segment elevation acute coronary syndromes	Eptifibatide, tirofiban
Followed by early revascularization[a]	Eptifibatide, tirofiban
Low-risk, elective percutaneous coronary intervention	Eptifibatide, abciximab
High-risk percutaneous coronary intervention	Abciximab
ST-segment elevation myocardial infarction	Abciximab

[a] 24–48 h after initiation of GP IIb/IIIa therapy.

the clinical presentation and preferred treatment strategy, clinicians can apply the available evidence to select the appropriate agent for use (Table 2).

Unresolved issues, such as the need for therapeutic monitoring and new potential indications, mandate further clinical trials to refine the place of these agents within a treatment algorithm for patients with ACS. Sufficient data to establish the use of GPIIb/IIIa inhibitors as a standard of care exists for patients undergoing PCI and for whom PCI is planned. Future studies will examine the role of these agents in the treatment of patients with heart failure and other vascular disorders.

REFERENCES

1. Tufts Center for the Study of Drug Development. Cost of a new prescription medicine. November 30, 2001. Available at http://www.tufts.edu/med/csdd/Nov30CostStudyPressRelease.html.
2. Fuster V, Badimon L, Badimon JJ, Chesebro JH. The pathogenesis of coronary artery disease and the acute coronary syndrome. N Engl J Med 1992;326:242–250, 310–318.
3. Lefkovits J, Plow EF, Topol EJ. Platelet glycoprotein IIb/IIIa receptors in cardiovascular medicine. N Engl J Med 1995;332:1553–1559.
4. Phillips DR, Charo IF, Parisi LV, Fitzgerald LA. The platelet membrane glycoprotein IIb-IIIa complex. Blood 1988;71:831–843.
5. Pytela R, Pierschbacher MD, Ginsberg MH, et al. Platelet membrane glycoprotein IIb/IIIa: member of a family of Arg-Gly-Asp specific adhesion receptors. Science 1986;231:1559–1562.
6. Coller BS, Peerschke EI, Scudder LE, Sullivan CA. A murine monoclonal antibody that completely blocks the binding of fibrinogen to platelets produces a thrombasthenic-like state in normal platelets and binds to glycoproteins IIb and/or IIIa. J Clin Invest 1983;72:325–338.
7. Adgey JAA. Overview of the results of clinical trials with glycoprotein IIb/IIIa inhibitors. Am Heart J 1998;135(Suppl):S43–S55.
8. Serruys PW, de Jaegere P, Kiemeneij F, et al. A comparison of balloon expandable stent implantation with balloon angioplasty in patients with coronary artery disease. N Engl J Med 1994;331:489–495.
9. Fischman DL, Leon MB, Baim DS, et al. A randomized comparison of coronary stent placement and balloon angioplasty in the treatment of coronary artery disease. N Engl J Med 1994;331:496–501.
10. Serruys PW, van Hout B, Bonnier H, et al. Randomised comparison of implantation of heparin-coated stents with balloon angioplasty in selected patients with coronary artery disease (BENESTENT II). Lancet 1998;352:673–681.
11. Kong DF, Califf RM, Miller DP, et al. Clinical outcomes of therapeutic agents that block the platelet glycoprotein IIb/IIIa integrin in ischemic heart disease. Circulation 1998;98:2829–2835.
12. The EPIC Investigators. Use of a monoclonal antibody directed against the platelet glycoprotein IIb/IIIa receptor in high-risk coronary angioplasty. N Engl J Med 1994;330:956–961.
13. The EPILOG Investigators. Platelet glycoprotein IIb/IIIa receptor blockade and low-dose heparin during percutaneous coronary revascularization. N Engl J Med 1997;336:1689–1696.

14. The CAPTURE Investigators. Randomised placebo-controlled trial of abciximab before and during coronary intervention in refractory unstable angina: the CAPTURE study. Lancet 1997;349:1429–1435.
15. The IMPACT-II Investigators. Randomised placebo-controlled trial of effect of eptifibatide on complications of percutaneous coronary intervention: IMPACT-II. Lancet 1997;349:1422–1428.
16. The RESTORE Study Group. Effects of platelet glycoprotein IIb/IIIa blockade with tirofiban on adverse cardiac events in patients with unstable angina or acute myocardial infarction undergoing coronary angioplasty. Circulation 1997;96:1445–1453.
17. The EPISTENT Investigators. Randomised placebo-controlled and balloon-angioplasty-controlled trial to assess safety of coronary stenting with use of platelet glycoprotein IIb/IIIa blockade. Lancet 1998;352:87–92.
18. The ESPRIT Investigators. Novel dosing regimen of eptifibatide in planned coronary stent implantation (Enhanced Suppression of the Platelet IIb/IIIa Receptor with Integrilin Therapy): a randomised, placebo-controlled trial. Lancet 2000;356:2037–2044.
19. O'Shea JC, Hafley GE, Greenberg S, et al., for the ESPRIT Investigators. Platelet glycoprotein IIb/IIIa integrin blockade with eptifibatide in coronary stent intervention. The ESPRIT trial: a randomized controlled trial. JAMA 2001;285:2468–2473.
20. O'Shea JC, Buller CE, Cantor WJ, et al. Long-term efficacy of platelet glycoprotein IIb/IIIa integrin blockade with eptifibatide in coronary stent intervention. JAMA 2002;287:618-621.
21. Roe MT, Ohman EM, Maas ACP, et al. Shifting the open-artery hypothesis downstream: the quest for optimal reperfusion. J Am Coll Cardiol 2001;37:9–18.
22. Anderson KM, Califf RM, Stone GW, et al. Long-term mortality benefit with abciximab in patients undergoing percutaneous coronary intervention. J Am Coll Cardiol 2001;37:2059–2065.
23. Gibson CM, Goel M, Cohen DJ, et al. Six-month angiographic and clinical follow-up of patients prospectively randomized to receive either tirofiban or placebo during angioplasty in the RESTORE trial. J Am Coll Cardiol 1998;32:28–34.
24. Neumann FJ, Kastrati A, Schmitt C, et al. Effect of glycoprotein IIb/IIIa receptor blockade with abciximab on clinical and angiographic restenosis rate after the placement of coronary stents following acute myocardial infarction. J Am Coll Cardiol 2000;35:915–921.
25. The ERASER Investigators. Acute platelet inhibition with abciximab does not reduce in-stent restenosis. Circulation 1999;100:799–806.
26. Topol EJ, Moliterno DJ, Herrmann HC, et al. Comparison of two platelet glycoprotein IIb/IIIa inhibitors, tirofiban and abciximab, for the prevention of ischemic events with percutaneous coronary revascularization. N Engl J Med 2001;344:1888–1894.
27. Coller BS. Monitoring platelet GP IIb/IIIa antagonist therapy. Circulation 1997;96:3828–3832.
28. Tcheng JE, Kereiakes DJ, Lincoff AM, et al. Abciximab readministration: results of the ReoPro Readministration Study. Circulation 2001;104:870–875.
29. Mark DB, Peterson ED. The health economics of acute coronary syndromes: clinical and economic potential of GP IIb/IIIa antagonists. J Thromb Thrombol 1998;5:5155–5162.
30. Brener SJ, Barr LA, Burchenal JE, et al. Randomized, placebo-controlled trial of platelet glycoprotein IIb/IIIa blockade with primary angioplasty for acute myocardial infarction. Circulation 1998;98:734–741.
31. Schomig A, Kastrati A, Dirschinger J, et al. Coronary stenting plus platelet glycoprotein IIb/IIIa blockade compared with tissue plasminogen activator in acute myocardial infarction. N Engl J Med 2000;343:385–391.
32. Neumann FJ, Blasini R, Schmitt C, et al. Effect of glycoprotein IIb/IIIa receptor blockade on recovery of coronary flow and left ventricular function after the placement of coronary-artery stents in acute myocardial infarction. Circulation 1998;98:2695–2701.
33. Montalescot G, Barragan P, Wittenberg O, et al., for the ADMIRAL Investigators. Platelet glycoprotein IIb/IIIa inhibition with coronary stenting for acute myocardial infarction. N Engl J Med 2001;344:1895–1903.
34. Stone GW, Grines CL, Cox DA, et al. A prospective, randomized trial comparing primary balloon angioplasty with or without abciximab to primary stenting with or without abciximab in acute myocardial infarction-primary endpoint analysis from the CADILLAC trial. Circulation 2000;18(Suppl 2):II–664.
35. Gold HK, Garabedian HD, Dinsmore RE, et al. Restoration of coronary flow in myocardial infarction by intravenous chimeric 7E3 antibody without exogenous plasminogen activators: observations in animals and humans. Circulation 1997;95:1755–1759.

36. Gold HK, Coller BS, Yasuda T, et al. Rapid and sustained coronary artery recanalization with combined bolus injection of recombinant tissue-type plasminogen activator and monoclonal antiplatelet GP IIb/IIIa antibody in a canine preparation. Circulation 1988;77:670–677.
37. Yasuda T, Gold HK, Fallon JT, et al. Monoclonal antibody against platelet glycoprotein (GP) IIb/IIIa receptor prevents coronary artery reocclusion after reperfusion with recombinant tissue-type plasminogen activator in dogs. J Clin Invest 1988;81:1284–1291.
38. Ohman EM, Kleiman NS, Gacioch G, et al., for the IMPACT-AMI Investigators. Combined accelerated tissue-plasminogen activator and platelet glycoprotein IIb/IIIa integrin receptor blockade with Integrilin in acute myocardial infarction: results of a randomized; placebo-controlled, dose-ranging trial. Circulation 1997;95:846–854.
39. Nicolini FA, Lee P, Rios G, et al. Combination of platelet fibrinogen receptor antagonist and direct antithrombin inhibitor at low doses markedly improves thrombolysis. Circulation 1994;89:1902–1809.
40. Harrington RA. Combining thrombolysis with the platelet glycoprotein IIb/IIIa inhibitor lamifiban: results of the platelet aggregation receptor antagonist dose investigation and reperfusion gain in myocardial infarction (PARADIGM) trial. J Am Coll Cardiol 1998;32:2003–2010.
41. Antman EM, Giugliano RP, McCabe CH, et al., for the TIMI–14 Investigators. Abciximab (ReoPro) potentiates thrombolysis in ST elevation myocardial infarction: results of the TIMI 14 trial. J Am Coll Cardiol 1998;31:191A.
42. Ohman EM, Lincoff AM, Bode C, et al. Enhanced early reperfusion at 60 minutes with low-dose reteplase combined with full-dose abciximab in acute myocardial infarction: preliminary results from the GUSTO-4 pilot (SPEED) dose-ranging trial. Circulation 1998;98(Suppl I):I–504.
43. Strategies for Patency Enhancement in the Emergency Department (SPEED) Group. Trial of abciximab with and without low-dose reteplase for acute myocardial infarction. Circulation 2000;101:2788–2794.
44. The Assessment of the Safety and Efficacy of a New Thrombolytic Regimen (ASSENT)-3 Investigators. Efficacy and safety of tenecteplase in combination with enoxaparin, abciximab, or unfractionated heparin: the ASSENT–3 randomised trial in acute myocardial infarction. Lancet 2001;358:605–613.
45. The GUSTO-V Investigators. Reperfusion therapy for acute myocardial infarction with fibrinolytic therapy or combination therapy with reduced fibrinolytic therapy and glycoprotein IIb/IIIa inhibition: the GUSTO-V randomised trial. Lancet 2001;357:1905–1914.
46. Ferguson JJ. Meeting highlights: highlights of the 21st Congress of the European Society of Cardiology. Circulation 1999;100:e126–e131.
47. Braunwald E, Antman EM, Beasley JW, et al. ACC/AHA guideline update for the management of patients with unstable angina and non–ST-segment elevation myocardial infarction. Updated March 17, 2002. Available at http://www.acc.org/clinical/guidelines/unstable/update/pdf/UA_update.pdf.
48. Cairns J, Theroux P, Armstrong P, et al. Unstable angina: report from a Canadian expert roundtable. Can J Cardiol 1996;12:1279–1292.
49. The TIMI IIIB Investigators. Effects of tissue plasminogen activator and a comparison of early invasive and conservative strategies in unstable angina and non–Q-wave myocardial infarction: results of the TIMI IIIB trial. Circulation 1994;89:1545–1556.
50. The GUSTO-IIb Investigators. A comparison of recombinant hirudin with heparin for the treatment of acute coronary syndromes. N Engl J Med 1996;335:775–782.
51. The PRISM Study Investigators. A comparison of aspirin plus tirofiban with aspirin plus heparin for unstable angina. N Engl J Med 1998;338:1498–1505.
52. The PRISM-PLUS Study Investigators. Inhibition of the platelet glycoprotein IIb/IIIa receptor with tirofiban in unstable angina and non–Q-wave myocardial infarction. N Engl J Med 1998;338:1488–1497.
53. The PARAGON Investigators. An international, randomized, controlled trial of lamifiban, a platelet glycoprotein IIb/IIIa inhibitor, heparin, or both in unstable angina. Circulation 1998;97:2386–2395.
54. Theroux P, Kouz S, Roy L, et al. Platelet membrane receptor glycoprotein IIb/IIIa antagonism in unstable angina: the Canadian lamifiban study. Circulation 1996;94:899–905.
55. Moliterno DJ. Patient-specific dosing of IIb/IIIa antagonists during acute coronary syndromes: rationale and design of the PARAGON B study. The PARAGON B International Steering Committee. Am Heart J 2000;139:563–566.
56. The PARAGON-B Investigators. Randomized, placebo-controlled trial of titrated intravenous lamifiban for acute coronary syndromes. Circulation 2002;105:316–321.
57. Newby LK, Ohman EM, Christenson RH, et al. Benefit of glycoprotein IIb/IIIa inhibition in patients with acute coronary syndromes and troponin T-positive status. Circulation 2001;103:2891–2896.

58. The PURSUIT Study Investigators. Inhibition of platelet glycoprotein IIb/IIIa with eptifibatide in patients with acute coronary syndromes. N Engl J Med 1998;339:436–443.

59. Schulman SP, Goldschmidt PJ, Topol EJ, et al. Effects of Integrilin, a platelet glycoprotein IIb/IIIa receptor antagonist, in unstable angina: a randomized multicenter trial. Circulation 1996;94:2083–2089.

60. The GUSTO IV-ACS Investigators. Effect of glycoprotein IIb/IIIa receptor blocker abciximab on outcome in patients with acute coronary syndromes without early coronary revascularization: the GUSTO-IV ACS randomised trial. Lancet 2001;357:1915–1924.

61. Boersma E, Harrington RA, Moliterno DJ, et al. Platelet glycoprotein IIb/IIIa inhibitors in acute coronary syndromes: a meta-analysis of all major randomised clinical trials. Lancet 2002;359:189-198.

62. Fredrickson BJ, Turner NA, Kleiman NS, et al. Effects of abciximab, ticlopidine, and combined abciximab/ticlopidine therapy on platelet and leukocyte function in patients undergoing coronary angioplasty. Circulation 2000;101:1122-1129.

63. Lincoff AM, Kereiakes DJ, Mascelli MA, et al. Abciximab suppresses the rise in levels of circulating inflammatory markers after percutaneous coronary revascularization. Circulation 2001;104:163-167.

64. Merlini PA, Bauer KA, Oltrona L, et al. Persistent activation of the coagulation system in unstable angina and myocardial infarction. Circulation 1994;90:61–68.

65. Van Belle E, Lablanche JM, Bauters C, et al. Coronary angioscopic findings in infarct-related vessel within 1 month of acute myocardial infarction: natural history and effect of thrombolysis. Circulation 1998;97:10–11.

66. Granger CB, Van de Werf F, Armstrong PW, et al., for the GUSTO-IIb Investigators. Hirudin reduces death and myocardial (re)infarction at 6 mo: follow-up results of the GUSTO-IIb trial. J Am Coll Cardiol 1998;31:79A.

67. Harrington RA, Lincoff AM, Berdan LG, et al. Maintenance of clinical benefit at six months in patients treated with the platelet glycoprotein IIb/IIIa inhibitor eptifibatide versus placebo during an acute ischemic event. Circulation 1998;98:I–359.

68. Cannon CP, McCabe CH, Borzak S, et al., for the TIMI 12 Investigators. A randomized trial of an oral glycoprotein IIb/IIIa antagonist, sibrafiban, in patients after an acute coronary syndrome: results of the TIMI 12 trial. Circulation 1998;97:340–349.

69. Kereiakes DJ, Kleiman NS, Ferguson JJ, et al. Pharmacodynamic efficacy, clinical safety, and outcomes after prolonged platelet glycoprotein IIb/IIIa receptor blockade with oral xemilofiban. Circulation 1998; 98:1268–1278.

70. O'Neill WW, Serruys P, Knudtson M, et al. Long-term treatment with a platelet glycoprotein-receptor antagonist after percutaneous coronary revascularization. N Engl J Med 2000;342:1316–1324.

71. The SYMPHONY Investigators. Comparison of sibrafiban with aspirin for prevention of cardiovascular events after acute coronary syndromes: a randomised trial. Lancet 2000;355:337–345.

72. The 2nd SYMPHONY Investigators. Randomized trial of aspirin, sibrafiban, or both for secondary prevention after acute coronary syndromes. Circulation 2000;103:1727–1733.

73. Cannon CP, McCabe CH, Wilcox RG, et al. Oral glycoprotein IIb/IIIa inhibition with Orbofiban in Patients with Unstable Coronary Syndromes (OPUS-TIMI 16) trial. Circulation 2000;102:149–156.

74. Topol EJ, Easton JD, Amarenco P, et al. Design of the blockade of the glycoprotein IIb/IIIa receptor to avoid vascular occlusion (BRAVO) trial. Am Heart J 2000;139:927–933.

75. Newby LK, Califf RM, White HD, et al. The failure of orally administered glycoprotein IIb/IIIa inhibitors to prevent recurrent cardiac events. Am J Med 2002;112:647–658.

76. Newby LK, McGuire DK. Oral platelet glycoprotein IIb/IIIa inhibition. Curr Cardiol Rep 2000;2:372–377.

77. Ault KA, Cannon CP, Mitchell J, et al. Platelet activation in patients after an acute coronary syndrome: results from the TIMI-12 trial. J Am Coll Cardiol 1999;33:634–639

78. Holmes MB, Sobel BE, Cannon CP, et al. Increased platelet reactivity in patients given orbofiban after an acute coronary syndrome: an OPUS-TIMI 16 substudy. Am J Cardiol 2000;85:491–493

79. Scarborough RM, Kleiman NS, Phillips DR. Platelet glycoprotein IIb/IIIa antagonists: what are the relevant issues concerning their pharmacology and clinical use? Circulation 1999;100:437–444.

80. Akkerhuis KM, Neuhaus KL, Wilcox RG, et al., for the FROST Investigators. Safety and preliminary efficacy of one month glycoprotein IIb/IIIa inhibition with lefradafiban in patients with acute coronary syndromes without ST-elevation; a phase II study. Eur Heart J 2000;21:2042–2055.

81. Antiplatelet Trialists' Collaboration. Collaborative overview of randomised trials of antiplatelet therapy. I. Prevention of death, myocardial infarction, and stroke by prolonged antiplatelet therapy in various categories of patients. BMJ 1994;308:81–106.

82. Hansson L, Zanchetti A, Carruthers SG, et al. Effects of intensive blood-pressure lowering and low-dose aspirin in patients with hypertension: principal results of the Hypertension Optimal Treatment (HOT) randomised trial. Lancet 1998;351:1755–1762.

83. Avanzini F, Palumbo G, Alli C, et al. Effects of low-dose aspirin on clinic and ambulatory blood pressure in treated hypertensive patients. Collaborative Group of the Primary Prevention Project (PPP)-Hypertension Study. Am J Hypertens 2000;13:611–616.

84. Steering Committee of the Physicians' Health Study Research Group. Final report on the aspirin component of the ongoing Physicians' Health Study. N Engl J Med 1989;321:129–135.

85. Cairns JA, Theroux P, Lewis DH, et al. Antithrombotic agents in coronary artery disease. Chest 2001; 119:228S–252S.

86. Antithrombotic Trialists' Collaboration. Collaborative meta-analysis of randomised trials of antiplatelet therapy for prevention of death, myocardial infarction, and stroke in high risk patients. BMJ 2002; 324:71–86.

87. Roderick PJ, Wilkes HC, Meade TW. The gastrointestinal toxicity of aspirin: an overview of randomised controlled trials. Br J Clin Pharmacol 1993;35:219–236.

88. Gent M, Blakely JA, Easton JD, et al. The Canadian American Ticlopidine Study (CATS) in thromboembolic stroke. Lancet 1989;1:1215–1220.

89. Balsano F, Rizzon P, Violi F, et al. Antiplatelet treatment with ticlopidine in unstable angina: a controlled multicenter clinical trial: the Studio della Ticlopidina nell'Angina Instabile Group. Circulation 1990;82:17–26.

90. Hass WK, Easton JD, Adams HP, et al. A randomized trial comparing ticlopidine hydrochloride with aspirin for the prevention of stroke in high-risk patients: Ticlopidine Aspirin Stroke Study Group. N Engl J Med 1989;321:501–507.

91. Leon M, Baim D, Popma J, Gordon P, et al. A clinical trial comparing three antithrombotic-drug regimens after coronary-artery stenting. N Engl J Med 1998;339:1665–1671.

92. Quinn MJ, Fitzgerald DJ. Cardiovascular drugs: ticlopidine and clopidogrel. Circulation 1999;100: 1667–1672.

93. The CAPRIE Steering Committee. A randomised, blinded, trial of clopidogrel versus aspirin in patients at risk of ischaemic events (CAPRIE). Lancet 1996;348:1329–1339.

94. The CURE Study Investigators. Effects of clopidogrel in addition to aspirin in patients with acute coronary syndromes without ST-segment elevation. N Engl J Med 2001;345:494–502.

95. Oler A, Whooley MA, Oler J, Grady D. Adding heparin to aspirin reduces the incidence of myocardial infarction and death in patients with unstable angina. JAMA 1996;276:811–815.

96. Lauer MA, Houghtaling PL, Peterson JG, et al. Attenuation of rebound ischemia after discontinuation of heparin therapy by glycoprotein IIb/IIIa inhibition with eptifibatide in patients with acute coronary syndromes: observations from the Platelet IIb/IIIa in Unstable Angina: Receptor Suppression Using Integrilin Therapy (PURSUIT) Trial. Circulation 2001;104:2772–2777.

97. Cohen M, Demers C, Gurfinkel EP, et al., for the Efficacy and Safety of Subcutaneous Enoxaparin in Non–Q-Wave Coronary Events Study Group. A comparison of low-molecular-weight heparin with unfractionated heparin for unstable coronary artery disease. N Engl J Med 1997;337:447–452.

98. Antman EM, Cohen M, Radley D, et al. Assessment of the treatment effect of enoxaparin for unstable angina/non–Q-wave myocardial infarction. TIMI 11B-ESSENCE meta-analysis. Circulation 1999;100: 1602–1608.

99. Klein W, Buchwald A, Hillis SE, et al. Comparison of low-molecular-weight heparin with unfractionated heparin acutely and with placebo for 6 wk in the management of unstable coronary artery disease. Circulation 1997;96:61–68.

100. The FRAXIS Study Group. Comparison of two treatment durations (6 d and 14 d) of a low molecular weight heparin with a 6-d treatment of unfractionated heparin in the initial management of unstable angina or non-Q wave myocardial infarction: FRAXIS. Eur Heart J 1999;20:1553–1562.

101. The Coumadin Aspirin Reinfarction Study (CARS) Investigators. Randomised double-blind trial of fixed low-dose warfarin with aspirin after myocardial infarction. Lancet 1997;350:389–396.

102. Fiore LD, Ezekowitz MD, Brophy MT, et al., for the Department of Veterans Affairs Cooperative Study Program. Clinical trial comparing combined warfarin and aspirin with aspirin alone in survivors of acute myocardial infarction. Circulation 2002;105:557-563.

103. The Organization to Assess Strategies for Ischemic Syndromes (OASIS) Investigators. Effects of long-term, moderate-intensity oral anticoagulation in addition to aspirin in unstable angina. J Am Coll Cardiol 2001;37:475–484.

104. Coletta AP, Cleland JGF. Clinical trials update: highlights of the scientific sessions of the XXIII Congress of the European Society of Cardiology—WARIS II, ESCAMI, PAFAC, RITZ-1 and TIME. Eur J Heart Failure 2001;3:747-750.

105. Simes RJ, Granger CB, Antman EM, Califf RM, Braunwald E, Topol EJ. Impact of hirudin versus heparin on mortality and (re)infarction in patients with acute coronary syndromes: a prospective meta-analysis of the GUSTO-IIb and TIMI 9b trials. Circulation 1996;94:I–430.

106. White H, for the Hirulog and Early Reperfusion or Occlusion (HERO)-2 Trial Investigators. Thrombin-specific anticoagulation with bivalirudin versus heparin in patients receiving fibrinolytic therapy for acute myocardial infarction: the HERO-2 randomised trial. Lancet 2001;358:1855-1863.

107. Bittl JA, Chaitman BR, Feit F, Kimball W, Topol EJ, for the Bivalirudin Angioplasty Study Investigators. Bivalirudin versus heparin during coronary angioplasty for unstable angina or postinfarction angina: final report reanalysis of the Bivalirudin Angioplasty Study. Am Heart J 2001;142: 952–959.

108. Kong DF, Topol EJ, Bittl JA, et al. Clinical outcomes of bivalirudin for ischemic heart disease. Circulation 1999;100:2049-2053.

109. The Direct Thrombin Inhibitor Trialists' Collaborative Group. Direct thrombin inhibitors in acute coronary syndromes: principal results of a meta-analysis based on individual patients' data. Lancet 2002; 359:294–302.

110. Eriksson BI, Bauer KA, Lassen MR, Turpie AGG, for the Steering Committee of the Pentasaccharide in Hip-Fracture Surgery Study. Fondaparinux compared with enoxaparin for the prevention of venous thromboembolism after hip-fracture surgery. N Engl J Med 2001;345:1298–1304.

111. Anonymous. Late breaking clinical trial abstracts. Circulation 2001;104:1B–4B.

112. Zoldhelyi P, McNatt J, Shelat HS, et al. Thromboresistance of balloon-injured porcine carotid arteries after local gene transfer of human tissue factor pathway inhibitor. Circulation 2000;101:289–295.

113. Steinhubl SR, Talley JD, Braden GA, et al. Point-of-care measured platelet inhibition correlates with a reduced risk of an adverse cardiac event after percutaneous coronary intervention. Results of the GOLD (AU-Assessing Ultegra) Multicenter Study. Circulation 2001;103:2572–2578.

114. Cannon CP, Weintraub WS, Demopoulos LA, et al., for the TACTICS-TIMI 18 Investigators. Comparison of early invasive and conservative strategies in patients with unstable coronary syndromes treated with the glycoprotein IIb/IIIa inhibitor tirofiban. N Engl J Med 2001;344:1879–1887.

115. Kereiakes DJ, Broderick TM, Roth EM, et al. Time course, magnitude, and consistency of platelet inhibition by abciximab, tirofiban, or eptifibatide in patients with unstable angina pectoris undergoing percutaneous coronary intervention. Am J Cardiol 1999;84:391–395.

116. Tam SH, Sassoli PM, Jordan RE, Nakada MT. Abciximab (ReoPro, chimeric 7E3 Fab) demonstrates equivalent affinity and functional blockade of glycoprotein IIb/IIIa and $\alpha_v\beta_3$ integrins. Circulation 1998; 98:1085–1091.

117. Neuman FJ, Zohlnhofer D, Fakhoury L, Ott I, Gawaz M, Schomig A. Effect of glycoprotein IIb/IIIa receptor blockade on platelet-leukocyte interaction and surface expression of the leukocyte integrin Mac-1 in acute myocardial infarction. J Am Coll Cardiol 1999;34:1420–1426.

118. McClure MW, Berkowitz SD, Sparapani R, et al. Clinical significance of thrombocytopenia during a non-ST-elevation acute coronary syndrome: the Platelet Glycoprotein IIb/IIIa in Unstable Angina: Receptor Suppression Using Integrilin Therapy (PURSUIT) trial experience. Circulation 2000;99:2892–2900.

119. Sane DC, Damaraju LV, Topol EJ, et al. Occurrence and clinical significance of thrombocytopenia during abciximab therapy. J Am Coll Cardiol 2000;36:75–83.

120. Boden WE, O'Rourke RA, Crawford MH, et al. Outcomes in patients with acute non–Q-wave myocardial infarction randomly assigned to an invasive as compared with a conservative management strategy. N Engl J Med 1998;338:1785–1792.

121. Mahaffey KW, Alexander JH, Roe MT, et al. Characterization of types of myocardial infarctions in two large acute coronary syndrome trials. Circulation 2001;104:II–697.

122. The FRISC II Investigators. Invasive compared with non-invasive treatment in unstable coronary artery disease: FRISC II prospective randomized multicentre study. Lancet 1999;354:708–715.

123. Mehta SR, Yusuf S, Peters RJG, et al., for the CURE Investigators. Effects of pretreatment with clopidogrel and aspirin followed by long-term therapy in patients undergoing percutaneous coronary intervention: the PCI-CURE study. Lancet 2001;358:526–533.

124. Stone GW, Cox D, Garcia E, et al. Normal flow (TIMI-3) before mechanical reperfusion therapy is an independent determinant of survival on acute myocardial infarction. Analysis from the Primary Angioplasty in Myocardial Infarction Trials. Circulation 2001;104:636–641.

125. Ross AM, Coyne KS, Reiner JS, et al. A randomized trial comparing primary angioplasty with a strategy of short-acting thrombolysis and immediate planned rescue angioplasty in acute myocardial infarction: the PACT trial. J Am Coll Cardiol 1999;34:1954–1962.
126. Morrison LJ, Verbeek PR, McDonald AC, et al. Mortality and prehospital thrombolysis for acute myocardial infarction: a meta-analysis. JAMA 2000;283:2686–2892.
127. Herrmann HC, Moliterno DJ, Ohman EM, et al. Facilitation of early percutaneous coronary intervention after reteplase with or without abciximab in acute myocardial infarction. Results from the SPEED (GUSTO-4 Pilot) Trial. J Am Coll Cardiol 2000;36:1489–1496.
128. Hamm CW, Heeschen C, Goldmann B, et al. Benefit of abciximab in patients with refractory unstable angina in relation to serum troponin T levels. N Engl J Med 1999;340:1623–1629.
129. Heeschen C, Hamm CW, Goldmann B, et al. Troponin concentrations for stratification of patients with acute coronary syndromes in relation to therapeutic efficacy with tirofiban. Lancet 1999;354:1757–1762.
130. Lincoff AM, Harrington RA, Califf RM, et al. Management of patients with acute coronary syndromes in the United States by platelet glycoprotein IIb/IIIa inhibition. Circulation 2000;102:1093–1100.
131. The CAST (Chinese Acute Stroke Trial) Collaborative Group. CAST: randomised, placebo-controlled trial of early aspirin use in 20 000 patients with acute ischemic stroke. Lancet 1997;349:1641–1649.
132. The Abciximab in Ischemic Stroke Investigators. Abciximab in acute ischemic stroke. A randomized, double-blind, placebo-controlled, dose-escalation study. Circulation 2000;31:601–609.
133. American Heart Association. 2001 Heart and Stroke Statistical Update. American Heart Association, Dallas, TX, 2001.
134. Gheorghiade M, Bonow RO. Chronic heart failure in the United States: a manifestation of coronary artery disease. Circulation 1998;97:282–289.
135. Al Khadra AS, Salem DN, Rand WM, Udelson JE, Smith JJ, Konstam MA. Antiplatelet agents and survival: a cohort analysis from the Studies of Left Ventricular Dysfunction (SOLVD) trial. J Am Coll Cardiol 1998;31:419–425.
136. Missov E, Calzolari C, Pau B. Circulating cardiac troponin I in severe congestive heart failure. Circulation 1997;96:2953–2958.
137. Hiatt WR. Drug therapy: management of peripheral arterial disease and claudication. N Engl J Med 2001;344:1608–1621.
138. Kapadia SR, Bajzer CT, Ziada KM, et al. Initial experience of platelet IIb/IIIa inhibition with abciximab during carotid stenting: a safe and effective adjunctive therapy. Stroke 2001;32:2328–2332.
139. Vorchheimer DA, Fuster V. Oral platelet glycoprotein IIb/IIIa receptor antagonists: the present challenge is safety. Circulation 1998;97:312–314.
140. Marso SP, Bhatt DL, Roe MT, et al. Enhanced efficacy of eptifibatide administration in patients with acute coronary syndrome requiring in-hospital coronary artery bypass grafting. Circulation 2000;102:2952–2958.
141. Michelson AD, Furman MI, Goldschmidt-Clermont P, et al. Platelet GP IIIa Pl(A) polymorphisms display different sensitivities to agonists. Circulation 2000;101:1013–1018.
142. Vijayan KV, Goldschmidt-Clermont PJ, Roos C, Bray PF. The Pl(A2) polymorphism of integrin beta(3) enhances outside-in signaling and adhesive functions. J Clin Invest 2000;105:793–802.
143. Goldschmidt-Clermont PJ, Coleman LD, Pham YM, et al. Higher prevalence of GPIIIa PlA2 polymorphism in siblings of patients with premature coronary heart disease. Arch Pathol Lab Med 1999;123:1223–1229.
144. Weiss EJ, Bray PF, Tayback M, et al. A polymorphism of a platelet glycoprotein receptor as an inherited risk factor for coronary thrombosis. N Engl J Med 1996;334:1090–1094.
145. Mikkelsson J, Perola M, Laippala P, et al. Glycoprotein IIIa/Pl(A) polymorphism associates with progression of coronary artery disease and with myocardial infarction in an autopsy series of middle-aged men who died suddenly. Arterioscler Thromb Vasc Biol 1999;19:2573–2578.
146. Walter DH, Schachinger V, Elsner M, Dimmeler S, Zeiher AM. Platelet glycoprotein IIIa polymorphisms and risk of coronary stent thrombosis. Lancet 1997;350:1217–1219.
147. Kastrati A, Koch W, Gawaz M, et al. PlA polymorphism of glycoprotein IIIa and risk of adverse events after coronary stent placement. J Am Coll Cardiol 2000;36:84–89.
148. Laule M, Cascorbi I, Stangl V, et al. A1/A2 polymorphism of glycoprotein IIIa and association with excess procedural risk for coronary catheter interventions: a case-controlled study. Lancet 1999;353:708–712.
149. Wheeler GL, Braden GA, Bray PF, Marciniak SJ, Mascelli MA, Sane DC. Reduced inhibition with abciximab in platelets with the Pl^{A2} polymorphism. Am Heart J 2002;143:76–82.

APPENDIX: LIST OF REFERENCED CLINICAL TRIALS

A to Z	Aggrastat to Zocor
ADMIRAL	Abciximab before Direct angioplasty and stenting in Myocardial Infarction Regarding Acute and Long-term follow-up
ADVANCE-MI	ADdressing the Value of facilitated Angioplasty after Combination therapy or Eptifibatide monotherapy in acute Myocardial Infarction
ASSENT-3	ASsessment of the Safety and Efficacy of a New Thrombolytic-3
BRAVO	Blockade of the IIb/IIIa Receptor to Avoid Vascular Occlusion
CADILLAC	Controlled Abciximab and Device Investigation to Lower Late Angioplasty Complications
CAPRIE	Clopidogrel versus Aspirin in Patients at Risk of Ischemic Events
CAPTURE	Chimeric 7E3 AntiPlatelet Therapy in Unstable angina REfractory to standard treatment
CARS	Coumadin and Aspirin Reinfarction Study
COMPARE	Comparison Of Measurements of Platelet aggregation with Aggrastat, ReoPro, and Eptifibatide
CURE	Clopidogrel in Unstable angina to prevent Recurrent Events
EPIC	Evaluation of c7E3 for the Prevention of Ischemic Complications
EPILOG	Evaluation in PTCA to Improve Long-term Outcome with abciximab GP IIb/IIIa blockade
EPISTENT	Evaluation of Platelet Inhibition in STENTing
ESPRIT	Enhanced Suppression of the Platelet IIb/IIIa Receptor with Integrilin Therapy
ESSENCE	Efficacy and Safety of Subcutaneous Enoxaparin in Non-Q wave Coronary Events
EXCITE	Evaluation of oral Xemilofiban in ControllIng Thrombotic Events
FINESSE	Facilitated InterventioN with Enhanced reperfusion Speed to Stop Events
FRISC-II	FRagmin and fast revascularization during InStability in Coronary artery disease-II
FROST	Fibrinogen Receptor Occupancy STudy
GOLD	AU-Assessing Ultegra Multicenter Study
GUSTO-IIb	Global Use of Strategies To Open occluded arteries in acute coronary syndromes
GUSTO-IV, -V	Global Use of Strategies To Open occluded coronary arteries
HERO-2	Hirulog and Early Reperfusion or Occlusion
HOT	Hypertension Optimal Treatment
IMPACT-II	Integrilin to Minimize Platelet Aggregation and Coronary Thrombosis

INTRO-AMI	INTegrilin and Reduced dose Of thrombolytics for Acute Myocardial Infarction
ISAR-2	Intracoronary Stenting and Antithrombotic Regimen
OASIS	Organization to Assess Strategies for Ischemic Syndromes
OPUS-TIMI 16	Orbofiban in Patients with Unstable coronary Syndromes
ORBIT	Oral glycoprotein IIb/IIIa Receptor Blockade to Inhibit Thrombosis
PACT	Primary Angioplasty Compatibility Trial
PAMI	Primary Angioplasty in Myocardial Infarction
PARAGON	Platelet IIb/IIIa Antagonists for Reduction of Acute coronary syndrome events in a Global Organization Network
PCI-CURE	Percutaneous Coronary Intervention-Clopidogrel in Unstable angina to prevent Recurrent Events
PRISM	Platelet Receptor inhibition in Ischemic Syndrome Management
PRISM-PLUS	Platelet Receptor inhibition for Ischemic Syndrome Management in Patients Limited by Unstable Signs and symptoms
PURSUIT	Platelet glycoprotein IIb/IIIa in Unstable angina: Receptor Suppression Using Integrilin Therapy
RAPPORT	ReoPro And Primary PTCA Organization and Randomized Trial
REPLACE-2	Randomized Evaluation in PCI Linking Angiomax to reduced Clinical Events
RESTORE	Randomized Efficacy Study of Tirofiban for Outcomes and REstenosis
SPEED	Strategies for Patency Enhancement in the Emergency Department
STOP-AMI	Stent versus Thrombolysis for Occluded coronary arteries in Patients with Acute Myocardial Infarction
SYMPHONY	Sibrafiban vs aspirin to Yield Maximum Protection from ischemic Heart events pOst acute coroNarY syndromes
SYNERGY	Superior Yield of the New strategy of Enoxaparin, Revascularization, and GlYcoprotein IIb/IIIa Inhibitors
TACTICS-TIMI 18	Treat angina with Aggrastat and determine Cost of Therapy with an Invasive or Conservative Strategy
TARGET	do Tirofiban And ReoPro Give similar Efficacy? Trial
TIMI	Thrombolysis In Myocardial Infarction
VANQWISH	Veterans Affairs Non-Q-Wave Infarction Strategies in Hospital
WARIS II	Warfarin Aspirin ReInfarction Study II

INDEX

A

Abciximab,
    acute myocardial infarction, percutaneous
        coronary intervention and abciximab
        therapy,
        ADMIRAL, 280–282
        CADILLAC, 281, 283
        clinical outcomes, 281–283
        contractile function recovery, 280
        ISAR-2, 279–281
        microvascular reperfusion, 278, 279
        myocardial salvage, 280
        prospects, 283, 284
        RAPPORT, 281
        rationale, 275, 276
        STOP-AMI, 280
        TIMI grade 3 flow establishment and
          adequacy, 276, 277
    antithrombin combination therapy, 348
    binding affinity for glycoprotein IIb/IIIa
        receptor, 84
    development,
        animal model studies of thrombosis,
          80, 81, 106
        chimeric antibody, 81
        overview, 105, 106
    duration of therapy, 85
    economic analysis,
        percutaneous coronary intervention,
        CAPTURE, 312
        EPIC, 309–311
        EPILOG, 311, 312
        EPISTENT, 312, 313
        ST-elevation myocardial infarction, 317
    epitope, 85, 383
    evidence-based selection, 450
    fibrinolysis, acute myocardial ischemia,
        and glycoprotein IIb/IIIa receptor
        blockade,
        ASSENT-3, 298, 300
        GUSTO-V, 295–297
        TAMI 8, 290

    low-molecular-weight heparin combination
        therapy, 352, 354, 355
    major adverse cardiac events, early vs
        late, 386, 387
    mechanisms of action,
    percutaneous carotid intervention adjunctive
        therapy, 400, 401
    percutaneous coronary intervention trials,
        EPIC,
        clinical efficacy, 111, 112, 114
        overview, 110, 111
        safety, 114, 115
        study design, 111
        EPILOG,
        clinical efficacy, 116, 117
        overview, 115
        safety, 117
        study design, 115, 116
        EPISTENT,
        clinical efficacy, 118–120
        overview, 117, 118
        safety, 120
        study design, 118
        overview of study design, 110
        phase II trials, 106, 107, 109, 110
        pooled trial findings,
        diabetes, 121, 122
        endpoints after 30 d, 113
        mortality, 120
        unstable angina, 121
    pharmacokinetics, 84–87, 106–110,
        168, 386
    receptor specificity, 82, 83, 168, 384–386
    stroke risks, 410–412, 415, 416
    trials, *see* ADMIRAL; CADILLAC;
        CAPTURE; EPIC; EPILOG;
        EPISTENT; GUSTO-IV; ISAR-2;
        RAPPORT; TARGET
    unstable angina trials, *see also* CAPTURE;
        GUSTO-IV,
        angiographic observations, 268, 269
        benefits, 264, 265

bleeding events, 252–254
clinical outcomes, 243
concomitant heparin therapy, 259
dosing, 258, 259
high-risk patient targeting, 265, 266
mortality, 248–252, 254
myocardial infarction, 251, 252, 254
overview, 237, 238
patient selection, 241, 242
primary therapy vs percutaneous
    intervention effect, 255–257
study designs, 241
ACS, *see* Acute coronary syndromes
ACUTE II, low-molecular-weight heparin
    use with glycoprotein IIb/IIIa receptor
    antagonists, 354
Acute coronary syndromes (ACS), *see also*
    specific diseases,
direct thrombin inhibitor trials, 355, 356
history of management, 4, 5
low-molecular-weight heparin therapy,
    glycoprotein IIb/IIIa receptor antagonist
        combination trials, 354, 355
    management, 348, 349
pathophysiology, 3, 4
percutaneous coronary intervention, *see*
    Percutaneous coronary intervention
plaque rupture, factors affecting,
    inflammatory markers, 10–12
    lipid content, 9
    overview, 8, 9
    thickness of fibrous cap, 10
    triggers, 12, 13
thrombosis components,
    atherosclerotic plaque, 6–13
    coagulation cascade, 16-18
    endothelium, 5, 6
    pathophysiology, 73–75
    platelets, 13–16
types, 3
ADMIRAL,
acute myocardial infarction, percutaneous
    coronary intervention, and abciximab
    therapy, 280–282
diabetic findings, 385
facilitated percutaneous coronary
    intervention, 445
intertrial comparison,
    clinical efficacy,
        endpoint at 30 d, 179–183
        general blockade effects, 190, 191

patient subgroups, 182
specific agent comparison, 191, 192
combination therapy, 178, 179
drug regimens, 177, 178
entry criteria, 177
heparin regimens and vascular access
    site management, 178
long-term efficacy,
    acute ischemic endpoints, 184, 185
    mortality, 185, 186
    overview, 182, 184
    safety, 187–189
    target vessel revascularization,
        186, 187
safety,
    bleeding, 192, 193
    emergency coronary bypass
        surgery, 193
    readministration, 194
    thrombocytopenia, 189, 193, 194
    trial conduct and endpoints, 179
ST-elevation myocardial infarction,
    431, 445
study design,
    algorithms, 170, 171
    entry criteria, 172
    heparin regimens and vascular sheath
        removal, 173
    overview, 176
ADP, receptors and signaling cross-talk, 49, 50
Angioguard, emboli protection device, 402,
    403, 405, 406
Antithrombin III,
heparin binding, 17
thrombin binding, 17
Argatroban,
acute coronary syndrome trials, 355, 356
percutaneous coronary intervention,
    glycoprotein IIb/IIIa receptor antagonist
        combination trials, 358, 359
    management, 356, 357
thrombin inhibition, 347, 348
Aspirin,
atherosclerosis benefits, 437, 438
dosing, 438
glycoprotein IIb/IIIa receptor antagonist
    interactions, 336
hemorrhagic stroke complication during
    acute ischemic stroke therapy,
    415, 416
history of use, 4

percutaneous carotid intervention
    adjunctive therapy, 400, 414
primary prevention, 438
resistance, 365
stroke benefits, 74, 75, 412, 413, 415
unstable angina management, 235
ASSENT-3, fibrinolysis, acute myocardial
    ischemia, and glycoprotein IIb/IIIa
    receptor blockade, 298, 300
Atherosclerotic plaque,
    classification of lesions, 7–9
    progression of disease, 7–9
    rupture, factors affecting,
        inflammatory markers, 10–12, 388, 389
        lipid content, 9
        overview, 8, 9, 427
        thickness of fibrous cap, 10
        triggers, 12, 13

B

Bivalirudin,
    acute coronary syndrome trials, 355, 356
    percutaneous coronary intervention,
        glycoprotein IIb/IIIa receptor antagonist
            combination trials, 358, 359
        management, 356, 357
    thrombin inhibition, 347, 348
Bleeding time, platelet function assay, 328
BRAVO, study design and outcomes, 372,
    377, 378, 437

C

CABG, *see* Coronary artery bypass grafting
CADILLAC,
    acute myocardial infarction, percutaneous
        coronary intervention and abciximab
        therapy, 281, 283
    intertrial comparison,
        clinical efficacy,
            endpoint at 30 d, 179–183
            general blockade effects, 190, 191
            patient subgroups, 182
            specific agent comparison, 191, 192
        combination therapy, 178, 179
        drug regimens, 177, 178
        entry criteria, 177
        heparin regimens and vascular access
            site management, 178
        long-term efficacy,
            acute ischemic endpoints, 184, 185
            mortality, 185, 186

overview, 182, 184
safety, 187–189
target vessel revascularization,
    186, 187
safety,
    bleeding, 192, 193
    emergency coronary bypass
        surgery, 193
    readministration, 194
    thrombocytopenia, 189, 193, 194
trial conduct and endpoints, 179
study design,
    algorithms, 170, 171
    entry criteria, 172
    heparin regimens and vascular sheath
        removal, 173
    overview, 176
Calcium, glycoprotein IIb/IIIa receptor
    binding, 47, 48
Calpain, activation in platelet aggregation, 54
CAPRIE, outcomes, 439
CAPTURE,
    economic analysis, 312
    intertrial comparison,
        clinical efficacy,
            endpoint at 30 d, 179–183
            general blockade effects, 190, 191
            patient subgroups, 182
            specific agent comparison, 191, 192
        combination therapy, 178, 179
        drug regimens, 177, 178
        entry criteria, 177
        heparin regimens and vascular access
            site management, 178
        long-term efficacy,
            acute ischemic endpoints, 184, 185
            mortality, 185, 186
            overview, 182, 184
            safety, 187–189
            target vessel revascularization,
                186, 187
    safety,
        bleeding, 192, 193
        emergency coronary bypass
            surgery, 193
        readministration, 194
        thrombocytopenia, 189, 193, 194
    trial conduct and endpoints, 179
    study design,
        algorithms, 170, 171
        entry criteria, 172

heparin regimens and vascular sheath
    removal, 173
  overview, 175
unstable angina trial of abciximab,
    angiogram assessment, 207–209, 211,
        212, 216, 222–225
    arteriography and angioplasty, 207,
        212, 213
    baseline characteristics of patients,
        215, 216
    comparison with other trials, 226–229
    electrocardiography, 206
    endpoints,
        4-yr follow-up, 219–221
        30 d, 216–218
    flow of patients, 214
    independent data reporting measures, 206
    patient selection, 204, 205
    pilot trial outcomes, 209–213
    prognostic factors, 219, 221, 222
    safety, 218, 219
    statistical analysis, 206, 207, 209
    study design, 205, 206
Carotid angioplasty and stenting,
  adjunctive therapy,
    abciximab, 400, 401
    aspirin, 400, 414
    clopidogrel, 400, 414
    heparin, 414
    ticlopidine, 400, 414
  advantages, 397
  emboli protection devices, 402–406
  historical perspective, 397, 413, 414
  stent studies and outcomes, 397–400, 414
CD11b/18,
  abciximab binding, 384
  acute coronary disease modulation, 384
  antiinflammatory effects of blocking, 389
CD40L,
  glycoprotein IIb/IIIa receptor binding, 40,
      42, 43, 47, 57, 58
  inflammation role, 57, 58
Citrate, eptifibatide interactions, 89, 90
Clopidogrel,
  CAPRIE trial, 439
  CURE trial, 439
  glycoprotein IIb/IIIa receptor antagonist
      interactions, 336, 337
  percutaneous carotid intervention
      adjunctive therapy, 400, 414
  stroke prevention trials, 413

unstable angina management, 236, 237
Clot Signature Analyzer (CSA), platelet
    function assay, 333, 334
Coagulation cascade,
  inhibition, 17, 18, 441, 442
  tissue factor-dependent pathway, 16, 17
Collagen,
  platelet,
    adhesion, 24, 25
    receptors, 31
  receptors and signaling cross-talk, 49–51
COMPARE, dosing, 442
Cone and platelet analyzer (CPA), platelet
    function assay, 332
Coronary artery bypass grafting (CABG),
  emergency surgery incidence with
      glycoprotein IIb/IIIa receptor
      blockade, 193
  glycoprotein IIb/IIIa receptor blockade
      indication, 448, 449
Cost-effectiveness, *see* Economic analysis
CPA, *see* Cone and platelet analyzer
C-reactive protein (CRP),
  atherosclerotic plaque rupture role, 11, 12
  glycoprotein IIb/IIIa receptor blockade
      effects, 387, 388
  risk assessment in CAPTURE trial,
      219, 221
  stent induction, 387
CRP, *see* C-reactive protein
CSA, *see* Clot Signature Analyzer
CURE, outcomes, 439

D

Diabetes,
  abciximab studies, 385
  pooled trial findings for glycoprotein IIb/
      IIIa receptor blockade, 121, 122

E

Economic analysis,
  abciximab in ST-elevation myocardial
      infarction, 317
  cost,
    classification, 306, 307
    clinical trial measurement, 309
    measurement, 307, 308
  cost-effectiveness analysis, definition and
      goals, 309
  eptifibatide in acute coronary syndromes,
      PURSUIT analysis, 315–317

percutaneous coronary intervention,
    abciximab,
        CAPTURE, 312
        EPIC, 309–311
        EPILOG, 311, 312
        EPISTENT, 312, 313
    eptifibatide,
        ESPRIT, 314, 315
        IMPACT II, 314
    tirofiban and RESTORE trial, 315
    prescription drug development and
        marketing costs, 425
    principles, 305–307
    secondary prevention, 317
    tirofiban and abciximab comparison in
        TARGET, 317, 318
EDRF, *see* Endothelium-derived relaxation
    factor
Electrical impedance aggregometry, platelet
    function assay, 327
Endothelium,
    platelet binding, 13, 14, 24, 25
    vasoactive substance production, 5–7,
        11, 24
Endothelium-derived relaxation factor
    (EDRF), *see* Nitric oxide
EPIC,
    economic analysis, 309–311
    intertrial comparison,
        clinical efficacy,
            endpoint at 30 d, 179–183
            general blockade effects, 190, 191
            patient subgroups, 182
            specific agent comparison, 191, 192
        combination therapy, 178, 179
        drug regimens, 177, 178
        entry criteria, 177
        heparin regimens and vascular access
            site management, 178
        long-term efficacy,
            acute ischemic endpoints, 184, 185
            mortality, 185, 186, 391–393
            overview, 182, 184
            safety, 187–189
            target vessel revascularization,
                186, 187
        safety,
            bleeding, 192, 193
            emergency coronary bypass
                surgery, 193
            readministration, 194

thrombocytopenia, 189, 193, 194
        trial conduct and endpoints, 179
    percutaneous coronary intervention trial
        of abciximab,
        clinical efficacy, 111, 112, 114
        overview, 110, 111
        pooled trial findings,
            diabetes, 121, 122
            endpoints after 30 d, 113
            mortality, 120
            unstable angina, 121
        safety, 114, 115
        study design, 111
    platelet inhibition levels and thrombotic
        event protection, 322, 323
    study design,
        algorithms, 170, 171
        entry criteria, 172
        heparin regimens and vascular sheath
            removal, 173
        overview, 169
EPILOG,
    economic analysis, 311, 312
    intertrial comparison,
        clinical efficacy,
            endpoint at 30 d, 179–183
            general blockade effects, 190, 191
            patient subgroups, 182
            specific agent comparison, 191, 192
        combination therapy, 178, 179
        drug regimens, 177, 178
        entry criteria, 177
        heparin regimens and vascular access
            site management, 178
        long-term efficacy,
            acute ischemic endpoints, 184, 185
            mortality, 185, 186, 391–393
            overview, 182, 184
            safety, 187–189
            target vessel revascularization,
                186, 187
        safety,
            bleeding, 192, 193
            emergency coronary bypass
                surgery, 193
            readministration, 194
            thrombocytopenia, 189, 193, 194
        trial conduct and endpoints, 179
    percutaneous coronary intervention trial
        of abciximab,
    clinical efficacy, 116, 117

overview, 115
safety, 117
study design, 115, 116
pooled trial findings,
    diabetes, 121, 122
    endpoints after 30 d, 113
    mortality, 120
    unstable angina, 121
study design,
    algorithms, 170, 171
    entry criteria, 172
    heparin regimens and vascular sheath
        removal, 173
    overview, 169
EPISTENT,
    economic analysis, 312, 313
    intertrial comparison,
        clinical efficacy,
            endpoint at 30 d, 179–183
            general blockade effects, 190, 191
            patient subgroups, 182
            specific agent comparison, 191, 192
        combination therapy, 178, 179
        drug regimens, 177, 178
        entry criteria, 177
        heparin regimens and vascular access
            site management, 178
        long-term efficacy,
            acute ischemic endpoints, 184, 185
            mortality, 185, 186, 391–393
            overview, 182, 184
            safety, 187–189
            target vessel revascularization,
                186, 187
        safety,
            bleeding, 192, 193
            emergency coronary bypass
                surgery, 193
            readministration, 194
            thrombocytopenia, 189, 193, 194
        trial conduct and endpoints, 179
    non-ST-elevation acute coronary
        syndromes, 429
    percutaneous coronary intervention trial
        of abciximab,
        clinical efficacy, 118–120
        overview, 117, 118
        safety, 120
        study design, 118
    pooled trial findings,
        diabetes, 121, 122, 385

endpoints after 30 d, 113
mortality, 120
unstable angina, 121
study design,
    algorithms, 170, 171
    entry criteria, 172
    heparin regimens and vascular sheath
        removal, 173
    overview, 174
Eptifibatide,
    calcium effects on glycoprotein IIb/IIIa
        receptor binding, 48
    citrate effect, 89, 90
    economic analysis,
        acute coronary syndromes, PURSUIT
            analysis, 315–317
        percutaneous coronary intervention,
            ESPRIT, 314, 315
            IMPACT II, 314
    evidence-based selection, 450
    fibrinolysis, acute myocardial ischemia,
        and glycoprotein IIb/IIIa receptor
        blockade,
        IMPACT-AMI, 291
        streptokinase studies, 291
    low-molecular-weight heparin combination
        therapy, 352, 354, 355
    mechanism of action, 125, 126
    percutaneous coronary intervention trials,
        ESPRIT,
            baseline characteristics of
                participants, 139, 140
            clinical efficacy, 140–145
            safety, 143, 144
            study design, 136–138
            subgroup analysis, 140
        IMPACT II,
            adverse events, 131
            clinical efficacy, 128–130
            composite endpoint components, 131
            dosing issues, 132, 134
            study design, 127, 128
            time to events, 130, 131
        phase II trials,
            IMPACT, 127
            IMPACT Hi/Low, 127
        PRIDE, 134, 136
        PURSUIT, 134
    pharmacokinetics, 88–90, 168, 386
    receptor selectivity, 88, 89
    trials, *see* ESPRIT; IMPACT II; PURSUIT

unstable angina trials, *see also*
PURSUIT,
angiographic observations, 268, 269
benefits, 264, 265
bleeding events, 252–254
clinical outcomes, 243
concomitant heparin therapy, 259
dosing, 258, 259
high-risk patient targeting, 265, 266
mortality, 248–252, 254
myocardial infarction, 251, 252, 254
overview, 245–247
patient selection, 241, 242
primary therapy vs percutaneous
intervention effect, 255–257
study designs, 241
ESPRIT,
baseline characteristics of participants,
139, 140
clinical efficacy, 140–145
economic analysis, 314, 315
intertrial comparison,
clinical efficacy,
endpoint at 30 d, 179–183
general blockade effects, 190, 191
patient subgroups, 182
specific agent comparison,
191, 192
combination therapy, 178, 179
drug regimens, 177, 178
entry criteria, 177
heparin regimens and vascular access
site management, 178
long-term efficacy,
acute ischemic endpoints, 184, 185
mortality, 185, 186
overview, 182, 184
safety, 187–189
target vessel revascularization,
186, 187
safety,
bleeding, 192, 193
emergency coronary bypass
surgery, 193
readministration, 194
thrombocytopenia, 189, 193, 194
trial conduct and endpoints, 179
non-ST-elevation acute coronary
syndromes, 429, 430
platelet inhibition levels and thrombotic
event protection, 323

safety, 143, 144
study design,
algorithms, 170, 171
entry criteria, 172
heparin regimens and vascular sheath
removal, 173
overview, 136–138, 174, 175
subgroup analysis, 140
EXCITE, study design and outcomes, 370,
373, 374, 436

F

Factor Xa, inhibitor therapy, 441
Fibrinogen,
glycoprotein IIb/IIIa receptor binding,
activated platelets, 40, 45, 46, 77
unstimulated platelets, 52
platelet adhesion, 25, 26
Fibrinolysis,
acute myocardial ischemia and glycoprotein
IIb/IIIa receptor blockade,
abciximab,
ASSENT-3, 298, 300
GUSTO-V, 295–297
TAMI 8, 290
eptifibatide,
IMPACT-AMI, 291
streptokinase studies, 291
lamifiban, PARADIGM trial, 291
limitations of tissue plasminogen
activator monotherapy, 289
rationale, 290
recommendations, 300, 301
reduced dose fibrinolysis trials,
phase II trials, 291–295
phase III trials, 295–300
ST-elevation myocardial infarction,
glycoprotein IIb/IIIa receptor
blockade, 431, 432
stroke management, *see* Stroke
Fibronectin,
glycoprotein IIb/IIIa receptor binding, 46
platelet adhesion, 24, 25
structure, 45
Flow cytometry, platelet function assay,
327, 328
FRISC-II, upstream therapy, 444
FROST,
outcomes, 437
platelet inhibition levels and thrombotic
event protection, 324

G

Gas-6, thrombus stability role, 42, 43
Glanzmann's thrombasthenia,
    clinical features, 75, 76
    glycoprotein IIb/IIIa receptor deficiency, 76
Glycoprotein Ib/IX receptor, platelet adhesion
    role, 30, 31
Glycoprotein IIb/IIIa receptor,
    antagonists, *see also* specific drugs,
        evidence-based selection, 450
        interaction with other antiplatelet
            agents, 335–337
        mechanisms of action, 15, 342
        platelet-derived growth factor effects,
            59, 60
        rationale for development, 23, 32, 39,
            40, 73, 79, 342, 343, 427
        structural overview, 47, 147
        thrombin formation reduction, 59
    calcium binding, 47, 48
    cytoskeletal interactions, 55
    deficiency in Glanzmann's
        thrombasthenia, 76
    inflammation role, 40, 42, 43, 47, 57–59
    ligand-induced binding site epitopes, 48, 49
    ligands, 31, 40, 45–47, 78
    platelets,
        abundance on platelet surface, 15, 41
        activation, 15, 16, 41
        adhesion role, 31, 32
        aggregation,
            outside-in signal transduction, 52–55
            role, 41, 42
            signaling, 40, 42, 49–51
            stimulus-induced activation, 49–52
    polymorphisms and cardiovascular risks,
        56, 57, 376, 449
    prospects for study, 60, 61
    recognition specificity, 15, 31, 45, 147
    shuttling, 41
    structure, 43–45
    thrombus stability role, 42, 43
    upregulation of expression, 41
GOLD,
    dosing, 442
    platelet inhibition levels and thrombotic
        event protection, 325
GUSTO-IV,
    abciximab unstable angina trial,
        angiographic observations, 268, 269

benefits, 264, 265
bleeding events, 252–254
clinical outcomes, 243
concomitant heparin therapy, 259
dosing, 258, 259
high-risk patient targeting, 265, 266
mortality, 248–252, 254
myocardial infarction, 251, 252, 254
overview, 237, 238
patient selection, 241, 242
primary therapy vs percutaneous
    intervention effect, 255–257
study designs, 241
facilitated percutaneous coronary inter-
    vention, 445, 446
non-ST-elevation acute coronary
    syndromes, glycoprotein IIb/IIIa
    receptor blockade, 435
GUSTO-V, fibrinolysis, acute myocardial
    ischemia, and glycoprotein IIb/IIIa
    receptor blockade, 295–297

H

Heart failure, glycoprotein IIb/IIIa receptor
    blockade, 447, 448
Heparin, *see also* Low-molecular-weight
    heparin,
    antithrombin complex, 344
    history of use, 4
    limitations, 346, 439
    percutaneous carotid intervention
        adjunctive therapy, 414
    stroke risks, 410–412, 415, 416
    structure, 344–346
    thrombin inhibition, 344–346
Hirudin,
    acute coronary syndrome trials, 355, 356
    percutaneous coronary intervention,
        glycoprotein IIb/IIIa receptor antagonist
            combination trials, 358, 359
        management, 356, 357
    thrombin inhibition, 347

I

ICAM, *see* Intercellular adhesion molecule
IL-1, *see* Interleukin-1
IL-6, *see* Interleukin-6
IMPACT, eptifibatide trial, 127
IMPACT II,
    adverse events, 131
    clinical efficacy, 128–130

Index

467

composite endpoint components, 131
dosing issues, 132, 134, 442
economic analysis, 314
intertrial comparison,
    clinical efficacy,
        endpoint at 30 d, 179–183
        general blockade effects, 190, 191
        patient subgroups, 182
        specific agent comparison, 191, 192
    combination therapy, 178, 179
    drug regimens, 177, 178
    entry criteria, 177
    heparin regimens and vascular access
        site management, 178
    long-term efficacy,
        acute ischemic endpoints, 184, 185
        mortality, 185, 186
        overview, 182, 184
        safety, 187–189
        target vessel revascularization,
            186, 187
    safety,
        bleeding, 192, 193
        emergency coronary bypass sur-
            gery, 193
        readministration, 194
        thrombocytopenia, 189, 193, 194
    trial conduct and endpoints, 179
platelet inhibition levels and thrombotic
    event protection, 323
study design,
    algorithms, 170, 171
    entry criteria, 172
    heparin regimens and vascular sheath
        removal, 173
    overview, 127, 128, 174
    time to events, 130, 131
IMPACT-AMI, fibrinolysis, acute myocardial
    ischemia, and glycoprotein IIb/IIIa
    receptor blockade, 291
IMPACT Hi/Low, eptifibatide trial, 127
Integrins, *see also* Glycoprotein IIb/IIIa
    receptor,
    platelet receptors, 27–30, 77, 79
    structure of adhesion receptors, 27, 28
INTERACT, low-molecular-weight heparin
    use with glycoprotein IIb/IIIa receptor
    antagonists, 355
Intercellular adhesion molecule (ICAM),
    atherosclerotic plaque rupture role, 11
    reperfusion limitation role, 278

Interleukin-1 (IL-1), atherosclerotic plaque
    rupture role, 11, 12
Interleukin-6 (IL-6),
    glycoprotein IIb/IIIa receptor blockade
        effects, 387, 388
    stent induction, 387
ISAR-2
    acute myocardial infarction, percutaneous
        coronary intervention, and abciximab
        therapy, 279–281
    intertrial comparison,
        clinical efficacy,
            endpoint at 30 d, 179–183
            general blockade effects, 190, 191
            patient subgroups, 182
            specific agent comparison, 191, 192
        combination therapy, 178, 179
        drug regimens, 177, 178
        entry criteria, 177
        heparin regimens and vascular access
            site management, 178
        long-term efficacy,
            acute ischemic endpoints, 184, 185
            mortality, 185, 186
            overview, 182, 184
            safety, 187–189
            target vessel revascularization,
                186, 187
        safety,
            bleeding, 192, 193
            emergency coronary bypass
                surgery, 193
            readministration, 194
            thrombocytopenia, 189, 193, 194
        trial conduct and endpoints, 179
    study design,
        algorithms, 170, 171
        entry criteria, 172
        heparin regimens and vascular sheath
            removal, 173
        overview, 175, 176

K

Klerval,
    pharmacology, 366, 367
    phase II trials, 367, 368

L

Lamifiban,
    fibrinolysis, acute myocardial ischemia,
        and glycoprotein IIb/IIIa receptor
        blockade,

unstable angina trials, *see also*
        PARAGON-A; PARAGON-B,
    bleeding events, 252–254
    clinical outcomes, 243
    concomitant heparin therapy, 259
    dosing, 258, 259
    mortality, 248–252, 254
    myocardial infarction, 251, 252, 254
    overview, 238–240
    patient selection, 241, 242
    primary therapy vs percutaneous
        intervention effect, 255–257
    study designs, 241
Laminin, platelet adhesion, 24
Lefradafiban,
    pharmacology, 366, 367
    phase II trials, 367, 368, 437
Lotrafiban,
    limitations, 379, 380
    meta-analysis of oral drugs, 378, 379
    pharmacology, 366, 367
    phase II trials, 367–369
    phase III trials,
        BRAVO, 372, 377, 378
        efficacy and safety, 377, 378
        overview, 366–368
        study design, 368–371
Low-molecular-weight heparin,
    acute coronary syndromes,
        glycoprotein IIb/IIIa receptor antagonist
            combination trials, 354, 355
        management, 348, 349
    advantages, 346, 439, 440
    percutaneous coronary intervention use,
        clinical studies, 350
        glycoprotein IIb/IIIa receptor antagonist
            combination trials, 352, 354
        hematologic considerations, 349, 350
        intravenous administration, 351, 352
    production, 346

M

MCSF, *see* Monocyte colony-stimulating
        factor
Monocyte colony-stimulating factor (MCSF),
    elevation in coronary disease, 389
    function, 390
Myocardial infarction, acute,
    direct thrombin inhibitor trials, 355, 356, 441
    fibrinolysis and glycoprotein IIb/IIIa
        receptor blockade,

abciximab,
    ASSENT-3, 298, 300
    GUSTO-V, 295–297
    TAMI 8, 290
eptifibatide,
    IMPACT-AMI, 291
    streptokinase studies, 291
lamifiban, PARADIGM trial, 291
limitations of tissue plasminogen
        activator monotherapy, 289
rationale, 290
recommendations, 300, 301
reduced dose fibrinolysis trials,
    phase II trials, 291–295
    phase III trials, 295–300
non-ST-elevation acute coronary syndromes,
    glycoprotein IIb/IIIa receptor blockade,
        428, 429, 433–435
    upstream therapy, 444, 445
percutaneous coronary intervention and
        abciximab,
    ADMIRAL, 280–282
    CADILLAC, 281, 283
    clinical outcomes, 281–283
    contractile function recovery, 280
    ISAR-2, 279–281
    microvascular reperfusion, 278, 279
    myocardial salvage, 280
    prospects, 283, 284
    RAPPORT, 281
    rationale, 275, 276
    STOP-AMI, 280
    TIMI grade 3 flow establishment and
        adequacy, 276, 277
platelets,
    pathophysiology role, 73–75
    reperfusion limitations, 277, 278
ST-elevation myocardial infarction,
    factor Xa inhibitor therapy, 441
    glycoprotein IIb/IIIa receptor blockade,
        facilitated percutaneous coronary
            intervention, 445, 446
        fibrinolysis, 431, 432
        percutaneous coronary intervention,
            429–431
stroke risks, *see* Stroke

N

NICE, low-molecular-weight heparin use
        with glycoprotein IIb/IIIa receptor
        antagonists, 352

Nitric oxide (NO), synthesis, 5, 6
NO, *see* Nitric oxide

O

OPUS-TIMI 16, study design and outcomes,
    370, 374–376, 437
ORBIT, outcomes, 436
Orbofiban,
    limitations, 379, 380
    meta-analysis of oral drugs, 378, 379
    pharmacology, 366, 367
    phase II trials, 367–369
    phase III trials,
        efficacy and safety, 374–376
        OPUS-TIMI 16, 370, 374–376
        overview, 366–368
        study design, 368–371

P

PAD, *see* Peripheral artery disease
PARADIGM, fibrinolysis, acute myocardial
    ischemia and glycoprotein IIb/IIIa
    receptor blockade, 291
PARAGON-A,
    bleeding events, 252–254
    clinical outcomes, 243
    concomitant heparin therapy, 259
    dosing, 258, 259
    mortality, 248–252, 254
    myocardial infarction, 251, 252, 254
    non-ST-elevation acute coronary
        syndromes, glycoprotein IIb/IIIa
        receptor blockade, 433, 434
    overview, 238–240
    patient selection, 241, 242
    platelet inhibition levels and thrombotic
        event protection, 323, 324
    primary therapy vs percutaneous
        intervention effect, 255–257
    study designs, 241
PARAGON-B,
    bleeding events, 252–254
    clinical outcomes, 243
    concomitant heparin therapy, 259
    dosing, 258, 259
    mortality, 248–252, 254
    myocardial infarction, 251, 252, 254
    non-ST-elevation acute coronary
        syndromes, glycoprotein IIb/IIIa
        receptor blockade, 434
    overview, 189, 190, 238–240

patient selection, 241, 242
platelet inhibition levels and thrombotic
    event protection, 324
primary therapy vs percutaneous
    intervention effect, 255–257
study designs, 241
PCI, *see* Percutaneous coronary intervention
PCI-CURE, upstream therapy, 444, 445
PDGF, *see* Platelet-derived growth factor
PercuSurge, emboli protection device, 402–404
Percutaneous carotid intervention, *see*
    Carotid angioplasty and stenting
Percutaneous coronary intervention (PCI),
    abciximab trials,
        acute myocardial infarction and
            abciximab therapy,
                ADMIRAL, 280–282
                CADILLAC, 281, 283
                clinical outcomes, 281–283
                contractile function recovery, 280
                ISAR-2, 279–281
                microvascular reperfusion, 278, 279
                myocardial salvage, 280
                prospects, 283, 284
                RAPPORT, 281
                rationale, 275, 276
                STOP-AMI, 280
                TIMI grade 3 flow establishment
                    and adequacy, 276, 277
        EPIC,
            clinical efficacy, 111, 112, 114
            overview, 110, 111
            safety, 114, 115
            study design, 111
        EPILOG,
            clinical efficacy, 116, 117
            overview, 115
            safety, 117
            study design, 115, 116
        EPISTENT,
            clinical efficacy, 118–120
            overview, 117, 118
            safety, 120
            study design, 118
        overview of study design, 110
        phase II trials, 106, 107, 109, 110
        pooled trial findings,
            diabetes, 121, 122
            endpoints after 30 d, 113
            mortality, 120
            unstable angina, 121

conjunctive heparin and vascular access
        site management, 195, 196
direct thrombin inhibitors,
        glycoprotein IIb/IIIa receptor antagonist
                combination trials, 358, 359
        management, 356, 357
economic analysis,
        abciximab,
                CAPTURE, 312
                EPIC, 309–311
                EPILOG, 311, 312
                EPISTENT, 312, 313
        eptifibatide,
                ESPRIT, 314, 315
                IMPACT II, 314
        tirofiban and RESTORE trial, 315
eptifibatide trials,
        ESPRIT,
                baseline characteristics of
                        participants, 139, 140
                clinical efficacy, 140–145
                safety, 143, 144
                study design, 136–138
                subgroup analysis, 140
        IMPACT II,
                adverse events, 131
                clinical efficacy, 128–130
                composite endpoint components, 131
                dosing issues, 132, 134
                study design, 127, 128
                time to events, 130, 131
        phase II trials,
                IMPACT, 127
                IMPACT Hi/Low, 127
        PRIDE, 134, 136
        PURSUIT, 134
facilitated percutaneous coronary
        intervention, 445, 446
glycoprotein IIb/IIIa receptor antagonists,
        agent selection, 195
        indications, 194, 195
        non-ST-elevation acute coronary
                syndromes, 428, 429
        rationale for use, 427, 428
        ST-elevation myocardial infarction,
                429–431
        trial designs,
                ADMIRAL, 176
                algorithms, 170, 171
                CADILLAC, 176
                CAPTURE, 175

entry criteria, 172
                EPIC, 169
                EPILOG, 169
                EPISTENT, 174
                ESPRIT, 174, 175
                heparin regimens and vascular
                        sheath removal, 173
                IMPACT II, 174
                ISAR-2, 175, 176
                RAPPORT, 175
                RESTORE, 175
                TARGET, 176
inflammatory response, 388–390
intertrial comparison,
        clinical efficacy,
                endpoint at 30 d, 179–183
                general blockade effects, 190, 191
                patient subgroups, 182
                specific agent comparison, 191, 192
        combination therapy, 178, 179
        drug regimens, 177, 178
        entry criteria, 177
        heparin regimens and vascular access
                site management, 178
        long-term efficacy,
                acute ischemic endpoints, 184, 185
                mortality, 185, 186
                overview, 182, 184
                safety, 187–189
                target vessel revascularization,
                        186, 187
        safety,
                bleeding, 192, 193
                emergency coronary bypass
                        surgery, 193
                readministration, 194
                thrombocytopenia, 189, 193, 194
        trial conduct and endpoints, 179
low-molecular-weight heparin therapy,
        clinical studies, 350
        glycoprotein IIb/IIIa receptor antagonist
                combination trials, 352, 354
        hematologic considerations, 349, 350
        intravenous administration, 351, 352
stroke risks, 410
tirofiban trials,
        dosing considerations, 158–160
        PRISM-PLUS,
                analysis, 162
                clinical efficacy, 161, 162
                study design, 160, 161

RESTORE,
    analysis, 153–155
    clinical efficacy, 152, 153
    study design, 151, 152
TACTICS-TIMI 18
    analysis, 163, 268
    clinical efficacy, 163, 266–268
    cost effectiveness, 269, 270
    study design, 162, 163, 266
TARGET,
    analysis, 158
    clinical efficacy, 156, 157
    study design, 155, 156
unstable angina, *see* Unstable angina
Peripheral artery disease (PAD), glycoprotein
    IIb/IIIa receptor blockade, 448
PFA-100, platelet function assay, 330–332
Pharmacokinetics,
    abciximab, 84–87
    eptifibatide, 88–90
    tirofiban, 87, 88
Phospholipase A2 (PLA2), signaling
    cross-talk, 51
Phospholipase C (PLC), signaling cross-talk, 51
PKC, *see* Protein kinase C
PLA2, *see* Phospholipase A2
PlA2, glycoprotein IIb/IIIa receptor poly-
    morphism and cardiovascular risks,
    56, 57, 376, 449
Plaque, *see* Atherosclerotic plaque
Platelet,
    adhesion,
      receptors, *see also* Glycoprotein IIb/IIIa
        receptor,
        collagen receptors, 31
        glycoprotein Ib/IX receptor, 30, 31
        integrins, 27–30
        overview, 26, 27
      substrate proteins,
        nonmatrix sources of matrix
          proteins, 25, 26
        shear effects on substrates, 26
        subendothelial matrix, 13, 14, 24, 25
    aggregation, *see also* Glycoprotein IIb/
      IIIa receptor,
    history of study, 77, 78
    inducers, 77
    measurement, 76, 77, 321, 322
    antiplatelet agent mechanisms in
      thrombosis, 13
    deposition in thrombosis, 79

granule content, 14
inhibition assays,
    bleeding time, 328
    Clot Signature Analyzer, 333, 334
    cone and platelet analyzer, 332
    electrical impedance aggregometry, 327
    flow cytometry, 327, 328
    PFA-100, 330–332
    platelet count ratio, 333
    precautions,
      calcium chelator effects, 334, 335
      inhibition level optimization, 335
      multiple agent studies, 334
    rapid platelet function assay, 328–330
    thromboelastography, 332, 333
    turbidimetric aggregometry, 326
inhibition levels,
    bleeding complications, 325, 326
    thrombotic event protection,
      animal studies, 322
      direct evidence from clinical trials,
        323–325
      indirect data from clinical trials,
        322, 323
integrin receptors, 27–30, 77, 79
myocardial infarction role,
    pathophysiology, 73–75
    reperfusion limitations, 277, 278
thrombogenic substances, 13
Platelet count ratio, platelet function assay, 333
Platelet-derived growth factor (PDGF),
    glycoprotein IIb/IIIa receptor antago-
    nist effects, 59, 60
PLC, *see* Phospholipase C
PRIDE, eptifibatide dosing, 134, 136
PRISM,
    non-ST-elevation acute coronary
      syndromes, glycoprotein IIb/IIIa
      receptor blockade, 433
    unstable angina trial,
      bleeding events, 252–254
      clinical outcomes, 243
      concomitant heparin therapy, 259
      dosing, 258, 259
      mortality, 248–252, 254
      myocardial infarction, 251, 252, 254
      overview, 240, 242, 244, 245
      patient selection, 241, 242
      primary therapy vs percutaneous
        intervention effect, 255–257
      study designs, 241

PRISM-PLUS,
    analysis, 162
    clinical efficacy, 161, 162
    non-ST-elevation acute coronary
        syndromes, glycoprotein IIb/IIIa
        receptor blockade, 433
    study design, 160, 161
    unstable angina trial,
        angiographic observations, 268, 269
        benefits, 264, 265
        bleeding events, 252–254
        clinical outcomes, 243
        concomitant heparin therapy, 259
        dosing, 258, 259
        high-risk patient targeting, 265, 266
        mortality, 248–252, 254
        myocardial infarction, 251, 252, 254
        overview, 189, 190, 240, 242, 244, 245
        patient selection, 241, 242
        primary therapy vs percutaneous
            intervention effect, 255–257
        safety, 269
        study designs, 241
Prostacyclin, synthesis, 5
Protein C, coagulation modulation, 18
Protein kinase C (PKC), signaling cross-talk, 51
Protein S, coagulation modulation, 18
P-selectin, platelet expression, 42, 278
PURSUIT,
    dosing of eptifibatide, 134, 442
    economic analysis, 315–317
    geographic differences in outcomes,
        446, 447
    non-ST-elevation acute coronary
        syndromes, glycoprotein IIb/IIIa
        receptor blockade, 435
    unstable angina trial,
        angiographic observations, 268, 269
        benefits, 264, 265
        bleeding events, 252–254
        clinical outcomes, 243
        concomitant heparin therapy, 259
        dosing, 258, 259
        high-risk patient targeting, 265, 266
        mortality, 248–252, 254
        myocardial infarction, 251, 252, 254
        overview, 189, 190, 245–247
        patient selection, 241, 242
        primary therapy vs percutaneous
            intervention effect, 255–257
        study designs, 241

R
Rapid platelet function assay (RPFA),
    overview, 328–330, 443
RAPPORT,
    acute myocardial infarction, percutaneous
        coronary intervention, and abciximab
        therapy, 281
    intertrial comparison,
        clinical efficacy,
            endpoint at 30 d, 179–183
            general blockade effects, 190, 191
            patient subgroups, 182
            specific agent comparison, 191, 192
        combination therapy, 178, 179
        drug regimens, 177, 178
        entry criteria, 177
        heparin regimens and vascular access
            site management, 178
        long-term efficacy,
            acute ischemic endpoints, 184, 185
            mortality, 185, 186
            overview, 182, 184
            safety, 187–189
            target vessel revascularization,
                186, 187
        safety,
            bleeding, 192, 193
            emergency coronary bypass
                surgery, 193
            readministration, 194
            thrombocytopenia, 189, 193, 194
        trial conduct and endpoints, 179
    ST-elevation myocardial infarction,
        430, 431
    study design,
        algorithms, 170, 171
        entry criteria, 172
        heparin regimens and vascular sheath
            removal, 173
        overview, 175
RESTORE,
    analysis, 153–155
    clinical efficacy, 152, 153
    dosing of tirofiban, 442
    economic analysis, 315
    intertrial comparison,
        clinical efficacy,
            endpoint at 30 d, 179–183
            general blockade effects, 190, 191
            patient subgroups, 182
            specific agent comparison, 191, 192

combination therapy, 178, 179
drug regimens, 177, 178
entry criteria, 177
heparin regimens and vascular access
        site management, 178
long-term efficacy,
        acute ischemic endpoints, 184, 185
        mortality, 185, 186
        overview, 182, 184
        safety, 187–189
        target vessel revascularization,
                186, 187
safety,
        bleeding, 192, 193
        emergency coronary bypass
                surgery, 193
        readministration, 194
        thrombocytopenia, 189, 193, 194
trial conduct and endpoints, 179
study design,
        algorithms, 170, 171
        entry criteria, 172
        heparin regimens and vascular sheath
                removal, 173
        overview, 151, 152, 175
Roxifiban,
limitations, 379, 380
meta-analysis of oral drugs, 378, 379
pharmacology, 366, 367
phase II trials, 367–369
phase III trials,
        overview, 366–368
        study design, 368–371
RPFA, *see* Rapid platelet function assay

S

Sibrafiban,
limitations, 379, 380
meta-analysis of oral drugs, 378, 379
pharmacology, 366, 367
phase II trials, 367–369
phase III trials,
        efficacy and safety, 377, 377
        overview, 366–368
        study design, 368–371
        SYMPHONY, 370, 372, 376, 377
SMC, *see* Smooth muscle cell
Smooth muscle cell (SMC), macrophage
        killing, 390
ST-elevation myocardial infarction, *see*
        Myocardial infarction, acute

STOP-AMI, acute myocardial infarction,
        percutaneous coronary intervention
        and abciximab therapy, 280
Streptokinase,
fibrinolytic therapy, *see* Fibrinolysis
history of use, 4
Stroke,
abciximab in acute stroke, 401
aspirin benefits, 74, 75, 412, 413, 415
cerebral angiograms of left middle
        cerebral artery occlusion and
        treatment, 418–420
clopidogrel prevention trials, 413
coronary artery disease and treatment
        complication,
        hemorrhagic stroke, 410–412
        ischemic stroke, 409, 410
fibrinolytic therapy, 447
hemorrhagic stroke complication during
        acute ischemic stroke therapy,
        415, 416
percutaneous carotid intervention, *see*
        Carotid angioplasty and stenting
ticlopidine prevention trials, 413
SYMPHONY, study design and outcomes,
        370, 372, 376, 377, 437

T

TACTICS-TIMI 18
tirofiban trial,
        analysis, 163, 268
        clinical efficacy, 163, 266–268
        cost effectiveness, 269, 270
        study design, 162, 163, 266
        unstable angina, 266–270
upstream therapy, 444
TAMI 8, fibrinolysis, acute myocardial
        ischemia, and glycoprotein IIb/IIIa
        receptor blockade, 290
TARGET,
analysis, 158
clinical efficacy, 156, 157
economic analysis, 317, 318
intertrial comparison,
        clinical efficacy,
                endpoint at 30 d, 179–183
                general blockade effects, 190, 191
                patient subgroups, 182
                specific agent comparison, 191, 192
        combination therapy, 178, 179
        drug regimens, 177, 178

entry criteria, 177
heparin regimens and vascular access
    site management, 178
long-term efficacy,
    acute ischemic endpoints, 184, 185
    mortality, 185, 186
    overview, 182, 184
    safety, 187–189
    target vessel revascularization,
        186, 187
safety,
    bleeding, 192, 193
    emergency coronary bypass
        surgery, 193
    readministration, 194
    thrombocytopenia, 189, 193, 194
trial conduct and endpoints, 179
non-ST-elevation acute coronary
    syndromes, 430
study design,
    algorithms, 170, 171
    entry criteria, 172
    heparin regimens and vascular sheath
        removal, 173
    overview, 155, 156, 176
TEG, see Thromboelastography
Thienopyridines, see Clopidogrel; Ticlopidine
Thrombin,
    direct inhibitors,
        acute coronary syndrome trials, 355, 356
        advantages, 440, 441
        percutaneous coronary intervention,
            glycoprotein IIb/IIIa receptor
                antagonist combination trials,
                358, 359
            management, 356, 357
        types, 347
    receptors and signaling cross-talk, 49, 50
    structure, 343, 344
    thrombosis role, 17, 18, 343, 344
Thrombocytopenia, glycoprotein IIb/IIIa
    receptor antagonist safety, 189, 193,
    194, 443, 444
Thromboelastography (TEG), platelet function
    assay, 332, 333, 348
Thrombomodulin, functions, 17, 18
Thrombospondin, platelet adhesion, 25, 26
Ticlopidine,
    adverse events, 439
    percutaneous carotid intervention
        adjunctive therapy, 400, 414

stroke prevention trials, 413
unstable angina management, 235, 236
TIMI-12, outcomes, 436
Tirofiban,
    abciximab comparison, 164
    antithrombin combination therapy, 348
    economic analysis,
        abciximab comparison in TARGET,
            317, 318
        percutaneous coronary intervention,
            RESTORE trial, 315
    evidence-based selection, 450
    low-molecular-weight heparin combination
        therapy, 352, 354, 355
    percutaneous coronary intervention trials,
        dosing considerations, 158–160
    PRISM-PLUS,
        analysis, 162
        clinical efficacy, 161, 162
        study design, 160, 161
    RESTORE,
        analysis, 153–155
        clinical efficacy, 152, 153
        study design, 151, 152
    TACTICS-TIMI 18
        analysis, 163
        clinical efficacy, 163
        study design, 162, 163
    TARGET,
        analysis, 158
        clinical efficacy, 156, 157
        study design, 155, 156
    pharmacodynamics, 87, 88, 148–151,
        168, 386
    pharmacology, 148
    receptor selectivity, 87
    structure, 148
    trials, see PRISM; PRISM-PLUS;
        RESTORE; TACTICS-TIMI 18;
        TARGET
    unstable angina trials, see also PRISM;
        PRISM-PLUS,
        angiographic observations, 268, 269
        benefits, 264, 265
        bleeding events, 252–254
        clinical outcomes, 243
        concomitant heparin therapy, 259
        dosing, 258, 259
        high-risk patient targeting, 265, 266
        mortality, 248–252, 254
        myocardial infarction, 251, 252, 254

overview, 240, 242, 244, 245
patient selection, 241, 242
primary therapy vs percutaneous
intervention effect, 255–257
study designs, 241
Tissue plasminogen activator, *see* Fibrinolysis
TNF-α, *see* Tumor necrosis factor-α
Troponin-T, risk assessment in CAPTURE
trial, 221, 222, 446
Tumor necrosis factor-α (TNF-α),
atherosclerotic plaque rupture role, 11, 12
Turbidimetric aggregometry, platelet function
assay, 326
Tyrosine kinase, glycoprotein IIb/IIIa receptor
outside-in signaling, 52–54

U

Ultegra-RPFA, *see* Rapid platelet function
assay
Unstable angina,
abciximab trials, *see also* CAPTURE;
GUSTO-IV,
angiographic observations, 268, 269
benefits, 264, 265
bleeding events, 252–254
clinical outcomes, 243
concomitant heparin therapy, 259
dosing, 258, 259
high-risk patient targeting, 265, 266
mortality, 248–252, 254
myocardial infarction, 251, 252, 254
overview, 237, 238
patient selection, 241, 242
primary therapy vs percutaneous
intervention effect, 255–257
study designs, 241
antiplatelet therapy,
aspirin, 235
clopidogrel, 236, 237
ticlopidine, 235, 236
CAPTURE trial of abciximab,
angiogram assessment, 207–209, 211,
212, 216, 222–225
arteriography and angioplasty, 207,
212, 213
baseline characteristics of patients,
215, 216
comparison with other trials, 226–229
electrocardiography, 206
endpoints,
4-yr follow-up, 219–221

30 d, 216–218
flow of patients, 214
independent data reporting measures, 206
patient selection, 204, 205
pilot trial outcomes, 209–213
prognostic factors, 219, 221, 222
safety, 218, 219
statistical analysis, 206, 207, 209
study design, 205, 206
classification of patients, 203, 233
eptifibatide trials, *see also* PURSUIT
angiographic observations, 268, 269
benefits, 264, 265
bleeding events, 252–254
clinical outcomes, 243
concomitant heparin therapy, 259
dosing, 258, 259
high-risk patient targeting, 265, 266
mortality, 248–252, 254
myocardial infarction, 251, 252, 254
overview, 245–247
patient selection, 241, 242
primary therapy vs percutaneous intervention effect, 255–257
study designs, 241
glycoprotein IIb/IIIa receptor antagonist
trials,
cost effectiveness, 269, 270
overview, 189, 190
treatment guidelines, 260
lamifiban trials, *see also* PARAGON-A;
PARAGON-B,
bleeding events, 252–254
clinical outcomes, 243
concomitant heparin therapy, 259
dosing, 258, 259
mortality, 248–252, 254
myocardial infarction, 251, 252, 254
overview, 238–240
patient selection, 241, 242
primary therapy vs percutaneous intervention effect, 255–257
study designs, 241
pathophysiology, 203, 233–235
tirofiban trials, *see also* PRISM;
PRISM-PLUS,
angiographic observations, 268, 269
benefits, 264, 265
bleeding events, 252–254
clinical outcomes, 243
concomitant heparin therapy, 259

dosing, 258, 259
high-risk patient targeting, 265, 266
mortality, 248–252, 254
myocardial infarction, 251, 252, 254
overview, 240, 242, 244, 245
patient selection, 241, 242
primary therapy vs percutaneous
intervention effect, 255–257
study designs, 241
Urokinase, *see* Fibrinolysis

V

Vascular cell adhesion molecule (VCAM),
atherosclerotic plaque rupture role, 11
VCAM, *see* Vascular cell adhesion molecule
Vitronectin,
glycoprotein IIb/IIIa receptor binding, 46
platelet adhesion, 25, 26
receptor,
abciximab binding, 83, 168, 384–386
animal studies of antagonism, 385
ligands, 77, 78

von Willebrand factor (vWF),
glycoprotein IIb/IIIa receptor binding,
46, 47
platelet adhesion, 24, 25
receptors and signaling cross-talk, 50, 51
shear effects, 26
vWF, *see* von Willebrand factor

W

Warfarin, clinical trials, 440

X

Xemilofiban,
limitations, 379, 380
meta-analysis of oral drugs, 378, 379
pharmacology, 366, 367
phase II trials, 367–369
phase III trials,
efficacy and safety, 373, 374
EXCITE, 370, 373, 374
overview, 366–368
study design, 368–371